WHAT'S NEW IN CARDIAC IMAGING?

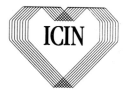

Developments in
Cardiovascular Medicine

VOLUME 133

What's New in Cardiac Imaging?

SPECT, PET, and MRI

Edited by

Ernst E. van der Wall,
and
Heinz Sochor,
Alberto Righetti,
Menco G. Niemeyer

Kluwer Academic Publishers

Dordrecht / Boston / London

Library of Congress Cataloging-in-Publication Data

What's new in cardiac imaging? : SPECT, PET, and MRI / edited by Ernst
E. van der Wall ... [et al.].
      p.   cm. -- (Developments in cardiovascular medicine ; v. 133)
   Includes index.
   ISBN 0-7923-1615-0 (hb : alk. paper)
   1. Heart--Imaging.   I. Series.
   [DNLM: 1. Coronary Disease--diagnosis.   2. Magnetic Resonance
Imaging--methods.   3. Tomography, Emission-Computed--methods.
4. Tomography, Emission-Computed, Single-Photon--methods.   W1
DE997VME v.133 / WG 300 W555]
RC683.5.I42W53   1992
616.1'207575--dc20
DNLM/DLC
for Library of Congress   92-3049

ISBN 0-7923-1615-0

Published by Kluwer Academic Publishers,
P.O. Box 17, 3300 AA Dordrecht, The Netherlands

Kluwer Academic Publishers incorporates
the publishing programmes of
D. Reidel, Martinus Nijhoff, Dr W. Junk and MTP Press.

Sold and distributed in the U.S.A. and Canada
by Kluwer Academic Publishers,
101 Philip Drive, Norwell, MA 02061, U.S.A.

In all other countries, sold and distributed
by Kluwer Academic Publishers Group,
P.O. Box 322, 3300 AH Dordrecht, The Netherlands

Printed on acid-free paper

Printed in the Netherlands

Contents

Positron emission tomography

Magnetic resonance imaging

Section two: Metabolism

Single photon imaging

Positron emission tomography

Section three: Infarct-avid imaging

Single photon imaging

Section four: Function

Single photon imaging, positron emission tomography

Single photon imaging

Section five: Sympathetic nerve system

Single photon imaging

Positron emission tomography

List of contributors

Douwe E. Atsma
Department of Cardiology
University Hospital Leiden
Building 1, C5-P25
Rijnsburgerweg 10
2333 AA LEIDEN
The Netherlands

Steven R. Bergmann
Cardiovascular Division
Washington University
School of Medicine, Box 8086
660 S. Euclid Avenue
ST LOUIS, MO 63110
USA

Co-author: Pilar Herrero

Albert V.G. Bruschke
Department of Cardiology
University of Hospital Leiden
Building 1, C5-P25
Rijnsburgerweg 10
2333 AA LEIDEN
The Netherlands

Manuel D. Cerqueira
Chief, Nuclear Medicine Section
Seattle, VA Medical Center
1660 South Columbian Way
SEATTLE, WA 98108
USA

Peter Cummins
Department of Physiology
University of Birmingham
BIRMINGHAM B15 2TJ
UK

Michael W. Dae
Radiology Service
Nuclear Medicine Section UCSF
Long 340
SAN FRANCISCO, CA 94143-0252
USA

Hans B.M.R. de Swart
Department of Cardiology
University Hospital Maastricht
P.O. Box 5800
6202 AZ MAASTRICHT
The Netherlands

Co-authors: Simon H. Braat, Joep R.L.M.
Smeets, Pierre Rigo, and Hein J.J. Wellens

Christian De Landsheere
Nuclear Medicine Department
Centre Hospitalier Universitaire B.35
Sart-Tilman
B-4000 LIEGE
Belgium

Co-authors: Luc Piérard, Pierre Melon,
Dominique Comar, Henri E. Kulbertus,
and Pierre Rigo

Mark A. Green
Division of Nuclear Pharmacy
Purdue University
Robert E. Heine Pharmacy Building
WEST LAFAYETTE, IN 47907
USA

Robert C. Hendel
Division of Cardiology
Northwestern University Medical School
250 East Superior Street
Suite 726
CHICAGO, IL 60611
USA

Brian Higley
Amersham International plc
White Lion Road
AMERSHAM, Buckinghamshire HP7 9LL
UK

Co-authors: Avijit Lahiri, and J. Duncan
Kelly

Abdulmassih S. Iskandrian
Director, Non-invasive Cardiac Imaging
Philadelphia Heart Institute
Presbyterian Medical Center
39th and Market Streets
PHILADELPHIA, PA 19104
USA

Ban An Khaw
Department of Radiology
Division of Nuclear Medicine
Harvard Medical School
Massachusetts General Hospital
BOSTON, MA 02114
USA

Co-authors: Jagat Narula, and Philip Nicol

Corinne Klöpping
Department of Cardiology
Heart Lung Institute
Heidelberglaan 100
3584 CX UTRECHT
The Netherlands

Co-author: Ernst E. van der Wall

René Lerch
Cardiology Center
University Hospital
24, Rue Michell-du-Crest
CH-1211 GENEVA 4
Switzerland

Pascal Merlet
Division of Nuclear Medicine
Service Hospitalier Frédéric Joliot
4, Place du Général-Leclerc
F-91406 ORSAY
France

Co-authors: Héric Valette, Michel H.
Bourguignon, Alain Castaigne, and André
Syrota

D. Douglas Miller
Director, Nuclear Cardiology
Divison of Cardiology
Saint Louis University Medical Center
P.O. Box 15250
ST. LOUIS, MO 63110-0250
USA

Menco G. Niemeyer
Department of Nuclear Medicine
University Hospital Leiden
Building 1, C4-Q-80
Rijnsburgerweg 10
2333 AA LEIDEN
The Netherlands

Co-authors: Aaf F.M. Kuijper, Eduard
G.M. D'Haene, and Ernst E. van der Wal

Richard M. Oliver
Cardiac Department
Middlesex Hospital
Mortimer Street
LONDON W1N 8AA
UK

Ernest K.J. Pauwels
Department of Nuclear Medicine
University Hospital Leiden
Building 1, C4-Q-75
Rijnsburgerweg 10
2333 AA LEIDEN
The Netherlands

Willem J. Remme
Department of Cardiology
Zuiderziekenhuis
Groene Hilledijk 315
3075 EA ROTTERDAM
The Netherlands

Alberto Righetti
Hôpital Cantonal Universitaire
Department of Cardiology
CH-1211 GENEVA
Switzerland

Pierre Rigo
Nuclear Medicine Department
Centre Hospitalier Universitaire B.35
Sart-Tilman
B-4000 LIEGE
Belgium

Co-authors: Marie-Paulie Larock, and
Simon H. Braat

Heinz Sochor
Department of Cardiology
University of Vienna
Garnisongasse 13
A-1090 VIENNA
Austria

Ann C. Tweddel
Department of Medical Cardiology
Royal Infirmary
Queen Elizabeth Building
10 Alexandra Parade
GLASGOW G31 2ER
Scotland

Co-author: William Martin

Neal G. Uren
MRC Cyclotron Unit
Hammersmith Hospital
Ducane Road
LONDON W12 0HS
UK

Co-author: Paolo G. Camici

Arnoud van der Laarse
Department of Cardiology
University Hospital Leiden
Building 1, C5-P25
Rijnsburgerweg 10
2333 AA LEIDEN
The Netherlands

Aren van Waarde
PET Center
University Hospital Groningen
P.O. Box 30.001
9700 RB GRONINGEN
The Netherlands

Co-authors: Paul K. Blanksma, Joan G.
Meeder, Gerben M. Visser, and Wiek H.
van Gilst

Paul R.M. van Dijkman
Department of Cardiology
University Hospital Leiden
Building 1, C5-P25
Rijnsburgerweg 10
2333 AA LEIDEN
The Netherlands

Co-author: Ernst E. van der Wall

Berthe L.F. van Eck-Smit
Department of Nuclear Medicine
University Hospital Leiden
Building 1, C4-Q-77
Rijnsburgerweg 10
2333 AA LEIDEN
The Netherlands

Co-author: Ernst E. van der Wall

Ernst E. van der Wall
Department of Cardiology
University Hospital Leiden
Building 1, C5-P25
Rijnsburgerweg 10
2333 AA LEIDEN
The Netherlands

Co-author: Berthe L.F. van Eck-Smit

Freek W.A. Verheugt
Department of Cardiology
Free University Hospital
P.O. Box 7057
1007 MB AMSTERDAM
The Netherlands

Frans C. Visser
Department of Cardiology
Free University Hospital
De Boelelaan 1117
1081 HV AMSTERDAM
The Netherlands

Co-authors Chapter 17: Gerrit W. Sloof,
and Furn F. Knapp
Co-authors Chapter 38: C. Jaap J. Teule,
Jacobus D.M. Herscheid, Guido R. van
Leeuwen, Arthur van Lingen, Hans
Huitink and Gerrit W. Sloof

Hubert W. Vliegen
Department of Cardiology
University Hospital Leiden
Building 1, C5-P25
Rijnsburgerweg 10
2333 AA LEIDEN
The Netherlands

Co-authors: Ernst E. van der Wall, Aaf
F.M. Kuijper, Paul R.M. van Dijkman,
Ernest K.J. Pauwels, and Albert V.G.
Bruschke

Mary Norine Walsh
Cardiovascular Division
Hospital of the Univ. of Pennsylvania
3400 Spruce Street
948 Gates Building
PHILADELPHIA, PA 19104-4283
USA

Donald M. Wieland
Director, Radiopharmaceutical Chemistry
3480 Kresge III Building
Box 0552
University of Michigan
ANN ARBOR, MI 48109-0552
USA

Kim A. Williams
Nuclear Cardiology
University of Chicago
5841 S. Maryland Avenue
Box 270
CHICAGO, IL 60637
USA

Christopher L. Wolfe
Division of Cardiology
University of California
Moffitt Hospital, M-1186
505 Parnassus Avenue
SAN FRANCISCO, CA 94141-0124
USA

Foreword

Nuclear cardiology has only a short history. With the commercial availability of the technetium-99m generator, nuclear medicine took off at the end of the sixties. With the discovery of thallium-201 as an agent for myocardial perfusion imaging, nuclear cardiology was born in the mid-seventies. Some of us with greyer hairs remember that we were all very reluctant to use this radionuclide, with an energy not too well suited for gamma cameras and with an unusually low photon yield, that reminded us of the pre-technetium era. In the following decade, we learned how to use this radionuclide from a technical and a clinical standpoint and, as a result, never have there been so many scientific publications appearing on one main theme in nuclear medicine as there have on thallium-201 myocardial scintigraphy.

One of the challenges of imaging is to identify viable myocardium after a serious cardiac event. For further patient management, the differentiation between reversible and irreversibly damaged tissue of crucial importance. Recently, using thallium-201, convincing evidence has been obtained concerning the identification of reversibly dysfunctional, but nevertheless viable myocardium. Among other things, this is new in cardiac imaging but more things are new and the overriding theme of this book is the emphasis on new developments in cardiac imaging. Throughout this book we encounter new intriguing radiopharmaceuticals such as technetium-99m labeled isonitrile, teboroxime and diphosphine. All these agents can be used to measure noninvasively myocardial infarct size. Also, magnetic resonance imaging (MRI) can fulfil a role to determine this important prognostic parameter. The development of contrast-enhanced MRI and – in the longer run – magnetic resonance spectroscopy in clinical routine, suggests that our goals can ultimately be realized.

Could one imagine a future in which nuclear cardiology and cardiac MRI do not live peacefully together? Even if one is certain about their synergistic

Ernst E. van der Wall et al. (eds), What's new in cardiac imaging?, xv–xvi.
© *1992 Kluwer Academic Publishers. Printed in the Netherlands.*

co-existence, one feels more sure after reading this book. This text convinces us that the available noninvasive imaging techniques will provide answers about the clinical status of the patient. This is fundamental progress and meets the needs of clinicians. It is reassuring to see that such techniques are already available in clinical practice. In this challenging new book, the editors have provided an elegant enumeration of the most important new imaging techniques in cardiovascular medicine.

Ernest K.J. Pauwels
Department of Nuclear Medicine
University Hospital Leiden
Leiden, The Netherlands

Preface

Since the introduction of myocardial perfusion imaging and radionuclide angiography in the mid-seventies, cardiovascular nuclear medicine has had an explosive growth. The use of nuclear cardiology techniques has become one of the cornerstones of the noninvasive assessment of coronary artery disease. During the past 15 years, major strides have been made from visual analysis to quantitative analysis, from planar imaging to tomographic imaging, from the detection of disease to prognosis, and from separate evaluations of perfusion, metabolism, and function to integrate assessment of myocardial viability.

Myocardial perfusion imaging using thallium-201 stress redistribution scintigraphy has become the most commonly performed procedure in nuclear cardiology. It allows the detection of coronary artery disease, the evaluation of patient prognosis, the assessment of the effect of therapy, and the determination of the hemodynamic significance of coronary artery stenosis. However, as thallium-201 has limitations in terms of a low energy and a relatively long half-life, attempts have been made to develop myocardial perfusion agents labeled with technetium-99m. At the end of 1990, two technetium labeled tracers were approved by the United States Food and Drug Administration (FDA), i.e. sestaMIBI and teboroxime. In Europe, a vast amount of experience was already available with these new agents in the detection of myocardial perfusion and viability. The clinical usefulness of sestaMIBI has been widely explored in various European and American studies. Most studies showed excellent quality sestaMIBI images and 80–90% agreement with thallium-201 imaging. The definite clinical role of the new agents, in particular of teboroxime, remains to be established.

Besides the approval of these new perfusion agents, intravenous use of dipyridamole as a pharmacological stress agent – which has been used for years in Europe – was recently approved by the US FDA. The diagnostic and

xvii

Ernst E. van der Wall et al. (eds), What's new in cardiac imaging?, xvii–xx.
© *1992 Kluwer Academic Publishers. Printed in the Netherlands.*

prognostic capabilities of the dipyridamole approach appear to be similar to the results of conventional exercise testing.

A recent interesting development in thallium-201 imaging was the reinjection approach, which allows the accurate assessment of myocardial viability. Redistribution thallium-201 imaging followed by reinjection of thallium-201 closely approximates the results of myocardial perfusion/metabolism mismatch employing the more expensive positron emission tomography. These findings have opened new doors for 'good old' thallium-201 imaging.

Apart from these eye-catching novelties (sestaMIBI, teboroxime, intravenous dipyridamole, and thallium reinjection), many more attainments have been achieved in cardiovascular nuclear imaging.

First, the development of new imaging agents in other dedicated fields of nuclear cardiology. In specific areas like function, metabolism, infarct-avid scintigraphy, neuronal imaging, etc., a large scale of new tracers has appeared on the horizon. Although the majority of these tracers await clinical validation, some of them are already being successfully applied in patients on a regular basis. In addition, relatively 'old' tracers such as krypton, xenon, ammonia, labeled fatty acids, etc., have found new clinical applications. Quantification of myocardial flow, measurement of coronary flow reserve, and assessment of tracer kinetics have widened the scope of the cardiac imaging agents to be of use in clinical practice.

Second, reevaluation and extension of existent procedures. Besides thallium reinjection, assessment of cardiac function has experienced a conspicuous revival. Although it seemed that cardiac function imaging had reached a plateau phase in clinical cardiology, a number of new developments have been recently launched such as new blood pool tracers, novel imaging devices (VEST), and new ways of analysis. Furthermore, combination of function with perfusion studies are presently receiving great attention.

Third, clinical applications have been broadened. Not only are patients manifesting coronary artery disease currently the sole focus of investigation, but also patients with small vessel disease, various forms of cardiomyopathies, metabolic muscle disorders, myocarditis, and dysfunction of the nervous system have become the present regions of research interest. Furthermore, new pharmacological stress agents such as dobutamine and adenosine have been suggested. Although still being considered by the FDA, much experience with these alternative stress agents has already been obtained in clinical practice.

These new achievements can be expected to serve the nuclear medicine community and, in particular, the clinical cardiologist.

The present book covers the most advanced developments in cardiovascular imaging within the domain of nuclear cardiology. Major emphasis has been laid on new cardiac imaging agents, reevaluation of existent procedures, and new clinical applications.

In preparing this textbook, several guiding principles have been followed.

First, contributors were selected because of their large expertise with the topic. Several outstanding centers from both Europe and the United States have put together their most recent knowledge in the investigative field of cardiovascular nuclear imaging.

Second, the topics should address either new imaging tracers/procedures or new developments/applications in clinical nuclear cardiology.

Third, the book has been divided into different sections and subsections related to the various physiological parameters that can be studied with the nuclear cardiology techniques. These sections are perfusion, metabolism, infarct-avid imaging, function, pharmacological stress imaging, neuronal imaging, viability, and imaging of thrombosis, leucocytes, and lipoproteins. In addition, one section on magnetic resonance was added, since this is a novel nuclear technique in cardiology. It was felt that a dedicated section on new contrast agents in magnetic resonance should be implemented in the book.

Fourth, each main section is preceded by an introductory chapter written by a contributor with a more generalist view. These introductory chapters can be considered as the combination of a comment and/or an editorial, a so-called 'commentorial'. The commentorials should facilitate the reader in interpreting the chapters in the particular sections. Finally, since the chief editor (EEvdW) reviewed the entire volume, duplication or overlap was avoided as much as possible.

The initiative to this book has been taken by the Officers' Board of the Working Group on Nuclear Cardiology and Magnetic Resonance belonging to the European Society of Cardiology, throughout the period 1990–1992. This Working Group has become a flourishing group of investigative people within Europe with highly scientific interests in cardiovascular nuclear medicine and in magnetic resonance. We though it therefore appropriate to compose a book on new aspects of cardiac imaging as a token of the firm position our Working Group has taken within the European Society of Cardiology. Apart from the superb chapters composed by investigators from the United States, excellent chapters have been written by many members of our Working Group. It is also noteworthy and gratifying that various chapters were written by Dutch investigators, several of whom are attached to the Interuniversity Cardiology Institute of the Netherlands (ICIN) or the Dutch Heart Foundation (NHS). Herewith, all contributors are very gratefully acknowledged for making great efforts in preparing their up-to-date chapters.

We hope that this book will assist the clinical cardiologist, the cardiology fellow, the nuclear medicine physician, and the radiologist in understanding the most recent attainments in clinical cardiovascular nuclear imaging.

On behalf of the Officers' Board of the Working Group on Nuclear Cardiology and Magnetic Resonance, 1990–1992,

Ernst E. van der Wall, *Chairman*
Heinz Sochor, *Vice-Chairman*
Alberto Righetti, *Treasurer*
Menco G. Niemeijer, *Secretary*

Introduction

1. What's new in cardiac imaging?

ERNST E. VAN DER WALL

Introduction

Nuclear cardiology is frequently used to detect, localize, and size the extent of damage to myocardial tissue. In combination with exercise or pharmacologic stress, it can also detect residual myocardial ischemia and thereby determine prognosis. New radionuclides have emerged that allow greater accuracy and feasibility for distinguishing viable from irreversible injury in patients with myocardial infarction, particularly after reperfusion therapy. A variety of new imaging approaches have emerged that employ both gamma- and positron-emitting tracers. This introductory chapter will briefly address the most important new cardiac imaging agents and the latest developments with the currently used tracers. Most of these attainments will be extensively discussed in the following chapters of this book.

Perfusion scintigraphy

A major topic of interest is the value of 24 hours delayed imaging [1] and, in particular, reinjection of thallium-201 at rest following redistribution [2].

Thallium-201

Conventional exercise/redistribution Tl-201 imaging may overestimate the extent of infarction because seemingly persistent defects may fill in on 24 hour delayed images after reinjection, indicating residual myocardial viability in

3

Ernst E. van der Wall et al. (eds), What's new in cardiac imaging?, 3–15.
© *1992 Kluwer Academic Publishers. Printed in the Netherlands.*

presumed necrotic areas. Dilsizian et al. [2] demonstrated improved or normal Tl-201 uptake after reinjection in 49% of apparently fixed defects, observed at redistribution. This phenomenon is important in patients after myocardial infarction to determine whether the infarcted tissue is completely necrotic or still contains viable, potentially jeopardized myocardial cells. There are also implications for patient management: a more conservative approach would be taken in the case of a definite necrotic area versus a more aggressive approach if viable myocardial tissue remains.

Technetium-99m SestaMIBI

To circumvent the radiophysical limitations of Tl-201 (low gamma-emission of 80 keV, long half life of 72 hours), Tc-99m labeled isonitrile complexes have been developed. The Tc-99m labeled isonitriles consist of lipophilic cationic Tc-99m complexes. Tc-99m methoxy-isobutyl-isonitrile (Tc-99m SestaMIBI) exhibits the best biological properties for clinical implications. Due to its short half-life of six hours, dosages up to 10 times as high as those of Tl-201 can be administered, resulting in better statistics.

Like Tl-201, Tc-99m SestaMIBI accumulates predominantly in the myocardium according to myocardial blood flow. Although the first-pass myocardial extraction of Tc-99m SestaMIBI is less efficient that that of Tl-201, the relative myocardial uptakes of both tracers are similar under physiologic flow conditions. In contrast to Tl-201, Tc-99m SestaMIBI has a slow washout with minimal myocardial redistribution. These features make Tc-99m SestaMIBI more suitable for SPECT imaging and allow more flexibility in the timing of the imaging procedure following tracer injection [3].

The tracer is particularly useful in patients with acute myocardial infarction for the immediate assessment of myocardial salvage in the reperfused regions without a delay in administration of thrombolytic therapy [4]. When subsequent comparative studies are performed after repeat injections, e.g. one of four days later, the zone of hypoperfusion representing the final infarct can be identified and compared to the perfusion defect of the initial risk zone [5].

Wackers et al. [6] showed a reduction of greater than 30% in defect size to be highly predictive of patency, while most patients with less than a 30% decrement in defect size on delayed imaging and an occluded infarct-related artery. This observation is important because there are few reliable noninvasive methods that predict successful reperfusion. In the future, Tc-99m SestaMIBI may be more effective than Tl-201 for predischarge assessment in patients after myocardial infarction because it will enable simultaneous assessments of exercise ejection fraction and exercise myocardial perfusion. The predischarge routine may eventually incorporate a first-pass analysis of ventricular function at rest, a delayed gated tomographic assessment of the size of the perfusion defect, and the performance of the first-pass and gated tomographic procedures with exercise.

It has been shown in patients with suspected coronary artery disease, that the results of exercise Tc-99m are comparable to those obtained with Tl-201. For Tc-99m SestaMIBI both a stress-rest sequence and a rest-stress sequence have proved suitable protocols, although a rest-stress sequence may be preferable when using a same-day protocol.

Technetium-99m SQ30217

Another new perfusion agent, Tc-99m SQ30217, a boronic adduct of technetium oxime (BATO), is a neutral lipophilic agent characterized by high myocardial extraction and rapid clearance kinetics. The myocardial first-pass retention fraction of this agent averages 90% in an open-chested canine model. Clearance of the tracer occurs in a biexponential manner with 67% of retained activity clearing with a half-time of 2.3 ± 0.6 minutes. An advantage of this agent is that it would allow repeated flow determinations within short time intervals.

Hendel et al. [7] described the initial use of Tc-99m teboroxime in 30 patients using a rapid dynamic planar imaging technique. Delayed postexercise images obtained five to 10 minutes after exercise demonstrated rapid disappearance of exercise-induced defects of ischemic heart disease within 10 minutes after tracer injection. Iskandrian et al. [8] reported a close (89%) agreement for Tc-99m teboroxime and Tl-201 in patients with coronary artery disease, both on planar and tomographic images. The image quality was improved by shorter acquisition times, upright positioning of the patient in planar imaging, and appropriate filtering for the tomographic images.

Rubidium-82 perfusion scintigraphy

Rubidium-82 represents the most practical flow marker for assessing myocardial perfusion. Gould et al. [9] were the first to show that the generator-produced positron-emitter Rb-82 (half-life 76 seconds) provides an accurate diagnosis of myocardial perfusion and flow reserve in patients with coronary artery disease. Williams et al. [10] examined the use of Rb-82 by planar positron imaging in the coronary care unit and clinical laboratory for detection of perfusion defects due to myocardial infarction. Their study of 22 patients with myocardial infarction showed similar sensitivity and specificity on the Rb-82 images as the Tl-201 images.

Nitrogen-13 ammonia

Ammonia labeled with the positron-emitter N-13 (half-life 10 minutes) has been successfully used to image relative myocardial flow under physiologic and pharmacologic conditions. The use of N-13 ammonia requires an on-site cyclotron. Its extraction by myocardial tissue is dependent both on flow and on metabolic trapping catalyzed by glutamine synthetase. Krivokapich et al. [11] performed rest and exercise studies in normal volunteers using N-13 ammonia. They found that an average blood flow reserve of 2.2 with exercise correlated well with invasively established values. It was concluded that N-13 ammonia may be used for determining absolute flows in patients with coronary artery disease.

Oxygen-15 water

In contrast to Rb-82 and N-13 ammonia, which show a nonlinear extraction at high flow rates, water labeled with the positron-emitter O-15 (half-life two minutes, on site cyclotron needed) is an ideal, freely diffusible perfusion tracer with an almost linear relation of extraction to blood flow. Bergmann et al. [12] showed that O-15 water allowed the measurement of absolute myocardial blood in normal volunteers. To validate this approach in patients before and after coronary angioplasty. Walsh et al. [13] noted a significant change in regional myocardial flow reserve following successful angioplasty. This finding demonstrates the utility of positron-emission tomography with O-15 water to assess the effects of interventions on flow and on flow reserve.

Copper-62-PTSM

Still under development, Cu-62 PTSM is a generator-produced positron tracer with a high myocardial extraction [14]. Further clinical testing and validation are needed.

Imaging-avid scintigraphy

Imaging of acute infarction with infarct-avid imaging agents allows definition of the zone of acute myocardial necrosis as an area of increased radio-activity ('hot spot'). A number of agents have been used, such as Tc-99m pyrophosphate and, more recently, indium-111-labeled antimyosin.

Technetium-99m pyrophosphate

First introduced as a means of diagnosing acute myocardial infarction in 1974, Tc-99m pyrophosphate proved to be highly sensitive for clinical diagnosis of acute infarct [15].

Tc-99m pyrophosphate forms a complex with calcium deposited in damaged myocardial cells. As myocardial uptake is flow-dependent, the uptake is poor in the center of low-flow areas of a large infarct, where the uptake is predominantly epicardial. It was shown in experimental studies with Tc-99m pyrophosphate that infarcts larger than 3 grams can be visualized by in vivo imaging [16]. Right ventricular infarction is especially easy to diagnose, as reported by Braat et al. [17].

The timing of the Tc-99m pyrophosphate study is of critial importance. Best results have been obtained 24 to 72 hours postinfarction, by which time any intervention to salvage myocardium should have taken place [18]. Although the sensitivity of pyrophosphate imaging is high, the specificity is low, because a number of different disease processes show radioisotope accumulation by the myocardium. Positive images have been observed in patients with myocardial trauma, ventricular aneurysm, and after radiation therapy. Additionally, the uptake of Tc-99m pyrophosphate in skeletal structures may restrict the proper interpretation of infarct size.

Although these disadvantages have prevented the wide clinical use of Tc-99m pyrophosphate, studies have again illustrated its utility in patients with acute myocardial infarction. Hashimoto et al. [19] performed early Tc-99m pyrophosphate tomographic imaging and showed that positive images were adequate in sizing myocardial infarction soon after coronary reperfusion as early as eight hours after the onset of infarction. In another study, Takeda et al. [20] reported that Tc-99m pyrophosphate and In-111 antimyosin antibody scintigraphy appear to be comparable methods for infarct detection.

Indium-111 antimyosin

The development of easily applicable infarct-avid agents is extremely important. These agents provide scintigrams, which become abnormal within shorter periods with closer correlation between tissue uptake and severity of necrosis. Radiolabeled In-111 antimyosin is a monoclonal antibody that binds to cardiac myosin exposed upon cell death.

Maximum uptake occurs in regions of lowest flow, and primarily in necrotic areas. Khaw et al. [21] performed the first application of radiolabeled antimyosin antibodies for in vivo imaging of myocardial infarction. Infarct size in grams can be calculated from transaxially reconstructed normalized and background-corrected In-111 antimyosin tomographic images [22]. By performing dual-isotope tomographic imaging with In-111 monoclonal antibodies and Tl-201, infarct size and percentage of infarcted myocardium can be estimated accurately [23]. Furthermore, the antimyosin images can then be superimposed on the perfusion images to distinguish between viable and necrotic tissue.

In-111 antimyosin has proved valuable not only for detection of myocardial necrosis, but also for assessment of prognosis. Follow-up for evaluation of major cardiac events was conducted in a large multicenter study to relate the extent of antimyosin uptake to the major event rate [24]. The incidence of cardiac events ranged from 5 to 8% in patients with negative or minimally positive scans, up to an event rate of about 40% in patients with extensive myocardial uptake of antimyosin. In a subsequent study, Johnson et al. [25] showed in 42 infarct patients that a mismatch pattern between Tl-201 defects and antimyosin uptake (i.e. regions with neither Tl-201 nor antimyosin uptake) identified patients at further ischemic risk. Van Vlies et al. [26] showed that the level and extent of In-111 antimyosin uptake in patients following reperfusion therapy could predict improvement of left ventricular wall motion.

Drawbacks of In-111 antimyosin are the blood pool contamination and interference from liver activity with In-111, its suboptimal imaging characteristics (gamma-emission 170 and 247 keV, half-life 68 hours), and the late moment of reliable infarct definition at about 48 hours after infarction.

Apart from the use of In-111 antimyosin in acute myocardial infarction, several studies have reported the value of antimyosin antibodies in the evaluation of myocarditis and heart transplant rejection. Carrio et al. [27] studied patients with suspected myocarditis and noticed a high myocardial uptake (heart/lung uptake ratio of two), suggesting a considerable incidence of ongoing cell damage, despite a small proportion of positive right ventricular endomyocardial biopsies. Ballester-Rodes et al. [28] analyzed the patterns of myocyte damage after transplantation in 21 patients 24, 48, and 72 hours after In-111 antimyosin administration. Differences in heart-to-lung ratio between absent and moderate rejection were significant. Dec et al. [29] showed that a normal In-111 antimyosin scintigram is associated with a very low rate (8%) of myocarditis on endomyocardial biopsy in patients with dilated cardiomyopathy and clinically suspected myocarditis. This finding may prompt reconsideration of the need for biopsy in such patients.

Metabolic imaging

Scintigraphy with radiolabeled metabolic substrates has become available for noninvasive studies of the normal and diseased myocardium. Metabolic imaging proves insight into the in vivo myocardial biochemistry and may assist in guiding and evaluating therapeutic interventions for acute ischemic states.

Carbon-11 palmitate, fluorine-18 deoxyglucose

Radioactive tracers derived specifically for imaging on the basis of their known biological activity have been extensively studied. Positron-emitters, such as C-11 palmitate (half-life 20 minutes) and F-18 deoxyglucose (half-life 108 minutes), and the single photon agents, radioiodinated free fatty acids and their analogs, are suitable for assessing infarct size and viable myocardial tissue [30, 31].

Positron emission tomography is valuable in delineating areas with reversible and irreversible injury, in assessing the feasibility of surgical revascularization, coronary angioplasty, or thrombolysis with respect to potentially salvageable tissue [32]. The potential benefits of interventions could be evaluated more precisely in patients after myocardial infarction with advanced coronary disease and severely impaired ventricular function. Clinical studies in infarct patients showed that areas with persistent Tl-201 perfusion defects have evidence of remaining metabolic activity in 47% of regions when studied with PET, indicating overestimation of irreversible injury [33]. This finding implies that the region is viable if glucose activity remains in areas with perfusion defects. Conversely, the area is likely to be infarcted or necrotic if such activity is absent. In case of remaining viability, patients are more likely to benefit from therapeutic interventions than patients with definite necrotic myocardial areas. Although the assessment of a (mis)match pattern is unique to PET, remaining myocardial viability can also be assessed by reinjection of Tl-201 immediately following the performance of the redistribution images. However, Tamaki et al. [34] showed that in comparison to F-18 deoxyglucose, Tl-201 still underestimates the extent of tissue viability. F-18 deoxyglycose seems to be the best accepted radionuclide indicator of viable tissue.

Iodine-123 fatty acids

Metabolic imaging has also been performed with single-photon radiopharmaceuticals using radioiodinated-free fatty acids. These can be imaged by both planar and tomographic techniques. Van der Wall et al. [35] demonstrated a regionally decreased uptake of I-123-labeled heptadecanoic acid in patients with acute myocardial infarction. In addition, altered fatty acid metabolism based on abnormal clearance rates was demonstrated in the infarcted regions.

Van Eenige et al. [36] demonstrated that myocardial time-activity curves allow the appreciation of fatty acid oxidation and storage. Visser et al. [37] showed restored fatty acid metabolism in acute infarct patients in myocardial areas that were successfully reperfused. Using I-123 phenylpentadecanoic acid (IPPA) and tomographic imaging, Hansen et al. [38] reported that this compound was suitable for identifying abnormalities in myocardial metabolism. IPPA was at least as sensitive as Tl-201 for detecting coronary artery disease using tomographic imaging and exercise testing. Additionally, it provides imaging not only of coronary flow but also of metabolic activity of myocardium and may thus be useful in identifying hibernating myocardium. Ugolini et al. [39] observed a more heterogeneous distribution of fatty acid uptake and a rapid myocardial clearance in patients with dilated cardiomyopathy.

Carbon-11 acetate

Carbon-11 acetate has emerged as a metabolic tracer capable of assessing metabolic activity, myocardial oxygen consumption, and viability independent of the metabolic environment. Armbrecht et al. [40] showed a close correlation between C-11 acetate clearance kinetics and myocardial oxygen consumption independent of glucose-loaded or fasting state. Buxton et al. [41] showed decreased myocardial oxygen consumption using C-11 acetate, together with enhanced F-18 deoxyglucose accumulation, early after reperfusion in a canine model. This was initially accompanied by regional wall motion abnormalities, which returned to normal four hours later after resumption of myocardial oxygen consumption.

Walsh et al. [42] showed a significant difference in regional myocardial oxygen consumption estimated from C-11 acetate in normal human myocardium compared to areas of myocardial infarction. The clearance of C-11 acetate was 6% of that in normal tissue within 48 hours of myocardial infarction and was unchanged seven days later. The use of C-11 acetate may broaden our knowledge of regional myocardial viability in the near future.

Fluorine-18 misonidazole

A new class of imaging agents, misonidazole derivatives, has been developed as tracers of tissue hypoxia. These compounds are selectively retained in hypoxic myocardial tissue. F-18 misonidazole diffuses across the cell membrane and undergoes enzymatic reduction, yielding a reactive enzyme radical. When oxygen is present, the compound is regenerated and diffuses out of the cell. In case of absence of oxygen, the reduced F-18 misonidazole remains in the cell.

Shelton et al. [43] observed a significant retention of F-18 misonidazole in ischemic myocardium in dogs within three hours after occlusion ($23 \pm 8\%$) versus $12 \pm 7\%$ and $5 \pm 2\%$ after six or more than 24 hours, respectively. Retention in normal myocardium is $2 \pm 1\%$. As marked tracer retention occurred only shortly after induction of ischemia, this agent holds promise for the noninvasive identification of jeopardized but salvageable myocardium. It may also assist in our understanding on the basic role of myocardial hypoxia in cardiac disease and its response to treatment.

Neuronal imaging agents

The noninvasive characterization of the cardiac sympathetic nervous system by radionuclide imaging techniques provides important pathophysiological information in various cardiac disease states. Imaging of the neuronal pathways may delineate the mechanisms by which neural discharge affects arrhythmogenesis and sudden cardiac death.

Iodine-123 metaiodobenzylguanidine

Iodine-123 metaiodobenzylguanidine (MIBG) can be used to depict adrenergic innervation of the heart. Kline et al. [44] were the first to demonstrate the value of I-123 MIBG for imaging the catecholamines stores of the myocardium. Focal denervation produced regional diminished uptake of I-123 MIBG [45].

In an experimental study in dogs, Dae et al. [46] showed that combined I-123 MIBG and Tl-201 functional maps display the regional distribution of sympathetic innervation. Stanton et al. [47] reported that by comparing I-123 MIBG and Tl-201, regional sympathetic denervation occurs in patients after myocardial infarction. Henderson et al. [48] observed reduced retention of I-123 MIBG in patients with congestive cardiomyopathy because of increased clearance of I-123 MIBG.

Carbon-11 hydroxephedrine

Positron-emitting radiopharmaceuticals specific to sympathetic neurons have also been developed. The myocardial distribution of C-11 hydroxyephedrine proved to be homogeneous throughout the normal heart, with a myocardial-to-blood-pool ratio exceeding five to 10 minutes after radioisotope administration. Schwaiger et al. [49] studied patients with recent cardiac transplants and observed that uptake of C-11 hydroxyephedrine was 82% less than in normal subjects.

Fluorine-18 dopamine

Goldstein et al. [50] used F-18 dopamine, a precursor of norepinephrine, and observed that this positron-emitter can be used to visualize the sites of sympathetic innervation and examine cardiac sympathetic function.

The new capability to noninvasively map the distribution of sympathetic nerves may provide important insights into mechanisms whereby an imbalance in sympathetic activity may relate to clinical disorders.

Conclusion

Radionuclide imaging with both gamma- and positron-emitting tracers remains a field with huge potential in nuclear cardiology. This holds particularly for imaging of myocardial tissue abnormalities. Although radionuclide angiography appears to have reached a phase of consolidation, new tracers for characterizing ventricular function (e.g. copper-62 labeled agents) are being developed which have to find clinical acceptance. A large scale of new tracers for myocardial perfusion and metabolism have been developed, but evaluation of tissue disorders is no longer restricted to patients with coronary artery disease only. Imaging of cardiac muscle disorders (cardiomyopathies), noninvasive detection of infectious disease of the myocardial cell (myocarditis, transplant rejection), and visualization of the sympathetic system of the heart (post-infarct arrhythmias) have become clinical realities.

References

1. Kiat H, Berman DS, Maddahi J et al. Late reversibility of tomographic myocardial thallium-201 defects: an accurate marker of myocardial viability. J Am Coll Cardiol 1988; 12: 1456–63.
2. Dilsizian V, Rocco T, Freedman NMT, Leon MB, Bonow RO. Enhanced detection of ischemic but viable myocardium by the reinjection of thallium after stress-redistribution imaging. N Engl J Med 1990; 323: 141–6.
3. Verzijlbergen JF, Cramer MJ, Niemeyer MG, Ascoop CAPL, Van der Wall EE, Pauwels EKJ. ECG—gated and static technetium-99m-SESTAMIBI planar myocardial perfusion imaging: a comparison with thallium-201 and study of observer variabilities. Am J Physiol Imaging 1990; 5: 60–7.

4. Santoro GM, Bisi G, Sciagrà R, Leoncini M, Fazzini PF, Meldolesi U. Single photon emission computed tomography with technetium-99m hexakis 2-methoxyisobutyl isonitrile in acute myocardial infarction before and after thrombolytic treatment: assessment of salvaged myocardium and prediction of late functional recovery. J Am Coll Cardiol 1990; 15: 301–14.

5. Kayden DS, Mattera JA, Zaret BL, Wackers FJ. Demonstration of reperfusion after thrombolysis with technetium-99m isonitrile myocardial imaging. J Nucl Med 1988; 29: 1865–7.

6. Wackers FJ, Gibbons RJ, Verani MS et al. Serial quantitative planar technetium-99m isonitrile imaging in acute myocardial infarction: efficacy for noninvasive assessment of thrombolytic therapy. J Am Coll Cardiol 1989; 14: 861–73.

7. Hendel RC, McSherry B, Karimeddini M, Leppo JA. Diagnostic value of a new myocardial perfusion agent, teboroxime (SQ 30,217), utilizing a rapid planar imaging protocol: preliminary results. J Am Coll Cardiol 1990; 16: 855–61.

8. Iskandrian AS, Heo J, Nguyen T, Mercuro J. Myocardial imaging with Tc-99m teboroxime: technique and initial results. Am Heart J 1991; 121: 889–94.

9. Gould KL, Goldstein RA, Mullani NA et al. Noninvasive assessment of coronary stenoses by myocardial perfusion imaging during pharmacologic coronary vasodilatation. VIII. Clinical feasibility of positron cardiac imaging without a cyclotron using generator-produced rubidium-82. J Am Coll Cardiol 1986; 7: 775–89.

10. Williams KA, Ryan JW, Resnekov L et al. Planar positron imaging of rubidium-82 for myocardial infarction: a comparison with thallium-201 and regional wall motion. Am Heart J 1989; 118: 601–10.

11. Krivokapich J, Smith GT, Huang SC et al. N-13 ammonia myocardial imaging at rest and with exercise in normal volunteers. Quantification of absolute myocardial perfusion with dynamic positron emission tomography. Circulation 1989; 30: 1328–37.

12. Bergmann SR, Herrero P, Markham J, Weinheimer CJ, Walsh MN. Noninvasive quantitation of myocardial blood flow in human subjects with oxygen-15-labeled water and positron emission tomography. J Am Coll Cardiol 1989; 14: 639–52.

13. Walsh MN, Geltman EM, Steele RL et al. Augmented myocardial perfusion reserve after coronary angioplasty quantified by positron emission tomography with oxygen-15 labeled water. J Am Coll Cardiol 1990; 15: 119–27.

14. Shelton ME, Green MA, Mathias CJ, Welch MJ, Bergmann SR. Assessment of regional myocardial and renal blood flow using copper-PTSM and positron emission tomography. Circulation 1990; 82: 990–7.

15. Willerson JT, Parkey RW, Stokely EM et al. Infarct sizing with technetium-99m stannous pyrophosphate scintigraphy in dogs and man; relationship between scintigraphic and precordial mapping estimates of infarct size in patients. Cardiovasc Res 1977; 11: 291–8.

16. Stokely EM, Buja LM, Lewis SE et al. Measurement of acute myocardial infarcts in dogs with 99m-Tc-stannous pyrophosphate scintigrams. J Nucl Med 1976; 17: 1–5

17. Braat SH, Brugada P, De Zwaan C, Coenegracht JM, Wellens HJJ. Value of electrocardiogram in diagnosing right ventricular involvement in patients with an acute inferior wall myocardial infarction. Br Heart J 1983; 49: 368–72.

18. Olson HG, Lyons KP, Butman S, Piters KM. Validation of technetium-99m stannous pyrophosphate myocardial scintigraphy for diagnosing acute myocardial infarction more than 48 hours old when serum creatine kinase-MB has returned to normal. Am J Cardiol 1983; 52: 245–51.

19. Hashimoto T, Kambara H, Fudo T et al. Early estimation of acute myocardial infarct size soon after coronary reperfusion using emission computed tomography with technetium-99m pyrophosphate. Am J Cardiol 1987; 60: 952–7.

20. Takeda K, LaFrance ND, Weisman HF, Wagner HN, Becker LC. Comparison of indium-111

antimyosin antibody and technetium-99m pyrophosphate localization in reperfused and nonreperfused myocardial infarction. J Am Coll Cardiol 1991; 17: 519–26.

21. Khaw BA, Beller GA, Haber E, Smith TW. Localization of cardiac myosin-specific antibody in myocardial infarction. J Clin Invest 1976; 58: 439–46.

22. Antunes ML, Seldin DW, Wall RM, Johnson LL. Measurement of acute Q-wave myocardial infarct size with single photon emission computed tomography imaging of indium-111 antimyosin. Am J Cardiol 1989; 63: 777–83.

23. Johnson LL, Lerrick KS, Coromilas J et al. Measurement of infarct size and percentage myocardium infarcted in a dog preparation with single photon emission computed tomography, thallium-201, and indium 111-monoclonal antimyosin Fab. Circulation 1987; 76: 181–90.

24. Johnson LL, Seldin DW, Becker LC et al. Antimyosin imaging in acute transmural myocardial infarctions: results of a multicenter clinical trial. J Am Coll Cardiol 1989; 13: 27–35

25. Johnson LL, Seldin DW, Keller AM et al. Dual isotope thallium and indium antimyosin SPECT imaging to identify acute infarct patients at further ischemic risk. Circulation 1990; 81: 37–45.

26. Van Vlies B, Baas J, Visser CA et al. Predictive value of indium-111 antimyosin uptake for improvement of left ventricular wall motion after thrombolysis in acute myocardial infarction. Am J Cardiol 1989; 64: 167–71.

27. Carrio I, Berna L, Ballester M et al. Indium-111 antimyosin scintigraphy to assess myocardial damage in patients with suspected myocarditis and cardiac rejection. J Nucl Med 1988; 29: 1893–1900.

28. Ballester-Rodes M, Carrio-Gasset I, Abadal-Berini L, Obrador-Mayol D, Berna-Roqueta L, Caralps-Riera JM. Patterns of evolution of myocyte damage after human heart transplantation detected by indium-111 monoclonal antimyosin. Am J Cardiol 1988; 62: 623–7.

29. Dec GW, Palacios I, Yasuda T et al. Antimyosin antibody cardiac imaging: its role in the diagnosis of myocarditis. J Am Coll Cardiol 1990; 16: 97–104.

30. Ter-Pogossian MM, Klein MM, Markham J, Roberts R, Sobel BE. Regional assessment of myocardial metabolic integrity in vivo by positron-emission tomography with C-11-labeled palmitate. Circulation 1980; 61: 242–55.

31. Sochor H, Schwaiger M, Schelbert HR et al. Relationship between TI-201, Tc-99m (Sn) pyrophosphate and F-18 2-deoxyglucose uptake in ischemically injured dog myocardium. Am Heart J 1987; 114: 1066–77.

32. Bergmann SR, Lerch RA, Fox KAA et al. Temporal dependence of beneficial effects of coronary thrombolysis characterized by positron tomography. Am J Med 1982; 73: 573–81.

33. Brunken R, Schwaiger M, Grover-McKay M, Phelps ME, Tillisch J, Schelbert HR. Positron emission tomography detects tissue metabolic activity in myocardial segments with persistent thallium perfusion defects. J Am Coll Cardiol 1987; 10: 557–67.

34. Tamaki N, Othani H, Yamashita K et al. Metabolic activity in the areas of new fill-in after thallium-201 reinjection: comparison with positron emission tomography using fluorine-18-deoxyglucose. J Nucl Med 1991; 32: 673–8.

35. Van der Wall EE, Den Hollander W, Heidendal GAK, Westera G, Majid PA, Roos JP. Dynamic myocardial scintigraphy with I-123 labeled free fatty acids in patients with myocardial infarction. Eur J Nucl Med 1981; 6: 383–9.

36. Van Eenige MJ, Visser FC, Duwel CMB, Karreman AJP, Van Lingen A, Roos JP. Comparison of 17-iodine-131 heptadecanoic acid kinetics from externally measured time-activity curves and from serial myocardial biopsies in an open-chest canine model. J Nucl Med 1988; 29: 1934–42.

37. Visser FC, Westera G, Van Eenige MJ, Van der Wall EE, Heidendal GAK, Roos JP. Free

fatty acid scintigraphy in patients with successful thrombolysis after myocardial infarction. Clin Nucl Med 1985; 10: 35–9.

38. Hansen CL, Corbett JR, Pippin JJ et al. Iodine-123 phenylpentadecanoic acid and single photon emission computed tomography in identifying left ventricular regional metabolic abnormalities in patients with coronary heart disease: comparison with thallium-201 myocardial tomography. J Am Coll Cardiol 1988; 12: 78–87.

39. Ugolini V, Hansen CL, Kulkarni PV, Jansen DE, Akers MS, Corbett JR. Abnormal myocardial fatty acid metabolism in dilated cardiomyopathy detected by iodine-123 phenyl-pentadecanoic acid and tomographic imaging. Am J Cardiol 1988; 62: 923–8.

40. Armbrecht JJ, Buxton DB, Schelbert HR. Validation of {1-11C}acetate as a tracer for noninvasive assessment of oxidative metabolism with positron-emission tomography in normal, ischemic, postischemic, and hyperemic canine myocardium. Circulation 1990; 81: 1584–1605

41. Buxton DB, Schwaiger M, Mody FV et al. Regional abnormality in oxygen consumption in reperfused myocardium assessed with {1-11C}acetate and positron emission tomography. Am J Card Imaging 1990; 3: 276–87.

42. Walsh MN, Geltman EM, Brown MA et al. Noninvasive estimation of regional myocardial oxygen consumption by positron emission tomography with carbon-11 acetate in patients with myocardial infarction. J Nucl Med 1989; 30: 1798–1808.

43. Shelton M, Dence CS, Hwang DR, Herrero P, Walsh MN, Bergmann SR. In vivo delineation of myocardial hypoxia during coronary occlusion using fluorine-19 fluoromisonidazole and positron emission tomography: a potential approach for identification of jeopardized myocardium. J Am Coll Cardiol 1990; 16: 477–85.

44. Kline RC, Swanson DP, Wieland DM et al. Myocardial imaging in man with I-123 meta-iodobenzylguanidine. J Nucl Med 1981; 22: 129–32.

45. Minardo JD, Tuli MM, Mock BH et al. Scintigraphic and electrophysiological evidence of canine myocardial sympathetic denervation and reinnervation produced by myocardial infarction or phenol application. Circulation 1988; 78: 1008–19.

46. Dae MW, O'Connell JW, Botvinick EH et al. Scintigraphic assessment of regional cardiac adrenergic innervation. Circulation 1989; 79: 634–44.

47. Stanton MS, Tuli MM, Radtke NL et al. Regional sympathetic denervation after myocardial infarction in humans detected noninvasively using I-123-metaiodobenzylguanidine. J Am Coll Cardiol 1989; 14: 1519–26.

48. Henderson EB, Kahn JK, Corbett JR et al. Abnormal I-123 metaiodobenzylguanidine myocardial washout and distribution may reflect myocardial adrenergic derangement in patients with congestive cardiomyopathy. Circulation 1988; 78: 1192–9.

49. Schwaiger M, Kalff V, Rosenspire K et al. Noninvasive evaluation of sympathetic nervous system in human heart by positron emission tomography. Circulation 1990; 82: 457–64.

50. Goldstein DS, Change PC, Eisenhofer G et al. Positron emission tomographic imaging of cardiac sympathetic innervation and function. Circulation 1990; 81: 1606–21.

2. Why new cardiac imaging agents?

D. DOUGLAS MILLER

Introduction

As with pharmaceutical agents in general, diagnostic radiopharmaceutical research and development is proceeding at a rapid pace [1]. A wide range of radiopharmaceuticals have been developed for evaluation of myocardial perfusion, ventricular function, myocardial viability, and substrate metabolism [2]. The first two decades of cardiovascular nuclear medicine has witnessed the experimental and clinical validation of thallium-201 myocardial perfusion imaging and technetium-99m (Tc-99m) radionuclide angiography, two techniques which are widely applied in medical practice for detection and prognostication of cardiac diseases. Single photon nuclear medicine camera-computer systems (both planar and tomographic) have been configured to accommodate the physical characteristics and biologic behavior of these two isotopes. Application of comparable image acquisition protocols, implementation of radiopharmacy preparation for dose preparation and quality control, and dissemination of validated quantitation software and standardized normal files have significantly enhanced the diagnostic utility of these radionuclide procedures.

Despite changing patient referral bases and laboratory utilization profiles, these radionuclide studies have persistently demonstrated high sensitivity for disease detection and significant positive predictive accuracy for adverse cardiac events, particularly in the setting of ischemic heart disease. Specificity values vary widely between 50 and 90%, principally due to post-test referral bias, which increasingly directs positive test responders for diagnostic cardiac catheterization. Industry-investigator collaborations have produced quantita-

17

Ernst E. van der Wall et al. (eds), What's new in cardiac imaging?, 17–30.

Table 1. Prerequisites for development of new diagnostic cardiovascular radiopharmaceuticals.

I	Radiopharmacy advances

I   Radiopharmacy advances
     1.   Dosimetry
        a. total body
        b. critical organ
     2.   Dose preparation
        a. labeling method (in vitro, in vivo, 'kit', etc.)
        b. quality control (labeling efficiency, detecting contaminants)
     3.   Dose availability
        a. radiochemistry
        b. source (cyclotron, generator, etc.)
        c. physical half-life (ultrashort, short, long)

II.   Imaging advantages
     1.   Resolution
        a. spatial
           i. biodistribution (target-to-background, tissue 'crosstalk', etc.)
           ii. gating (possible?)
        b. temporal
           i. dynamic vs. static acquisition
           ii. tissue clearance ('washout') kinetics
     2.   Radiotracer properties
        a. tissue extraction (from blood pool, low-flow to hyperemia)
        b. tissue retention (vs. clearance)
        c. isotope (positron vs. single photon emittor, photopeak, etc.)
     3.   Patient 'throughput':
        a. single vs. multiple doses (reinjection nec.?)
        b. rest vs. stress (vs. both) studies
        c. minimum interstudy 'window' (physical and biologic clearance rates)
        d. post-injection 'window' for acquisition
        e. 'delayed' study (4 hr, 24 hr, > 24 hr)
        f. counts statistics (activity/dose, acquisition time/study)
        g. 'dual purpose' study (i.e. flow, function)

III.   Physiology/pharmacologic-driven
     1.   Metabolic pathways (de novo, response to anaerobic stress, etc.)
     2.   Neuro-adrenergic/cholinergic pathways
        a. receptor (binding, processing, up- and down-regulation)
        b. en/denervation (response to injury)
        c. humoral effects
        d. drug effects
     3.   'Pre-clinical' diagnosis (occult disease, early recovery, early dysfunction, etc.):
        a. atherosclerosis (platelets, thrombosis, plaque components)
        b. 'silent' myocardial ischemia
        c. tissue viability (pre-infarction/pre-necrotic injury phase)

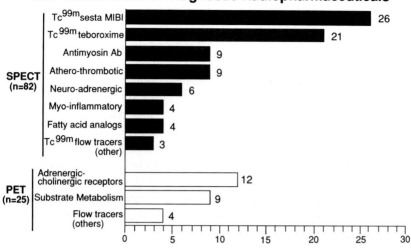

Figure 1. Distribution of abstract topics on 'new' cardiovascular radiotracers at the 38th Annual Society of Nuclear Medicine Meeting, 1991 [3].

tive image analytic techniques which demonstrate excellent transportability between medical centers, and high reproducibility between studies. In this setting, newly developed cardiovascular radiopharmaceuticals must offer improved dosimetry or image resolution (temporal or spatial), or provide diagnostic information on a previously unmeasurable but relevant biologic parameter. An expanded summary of the prerequisites for new cardiovascular radiopharmaceutical development is given in Table 1.

State-of-the-art 1992

The Proceedings of the 38th Annual Meeting of the Society of Nuclear Medicine [3] produced an interesting survey of the current international trends in cardiovascular radiopharmaceutical development (Figure 1). Despite the significant continued presence of papers on the use of thallium-201 for single photon perfusion imaging and viability assessment (7%) and PET studies of cardiac flow and metabolism with rubidium-82, nitrogen-13 ammonia and fluorine-18 deoxyglucose (5%), 107 of the 843 general and cardiovascular papers accepted for this meeting (13%) provided information on the radiochemistry and applications of new tracers for cardiovascular imaging. Of these papers, 77% evaluated single photon emitting radionuclides, while 23% presented data on positron emitting radiotracers.

Studies of the recently approved myocardial perfusion tracers, Tc-99m sestaMIBI (24%) and Tc-99m teboroxime (20%), were most numerous among these novel radiopharmaceuticals. Single photon and positron emitting isotope labeled radioligands for receptor binding (alpha and beta adrenergic, cholinergic/muscarinic) also constituted a significant percentage (17%) of 'new agent' papers. These tracers included iodine-125 labeled hydroxy-phenyl-ethyl-amino-methyl-tetralone (HEAT) for studies of the alpha-I receptor, carbon-11 (S) CGP-12177, iodine-125 iodocyanopindolol and carbon-11 carazolol (for beta-adrenergic receptor studies, carbon-11 epinine (a dobutamine derivative), and 6-(F-18) fluorodopamine (for dopaminergic receptors), carbon-11 benzovesamicols (for acetylcholine receptors), and iodine-123 3-quinuclidinyl benzilate (QNB) analogs (for muscarinic receptors). Previously evaluated tracers of adrenergic neuronal function including iodine-123 meta-iodo-benzyl-guanidine (MIBG), and carbon-11 (meta) hydrox-yephedrine (MHED) were the subject of further study.

Useful clinical applications for the antimyosin antibody scan for myocardial necrosis were presented (99%), including molecular modifications of anti-myosin to produce sFv fragments for rapid blood pool clearance, fluorine-18 labeling for PET studies and indium-111 liposomes for antimyosin delivery. Radiotracers for detection of thrombosis and early atherosclerosis, Tc-99m labeled antifibrin (T_2G_2) and antiplatelet monoclonal antibodies (S12), were represented. In addition, studies of radiolabeled low density lipoprotein (LDL), indium-111 Z_2D_3(IgM) antibody directed against atheromatous ground substance, and a placental anticoagulant protein I ligand for platelet imaging were reported. Single photon agents for atheroma and thrombus imaging totalled 8% of new studies.

Single photon labeled modified fatty acid analogs for studies of cardiac metabolism made up 4% of studies, including new reports on iodine-123 beta-methyl IPPA and Tc-99m N_2S_2 derivatized analogs. Modified fluorine-18 FTHA (fluoro-6-thia-heptadecanoic acid) studies of a long chain fatty acid designed to undergo beta-oxidation and subsequently be metabolically 'trapped' in the myocardium were also reported (2%). Other novel metabolic tracers, in particular positron-emitting copper-62 PTSM (pyruvaldehyde-bis--N$_4$methyl thiosemicarbozone), represented 5% of new studies. This generator-produced PET imaging agent may be an alternative to cyclotron-produced carbon-11 (C-11) acetate, which was the subject of 3% of papers presented.

New single photon emitting myocardial flow markers (3%) and potential positron emitting perfusion tracers (4%) were a significant component of new studies. These tracers included technetium-94, gallium-68 (Ga-68) BAT-TECH (a lipid soluble agent), Tc-99m (III) cationic diphosphines (Q12, P53) and fluorine-18 fluoromisonidazole (FMISO), which concentrates in ischemic tissue.

Each of these novel radiotracers fulfills one or more of the specifications for cardiovascular radiopharmaceutical development outlined in Table 1. A range of pre-clinical to post-release (phase IV) studies are represented in these abstracted papers. A significant percentage of these agents may never achieve widespread clinical utilization, while others have already become significantly entrenched in modern cardiovascular nuclear medicine practice.

Published studies: 1990–1991

In the preceding year (August 1990 to July 1991), a total of 30 manuscripts have been published in the *Journal of Nuclear Medicine* dealing with the experimental and clinical validation of novel cardiovascular radioisotopes. Nineteen of these articles (63%) reported studies on single photon radiotracers, while the remaining 11 manuscripts (37%) dealt with applications of new positron emitting radiotracers. A significant number of both single photon and positron emitting radiotracers were studied for myocardial perfusion imaging applications. In addition to further studies of the Tc-99m perfusion agents sestaMIBI [4–7] and teboroxime [8], iodine-123 9-methyl PPA [9–13], C-11 acetate [14–18], and Ga-68 BAT TECH [19, 20] were evaluated as myocardial perfusion radiotracers. Fluorine-18 misonidazole uptake is also reported to be increased in studies of acute reversible myocardial ischemia due to changes in glycolytic metabolism [52]. Several reports dealt with the myocardial uptake of indium-111 antimyosin antibody in previously untested clinical subgroups [21–24], including patients with dilated hypertrophic cardiomyopathy, doxorubicin cardiac toxicity, and non-Q wave myocardial infarction. A new Tc-99m based carbohydrate ligand, Tc-99m glucaric acid, demonstrates increased uptake in experimental zones of infarction reflecting alternative metabolism [53].

Perfusion imaging agents

A new generator produced positron admitting myocardial perfusion agent, copper-62 pyruvaldehyde bis (N^4-methythiosemicorbazone) (Cu-62-PTSM) has been extensively studied [25–27]. The capacity to produce this compound from a zinc-62/copper-62 generator may provide a more convenient source of positron radiopharmaceutical for regional blood flow determinations in both the heart (Plate 2.1) and brain. The half life the parent compound (9 hours) and daughter (9 minutes) may limit the clinical utility due to a generator life span of 2 days. Radiochemical complexing of Cu-62 with PTSM produces a neutral, lipid soluble compound which rapidly passes through cell membranes and subsequently decomposes intracellularly after interacting with sulfhydril groups. This agent is analogous to Tc-99m teboroxime in this regard, with some properties of a 'chemical microsphere'. The short physical half life of the Cu-62 daughter permits repeat imaging studies over short time intervals as well as 'kit' chemical synthesis of radiopharmaceuticals. When administered intravenously, Cu-62 PTSM is highly extracted by myocardial tissues with good myocardial retention and no recognized toxicity. Additional copper-62 based radiotracers produced from this generator include Cu-62 benzyl TETA-human serum albumin (HSA) for blood pool imaging [27]. This agent is well retained within the intravascular space and has suitable radiation dosimetry. A zinc-62/copper-62 positron generator can produce radionuclide for both blood pool imaging with Cu-62 benzyl TETA-HSA and perfusion studies with Cu-62 PTSM. Subtraction imaging of blood pool and myocardial perfusion phases would also be possible with these agents at laboratories that do not possess an on site cyclotron. PET blood pool images obtained with this agent are comparable to those generated with Carbon-15 Oxyole. Gated right and left ventricular blood pool function studies can be produced with this agent in combination with traditional PET perfusion agents (i.e. rubidum-82, nitrogen-13 ammonia, etc.).

Another potentially useful positron generator system is the germanium-68/gallium-68 generator [20, 27]. The parent compound has a half life of 287 days and is useful for approximately 1 year, while the daughter has a half life of 68 minutes, making it suitable for complex radiochemical labeling studies. A series of lipid soluble Ga-68 complexes of potential utility for myocardial perfusion imaging have been investigated, but have significant limitations for this application. Other neutral lipid soluble Ga-68 complexes have been studied for cerebral perfusion imaging. Ga-68 BAT TECH is a complex of Ga^{3+} with bis-amino-ethanethiol-tetra-ethyl-cyclohexyl (BAT TECH) ligand. PET myocardial perfusion imaging studies with this novel agent have beem reported (Plate 2.2). Ga-68 transferrin has been produced from the same generator system for blood pool imaging studies. The percent of the initial dose retained by the myocardium 2 minutes following injection of Ga-68 BAT TECH is 1.68% (in rats). Rapid myocardial clearance of BAT TECH and other agents limits image quality over time, since the rate of radiotracer clearance is likely to be greater in hyperemic than ischemic myocardial regions. Tracer clearance will enforce abbreviated imaging acquisition times in order to assure a constant relationship between tissue counts and relative regional myocardial perfusion. Thus, the pharmokinetics of these agents may be unsuitable for clinical applications. Heart-to-blood activity ratios obtained

2 minutes following injection of Ga-68 BAT TECH are 3.5, decreasing to 3.1 at 30 minutes and 1.2 at 60 minutes in a rat model. Comparable heart-to-blood activity ratios for Cu-62 PTSM at 1 minute, 5 minutes and 120 minutes are 5.9, 9.8, and 9. Thus, Cu-62 PTSM myocardial activity is better suited to cardiac imaging PET studies.

Metabolic imaging agents

A series of iodinated fatty acid molecules have been under evaluation over the last decade for detection of myocardial metabolic rates and viability with single photon imaging systems [9–13]. Analogs of phenyl pentadecanoic acid (PPA) have demonstrated the capacity for perfusion assessment based on initial uptake, and fatty acid metabolism based on differential clearance from the myocardium. Difficulties in obtaining iodine-123 for labeling to this moiety have reduced its clinical application. The desire to provide this metabolic information without the need for expensive PET detector systems and cyclotrons has fueled this line of investigation. Most recently, iodine-131 ortho-PPA has been compared to fluorine-18 deoxyglucose in 'fixed' thallium-201 defects, and has demonstrated a reasonable correlation with FDG data ($r = 0.51$) for detection of viability in these zones [13]. Additional studies have correlated modified fatty acids including 9-methyl iodine-123 PPA with thallium uptake in patients with coronary artery disease induced myocardial ischemia [12]. Compartmental 15-ortho/para iodine-123/131 PPA myocardial uptake has been fractionated in experimental studies [9]. The ortho-PPA compound is bound to co-enzyme A and remains principally within the free fatty acid pool, while para-PPA enters mitochondrial beta oxidation. The implications of these metabolic fates for detection of myocardial viability, and the relationship to myocardial ATP content have been evaluated in further basic studies [10]. The search for a single photon emitting fatty acid metabolic tracer for the detection of viability is ongoing.

PET imaging studies utilizing C-11 acetate as a metabolic marker of aerobic metabolism via the tricarboxylic acid (TCA) cycle have increased [14–18]. The myocardial uptake of this agent at steady state is proportional to the cellular generation of carbon dioxide. The agent is avidly abstracted by the myocardium, in response to increased myocardial oxygen consumption where mitochondria convert it to C-11 acetyl-CoA prior to entering the TCA cycle. As compared to C-11 palmitate, C-11 acetate is rapidly and completely oxidatively metabolized. Its clearance from the myocardium is closely related to myocardial oxygen consumption over a range of physiologic conditions and cardiac workloads in experimental studies. The metabolism of carbon-11 acetate is not significantly affected by circulating levels of other competitive substrates, as opposed to the dependance of C-11 palmitate and fluorine-18 FDG on metabolic conditions. Modeling of C-11 acetate clearance kinetics provides the potential for future absolute quantification of myocardial oxygen consumption using PET imaging data derived with this radiotracer. In addition to the value of clearance data following injection of this agent, preliminary studies indicate a direct proportionality between initial uptake and myocardial blood flow in coronary artery disease patients. Despite its relatively complex radiochemistry, C-11 acetate will be widely evaluated as a clinical tool in the near future.

Neuro-humoral imaging agents

Cardiac adrenergic and muscarinic receptors continue to be the focus of new radiotracer studies [30–34]. In particular, the myocardial beta adrenergic receptor can be characterized by PET imaging with C-11 CGP 12177 and C-11 metahydroxyephedrine (MHED). Fluorine-18 labeling of the norepinephrine analog metaraminol, provides an indirect approximation of tissue NE levels from PET images. C-11 CGP 12177 is a potent high affinity hydrophilic beta adrenergic receptor ligand which couples to adenylate cyclase [33]. This agent has significant image advantages over C-11 propranolol which is confounded by excessive background lung uptake. C-11 MHED has been utilized to detect myocardial innervation and denervation in response to a variety of insults including myocardial infarction, congestive heart failure and chronic hypoxia [30, 34] (Plate 2.3). Use of this sympathetic nervous system probe provides for competitive uptake between the radiolabeled drug (C-11 MHED) and the endogenous neurotransmitter, norepinephrine (NE). Mathematical modeling has been developed for quantification of the uptake of this agent. Another radiolabeled catecholamine analog, fluorine-18 metaraminol (FMR), can be used to assess the cardiac sympathetic nervous system response to regional ischemia [31]. Experimental studies have demonstrated significantly reduced F-18 metaraminol activity in post occlusive zones with 87% flow reduction and 18% reduction of tissue NE concentration. Transient disturbances of sympathetic neuronal function may occur in response to ischemia, and may be dynamically assessed by FMR imaging. Pharmacologic blocking studies of this agent in vivo confirm neuronal localization by the uptake I carrier system and subsequent vesicular storage. The relationship between regionally depressed post-ischemic FMR concentrations derived by PET imaging and electrophysiologic instability and arrhythmogenesis remain to be proven. Additional studies of muscarinic receptor binding agents including 4-iodine-125-iododexetimide [32] and C-11 MQNB have been reported. The potential for single photon or PET imaging of muscarinic cholinergic (ACH) receptors may be valuable in the assessment of cardiac dysfunction due to diabetes, aging, congestive heart failure and anti-arrhythmic therapy. Fluorine-18 fluorodopamine has been utilized experimentally to assess cardiac sympathetic innervation in animals [51]. Cardiac uptake of this positron emitting neuronal radiotracer can be significantly diminished by pre-treatment with the competitive antagonist desipramine. Clinical studies with these and other radioisotope markers of neuronal function are proceeding with the goal of defining the cardiac response to pharmocalogic interventions and disease states.

Myocardial perfusion imaging with technetium based radionuclides

The relative advantages and disadvantages of thallium-201 and Tc-99m sesta-MIBI (Cardiolite®) and Tc-99m teboroxime (Cardiotec®) have been extensively reviewed [35]. Prior approval of the technetium-based perfusion compounds by licensing bodies in Europe and Canada has been followed by recent approval in the United States. However, insufficient time has elapsed to determine what impact these novel perfusion agents will have on the day-to-day practice of clinical nuclear cardiology. Whether these agents will replace thallium-201 in the detection and assessment of patients with known or suspected coronary artery disease is unclear. Tc-99m sestaMIBI (Cardiolite®) offers significant advantages for SPECT imaging over results achieved with thallium-201, with improved diagnostic accuracy in most clinical validation trials. Thallium-201 activity distribution over time, in particular detection of defect 'redistribution' by thallium-201 reinjection or delayed (18–24 hour) imaging, is highly correlated with myocardial viability. The relationship between Tc-99m perfusion agent distribution and perfusion is better validated than is the distribution of these agents to tissue viability [36]. Dual isotope imaging studies with indium-111 antimyosin and thallium-201 will permit clarification of this unresolved aspect of Tc-99m perfusion agent imaging. Positron emission tomography correlates will also be useful in this regard. Technical methods for reconstruction and quantitative analysis of Tc-99m sestaMIBI images remain challenging, and cannot be directly extrapolated from techniques of thallium image analysis [4].

Despite the rapid myocardial clearance of Tc-99m teboroxime, it appears that high quality planar and tomographic images can be generated with this perfusion agent, and that differential clearance from ischemic and normal myocardial zones may permit detection of early perfusion defect 'redistribution' within 10 minutes of stress injection [37, 38].

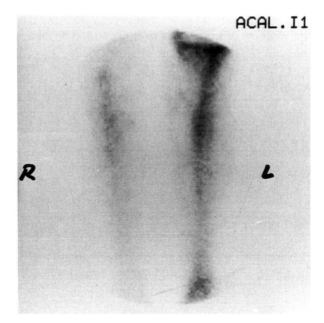

Figure 2. A Tc-99m labeled antifibrin antibody image acquired in a planar anterior projection from a 71-year-old patient who developed acute deep venous thrombosis 11 days following left total knee replacement. Uptake of the radiolabeled antibody is observed in the left calf area in a location confirmed by contrast venography. These antifibrin antibody images were acquired 6 hours following injection of the radiotracer figure (supplied by Dr. Peter Daddona, Centocor, Inc., Malvern, PA).

The evolution of thallium-201 myocardial perfusion imaging from its inception in 1977 [39] to the tomographic description of persistent fluorine-18 deoxyglucose in persistent thallium perfusion defects [40] and delayed (8–24 hour) tomographic defect redistribution [41], required a decade of intensive experimental and clinical evaluation. Despite tremendous interest and enthusiasm, a full understanding of the scope and importance of myocardial perfusion imaging with Tc-99m isonitrile [42] and teboroxime [43] may not be achieved without a similar duration of intensive investigation and validation. At present, these Tc-99m based myocardial perfusion radiotracers may be classified in a grey zone between 'new' and 'established' clinical radiopharmaceuticals.

Indicators of atherosclerotic plaque instability

A significant future challenge for cardiovascular radionuclide imaging is the detection of insipient subclinical atherosclerotic plaque instability. The local metabolic activity of atheroma and activated platelets can now be assessed in vivo using radiolabeled plaque components and monoclonal antibodies. For example, monoclonal antibodies specific for the platelet surface membrane glycoprotein IIB-IIIA, indium-111 P256 antibody, has been utilized to image canine vascular thrombi. Another monoclonal antibody within this cluster of differentiation with specificity for translocated α-granule membrane proteins, iodine-123 anti-PADGEM, has been utilized to detect baboon deep venous thrombi [44]. A novel Tc-99m monoclonal antibody with specificity for the α-granule GMP-140 membrane glycoprotein expressed on the surface of activated platelets, Tc-99m S12, has been successfully imaged in animals and man following arterial angioplasty injury [45, 46] (Plate 2.4). These highly specific radiolabeled monoclonal antibodies demonstrate favorable biodistribution and imaging characteristics with minimal contamination of blood pool usually associated with autologous platelet imaging studies.

Other components of atherosclerotic lesions [47] and local thrombi [48] can be directly imaged following Tc-99m labeling of low density lipoproteins and thrombus-specific monoclonal antibodies. Thrombus components including recombinant tissue plasminogen activator (t-PA) and factor-XIII have also been radiolabeled for noninvasive in vivo imaging studies of experimental thrombi [49, 50]. The incorporation of various thrombus components has been studied in vivo with radiotracers including indium-111 antifibrin monoclonal antibody (for deep venous thrombosis) [28] (Figure 2) and indium-111 'inhibited' recombinant tissue plasminogen activator (rt-PA) [29]. The role of cardiovascular nuclear medicine studies of thrombotic and thrombolytic proteins is being evaluated during the preclinical and therapeutic phases of thrombogenesis and fibrinolysis.

Acknowledgement

I would like to thank Dr. H. William Strauss for his expert editorial assistance and Ms. Lori Gallini Meeker for her secretarial assistance.

References

1. Miller DD, Gill JB, Fischman AJ et al. New radionuclides for cardiac imaging. Prog Cardiovasc Dis 1986; 28: 419–34.
2. Miller DD, Elmaleh DR, McKusick KA, Boucher CA, Callahan RJ, Strauss HW. Radiopharmaceuticals for cardiac imaging. Radiol Clin North Am 1985; 23: 765–81.

3. Proceedings of the 38th Annual Meeting, Society of Nuclear Medicine. Cincinatti, OH; June 11–14, 1991. J Nucl Med 1991; 32 Suppl: 909–1155.

4. Koster K, Wackers FJT, Mattera JA, Fetterman RC. Quantitative analysis of planar technetium-99m-sesamibi myocardial perfusion images using modified background subtraction. J Nucl Med 1990; 31: 1400–8.

5. Pellikka PA, Behrenbeck T, Verani MS, Mahmarian JJ, Wackers FJ, Gibbons RJ. Serial changes in myocardial perfusion using tomographic technetium-99m-hexakis-2-methoxy-2-- methylpropyl-isonitrile imaging following reperfusion therapy of myocardial infarction. J Nucl Med 1990; 31: 1269–75.

6. Tartagni F, Dondi M, Limonetti P et al. Dipyridamole technetium-99m-2-methoxy isobutyl isonitrile tomoscintigraphic imaging for identifying diseased coronary vessels: comparison with thallium-201 stress-rest study. J Nucl Med 1991; 32: 369–76.

7. De Puey EG, Jones ME, Garcia EV. Evaluation of right ventricular regional perfusion with technetium-99m-sestamibi SPECT. J Nucl Med 1991; 32: 1199–1205.

8. Nakajima K, Taki J, Bunko H et al. Dynamic acquisition with a three-headed SPECT system: application to technetium-99m-SQ30217 myocardial imaging. J Nucl Med 1991; 32: 1273–7.

9. Kaiser KP, Geuting B, Grossmann N. et al. Tracer kinetics of 15-(ortho-[123/131]-phenyl)-- pentadecanoic acid (oPPA) and 15-(para-[123/131]-phenyl)-pentadecanoic acied (pPPA) in animals and man. J Nucl Med 1990; 31: 1608–16.

10. Fujibayashi Y, Yonekura Y, Takemura Y et al. Myocardial accumulation of iodinated beta-methyl-branched fatty acid analogue, iodine-125-15(p-iodophenyl)-3-(R,S)methyl- pentadecanoic acid (BMIPP), in relation to ATP concentration. J Nucl Med 1990; 31: 1818–22.

11. Fink GD, Montgomery JA, David F et al. Metabolism of beta-methyl-heptadecanoic acid in the perfused rat heart and liver. J Nucl Med 1990; 31: 1823–30.

12. Chouraqui P, Maddahi J, Henkin R, Karesh SM, Galie E, Berman DS. Comparison of myocardial imaging with iodine-123-iodophenyl-9-methyl pentadecanoic acid and thallium-201-chloride for assessment of patients with exercise-induced myocardial ischemia. J Nucl Med 1991; 32: 447–52.

13. Heinrich MM, Vester E, von der Lohe E et al. The comparison of a 2-^{18}F-2-deoxyglucose and 15-(ortho-^{131}I-phenyl)-pentadecanoic acid uptake in persisting defects on thallium-201 tomography in myocardial infarction. J Nucl Med 1991; 32: 1353–7.

14. Hicks RJ, Herman WH, Kalff V et al. Quantitative evaluation of regional substrate metabolism in the human heart by positron emission tomography. J Am Coll Cardiol 1991; 18: 101–11.

15. Kotzerke J, Hicks RJ, Wolfe E et al. Three-dimensional assessment of myocardial oxidative metabolism: a new approach for regional determination of PET-derived Carbon-11 acetate kinetics. J Nucl Med 1990; 31: 1876–83.

16. Gropler RJ, Siegler BA, Geltman EM. Myocardial uptake of carbon-11-acetate as an indirect estimate of regional myocardial blood flow. J Nucl Med 1991; 32: 245–51.

17. Schwaiger M, Hicks R. The clinical role of metabolic imaging of the heart by positron emission tomography. J Nucl Med 1991; 32: 565–78.

18. Chan SY, Brunken RC, Phelps ME, Schelbert HR. Use of the metabolic tracer carbon-11- acetate for evaluation of regional myocardial perfusion. J Nucl Med 1991; 32: 665–72.

19. Kung HF, Liu BL, Mankoff D et al. A new myocardial imaging agent: synthesis, characterization, and biodistribution of gallium-68-BAT-TECH. J Nucl Med 1990; 31: 1635–40.

20. Green MA. The potential for generator-based PET perfusion tracers [editorial]. J Nucl Med 1990; 31: 1641–5.

21. Hendel RC, McSherry BA, Leppo JA. Myocardial uptake of indium-111-labeled antimyosin

in acute subendocardial infarction: clinical, histochemical, and autoradiographic correlation of myocardial necrosis. J Nucl Med 1990; 31: 1851–3.

22. Estorch M, Carrio I, Berna L et al. Indium-111-antimyosin scintigraphy after doxorubicin therapy in patients with advanced breast cancer. J Nucl Med 1990; 31: 1965–9.

23. Nakata T, Sakakibara T, Noto T et al. Myocardial distribution of indium-111-antimyosin fab in acute inferior and right ventricular infarction: comparison with technetium-99m-pyrophosphate imaging and histologic examination. J Nucl Med 1991; 32: 865–7.

24. Nishimura T, Nagata S, Uehara T, Hayashida K, Mitani I, Kumita SI. Assessment of myocardial damage in dilated-phase hypertrophic cardiomyopathy by using indium-111-antimyosin fab myocardial scintigraphy. J Nucl Med 1991; 32: 1333–7.

25. Green MA, Mathias CJ, Welch MJ et al. Copper-62-labeled pyruvaldehyde *Bis* (N⁴--methylthiosemicarbazonato) copper (II): synthesis and evaluation as a positron emission tomography tracer for cerebral and myocaridal perfusion. J Nucl Med 1990; 31: 1989–96.

26. Mathias CJ, Welch MJ, Green MA et al. In vivo comparison of copper blood-pool agents: potential radiopharmaceuticals for use with copper-62. J Nucl Med 1991; 32: 475–80.

27. Subramanian KM. Cardiac blood-pool tracers [editorial]. J Nucl Med 1991; 32: 480–2.

28. De Faucal P, Peltier P, Planchon B et al. Evaluation of indium-111-labeled antifibrin monoclonal antibody for the diagnosis of venous thrombotic disease. J Nucl Med 1991; 32: 785–91.

29. Butler SP, Kader KL, Owen J, Wang TS, Fawwaz RA, Alderson PO. Rapid localization of indium-111-labeled inhibited recombinant tissue plasminogen activator in a rabbit thrombosis model. J Nucl Med 1991; 32: 461–7.

30. Rosenspire KC, Haka MS, Van Dort ME et al. Synthesis and preliminary evaluation of carbon-11-meta-hydroxyephedrine: a false transmitter agent for heart neuronal imaging. J Nucl Med 1990; 31: 1328–34.

31. Schwaiger M, Guibourg H, Rosenspire K et al. Effect of regional myocardial ischemia on sympathetic nervous system as assessed by fluorine-18-metaraminol. J Nucl Med 1990; 31: 1352–7.

32. Matsumura K, Uno Y, Scheffel U et al. In vitro and in vivo characterization of 4-[¹²⁵I]Iododexetimide binding to muscarinic cholinergic receptors in the rat heart. J Nucl Med 1991; 32: 76–80.

33. Delforge J, Syrota A, Lambon JP et al. Cardiac beta-adrenergic receptor density measured in vivo using PET, CGP 12177, and a new graphical method. J Nucl Med 1991; 32: 739–48.

34. Schwaiger M, Kalff V, Rosenspire K et al. Noninvasive evaluation of sympathetic nervous system in human heart by positron emission tomography. Circulation 1990; 82: 457–64.

35. Berman DS. A symposium: Technetium-99m myocardial perfusion imaging agents and their relationship to thallium-201. Am J Cardiol 1990; 66 (13): 1E–96E.

36. De Coster PM, Wijns W, Cauwe F, Robert A, Beckers C, Melin JA. Area-at-risk determination by technetium-99m-hexakis-2-methoxyisobutyl isonitrile in experimental reperfused myocardial infarction. Circulation 1990; 82: 2154–62.

37. Hendel RC, McSherry B, Karimeddini M, Leppo JA. Diagnostic value of a new myocardial perfusion agent, teboroxime (SQ 30,217), utilizing a rapid planar imaging protocol: preliminary results. J Am Coll Cardiol 1990; 16: 855–61.

38. Stewart RE, Heyl B, O'Rourke RA, Blumhardt R, Miller DD. Demonstration of differential post-teboroxime clearance kinetics after experimental ischemia and hyperemic stress. J Nucl Med 1991; 32: 2000–8.

39. Strauss HW, Pitt B. Thallium-201 as a myocardial imaging agent. Semin Nucl Med 1977; 7: 49–58.

40. Brunken R, Schwaiger M, Grover-McKay M, Phelps ME, Tillisch J, Schelbert HR. Positron

emission tomography detects tissue metabolic activity in myocardial segments with persistent thallium perfusion defects. J Am Coll Cardiol 1987; 10: 557–67.

41. Cloninger KG, DePuey EG, Garcia EV et al. Incomplete redistribution in delayed thallium-201 single photon emission computed tomographic (SPECT) images: an overestimation of myocardial scarring. J Am Coll Cardiol 1987; 12: 955–63.

42. Jones AG, Abrams MJ, Davison A et al. Biological studies of a new class of technetium complexes: the hexakis(alkyl/isonitrile)technetium(I) cations. Int J Nucl Med Biol 1984; 11: 225–34.

43. Treher EN, Gougoutas J, Malley M, Nunn AD, Unger SE. New technetium radiopharmaceuticals: boronic acid adducts of vicinal dioxine complexes. J Label Compounds Radiopharm 1986; 23: 1118–20.

44. Palabrica TM, Furie BC, Konstam MA et al. Thrombus imaging in a primate model with antibodies specific for an external membrane protein of activated platelets. Proc Natl Acad Sci USA 1989; 86: 1036–40.

45. Miller DD, Boulet AJ, Tio FO et al. In vivo technetium-99m S12 antibody imaging of platelets alpha-granules in rabbit endothelial neointimal proliferation after angioplasty. Circulation 1991; 83: 224–46.

46. Miller DD, Palmaz JC, Garcia OJ et al. Platelet activation at human angioplasty sites: noninvasive detection by specific S12 monoclonal antibody imaging [abstract]. Circulation 1990; 82 (4 Suppl III): III 650.

47. Lees AM, Lees RS, Schoen FJ et al. Imaging human atherosclerosis with 99mTc labeled low density lipoproteins. Arteriosclerosis 1988; 8: 461–70.

48. Rosebrough SF, McAfee JG, Grossman ZD et al. Thrombus imaging: a comparison of radiolabeled GC4 and T2G1s fibrin-specific monoclonal antibodies. J Nucl Med 1990; 31: 1048–54.

49. Ord JM, Daugherty A, Thorpe SR, Bergmann SR, Sobel BE. Detection of thrombi with modified t-PA coupled to a residualizing radiolabel [abstract]. Circulation 1990; 82 (4 Suppl III): III 320.

50. Cergueira MD, Edwards M, Bishop P, Curtis D, Stratton JR, Ritchie JL. In vivo arterial thrombus labeling with recombinant factor-XIII [abstract]. Circulation 1990; 82 (4 Suppl III): III 650.

51. Goldstein DS, Chang PC, Eisenhofer G et al. Positron emission tomographic imaging of cardiac sympathetic innervation and function. Circulation 1990; 81: 1606–21.

52. Shelton ME, Dence CS, Hwang DR, Herrero P, Welch MJ, Bergmann SR. In vivo delineation of myocardial hypoxia during coronary occlusion using fluorine-18 fluoro-misonidazole and positron emission tomography: a potential approach for identification of jeopardized myocardium. J Am Coll Cardiol 1990; 16: 477–85.

53. Orlandi C, Crane PD, Edwards S et al. Early scintigraphic detection of experimental myocardial infarction in dogs with technetium-99m-glucaric acid. J Nucl Med 1991; 32: 263–8.

SECTION ONE

Perfusion

3. The value of measuring myocardial perfusion in coronary artery disease

ALBERT V.G. BRUSCHKE

In the vast majority of cases, the underlying cause of coronary artery disease is coronary atherosclerosis. This is essentially an asymptomatic disease process which becomes manifest when the coronary artery obstructions lead to a reduction of coronary flow and consequently myocardial ischemia. Thus, the following sequence can be reconstructed:

Coronary atherosclerosis
↓
Coronary artery narrowing
↓
Coronary flow reduction
↓
Myocardial metabolic changes
↓
Impairment of ventricular function
(transient or permanent)

These steps in the process are not entirely independent, for example metabolic changes and left ventricular dilatation may, in turn, reduce coronary flow.

In the following discussion, we will in particular highlight the relation between coronary artery narrowing and flow reduction, and flow regulation at microvascular level.

33

Ernst E. van der Wall et al. (eds), What's new in cardiac imaging?, 33–39.
© *1992 Kluwer Academic Publishers. Printed in the Netherlands.*

Assessment of coronary artery narrowings

At present, coronary arteriography is still the only diagnostic method which allows accurate visualization of the coronary vasculature. Quantitative methods, ranging from simple caliper systems to sophisticated computer-assisted systems, have made it possible to analyze with great precision atherosclerotic lesions [1–3]. Recently, digital angiographic systems have provided the possibility to obtain these quantitative assessments on-line during the catheterization procedure [4]. It may be expected that in the near future the number of catheterization laboratories equipped with digital systems will rapidly increase which will eventually bring the possibilities of quantitative assessments within the reach of the majority of the practicing cardiologists.

Quantitative assessment of the morphology of coronary obstructions allows, with some accuracy, calculation of the hemodynamic significance of narrowing lesions [5, 6]. However, this approach is subject to several limitations. In the first place, currently available systems assume relatively simple geometric dimensions of the luminal cross-section, whereas in reality the geometry of the residual lumen is often very complex. Further, even if a reliable reconstruction were possible, it would still be practically impossible to accurately determine the resistance to flow caused by complex lesions involving long segments of the arteries. In the second place, the diameter size of the smallest arteries that can be visualized is between 0.5 and 1 mm [7], which is well above the size of the resistance vessels and other vessels considered to constitute the coronary microcirculation.

Consequently, if an accurate assessment of the coronary circulation is required, flow data are needed in addition to arteriographic data. This information should be interpreted in conjunction with left ventricular function parameters and, in some cases, it may be desirable to obtain metabolic data as well.

Methods to determine myocardial perfusion

Understanding the value of various methods and determining myocardial perfusion requires a basic understanding of the physiology of the coronary circulation.

Since the extraction of oxygen from the coronary blood varies only slightly, the balance between myocardial oxygen demand and supply must be mainly maintained by regulation of coronary blood flow. Coronary flow is controlled by constriction and dilatation of the coronary resistance vessels. This appears to include a wide size range of arterioles which is in the order of 25 to 200 μm.

Regulatory mechanisms of the coronary circulation may be divided into metabolic regulation and autoregulation [8]. The first mechanism refers to regulation of flow according to metabolic requirements, while autoregulation refers to the mechanism by which a constant coronary flow is maintained over a wide range of perfusion pressures in conditions in which oxygen demand is constant. Coronary atherosclerosis eventually leads to a significant pressure drop across obstructive lesions, which results in a drop in perfusion pressure and would lead to a reduction of myocardial perfusion if it were not for the coronary autoregulation which compensates for the reduced pressure by dilatation of the resistance vessels. When the point of maximal vasodilation is reached, the compensatory possibilities provided by autoregulation are exhausted. Beyond this threshold, coronary flow begins to decline and ischemia sets in.

To express, in a quantitative manner, the capacity of the heart to increase coronary flow by vasodilation, the concept 'coronary flow reserve (CFR)' is very convenient. CFR can be defined as the ratio maximal coronary flow/ resting coronary flow [9, 10]. To determine CFR, maximal flow is usually obtained by pharmacological coronary vasodilation.

In the presence of obstructive lesions in the epicardial coronary arteries and compensatory dilatation of the resistance vessels, the reserve to further increase coronary flow declines. In other words CFR decreases as a function of increasing severity of narrowing until autoregulation is exhausted; at this point CFR = 1. This may suggest that CFR is an ideal measure of the functional significance of narrowing lesions. However, in clinical practice, CFR determinations should be interpreted cautiously because several factors that are unrelated to the status of the coronary vasculature may influence both the denominator and the numerator of the quotient. Resting flow may be increased in various conditions, for example, in the presence of anemia or tachycardia, while maximal flow, representing flow with abolished autoregulation, is characterized by being pressure dependent and is consequently strongly influenced by the aortic pressure. Therefore, if a drug used for coronary vasodilation at the same time causes a decrease of blood pressure, the CFR determination will be unreliable. For the same reasons, it is hazardous to compare CFR determination in a patient acquired on different occasions. In the evaluation of coronary atherosclerosis with typical regional flow deficits, assessment of global CFR is practically useless but assessment of regional CFR may be also misleading if one only looks at the entire wall thickness and not separately at different layers. It has since long been recognized that CFR is not the same throughout the myocardium. In dogs, Guyton et al. [11] demonstrated that, in the subendocardium, flow decreased linearly with pressure, if the pressure was below 70 mmHg, whereas in the subepicardium, flow was still constant down to a pressure of 40 mmHg [11]. The finding that the subendocardium, i.e., the deepest one-quarter or one-third of the ventricular wall, is at greatest risk of ischemia has been confirmed by several other investigators [8, 12–14]. Mechanisms which may explain the transmural differences include:

(1) Differential systolic intramyocardial pressures causing differential systolic flows across the wall.
(2) Differential diastolic intramyocardial pressures and back pressures.
(3) Interactions between systole and diastole.
(4) Differences in vascular density across the ventricular wall [8, 14].

Another pitfall is presented by the inhomogeneity of regional ischemia. Hoffman et al. [14] showed that, in all layers of the left ventricular wall at low perfusion pressures, some small pieces of muscle have no flow reserve left, while other pieces nearby can have substantial reserve. The findings may explain the apparent inability of ischemia to maximally dilate myocardial vessels. Another confounding factor is the heterogeneity of responses of different sized small vessels to various stimuli. For example, adenosine only dilates microvessels of less than 150 μm in diameter, whereas serotonin constricts microvessels greater than 100 μm in diameter and simultaneously dilates vessels of less than 100 μm in diameter [15]. Similar complex reactions have been described for various drugs.

Methods to assess myocardial perfusion

Based upon physiological principles the following desiderata for methods to assess myocardial perfusion in clinical practice may be formulated:

(1) In the evaluation of atherosclerotic coronary artery disease, the method used should provide information about regional flow. A high spatial resolution is desirable and methods which provide information about transmural flow gradients (e.g. by tomographic techniques) merit preference.
(2) The method should allow assessment of flow during interventions such as pharmacological coronary vasodilation. This requires that the method be fast enough to complete measurements during the short period of time that the maximal effect of the intervention is maintained.
(3) Preferably, coronary flow, both global and regional, should be determined in absolute values as volume per gram of myocardium. Currently, none of the readily accessible techniques fulfills this desideratum. Therefore, it is more realistic to require that the method allow quantitative comparisons

of perfusion in different areas of the myocardium and assessments at rest versus assessments during interventions.

(4) Methods which allow simultaneous measurements of perfusion and metabolism will be of great clinical value.

(5) As is true for any diagnostic method, the method used to assess myocardial perfusion should neither present significant risk to the patients nor cause much discomfort.

The methods currently used in clinical practice may, for practical reasons, be divided into those which require cardiac catheterization and so-called noninvasive techniques. Obviously, methods of the latter category should be preferred if the patient does not have to undergo cardiac catheterization anyway. The merits and limitations of several methods from this category are discussed elsewhere in this volume. Of the methods employed at cardiac catheterization, currently mainly the Doppler technique and angiographic techniques are being used. It is beyond the scope of this chapter to discuss these methods in any detail; the interested reader may find this information elsewhere [16–18]. Suffice it to say that neither of the two methods measures absolute flow or flow in different layers of the myocardium but both methods allow adequate determination of CFR while angiographic methods also provide good spatial resolution.

Clinical application of assessment of myocardial perfusion

The oldest and probably still most common indication for assessment of myocardial perfusion is risk stratification in patients with proven or suspected coronary artery disease. Within this context, risk stratification ranges from determining whether a patient with chest pain has or does not have obstructive coronary artery disease to risk assessment in patients who have recently sustained an acute myocardial infarction. The risk stratification thus obtained may serve as a basis for further management, in particular, to decide whether a patient should undergo coronary arteriography and, if feasible, surgical or catheter revascularization.

However, assessment of myocardial perfusion also has its own unique place in the evaluation of patients with coronary disease. During the last decade, knowledge about the mechanisms governing coronary circulation has improved tremendously, and has just begun to influence clinical thinking. This research has clearly demonstrated the importance of the coronary microcirculation. The sizes of the vessels constituting the microcirculation are well below the threshold of visualization by coronary arteriography but useful indirect evidence about their status may be obtained by assessment of myocardial perfusion. This may not always be necessary in relatively straightforward cases, for example, patients with severe angina pectoris and typical proximal coronary atherosclerosis, but this information may be of crucial importance in complex cases of coronary atherosclerosis or when small vessel disease (with or without obstructive atherosclerosis) is suspected to be present. Indeed, in small vessel disease, which occurs in a variety of conditions with much greater frequency than has long been thought, assessment of perfusion is the only method which may substantiate the diagnosis [19–21].

In conclusion, methods (such as radionuclide and magnetic resonance techniques) which provide information about myocardial perfusion will be increasingly important in clinical diagnosis and the process of clinical decision making. Efforts should be directed towards developing these methods to the point that they satisfy the desiderata mentioned above and can be performed in most institutions dedicated to the care of patients with coronary artery disease.

References

1. Reiber JHC, Serruys PW, Slager CJ. Quantitative coronary and left ventricular cineangiography: methodology and clinical applications. Dordrecht, The Netherlands: Martinus Nijhoff Publishers, 1986.
2. Bruschke AVG, Buis B. Quantitative angiography. Curr Opin Cardiol 1988; 3: 881–6.
3. Reiber JHC. Morphologic and densitometric analysis of coronary arteries. In: Heintzen PH, Bürsch JH, editors, Progress in digital angiocardiography. Dordrecht, The Netherlands: Kluwer Academic Publishers 1988: 137–58.
4. Mancini GBJ. Digital coronary angiography: advantages and limitations. In: Reiber JHC, Serruys PW, editors, Quantitative coronary arteriography. Dordrecht, The Netherlands: Kluwer Academic Publishers 1991: 23–42.
5. Kirkeeide RL, Gould KL, Parsel L. Assessment of coronary stenoses by myocardial perfusion imaging during pharmacologic coronary vasodilation. VII. Validation of coronary flow reserve as a single integrated functional measure of stenosis severity reflecting all its geometric dimensions. J Am Coll Cardiol 1986; 7: 103–13.
6. Wilson RF, Marcus ML, White CW. Predictions of the physiologic significance of coronary arterial lesions by quantitative lesion geometry in patients with limited coronary artery disease. Circulation 1987; 75: 723–32.
7. Bruschke AVG, Padmos I, Buis B, Van Benthem A. Arteriographic evaluation of small coronary arteries. J Am Coll Cardiol 1990; 15: 784–90.
8. Dole WP. Autoregulation of the coronary circulation. Prog Cardiovasc Dis 1987; 29: 293–323.
9. Hoffman JIE. Maximal coronary flow and the concept of coronary vascular reserve. Circulation 1984; 70: 153–9.
10. Hoffman JIE. Coronary flow reserve. Curr Opin Cardiol 1988; 3: 874–80.
11. Guyton RA, McClenathan JH, Newman GE, Michaelis LL. Significance of subendocardial S-T segment elevation caused by coronary stenosis in the dog. Am J Cardiol 1977; 40: 373–80.

12. Rouleau J, Boerboom LE, Surjadhana A, Hoffman JIE. The role of autoregulation and tissue diastolic pressures in the transmural distribution of left ventricular blood flow in anesthetized dogs. Circ Res 1979; 45: 804–15.
13. Grattan MT, Hanley FL, Stevens MB, Hoffman JIE. Transmural coronary flow reserve patterns in dogs. Am J Physiol 1986; 250: H276–88.
14. Hoffman JIE. Transmural myocardial perfusion. In: Kajiya F, Klassen GA, Spaan JAE, Hoffman JIE, editors, Coronary Circulation. Tokyo: Springer-Verlag 1990: 141–52.
15. Marcus ML, Chilian WM, Kanatsuka H, Dellsperger KC, Eastham CL, Lampint KG. Understanding the coronary circulation through studies at microvascular level. Circulation 1990; 82: 1–7.
16. Bruschke AVG. Coronary circulation. In: Van der Wall EE, De Roos A, editors, Magnetic resonance imaging in coronary artery disease. Dordrecht, The Netherlands: Kluwer Academic Publishers 1991: 35–48.
17. Marcus ML, Wilson RF, White CW. Methods of measurement of myocardial blood flow in patients: a critical review. Circulation 1987; 76: 245–53.
18. Serruys PW, Laarman GH, Reiber HC, Beatt K, Roelandt J. A comparison of two methods to measure coronary flow reserve in the setting of coronary angioplasty: intracoronary blood flow velocity measurements with a Doppler catheter, and digital subtraction cineangiography. Eur Heart J 1989; 10: 725–35.
19. James TN. The spectrum of diseases of small coronary arteries and their physiologic consequences. J Am Coll Cardiol 1990; 15: 763–74.
20. James TN, Bruschke AVG. Seminar on small coronary artery disease. (Guest editors James TN, Bruschke AVG) Introduction. Structure and function of small coronary arteries in health and disease. J Am Coll Cardiol 1990; 15: 511–2.
21. Strauer B-E. The significance of coronary reserve in clinical heart disease. J Am Coll Cardiol 1990; 15: 775–83.

4. Myocardial perfusion imaging with xenon-133

ANN C. TWEDDEL and WILLIAM MARTIN

Introduction

In 1948, Eckenhoff et al. [1] described a method of measuring coronary flow based on the principle that an inert gas (nitrous oxide) diffuses across the capillary membrane in proportion to the rate of coronary flow. A concentration curve was obtained by sampling from the coronary sinus and by applying the Fick principle, myocardial flow may be calculated. Several different gases have been employed (H-2 helium, argon and radioactive xenon-133) with arterial or coronary venous sampling to construct desaturation curves.

The first assessments of global myocardial flow, with external precordial counting were developed by Herd et al. for krypton-85 [2] and Ross et al. for xenon-133 [3]. External precordial counters have been replaced by more sophisticated detectors, in the form of gamma cameras, with increased computing 'power' but the principles are identical.

Principles of measurement

Following direct intracoronary injection, of typically 1 400 MBq of xenon-133, dissolved in saline, there is a rapid diffusion into the myocardium subtended by the artery. Subsequent washout is in proportion to the local blood flow. Xenon emits low energy gamma emission (81 keV) (that is readily imaged by a gamma camera) and 95% is eliminated from the lungs on first pass resulting in a low radiation exposure to the patient. The radioisotope washout curve can be analyzed by applying a mono-exponential model to the initial slope, according to the Kety Schmidt formula [4].

41

Ernst E. van der Wall et al. (eds), What's new in cardiac imaging?, 41–48.
© *1992 Kluwer Academic Publishers. Printed in the Netherlands.*

$$F/\omega = \frac{k \lambda 100}{\varrho},$$

where F = myocardial flow rate per 100 g myocardium = ω
        λ = myocardial: blood partition coefficient (obtained by Conn in normal dog 0.72) [5]
        ϱ = the specific gravity of heart (1.05) [6]
        k = the rate constant, is calculated by $k = \ln 2/t^{1}/_{2}$ is the time, in minutes required for the count rate to be reduced by 50%.

Measurements of flow can be performed at rest and during interventions. Measurements can normally be repeated after 5 minutes to allow adequate lung clearance, but by scaling the doses injected (1/3 then 2/3), repeat measurements may be made after 3 minutes. Since regional washout rates are largely independent of xenon concentration, assessment of flow is not critically dependent on perfect mixing within the coronary artery, which is fortunate as this is difficult to ensure. However, the intracoronary injection technique must be standardized to allow comparisons of sequential measurements. Although flow, or washout, is independent of the delivery, the volume of myocardium supplied is critically dependent on the injection pressure (high injection pressures may 'open up' collateral beds that would not otherwise be seen). By ensuring careful standardization of the technique, the reproducibility was $\pm 6\%$, $n = 50$ which is similar to that reported by other workers [7].

Analysis

Intracoronary injection of xenon-133 provides two types of complementary information.
(a) Distribution of myocardium subtended by the artery injected, from the initial delivery of xenon-133.
(b) Washout (or flow) of isotope from the myocardium; clearance of tracer from identifiable areas of myocardium which is directly related to regional myocardial blood flow.

(a) *Distribution:* In 85% of patients, the myocardial circulation is termed right dominant, with a large right coronary artery, which supplies a substantial proportion of the posterior wall of the heart [8]. In approximately 10%, the right coronary artery is small and the left circumflex artery is 'dominant'. There is a spectrum of normal, ranging from the right coronary artery supplying none of the left ventricle, to virtually the whole of the posterior wall (Plate 4.1). In addition, the inferior surface and lower end of the septum has a dual blood supply, depicted in yellow (Plate 4.1).

(b) *Flow:* (i) Ventricular flow: Total left ventricular flow can be obtained by summing the contributions from the left and right coronary artery injections. Right ventricular flow is supplied exclusively by the right coronary artery. (ii) Regional flow: By drawing regions of interest over the appropriate areas of myocardium, regional flow can be obtained from, e.g. the septum or posterior wall.

Background subtraction
Xenon-133 is excreted in the lungs, with little recirculation ($< 10\%$). Thus, the lung activity increases, especially with repeated measurements. To obviate this, a background region of interest is drawn which, when subtracted from the initial flow data, produces a curve that is acceptable as a monoexponential decay. Restricting data analysis from the peak activity to 30 or 40 seconds afterwards obviates some of the problems associated with assessment of regional flow rates, since detailed analysis suggests curves better fitted by dual or triple exponentials (with a fast initial phase, with other considerably longer half life phases). In practice, however, reproducible results are obtained by monoexponential analysis, if suitable background subtraction is incorporated (Plate 4.2).

Technical improvements in the technique
In most cases, previous reported work using the intracoronary xenon-133 technique has employed a 40° LAO projection to obtain dynamic image data, with relatively fast (2–5 seconds) framing rates to allow assessment of washout rates. Overlapping areas of myocardium and the mixture of scar/nonscar tissue lead to difficulties in assessing the distribution images and washout rates. We have introduced two simple technical modifications in the method of data acquisition, which enhance the clinical information.
(a) Biplane collimation: The use of a biplane collimator permits the simultaneous acquisition of 30° and 70° left anterior oblique projections. Assessment of the posterior wall is inadequate using a single projection in the 40° left anterior oblique.
(b) Listmode acquisition: By acquiring data in listmode, gated to the electrocardiogram, it is possible to utilize the image data more flexibly. The listmode data can be retrospectively reconstructed into standard framed data, to allow washout rates to be evaluated. However, the listmode data can also be retrospectively reconstructed into a representative gated cardiac cycle, which may be viewed in a cine display or by using functional images to allow an assessment of regional wall motion, in addition to the distribution and flow information.

Limitations of the technique

Xenon's gamma ray emission at 81 keV are low energy, which limits the spatial resolution of the images. Xenon also has different solubility in muscle, scar and fat, for example although the partition coefficient of xenon in myocardium is taken as 0.72, that for fat is 8.0 [7]. Therefore, if the myocardium is composed of a mixture of tissues, as may occur post-infarction, this results in inhomogeneous flow. In common with other imaging techniques, it is also impossible to differentiate subendocardial and subepicardial, which may differ with changing pathophysiological situations. At very high flow rates, as may be produced with pharmacological challenges, there is some question as to the ability of xenon to adequately diffuse into the myocardium [3, 7].

Clinical applications of the technique

Normal flow

Total left ventricular flow in patients with angiographically normal coronary arteries in our laboratory was 75.5 ± 8.8 ml/100 g/min, which is similar to that quoted by Engel et al. [9], 65.9 ± 17.8 ml/100 g/min ($n = 39$), and by Cannon et al. [6], $61.0 \pm 8\%$.

In response to stress, total left ventricular flow increases, as expected. In 10 patients with arteriographically normal right dominant coronary systems, and normal left ventricular function, xenon was injected into the left and right coronary arteries during atrial pacing (90 and 110 beats/minute) and immediately post-maximal symptom limited supine exercise (see Table 1). The distribution of the flow to the left ventricle from each artery varied very little (mean ± 8%). Flows calculated from the washout curves suggest that during

Table 1. Percentage changes in flow with atrial pacing and dynamic exercise.

	Atrial pacing 90 beats/min	Atrial pacing 110 beats/min	Immediately post-exercise
LV	$14.3 \pm 2\%$[a]	45.8 ± 16[a]	18.5 ± 5[b]
LAD	$13.0 \pm 2\%$[a]	40.0 ± 1[a]	18.0 ± 7[a]
Cx	$16.0 \pm 3.6\%$[a]	51.0 ± 14.6[a]	24.0 ± 6[a]
RCA	$-3.6 \pm 1\%$	$+0.4 \pm 2$	-18.0 ± 5

[a] $p < 0.02$, [b] $p < 0.05$.

stress the increased left ventricular flow is supplied predominantly by the left coronary artery.

Microvascular angina

Patients with arteriographically normal arteries, with effort related angina, are thought to have a functional abnormality of the micro-vasculature. This can be demonstrated in the flow response to atrial pacing stress and to a vasodilator challenge. Coronary flow reserve has not been calculated as absolute flow at high flow rates is unreliable [7]. Scans from a patient with microvascular angina are illustrated in Plate 4.3. Atrial pacing at 135 beats/minute induced angina, electrocardiographic ST changes and reduced flow distribution and no increase in flow rate at the lower septum (a mean fall in flow of 30%, $n = 18$, where atrial pacing produced angina). A new wall motion abnormality was seen on the gated image. Vasodilator stress produced a substantial increase in flow (250%) in the circumflex distribution but no change in flow in the lower septum.

These changes are in keeping with some previous reports of wall motion abnormalities with stress [10], but not with recent work published in the *Journal of American College of Cardiology,* which demonstrated abnormalities in carbohydrate metabolism [11].

Similar flow abnormalities are seen within the myocardium post infarction, where the subtending vessel is patent. In 10 patients, 36–48 hours post myocardial infarction, the flow response to intracoronary nifedipine at the infarct site was a mean fall in flow of 8%, whereas in normal myocardium, flow increased by $95 \pm 21\%$.

Coronary artery disease

At rest, flow is not diminished unless the vessel has a subtotal or total obstruction. This is similar to other published reports [7, 12], and in keeping with the absence of clinical symptoms. Engel [7] has suggested that post stenotic flow is not significantly reduced in patients with normal wall motion, irrespective of the severity of the coronary obstruction. Patients with lesions >75% of the luminal diameter, with normal wall motion, had collaterals present and normal flow rates were thought to reflect the adequacy of the collaterals (see Plate 4.4). Where the left ventricular wall was akinetic or hypokinetic, flow was reduced. At the time of surgery in patients with ECG evidence of myocardial infarction, flow within akinetic areas was 10 times faster than that recorded within fibrous tissue and fat, suggesting the presence of areas of viable myocardium, and indeed this has been demonstrated macroscopically and microscopically at the time of surgery and at post mortem.

The response of the myocardium to stress where it is supplied by a coronary artery with a significant stenosis, is as one would expect, a reduction in flow but often also in distribution. A patient with isolated left anterior descending disease is demonstrated in Plate 4.5, showing reduced distribution and flow, and with the induction of angina a new wall motion abnormality of the lower septum.

Collaterals

Contrast angiography may only delineate vessels down to 50–100 microns in diameter and many collateral channels are smaller than this. Collateral flow can be demonstrated at rest in response to changing distributions in flow, as shown by Rentrop et al. [13] during angioplasty and Matsuda [14] in patients with coronary artery spasm. Xenon, with its small molecular size, can demonstrate distribution from even these small vessels that are beyond angiographic resolution. In 50 patients, at the time of angiography, we have demonstrated that the presence of collateral flow, that is capable of responding to exercise, is associated with preserved regional wall motion, measured by percentage shortening. In addition, using xenon, we were able to identify areas of myocardium, supplied by collateral flow, which were not seen angiographically but whose response to stress varied in a similar way, reflecting their adequacy to

Table 2. Left ventricular function.

Collaterals identified	Angiographically	Xenon-133	Both
Collateral flow on exercise	Ejection fraction %		
Increased	37.5 ± 2.6	45.7 ± 2.9	37.9 ± 2.5
Maintained	50.2 ± 2.8	39.1 ± 2.7	42.1 ± 2.5
Decreased	34.0 ± 2.0	41.0 ± 2.0	38.4 ± 2.7
	Percentage shortening %		
Increased	35.0 ± 8.2[a]	43.5 ± 6.0[a]	38.9 ± 3.9[a]
Maintained	45.7 ± 9.3[b]	34.2 ± 6.6[a]	38.8 ± 4.0[a]
Increased and maintained	39.8 ± 8.8[b]	38.9 ± 6.3[a]	38.3 ± 2.8[b]
Decreased	18.5 ± 6.1	29.9 ± 3.0	25.6 ± 2.8

[a] $p < 0.05$, [b] $p < 0.001$.

supply myocardial flow and also associated with preservation of regional left ventricular function [15] (see Table 2).

Grafts, saphenous vein and internal mammary

We have found that using xenon is of inestimable value in assessing graft flow. Angiographic patency provides very little information as to the distribution of graft flow to the myocardium, or the adequacy of this flow. By selectively cannulating each native vessel and each graft, total left ventricular flow can be assessed (Plate 4.6), as can regional flow. This may give surprising results – in what looks angiographically as a very adequate graft, myocardial flow may be reduced, suggesting that the graft although patent subtends myocardium with an abnormal micro-vasculature (Plate 4.7).

The response of graft flow to stress can also be assessed. In 20 patients with internal mammary artery grafts to the left anterior descending coronary artery, flow in response to atrial pacing increased in the septum in 10 (46.2 ± 5.4 → 55.1 ± 5.3 ml/100 g/min) and decreased in 10 (45.6 ± 4.7 → 38.4 ± 6.0 ml/100 g/min), reflecting the quality of the native vessels (Plate 4.8).

Conclusion

In summary, intracoronary xenon performed at the time of routine angiography can provide information as to regional myocardial flow, distribution and function, which in selected situations may be of inestimable clinical value. The technique uses a standard gamma camera and is of relatively low cost. It requires selective cannulation of the coronary arteries, which is invasive, and therefore is unlikely to be used routinely in patient assessment. However, the technique does provide a unique regional myocardial assessment.

References

1. Eckenhoff JE, Hafkenschiel JH, Harmer MH et al. Measurement of coronary blood flow by nitrous oxide method. Am J Physiol 1948; 152: 356–64.
2. Herd JA, Hollenberg M, Thronburn GD, Kopald HH, Barger AC. Myocardial blood flow determined with Krypton 85 in unanesthetised dogs. Am J Physiol 1962; 203: 122–4.
3. Ross RS, Ueda K, Lichtlen PR, Rees JR. Measurement of myocardial blood flow in animals and man by selective injection of radioactive inert gas into the coronary arteries. Circ Res 1964; 15: 28–41.
4. Kety SS. Theory and applications of exchange of inert gas at lungs and tissues. Pharmacol Rev 1951; 3: 1–41.

5. Conn HL Jr. Equilibrium distribution of radioxenon in tissue: Xenon-hemoglobin association curve. J Appl Physiol 1961; 16: 1065–70.

6. Cannon PJ, Dell RB, Dwyer EM Jr. Measurement of regional myocardial perfusion in man with 133 xenon and a scintillation camera. J Clin Invest 1971; 51: 964–77.

7. Engel HJ. Assessment of regional myocardial blood flow by the precordial 133-Xenon clearance technique. In: Schaper W, editor, The pathophysiology of myocardial perfusion, 1979: 58–92

8. Gensini GG. Coronary arteriography. In: Braunwald E, editor, Heart disease, textbook of cardiovascular medicine. Philadelphia: Saunders 1980: 308–62.

9. Engel HJ, Hein R, Liese W, Hundeshagen H, Lichtlen P. Regional myocardial perfusion at rest in coronary disease assessed by microsphere scintigraphy and inert gas clearance [abstract]. Am J Cardiol 1976; 37: 134.

10. Cannon RD, Bonow RO, Bacharach SL et al. Left ventricular dysfunction in patients with angina pectoris, normal epicardial coronary arteries, and abnormal vasodilator reserve. Circulation 1985; 71: 218–26.

11. Maseri A. Syndrome X: still an appropriate name [editorial]. J Am Coll Cardiol 1991; 17: 1471.

12. Klocke FJ. Measurements of coronary blood flow and degree of stenosis: current clinical implications and continuing uncertainties. J Am Coll Cardiol 1983; 1: 31–41.

13. Rentrop KP, Cohen M, Blarke H, Philips R. Changes in collateral channel filling immediately after controlled coronary artery occlusion by an angioplasty balloon in human subjects. J Am Coll Cardiol 1985; 5: 587–92.

14. Matsuda Y, Ogawa H, Moritoni K et al. Transient appearance of collaterals during vasospastic occlusion in patients without obstructive coronary atherosclerosis. Am Heart J 1985; 109: 759–63.

15. Tweddel AC, Martin W, Hutton I. Perfusion imaging. Br Med Bull 1989; 45: 896–921.

5. Myocardial perfusion and krypton-81m

WILLEM J. REMME

Introduction

In humans, myocardial ischemia may be induced by various different mechanisms. Besides the classic concept of a disturbed ratio between myocardial oxygen demand versus supply, whereby a fixed epicardial coronary stenosis prevents sufficient oxygen and substrate supply to the heart in relation to its instantaneous need, abnormal coronary vasomotor regulation may significantly affect myocardial perfusion and oxygen supply irrespective of demand. Such abnormalities in vasomotor control may range from severe vasospasm to merely reduced coronary vasodilatation following an appropriate stimulus. Moreover, abnormal vasomotor regulation is not restricted to severe coronary lesions, but may also occur in apparently normal epicardial arteries or microvessels when hypercholesterolemia is present.

The realization that abnormal dynamic changes in coronary diameter do occur during normal daily stimuli, such as exercise or cold, and may be involved in the induction of ischemia, underlines the importance of monitoring regional myocardial perfusion to establish the functional significance of such changes in coronary diameter.

As stimuli involved in vasomotor deregulation, whether endothelium- or platelet-derived or neurohumoral by nature, are often short-acting, methods are clearly needed which allow continuous recording of changes in myocardial perfusion at short time intervals.

Besides digital coronary angiography, intracoronary Doppler methods, contrast echocardiography and, possibly, magnetic resonance techniques, several radionuclide methods allow for the determination of coronary flow. Of

Ernst E. van der Wall et al. (eds), What's new in cardiac imaging?, 49–68.
© *1992 Kluwer Academic Publishers. Printed in the Netherlands.*

the latter, krypton-81m may be the isotope of choice where the continuous monitoring of fast changes in myocardial perfusion is concerned.

Characteristics and production of krypton-81m

Krypton-81m is a chemically and biologically inert gas, formed by isomeric transition from unstable rubidium-81 to stable krypton-85. It is eluted in solubilized form in 5% glucose from a generator system in which the parent compound rubidium-81 is absorbed on an ion exchange column [1–3]. The 4.7 hr half-life mother compound rubidium-81 is cyclotron-produced following alpha particle irradiation of natural bromine (Na Br), cuprous bromide or bromide-79 or after bombardment of natural krypton gas [4]. The latter results in a rubidium-81 production rate of 3 mCi/μ A.h., of which > 95% us recovered in aqueous solution. Elution of the ^{81}Rb^{81m}Kr generator with 5% glucose yields only krypton-81m. Contamination by rubidium-81 is negligible if no ionic substances are present in the elution solvent, even at high perfusion rates of 25 ml/minute.

However, optimal perfusion rates to achieve sufficient and a constant delivery of krypton-81m from the generator are between 12 and 15 ml/minute.

Krypton-81m has a very short half-life of 13.6 seconds and emits 190 keV gamma rays (65% abundance). Both the generator system and its short half-life makes this radionuclide more suitable for continuous perfusion studies than for bolus administrations. As such, krypton-81m has been used for the determination of cerebral blood flow [5], right ventricular function studies [6, 7] and venous scintigraphy [8]. Moreover, as a gas, it is widely applied to assess pulmonary ventilation abnormalities [9].

Krypton-81m as a marker for myocardial blood flow

Its usefulness in coronary flow studies relates to its 13.6 second half-life, which is short in relation to myocardial transit time, and to the fact that in eluted form krypton-81m is soluble in plasma and diffuses freely through capillary membranes [10]. When the isotope is continuously administered in a constant amount, e.g. by intracoronary infusion, it distributes through the myocardium in relation to regional coronary blood flow. Subsequent equilibration in the vascular and extravascular compartments occurs rapidly. Approximately 30–60 seconds after onset of infusion a stable distribution pattern is obtained as local supply and decay of the isotope get into equilibrium. Subsequent alterations in krypton-81m distribution depend on its regional supply rate and, hence, on changes in local coronary perfusion. When the isotope is administered at a constant rate, alterations in regional coronary blood flow can be measured by calculating the percentage change in local krypton distribution from the control situation. As a result of its short half-life, tracer washout in the right atrium is neglegible. Both the relative absence of background counts and the 190 keV radiation spectrum ensure optimal imaging.

The potential of the isotope to define changes in regional coronary perfusion was demonstrated in several canine models of coronary artery occlusion, both with a direct intracoronary infusion technique as well as by nonselective administration of krypton-81m in the aortic root [11–13]. These studies already emphasized the capability of this isotope to assess fast sequential alterations in myocardial perfusion. Moreover, a good correlation was observed when krypton-81m myocardial blood flow studies were compared with electromagnetic flow probe measurements [13].

Krypton-81m myocardial perfusion studies in man

In the first coronary flow studies with krypton-81m reported in humans, the isotope was administered continuously in the aortic sinus through a modified Paulin ring catheter, designed for constant administration of krypton-81m in both the left and right aortic cusp [14, 15]. With this approach, Selwyn et al. [15] demonstrated coronary flow reductions in myocardial areas supplied by coronary arteries with significant diameter stenoses. In their studies, regional perfusion abnormalities were observed in the majority of patients with coronary artery disease during pacing-induced stress. During pacing, krypton-81m perfusion decreased in most, but not in all areas with > 70% diameter stenoses, whereas count rates increased in normal regions. However, various areas with significant lesions were not described as abnormal in patients with multivessel disease.

This nonselective approach, i.e. the administration of krypton-81m in the aortic sinuses rather than direct in the coronary arterial system, may result in a number of restrictions.

Even when catheters are designed to deliver the isotope at various preselected locations in the aortic sinuses simultaneously, the total amount of radioactivity which reaches the left ventricle will be proportionally small compared with the direct intracoronary administration. In our experience, reliable data were difficult to obtain when a nonselective method of administration in the aortic sinuses was applied, irrespective of whether specially designed catheters

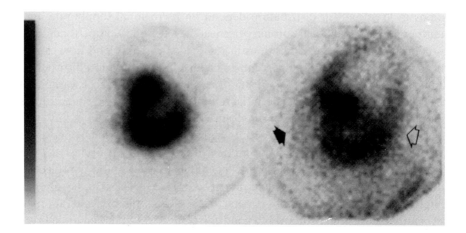

Figure 1. An example of the difference between direct intracoronary infusion of krypton-81m (left image) and nonselective administration of the isotope in the aortic sinuses via a modified Paulin catheter (right image) with respect to imaging quality in the same patient. Activity over the heart is clearly more pronounced with the intracoronary technique. Moreover, with the nonselective method concomitant perfusion of the right coronary artery occurs (closed arrow), which may lead to overlap with left coronary artery distribution in the inferoapical region. Also, overprojection of counts from the descending thoracic aorta in the circumflex area occurs with the nonselective method (open arrow).

or standard angiographic catheters were used [16]. In contrast, selective intracoronary infusion of krypton-81m in the same patient provided acceptable information.

An additional problem with the nonselective infusion technique is that both coronary arteries are simultaneously perfused which leads to overprojection during planar imaging. Both the overprojection and relatively high background activity of the descending aorta, which in the 45° left anterior oblique (LAO) projection, commonly applied during these invasive studies, concerns the left circumflex or right posterolateral regions, present problems defining krypton-81m perfusion changes in these areas (Figure 1), problems which do not arise with the selective intracoronary infusion technique.

Selective intracoronary administration of krypton-81m

We have focused on the value of continuous intracoronary infusion of krypton-81m to assess functionally significant coronary artery lesions in humans

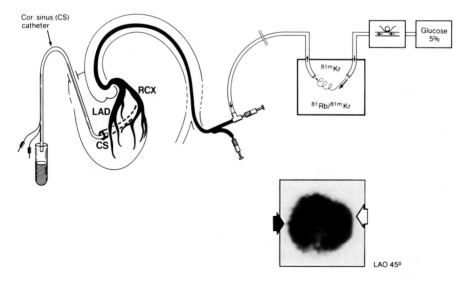

Figure 2. Schematic representation of the intracoronary krypton-81m study design. Krypton-81m is eluted from the ^{81}Rb/^{81m}Kr generator in glucose 5% and administered directly through a left coronary artery catheter into the coronary system, where it distributes over the left anterior descending (LAD, closed arrow) and left circumflex artery (LCX, open arrow) perfusion areas. Studies were performed in the 45° LAO position. An example of krypton distribution in a patient without coronary artery disease is given at the bottom.

[17–19]. Studies were carried out during elective cardiac catheterization in patients with suspected or confirmed ischemic heart disease.

Catheterizations were performed in the morning after an overnight fast and without pre-medication using the Seldinger technique, but before routine coronary and left heart angiography. Typically, a 7F Judkins or Amplatz left coronary artery catheter was positioned in the left coronary main stem and the length of the latter examined in relation to the position of the catheter tip. Next, the occurrence of selective injections in one of the branches of the left coronary artery were determined by slow and fast manual contrast injections in both the 45° LAO and 30° right inferior oblique (RIO) positions. When the possibility of streaming could not be excluded, different catheter types and sizes were tried. Finally, any fluctuation in isotope distribution over the left ventricle was assessed during a 10-minute control infusion period with krypton-81m before initiation of the study.

A schematic representation of the investigational set-up is given in Figure 2. During our studies, a constant perfusion rate of 13.3 ml/minute 5% glucose was achieved by way of a peristaltic infusion pump, resulting in approximately 15 mCi total radioactivity per minute with a 20 mCi generator. The eluate was then passed through a sterile 200 nm membrane filter and continuously infused into the left coronary artery at a rate of 800 ml/hour.

Imaging was performed with a 1/2 inch single crystal gamma camera (General Electrics Portacamera) connected on-line with a Medical Data System A² computer. Energy detection was set on 190 keV ± 20%. In a small number of patients imaging was carried out with a 1/4 inch crystal camera (Siemens LEM portable camera). Using similar data processing techniques total counts over the heart/min averaged ± 250,000 for the 1/2 inch and ± 180,000 for the 1/4 inch crystal camera. Consequently, all krypton-81m studies in patients were carried out with the General Electric Portacamera during imaging periods of 15 seconds each.

Continuous determination of regional myocardial blood flow with intracoronary krypton-81m

The usefulness of continuous intracoronary krypton-81m infusion to delineate abnormalities in regional coronary flow was studied during incremental atrial pacing in 25 patients, 21 with significant (> 50% diameter stenosis) left coronary artery disease (L-CAD) and four without coronary lesions (N-CAD) [20]. In the L-CAD group 15 regions with a > 90%, eight with a 70–90% and seven with a 50–70% coronary artery stenosis were present.

Krypton-81m distribution at rest before pacing

After instrumentation, a 20-minute resting period was allowed before pacing was initiated. Krypton infusion was started during the last 10 minutes of this control period.

Baseline krypton-81m distribution was stable with only minor fluctuations over heart and aorta (< 5%) and negligible background counts. Although none of the patients had signs of ischemia before pacing, krypton-81m perfu-

→

Figure 3a. Krypton-81m study in a patient with a recent (< one week) occlusion of the proximal left circumflex artery (LCX, closed arrow) and a 50–70% stenosis halfway the left anterior descending (LAD) artery. No anterograde collaterals have formed. Consequently, krypton-81m distribution is absent in the post-stenotic LCX area. Also, during pacing and ischemia no distribution changes occur in the LAD region.
Figure 3b. A subsequent study is performed after 30 minutes in the same patient, but now krypton is administered in the right coronary artery, which is normal and has formed retrograde collaterals (closed arrow upper image). During pacing retrograde collateral perfusion increases and krypton-81m distribution in the LCX area develops (arrow lower image).

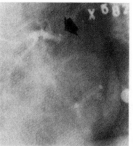

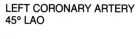

LEFT CORONARY ARTERY
45° LAO

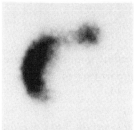 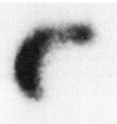 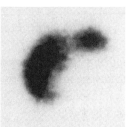

| CONTROL | ANGINA PECTORIS 130 B/MIN | 5 MIN P-P |

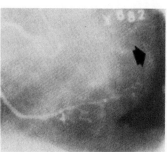

RIGHT CORONARY ARTERY
45° LAO

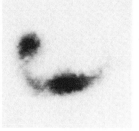 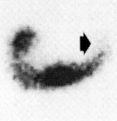 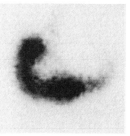

| CONTROL | ANGINA PECTORIS 130 B/MIN | 5 MIN P-P |

sion at rest had already decreased, although stable in five areas, all with > 90% lesions. In four such regions which corresponded with a documented previous myocardial infarction, anterograde collaterals were present. In contrast, in the fifth patient who was studied twice within one week, the left circumflex artery, which initially had a 99% proximal stenosis, had closed without anterograde collaterals and, consequently, absent krypton-81m perfusion of the circumflex region (Figure 3a). However, retrograde collaterals had formed from the right coronary artery, resulting in perfusion of the left circumflex area, as shown by subsequent krypton-81m infusion of the right coronary artery (Figure 3b) [16].

Krypton-81m distribution in patients without coronary artery disease

During pacing, heart rate was increased by 10 beats/2 minutes until moderate to severe angina, atrioventricular block or a maximal heart rate of 170 beats/ minute was reached. Maximal heart rates were comparable in groups L-CAD and N-CAD.

Nevertheless, patients without significant coronary lesions did not develop signs of ischemia during pacing.

Also, krypton-81m distribution did not change in areas with or without only minimal (< 50%) coronary lesions, although minor fluctuations (< 5%) were present throughout the study.

Krypton-81m distribution in areas with significant coronary lesions

In all regions with > 70% coronary diameter stenoses, krypton distribution decreased during the pacing stress test. However, both the onset and the degree of distribution changes were different in > 90% versus 70–90% lesion

Table 1. Krypton-81m distribution changes during and after pacing.

Areas	Pacing period			Post-pacing period		
	100 beats/min	120 beats/min	AP	15 sec	1 min	5 min
L-CAD						
≥ 90% (n = 15)	81 ± 4[a]	77 ± 7.5[a]	69 ± 6[a]	79 ± 6[a]	81 ± 7[a]	84 ± 4[a]
71–90% (n = 18)	97 ± 2[a]	87 ± 4[a]	81 ± 4[a]	81 ± 3[a]	83 ± 5.5[a]	87 ± 2[a]
Normal						
(n = 21)	110 ± 3[a]	116 ± 3[a]	132 ± 7[a]	121 ± 7[a]	119 ± 7[a]	113 ± 5[a]

[a] $p < 0.05$ vs control values. AP = anginal pain; L-CAD = left coronary artery disease.

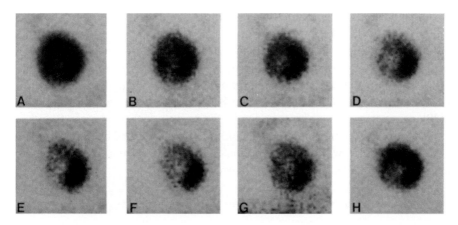

Figure 4. Representative example of krypton-81m distribution changes during incremental pacing and the temporal relation with electrocardiographic, metabolic and subjective symptoms of ischemia in a patient with a proximal 90% left anterior descending coronary artery stenosis. At rest, there is normal krypton-81m distribution (A). Early during pacing (100 b/min), a decrease of krypton-81m perfusion is observed over the LAD area without signs of ischemia (B). A progressive reduction is observed at higher pacing rates accompanied by ST-segment changes (C, 120 b/min), lactate production (D, 140 b/min) and angina (E, 160 b/min). No changes immediately after pacing (F), but still significantly reduced krypton-81m distribution at 5 and 15 minutes post-pacing (G and H, resp.), long after signs of ischemia have disappeared.

areas. In severe lesions, krypton-81m perfusion started to decrease early after the onset of pacing with a significant reduction to 81% of control at 100 beats/minute, followed by a progressive decline to 69% at maximal pacing rates (Table 1). In contrast, in 70–90% stenosis areas changes occurred later, in some instances at the end of the test. In the latter regions, maximal reduction in krypton-81m perfusion was 81 ± 4%, significantly different from the changes in > 90% stenosis areas. Collateralized areas generally showed reductions in krypton distribution comparable to noncollateralized regions, although changes tended to be more abrupt in the presence of collaterals. Only in one area with a 100% occlusion and anterograde collaterals, a late increase in krypton-81m perfusion was observed towards the end of the pacing procedure.

Persistence of coronary flow reductions after pacing

An interesting and, at that time, unexpected finding in these krypton studies, was the observation that coronary flow reductions persisted for relatively long periods after pacing [16, 19, 20]. Although per protocol 5-minute post-pacing values were available in all patients, studies were extended in several others.

These indicated that coronary flow reductions could persevere for as long as 15 minutes after the stress test, long after signs and symptoms of ischemia had disappeared (Figure 4). As overall myocardial blood flow is back to control in approximately 1–2 minutes after pacing [21], this implies a persistent absolute flow reduction in the ischemia area. In our studies, coronary flow only returned to normal in 30% of >70% stenosis areas within 5 minutes after pacing [20].

Prolonged reductions in regional coronary flow have also been reported by Selwyn et al. [22], who observed diminished rubidium-82 uptake which persevered for as long as 20 minutes after stress testing.

Krypton-81m distribution changes in 50–70% stenosis areas

In contrast to the consistent observations with respect to krypton-81m distribution in >70% stenosis areas during and after pacing, changes were more variable in regions with 50–70% coronary diameter narrowings. Irrespective as to whether single- or multivessel disease was studied, krypton distribution either remained unchanged or increased in the majority of lesions. However, in two instances, krypton perfusion did decrease, indicative of the functional significance of these lesion areas.

Temporal relation of krypton distribution changes and myocardial ischemia

The continuous determination of krypton-81m distribution changes makes it possible to assess the temporal relation between alterations in regional coronary flow and the occurrence of ischemia in man. This probably reflects one of the more important advantages of the technique.

Combined krypton-81m and metabolic studies were carried out in 17 patients with >70% diameter stenosis in at least one branch of the left coronary artery [23]. The metabolic studies implied simultaneous blood sampling from a coronary sinus catheter (7F Zucker or Wilton Webster flow catheter) and the side line of the arterial Desilet introducer system. Consequently, only those coronary lesions which were in the sampling area of the coronary sinus catheter were accepted in this study. The pacing protocol was identical to that described before. However, emphasis was on the immediate pacing period, as previous studies had indicated that the optimal timing for the determination of the metabolites to be studied, lactate and the nucleoside hypoxanthine [24, 25], is in the first minute post-pacing [26, 27]. The techniques for blood collection and metabolic assays have been described before [23, 26].

Continuous determination of krypton-81m distribution and sampling at fixed intervals during pacing indicated that coronary flow reductions in severe

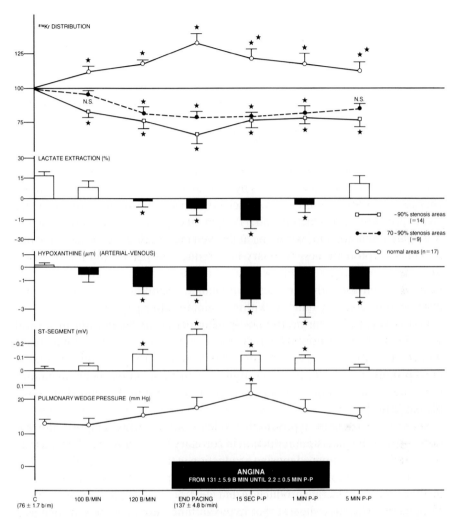

Figure 5. Temporal relation of krypton-81m distribution changes and metabolic, electrocardiographic, hemodynamic and subjective signs of ischemia. In areas with severe (> 90%) coronary lesions krypton perfusion is already reduced before myocardial ischemia is objectivated. In less severe stenosis areas perfusion abnormalities are of later onset, coinciding with myocardial lactate and hypoxanthine release and ST segment depression. Angina is a late phenomenon. After pacing, krypton-81m distribution abnormalities persevere for at least 5 minutes after the stress test, indicating a sustained reduction in myocardial perfusion. In contrast, most signs of ischemia disappear between 1 and 5 minutes post-pacing. Only hypoxanthine release from the heart persists, indicating ongoing ischemia besides coronary flow reduction.

→

Figure 6a. The usefulness of performing repetitive studies in different imaging positions is indicated in this patient who had 90% diameter stenoses in the left anterior descending (LAD, closed arrow) and first marginal branch (open arrow, Figure 5b). During the first study in the 45° LAO position diminished krypton-81m distribution over the LAD area is present, but not clear in the LCX region, possibly due to overlap of adjoining normal marginal branches.
Figure 6b. The functional significance of the LCX lesion becomes clear when a second study is performed in the 30° right inferior oblique position. A krypton-81m perfusion defect is visible during the second pacing test in the post-stenotic marginal area (arrows).

lesion areas (>90% stenosis) preceded metabolic, hemodynamic, and electrocardiographic ischemic changes by several minutes (Figure 5). In contrast, changes in 70–90% lesion areas coincided with significant myocardial lactate and hypoxanthine production and ST-segment depression. Of interest, angina was a late phenomenon, occurring at an even later period. As observed in our previous krypton studies, coronary flow reductions persevered for at least 5 minutes after pacing together with sustained hypoxanthine release from the heart. In contrast, other indices of ischemia, including lactate production, disappeared relatively quickly, within 2 minutes after pacing.

Our observations during the post-pacing period are important in several ways. First, coronary flow in the ischemic regions apparently does not increase immediately after cessation of pacing when lactate and hypoxanthine release is most prominent [21, 26, 27]. This argues against a wash-out phenomenon of these metabolites from the ischemic part of the heart in the immediate post-pacing period.

Secondly, sustained hypoxanthine release after pacing supports the hypothesis that the persistent reduction in coronary flow following ischemia may be caused by continuing adenosine production in the ischemic area [25, 28, 29].

Significant krypton distribution changes and hypoxanthine release occurred in all patients, but lactate production and electrocardiographic changes only in 15 patients. This may suggest that hypoxanthine may be more sensitive as a metabolic marker of ischemia than lactate. Also, in this study four patients had reduced krypton perfusion at rest without angina or electrocardiographic signs of ischemia. However, in two patients significant hypoxanthine release was present as the only indication that (silent) ischemia did accompany this reduction in regional coronary flow [23].

Usefulness of repetitive krypton-81m imaging in different positions

Krypton-81m studies were typically performed in the 40–45° LAO position with or without ≤ 10° cranial tilt. This allowed clear separation of the left

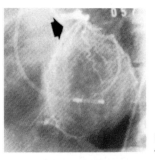

**LEFT CORONARY ARTERY
45° LAO**

  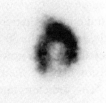

CONTROL   110 B/MIN   ANGINA PECTORIS
                                                130 B/MIN

Figure 6a

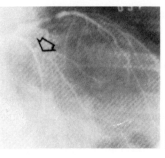

**LEFT CORONARY ARTERY
30° RIO**

 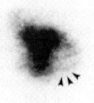 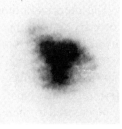

CONTROL   ANGINA PECTORIS   2 MIN P-P
                  130 B/MIN

Figure 6b

anterior descending and circumflex regions. In addition, right coronary artery perfusion studies were conducted from this position. In most patients with multivessel disease and in all with single vessel disease, one study in the LAO position was sufficient to obtain the information required.

Occasionally, however, a second study from a different angle was needed to separate overlapping areas in the left circumflex area. The position which best suited this was the 30 degree right inferior oblique. Repeated pacing was carried out after a 30-minute interval. An example is given in Figure 6a. The patient concerned had both a 90% lesion of the left anterior descending (LAD) artery and of the left obtuse marginal branch. During the first pacing test in the 45° LAO position, the reduction in krypton perfusion in the LAD region was obvious, but less clear in the circumflex area, probably through simultaneous hyperemia in overlapping areas with normal marginal branches. However, in the 30° RIO position, the different marginal branches were better separated and now the functional significance of the 90% obtuse marginal lesion became clear (Figure 6b).

This indicates another advantage of krypton-81m studies, the possibility to perform repetitive investigations at relatively short intervals without tracer accumulation in the organ under study or in the background. The latter may be a matter of concern with other tracer techniques.

Comparison of krypton-81m studies with other methods of coronary flow determinations

In humans, coronary blood flow can be determined in several ways. In open-chest conditions during surgery, electromagnetic flow probes allow excellent recordings of single vessel coronary flow. However, in the intact individual, matters are different, however. Although a number of techniques are available, there is no universally applicable method to accurately assess regional coronary flow changes at short intervals over a prolonged period of time in absolute terms.

The thermodilution [30] and inert gas washout methods [31–33] require coronary sinus catheterization and then only indicate overall left ventricular myocardial flow. This limits their use in coronary artery disease, which is essentially a regional problem. Although multiple thermistor catheters allow flow measurements in one subregion [34, 35], more or less the LAD area, our krypton studies have indicated that flow changes distal to LAD lesions may be compensated by increased flow in the LAD area proximal of the lesion. Also, to achieve a stable position with these types of catheter, they have to be advanced into the middle part of the coronary sinus, thereby bypassing the posterolateral region of the left coronary artery.

Doppler flow catheter techniques allow continuous recording of flow velocity changes, however, they are also limited to the proximal coronary system or to one coronary branch only. Other new developments include contrast echocardiography and magnetic resonance spectroscopy. At present, insufficient data are available with respect to their usefulness as methods to determine regional coronary flow changes.

In addition, various radionuclide methods exist which, to some extent, may provide information on regional coronary flow or myocardial perfusion changes.

Radionuclide techniques to determine coronary flow changes

Labelled microspheres of approximately $15\,\mu$, particularly useful in animal studies [36], can be safely applied in man, using macroaggregated albumen, provided that no more than 200,000 particles are administered intracoronary at a slow rate [37, 38]. The obvious disadvantage is that only a few investigations per patient can be performed. Moreover, a potential risk of an allergic response and embolization remains.

Noninvasive studies with thallium-201 or technetium-99m-MIBI or -teboroxime only allow one registration of perfusion changes during ischemia and do not afford a continuous recording of regional coronary flow changes during ischemia.

In contrast, rapid sequential noninvasive estimation of relative regional myocardial flow is obtained by PET scanning using short-lived isotopes as $H_2^{15}O$ [40], nitrogen-13 [39] or rubidium-82 [22, 41]. Although these techniques are well-suited for simultaneous, noninvase monitoring of myocardial perfusion and metabolism in man in specialized centres, the necessary availability of PET scanning equipment precludes general use of these isotopes. One advantage of rubidium-82 is that it is generator-produced. A potential disadvantage of rubidium-82 is that it is dependent on myocardial cellular uptake mechanisms which may be affected by ischemia. In contrast, inert gases such as krypton and xenon are freely diffusable and not dependent on membrane-active uptake mechanisms.

Precordial mapping of inert, radioactive gases

Several solubilized, inert, radioactive gases, such as xenon-133, krypton-85 and xenon-127 diffuse rapidly and freely over capillary membranes into cardiac cells [10]. Besides blood flow, their distribution depends on capillary and cell membrane permeability. Myocardial to blood partition coefficients are 1 and 0.72 for krypton and xenon, respectively [42]. These gases are theoretically capable of estimating regional blood flow during precordial mapping [43, 44]. Of these, xenon-133 has been used most intensively in humans [44–49].

Like our krypton-81m studies, the gas is administered intracoronary in solution. However, in contrast, xenon-133 is administered as a bolus injection and regional wash-out curves measured rather than regional distribution changes. To this purpose, multicrystal cameras are preferentially used due to their fast count rate capabilities. Such fast count rates (up to 200,000–500,000 cts/sec) are unnecessary in krypton-81m studies in view of the limited production of the isotope by the generator. In contrast, the single crystal used in our studies allows for better spatial resolution, important when flow changes in small cardiac areas are determined.

Although several xenon-133 studies with an interval of 6–8 minutes can be performed, background accumulation of the isotope occurs as a result of its affinity for fat tissue (partition coefficient 8). Also, some recirculation may be present ($\pm 5\%$), whereas its relatively low energy spectrum facilitates Compton scatter.

Limitations of krypton-81m in the determination of myocardial flow

An obvious limitation of the technique is its invasive nature. Moreover, in contrast to other invasive precordial mapping techniques, e.g. xenon-133, only distributional changes and not coronary flow alterations in absolute quantities are measured during continuous intracoronary administration of a fixed amount of the isotope. It, therefore, is not always possible to know whether the observed alterations reflect an absolute change in flow or redistribution from areas with a limited vasodilator reserve to normal regions. Also, streaming may occur during any form of intracoronary administration. This, however, is easily assessed before the stress test is applied. The fact that, in our studies, coronary flow changes persisted after pacing, strongly suggests that the observed changes were real and not induced by changes in catheter tip position during fast pacing rates.

Clinical implications

It should be realized that, as the procedure is, through necessity, invasive of nature, it is not suitable for use as a routine procedure. However, the valuable information which may be derived from this method and which otherwise may be difficult to obtain, underlines its potential usefulness in particular situations both from a clinical and investigational standpoint.

When potential errors are carefully excluded, the continuous intracoronary administration of krypton-81m may enable the clinician to understand better the functional significance of coronary lesions and the appropriate therapeutic approach in the individual patient. This may be particularly useful when 50–70% coronary stenoses diameters are present.

Also, the functional significance of collateral circulation may be determined. Our present knowledge that in stenosis areas of 70% or more, krypton-81m distribution generally declines during a stress test such as atrial pacing indicates that the collateral circulation is well-functioning when myocardial perfusion is preserved in a collateralized area. Moreover, the technique may help clarify the temporal relation between regional post-stenotic changes in coronary flow and manifestations of myocardial ischemia. Furthermore, it may help identify the significance of abnormal vasomotor regulation following endothelium-dependent or independent stimuli.

Finally, the effect of pharmacological interventions on coronary flow and ischemia may be defined during repetitive stress tests in the setting of cardiac catheterization. The short half-life of krypton-81m makes it feasible to carry out several successive studies in the same patient without extra exposure to radiation other than necessary for the instantaneous investigational procedure.

References

1. Jones T, Clark JC. A cyclotron produced 81Rb-81m Kr generator and its uses in gamma-camera studies. Br J Radiol 1969; 42: 237.
2. Yano Y, Anger HO. Ultrashort-lived radioisotopes for visualizing blood vessels and organs. J Nucl Med 1969; 9: 2–6.
3. Colombetti LG, Mayron LW, Kaplan E, Barnes WE, Friedman AM, Gindler JE. Continuous radionuclide generation. I. Production and evaluation of a 81m Kr minigenerator. J Nucl Med 1974; 15: 868–73.
4. Guillaume M, Czichisz R, Richard P, Fagard E. Krypton-81m generator for ventialtion and perfusion. Dosimetry, routine production, methodology for medical applications. Bull Soc Sci Lièges 1983; 52: 214–81.
5. Schroth HJ, Bialy J, Hans FJ et al. Bestimmung des zerebralen Blutflusses mittels des 81Rb/81mKr-Generatorsystems. Nuklearmedizin 1990; 29: 7–12.
6. Oliver RM, Gray JM, Challenor VF, Fleming JS, Waller DG. 81mKr equilibrium radionuclide ventriculography for the assessment of right heart function. Eur J Nucl Med 1990; 16: 89–95.

7. Caplin JL, Flatman WD, Dymond DS. Gated right ventricular studies using krypton-81m: comparison with first-pass studies using gold 195-m. J Nucl Med 1986; 27: 602–8.

8. Zicot M, Guillaume M, Ham H, Redote R. Dynamic isotopic phlebography using soluble krypton-81m. Eur J Nucl Med 1986; 12: 192–6.

9. Hicks IP, Barter SJ, Carr DH, Joyce H, Pride NB, Lavender JP. Abnormal regional distribution of ventilation in middle-aged smokers: comparison of changes in 81Krm ventilation scans and computed tomography of the lung. Clin Radiol 1990; 41: 347–52.

10. Kety SS. The theory and applications of the exchange of inert gas at the lungs and tissues. Pharmacol Rev 1951; 3: 1–41.

11. Kaplan E, Mayron LW, Friedman AM et al. Definition of myocardial perfusion by continuous infusion of krypton-81m. Am J Cardiol 1976; 37: 878–84.

12. Turner JH, Selwyn AP, Jones T, Evans TR, Raphael MJ, Lavender JP. Continuous imaging of regional myocardial blood flow in dogs using krypton-81m. Cardiovasc Res 1976; 10: 398–404.

13. Selwyn AP, Jones T, Turner JH, Pratt T, Clark J, Lavender P. Continuous assessment of regional myocardial perfusion in dogs using krypton-81m. Circ Res 1978; 42: 771–7.

14. Selwyn AP, Steiner R, Kivisaari A, Fox KM, Forse G. Krypton-81m in the physiologic assessment of coronary artery stenosis in man. Am J Cardiol 1979; 43: 547–53.

15. Selwyn AP, Forse G, Fox KM, Jonathan A, Steiner P. Patterns of disturbed myocardial perfusion in patients with coronary artery disease. Circulation 1981; 64: 83–90.

16. Remme WJ, Cox PH, Krauss XH, Kruijssen HACM, Storm CJ, Van Hoogenhuyze DCA. Visualization of myocardial blood-flow changes with intracoronary 81mKr. In: Biersack HJ, Cox PH, editors, Radioisotope studies in cardiology. Dordrecht, The Netherlands: Martinus Nijhoff 1985: 263–8.

17. Remme WJ, Cox PH, Krauss XH. Continuous myocardial bloodflow distribution imaging in man with krypton 81m intracoronary [abstract]. Am J Cardiol 1982; 49: 979.

18. Remme WJ, Kruijssen HA, Cox PH, Krauss XH. Assessment of functionally significant coronary artery disease during continuous intracoronary administration of krypton-81m [abstract]. Eur Heart J 1983; 4 Suppl E: 32.

19. Remme WJ, Cox PH, Krauss XH, Van der Kemp P, Storm CJ, Van Hoogenhuyze DCA. Continuous myocardial blood flow imaging with krypton-81m selective intracoronary. In: Salvatore M, Porta E, editors, Radioisotopes in cardiology. New York: Plenum Press 1983: 155–63.

20. Remme WJ, Krauss XH, Van Hoogenhuyze DCA, Cox PH, Storm CJ, Kruijssen HACM. Continuous determination of regional myocardial blood flow with intracoronary krypton-81m in coronary artery disease. Am J Cardiol 1985; 56: 445–51.

21. Remme WJ, Van Hoogenhuyze DCA, Krauss XH, Hofman A, Kruijssen HACM, Storm CJ. Acute hemodynamic and antiischemic effects of intravenous amiodarone. Am J Cardiol 1985; 55: 639–44.

22. Selwyn AP, Allan RM, l'Abbata A et al. Relation between regional myocardial uptake of rubidium-82 and perfusion: absolute reduction of cation uptake in ischemia. Am J Cardiol 1982; 50: 112–21.

23. Remme WJ, Van de Berg MD, Mantel M et al. Temporal relation of changes in regional coronary flow and myocardial lactate and nucleoside metabolism in humans during pacing-induced ischemia. Am J Cardiol 1986; 58: 1188–94.

24. Remme WJ, De Jong JW, Verdouw PD. Effects of pacing induced myocardial ischemia on hypoxanthine efflux from the human heart. Am J Cardiol 1977; 40: 55–62.

25. Remme WJ. Myocardial ischemia: a profile of its pathophysiological basis and its detection by

nuclear cardiology. In: Biersack HJ, Cox PH, editors, Radioisotope studies in cardiology. Dordrecht, The Netherlands: Martinus Nijhoff 1985: 3–48.

26. Remme WJ, Krauss XH, Storm CJ, Kruijssen HACM, Van Hoogenhuyze DCA. Improved assessment of lactate production during pacing induced ischemia [abstract]. J Moll Cell Cardiol 1981; 13 suppl 1: 76.

27. Remme WJ, Kruijssen HACM, Krauss XH, Storm CJ, Van Hoogenhuyze DCA. Myocardial metabolism during pacing-induced ischemia in man. Temporal relationship with changes in post-stenotic coronary flow. In: Mohl W, Faxon D, Wolner E, editors, Progress in coronary sinus interventions. Vol II. Darmstadt: Clinics of CSI, Steinkopff 1986.

28. Olsson RA. Changes in content of purine nucleoside in canine myocardium during occlusion. Circ Res 1970; 26: 301–6.

29. Fox AC, Reed GE, Glassman E, Kaltman AJ, Silk BB. Release of adenosine from human hearts during angina induced by rapid atrial pacing. J Clin Invest 1974; 53: 1447–57.

30. Ganz W, Tamura K, Marcus HS, Donoso R, Yoshida S, Swan HJC. Measurement of coronary sinus blood flow by continuous thermodilution in man. Circulation 1971; 44: 181–95.

31. Weisse AB, Regan TJ. A comparison of thermodilution, coronary sinus blood flows and krypton myocardial blood flows in the intact dog. Cardiovasc Res 1974; 8: 526–33.

32. Rau G. Messung der Koronardurchblutung mit der Argon-Femdgasmethode. Tierexperimenten und Untersuchungen am Patienten bei niedriger und hoher Durchblutung. Arch Kreislaufforsch 1969; 58: 322–98.

33. Tauchert M, Kochsiek K, Heiss HW, Rau G, Bretschneider HJ. Technik der Organdurchblutungsmessung mit der Argon-methode. Z Kreislaufforsch 1971; 60: 871–80.

34. Pepine CJ, Mehta J, Webster WW, Nichols WW. In vivo validation of a thermodilution method to determine regional left ventricular blood-flow in patients with coronary disease. Circulation 1978; 58: 795–802.

35. Feldman RL, Pepine CJ, Whittle JL, Curry RC, Conti CR. Coronary hemodynamic findings during spontaneous angina in patients with variant angina. Circulation 1981; 64: 76–82.

36. Domenech RJ, Hoffman JI, Noble MI, Saunders KB, Henson JR, Subijanto S. Total and regional coronary blood flow measured by radioactive microspheres in conscious and anesthetized dogs. Circ Res 1969; 25: 581–96.

37. Ashburn WL, Braunwald E, Simon AL, Peterson KL, Gault JH. Myocardial perfusion imaging with radioactive labeled particles injected directly into the coronary circulation of patients with coronary artery disease. Circulation 1971; 44: 581–96.

38. Weller DA, Adolph RJ, Wellman NH, Caroll RG, Kim O. Myocardial perfusion scintigraphy after intracoronary injection of 99m Tc-labeled human albumin microspheres. Circulation 1972; 46: 963–75.

39. Bergmann SR, Fox KAA, Rand AL et al. Quantification of regional myocardial blood flow in vivo with $H_2{}^{15}O$. Circulation 1984; 70: 724–33.

40. Schelbert HR, Phelps ME, Hoffman EJ, Huang SC, Selin CE, Kuhl DE. Regional myocardial perfusion assessed with N-13 labelled ammonia and positron emission computerized axial tomography. Am J Cardiol 1979; 43: 209–18.

41. Budinger TF, Yano Y, Hoop B. A comparison of ^{82}Rb and $^{13}NH_3$ for myocardial positron scintigraphy. J Nucl Med 1975; 16: 429–31.

42. Parkey RW, Lewis SE, Stokely EM, Bonte FJ. Compartmental analysis of the 133Xe regional myocardial blood-flow curve. Radiology 1972; 104: 425–6.

43. Herd JA, Hollenberg M, Thorburn GD, Kopala HH, Barger AC. Myocardial blood flow determined with krypton 85 in unanaesthetized dogs. Am J Physiol 1962; 203: 122–4.

44. Ross RS, Ueda K, Lichtlen PR et al. Measurement of myocardial blood flow in animals and

man by selective injection of radioactive inert gas into the coronary arteries. Circ Res 1964; 15: 28–41.

45. Cannon PJ, Dell RB, Dwyer EM Jr. Measurement of regional myocardial perfusion in man with 133 Xe and a scintillation camera. J Clin Invest 1972; 51: 964–77.

46. Maseri A, Mancini P. The evaluation of regional myocardial perfusion in man by a scintillation camera computer system. In: Maseri A, editor, Myocardial blood flow in man. Torino: Minerva Medica 1972: 219–29.

47. Holman BL, Adams DF, Jewitt D et al. Measuring regional myocardial blood flow with 133Xe and the Anger camera. Radiology 1974; 112: 99–107.

48. Schmidt DH, Weiss MB, Casarella WJ, Fowler DL, Sciacca RR, Canron PJ. Regional myocardial perfusion during atrial pacing in patients with coronary artery disease. Circulation 1976; 53: 807–19.

49. Maseri A, l'Abbate A, Pesola A, Michelassi C, Marzilli M, De Nes M. Regional myocardial perfusion in patients with atherosclerotic coronary artery disease at rest and during angina pectoris induced by tachycardia. Circulation 1977; 55: 423–33.

6. Myocardial perfusion imaging with technetium-99m isonitriles: Attractive thallium substitutes?

PIERRE RIGO, MARIE-PAULIE LAROCK and SIMON H. BRAAT

Introduction

Myocardial imaging has been used extensively over the past 20 years to assess the repercussions of coronary artery disease on regional myocardial perfusion, function, and viability, and to evaluate the patients' prognosis [1]. Thallium-201 has been the tracer of choice for most of these years after less satisfactory initial experiences using cesium-131, potassium-43, or isotopes of rubidium [2–4]. However, the physical and biological characteristics of thallium-201 are less than ideal; its energy of 68 to 80 keV makes it suboptimal to use with a scintillation camera, while its half-life of 73 hours increases the dose of radiation delivered and limits the applicable activity. Furthermore, thallium redistribution creates logistic problems.

The impetus to develop a technetium-99m labeled perfusion agent has therefore remained high considering the demonstrated value of myocardial imaging and the potential improvement resulting from such a tracer. After several unsatisfactory trials, success has first been met with the development of technetium isonitrile compounds by Jones et al. at Harvard University [5–7].

Methoxyisobutyl isonitrile or sestaMIBI or Cardiolite® has emerged as the most satisfactory compound among several alternatives [8]. It has undergone extensive clinical trials and is now clinically available.

Kinetics and pathophysiological characteristics of technetium sestaMIBI in comparison to thallium

Hexakis alkylisonitrile technetium complexes are monovalent cations with a

69

Ernst E. van der Wall et al. (eds), What's new in cardiac imaging?, 69–85.
© *1992 Kluwer Academic Publishers. Printed in the Netherlands.*

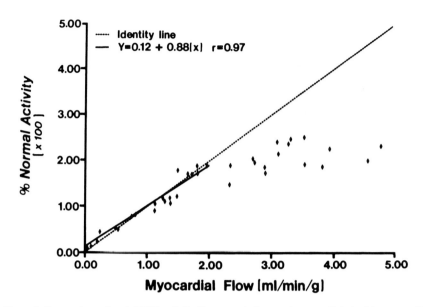

Figure 1. Comparison of sestaMIBI activity (in percent of normal zone activity) with myocardial blood flow determined by microsphere under hyperemic conditions induced by dipyridamole infusion. SestaMIBI distribution is linearly related to flow up to 2.0 ml/min/g. At higher flow rates sestamibi distribution underestimated flow (from Glover and Okada (1990) *Circulation* 81: 628–636, by permission of the American Heart Association).

central technetium core octahedrally surrounded by six identical ligands coordinated through the isonitrile carbon. The terminal alkyl groups, when bound to technetium, encase the metal with a sphere of lipophilicity. The capillary membrane permeability of sestaMIBI is smaller than that of thallium but the opposite is true at the parenchymal cell level [9].

Net retention in the early phase (extraction) is larger for thallium but later this phenomenon reverses due to thallium redistribution. The mechanism of uptake of both tracers differs. It is likely that thallium uptake uses a potassium-like mechanism (adenosine triphosphatase and others) although depression of thallium-201 influx with ouabain was only clearly demonstrated in erythrocyte membranes [10] and not in cultured heart cell [11]. Technetium sestaMIBI uptake is related to its lipophilicity but probably also involves distribution across biological membranes in response to membrane potential, as previously demonstrated for carbon-11 triphenylmethylphosphonium [12]. Chiu et al. [13] tested that hypothesis in cultured mouse fibroblasts as well as in cultured chicken embryo heart cells. Depolarization of plasma membrane potential or of mitochondrial membrane potential inhibited net uptake and retention while hyperpolarization increases net uptake of technetium sestaMIBI. These re-

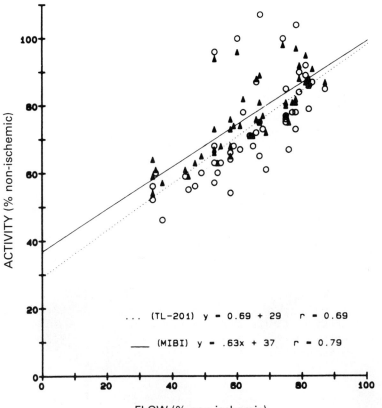

Figure 2. Comparison of thallium and technetium sestaMIBI activity and myocardial blood flow in regions rendered ischemic by restricting coronary flow to ≤ 60% of preocclusion flow. Activity is expressed in percent of non-ischemic values. A good correlation is observed for both tracers in these low flow conditions (from Sinusas et al. (1989) *J Am Coll Cardiol* 14: 1785–1793, by permission of the American College of Cardiology).

sults suggest that sestaMIBI is a lipophilic cation responsive to changes in mitochondrial or plasma membrane potentials, raising the possibility of monitoring membrane potential in vivo in addition to assessing myocardial perfusion. This probably explains why sestaMIBI uptake is influenced by profound hypoxia or metabolic poisoning. It should finally be pointed out that such a mechanism of uptake has never been adequately assessed for thallium and cannot be ruled out in the case of that tracer.

Fundamental to the measurement of myocardial perfusion with tracers is their characteristics to accumulate in the myocardium in proportion to blood flow. This requires a constant extraction sufficiently high to be completed

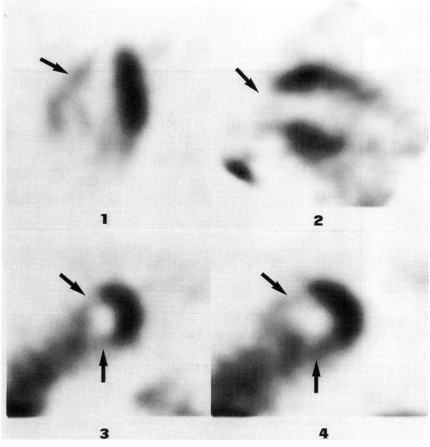

Figure 3(a)

during the time frame (few seconds or minutes) of the hemodynamic conditions to be measured. Although as mentioned before, technetium sestaMIBI is only partially extracted (± 60%) and its extraction fraction decreases with increasing flow, the tissue tracer content is proportional to blood flow measured, for instance, by microspheres (Figures 1 and 2). Among several studies, Okada et al. [14] demonstrated a good correlation between microsphere determined blood flow and technetium sestaMIBI distribution in a dog model with partial left circumflex coronary occlusion. This relation was maintained when coronary blood flow was increased by intravenous perfusion of dipyridamole [15]. Tomographic evaluation of technetium sestaMIBI also correlated with regional myocardial perfusion evaluated by microspheres during coronary occlusion and after reperfusion [16]. However, after injection during

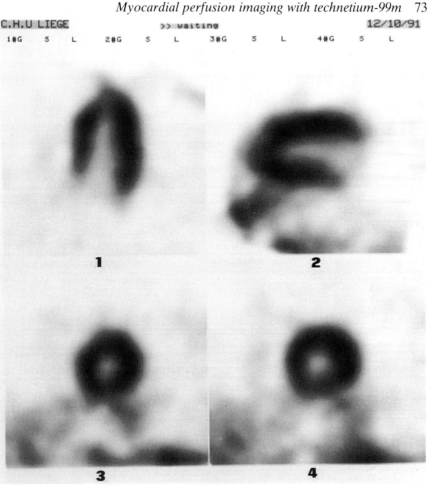

Figure 3(b)

Figure 3. Detection of multiple vessel coronary disease. The comparison of dipyridamole (a) and rest (b) tomograms shows the presence of reversible sestaMIBI defects in the anteroseptal and in the posteroinferior walls of the left ventricle (arrows), corresponding to myocardial ischemia in the LAD and RCA vessel territories. 1: Horizontal long axis view. 2: Vertical long axis view. 3, 4: Short axis view.

occlusion followed by 3 hours of reperfusion, some slight redistribution was observed by Li et al. [17], but to a much smaller degree than thallium. This slight redistribution has to be related to the low blood levels of technetium sestaMIBI and the slow myocardial release of accumulated tracer. This observation can partly explain that myocardial uptake of technetium sestaMIBI in a low-flow region is higher than expected on the basis of regional blood flow. Increased extraction of MIBI at low flow, a phenomenon observed with all the other cationic tracers, is an additional or alternative explanation. This in-

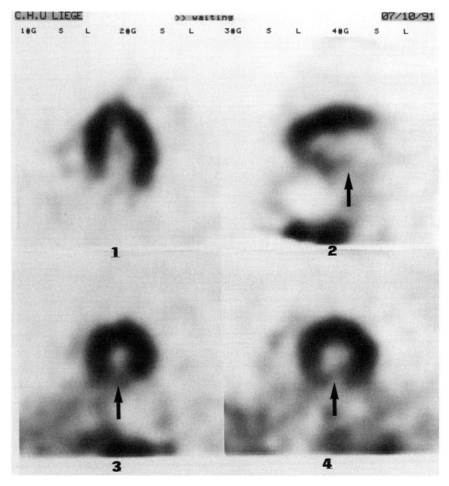

Figure 4(a)

creased extraction is not evident, however, when flow is decreased to between 0 and 10% of control, suggesting the need for persisting viable myocardium to extract the tracer [18].

Clinical applications

Detection of coronary artery disease

Myocardial scintigraphy with thallium has established the value of perfusion imaging for the diagnosis and assessment of patients with suspected or definite

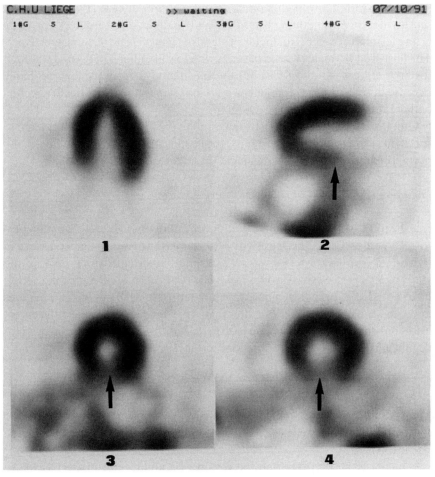

Figure 4(b)

Figure 4. Detection of myocardial infarction. Tomography performed both at stress (a) and rest (b) demonstrates the presence of sestaMIBI defects, identical in extent and severity, in the inferior wall of the left ventricle. These correspond to a myocardial scar. 1, 2, 3, 4: see Figure 3.

coronary artery disease. Demonstration of a reversible perfusion defect confirms the presence of coronary artery disease and of exercise-induced myocardial ischemia due to a functionally significant coronary artery stenosis (Figure 3). The presence of a fixed defect also confirms coronary artery disease but suggests the presence of a myocardial scar (Figure 4). The diagnostic accuracy of technetium sestaMIBI and thallium has been evaluated by several studies. The North American Multicenter Trial has evaluated 192 patients with suspected coronary artery disease submitted to coronary angiography as well as

86 patients with a low likelihood of coronary artery disease [19]. The overall sensitivities of technetium sestaMIBI and thallium-201 to detect coronary artery lesions (of > 50% diameter of stenosis) were 89 and 90%, respectively. The observed normalcy rate in patients with low likelihood of disease was high for both tracers (81 and 82%) but the specificity values were low, probably because of selection bias (patients with scintigraphic abnormalities are preferentially referred to coronary angiography).

Other studies have demonstrated similar sensitivity data with adequate specificity values [20]. Furthermore, the sectorial specificity evaluated in the normal regions of patients with single vessel disease is also excellent [21].

Detection of the extent of coronary artery disease

Localization of lesions and recognition of multivessel disease is better performed with SPECT. The sensitivity of sestaMIBI SPECT to detect disease in individual coronary arteries was 89%, while the specificity was 86% in the study of Kiat [20]. Several groups following the French Multicenter study [22], have noted that on planar images technetium sestaMIBI defects sometimes appeared less pronounced or smaller than thallium defects. These differences, also confirmed by Maddahi, do not persist with SPECT as this procedure significantly improves the technetium sestaMIBI defect contrast [23].

Detection and quantification of myocardial infarction

Myocardial imaging has been used not only to recognize the presence and location of old or recent myocardial infarction but also to assess the size of the perfusion defect.

Boucher et al. [24] reported the results of a multicenter phase III clinical trial to test the efficacy of sestaMIBI in the localization and detection of myocardial infarction. A total of 122 patients were enrolled in the study, 50 patients with recent infarction (less than 14 days old), 61 with an old infarction, and 11 with both. The diagnosis of myocardial infarction was made on clinical grounds based on appropriate history and electrocardiographic and/or enzymatic documentation of myocardial infarction. Twenty-four normal subjects served as control.

Of the 122 patients, 115 had Q waves on the electrocardiogram and 113 (98%) of these individuals had a abnormal technetium-99m sestaMIBI study. Two patients without Q waves also had normal perfusion images. Concordance between perfusion and wall motion abnormalities were recorded in 116 patients (95%). These data attest to the high degree of accuracy of sestaMIBI images to detect and localize myocardial infarction. The uptake of sestaMIBI in the affected territory has been quantified in relative terms by Dilsizian et al. [25] and compared to the results of coronary angiography. Uptake was $87 \pm 10\%$ of maximum in normal regions but decreased to $42 \pm 21\%$ in regions supplied by occluded vessels and poor collaterals and to $61 \pm 23\%$ in the territories of occluded arteries supplied by good collaterals. It thus seems that quantitative measurement of perfusion can give an insight into the severity of the disease. Another important aspect of quantitative analysis relates to the sizing of perfusion defects. These data are known to have important prognostic implications. Several studies in experimental animals have compared the myocardial SPECT images and pathologic data for assessment of infarct size. Verani et al. [26], Gibbons et al. [27], Bergin et al. [28] and Prigent et al. [29] all reported high correlation between SPECT and pathology. Experimental studies have also explored the possibility to evaluate the area at risk after a coronary occlusion together with the evolved infarct size.

Studies in the coronary care unit

Use of thallium in the coronary care unit has been hampered by logistical problems. Indeed, thallium on top of its physical disadvantages and relatively long half-life, demonstrates redistribution and requires imaging to be performed shortly after injection. This is frequently a problem, as many patients in the coronary care unit are unstable and not transportable to the nuclear cardiology laboratory, and as camera availability cannot be guaranteed at all times, Technetium sestaMIBI demonstrates no or only minimal redistribution and therefore offers the potential of overcoming these problems.

Uses in unstable angina

Grégoire et al. [30] investigated the value of sestaMIBI as a tool to diagnose myocardial ischemia in spontaneous chest pain. Forty-five patients with pain suggestive of myocardial ischemia were injected during the episode of pain. Injection and imaging were repeated when the patients were free of complaint. No patient in this group had evidence of previous myocardial infarction. Coronary angiography was performed in all patients and a stenosis of $> 50\%$ was considered to be significant. Using single photon emission tomography, technetium sestaMIBI during chest pain had a sensitivity of 96% and a specificity of 79% to detect significant coronary artery disease. If the criterion for positivity was a larger defect during pain as compared to control, sensitivity and specificity values were 81 and 84%, respectively. In contrast, transient electrocardiographic ischemic changes during pain only had figures of 35%

(sensitivity) and 68% (specificity), although ECG changes were sometimes also observed outside episodes of pain.

The authors concluded that technetium-99m sestaMIBI SPECT is a reliable noninvasive diagnostic tool that could aid in the diagnosis of unstable angina and provide additional information to that provided by electrocardiogram.

Assessment of the efficacy of thrombolytic therapy for myocardial infarction

The feasibility of technetium-99m sestaMIBI to assess the myocardial area at risk and the effect of reperfusion was first studied experimentally. After injection during coronary occlusion, the size of sestaMIBI perfusion defect was shown to correlate with the size of the monastral blue defect injected in similar conditions in the arrested heart which represents the size of the area at risk. On the contrary, when sestaMIBI is injected after reperfusion, the defect size corresponds to that observed with triphenyl tetrazolium chloride (TTC) staining that is the size of the pathologic infarct [26].

Assessment of the potential of technetium sestaMIBI to evaluate the area at risk was also performed in man during transient coronary occlusion in the course of balloon angioplasty [31, 32]. Larock et al. [32] compared estimates of perfusion defects as measured by sestaMIBI Spect 2–3 hours after injection with the degree of functional impairment observed during a per-occlusion angiogram. The size of perfusion defects correlated both with the drop in global ejection fraction and with the extent of wall motion abnormalities in these patients. Two to three hours after intravenous injection during coronary occlusion, the defect contrast remained extremely high, confirming the absence of redistribution. Finally, in all patients, a repeated sestaMIBI scintigram confirmed the success of angioplasty.

Several clinical studies [33, 34] have confirmed in humans the possibility of imaging the area at risk and the success of thrombolytic therapy in acute myocardial infarction. In these studies, technetium-99m sestaMIBI was injected intravenously within 4 hours of the onset of chest pain and before treatment with thrombolytic therapy. Imaging was performed 1 to 6 hours later but as soon as therapy was completed and the patient stabilized. A second study was performed several days later. A control group of patients in whom thrombolytic therapy was considered contraindicated was also studied. The initial area at risk varied considerably both in patients treated with thrombolysis and in those treated conventionally; however, there was a significant decrease in the area of hypoperfused myocardium between the initial and control studies in patients who received thrombolytic therapy as compared with an insignificant increase in the patients treated conventionally. Furthermore, irrespective of therapy, improvement was related to the early patency of the artery responsible for the infarct.

This imaging approach thus enables us to document the results of therapy in individual patients, but, currently, no data are available to support the concept that patients with large area at risk should be treated differently, for instance, with early interventions such as PTCA or coronary artery bypass grafting.

Assessment of myocardial viability

Little data is currently available regarding the value of sestaMIBI to assess myocardial viability. Studies mentioned earlier indicate the value of quantitative imaging to assess the severity of disease and the quality of collateral perfusion. As a tracer of flow, however, sestaMIBI is likely to overestimate the severity of myocardial damage and should recognize only with difficulty regions of low flow but persisting viability only recognized by metabolic imaging or rest-redistribution thallium studies. The possibility of improving the recognition of viable myocardium by pretreating patients with nitrates prior to rest sestaMIBI injection, has been mentioned but its efficacy has not been documented.

The combined assessment of perfusion and function should also be of value to better characterize myocardial viability and differentiate by instance stunned myocardium from acute ischemia or hibernating myocardium. Several authors have indicated the feasibility of concomitant function and perfusion evaluation. First-pass measurement of ejection fraction followed by SPECT evaluation of perfusion has been performed by Borges-Neto et al. [35] and Larock et al. [36]. Gated scintigraphic planar acquisitions have been proposed by Najm and found to provide functional information well correlated to the ejection fraction [37]. Finally, gated tomographic acquisitions have been performed by Corbett et al. [38] and by Larock et al. [39]. This approach enables simultaneous evaluation of perfusion and wall motion or better wall thickening on a regional basis.

Situations of restored flow but persistent wall motion abnormalities in the course of reperfusion are typical of stunned myocardium. The occurrence of abnormal flow in the absence of wall motion abnormality usually represent a temporal dissociation between the perfusion pattern corresponding to the time of injection and the functional pattern corresponding to the time of acquisition. Myocardial ischemia at the time of injection having resolved before acquisition is such a situation.

Normal wall motion is also sometimes observed in the apical region, where a

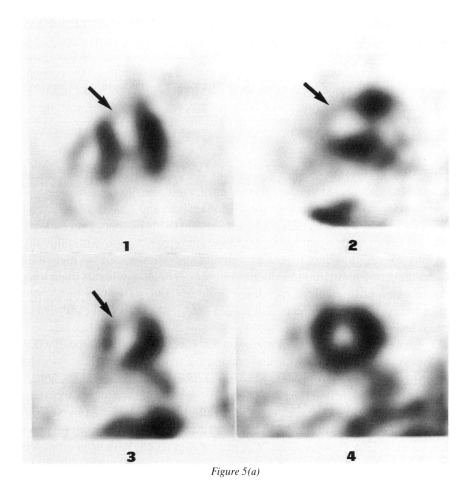

Figure 5(a)

somewhat decreased uptake is a normal variant. In this case, the wall motion pattern helps to recognize the absence of perfusion abnormality.

Results of revascularization therapy

Myocardial perfusion imaging with thallium has taken an important role in the pre- and post-intervention assessment of patients with PTCA and bypass. No intervention should be performed solely on the basis of an angiographic abnormality without concomitant proof that that lesion is responsible for myocardial ischemia. Documentation of the results of intervention and detection of restenosis during later follow-up are also best performed by myocardial imaging [40] (Figure 5).

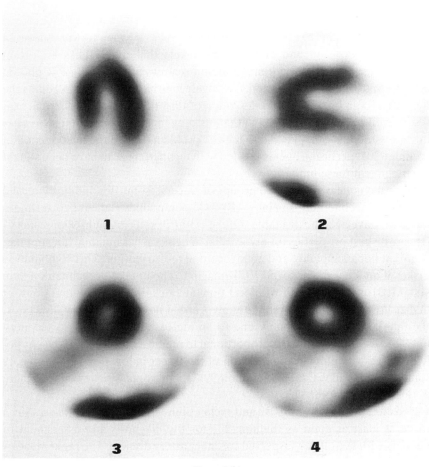

Figure 5(b)

Figure 5. Reperfusion after transluminal angioplasty. Comparison between tomography performed at stress before (a) and after (b) angioplasty allows to visualize the improvement of sestaMIBI
myocardial uptake in the anteroseptal wall of the left ventricle after PTCA. Successful reperfusion
of the LAD vessel territory after angioplasty is thereby demonstrated. 1, 2, 3, 4: see Figure 3.

The place of sestaMIBI in these indications has not yet been fully documented, but preliminary data indicate that it will provide similar information to that
obtained by thallium.

Conclusion

Thallium-201 is and has been used for more than 15 years for measuring of myocardial perfusion and viability. However, thallium-201 has important disadvantages, soft tissue attenuation and scatter caused by the low photon energy emission (68–80 keV) and a relatively long half-life (73 hours) limits the dose which can be administered. On top of this, thallium-201 redistributes at rest as well as during exercise, so that imaging must be performed soon after injection and this can give rise to logistic problems. Since the introduction of thallium-201, perfusion agents labeled with technetium-99m have been sought to circumvent these limitations.

Since a couple of years, two groups of tracers, isonitriles and boronic acid adducts of technetium dioximes (BATO) compounds, labeled to technetium-99m, have become available. Of the isonitriles, technetium-99m sestaMIBI has the best properties for myocardial imaging, it has minimal lung uptake, transient hepatic uptake, and no myocardial redistribution. This combination makes it an ideal tracer for SPECT imaging. The uptake of technetium-99m sestaMIBI is proportional to blood flow at rates up to 2.0 ml/mm/g but, at higher flow rates, it underestimates myocardial flow while, at low flow rates, the uptake is higher probably due to an increased extraction. So technetium-99m sestaMIBI uptake is proportional to regional blood flow in the physiologic range with enhanced extraction of the tracer in low flow regions where some tissue is still viable. Technetium-99m teboroxime is reviewed elsewhere in this book (Chapter 9).

Technetium-99m sestaMIBI and technetium-99m teboroxime have shown to be at least as good as thallium-201 for the diagnosis and assessment of patients with definite or suspected coronary artery disease. The rapid myocardial washout of technetium teboroxime necessitates brief imaging protocols. Technetium-99m sestaMIBI does not redistribute, therefore it can be injected in the coronary care unit or catheterization laboratory and imaging can be performed later at a convenient time in the nuclear cardiology laboratory. Using this possibility, technetium-99m sestaMIBI has been shown to be not only of value to detect and localize myocardial ischemia and infarction, but also to be able to assess the efficacy of thrombolytic therapy and to determine the size of the myocardial area perfused by a coronary artery.

While several questions regarding the role of sestaMIBI remain to be answered, the gathering of information regarding this tracer has been much faster than in the past and it has demonstrated several physical and biological characteristics that constitute a definite improvement over thallium.

References

1. Brown KA. Prognostic value of thallium-201 myocardial perfusion imaging. Circulation 1991; 83: 363–81.
2. Carr EA Jr, Gleason G, Shaw J et al. The direct diagnosis of myocardial infarction by photoscanning after administration of cesium-131. Am Heart J 1964; 68: 627–36.
3. Hurley PJ, Cooper M, Reba RC, Poggenburg KJ, Wagner HN Jr. 43KCl: a new radiopharmaceutical for imaging of the heart. J Nucl Med 1971; 12: 516–9.
4. Rigo P, Schelbert HR, Henning H, Khullar S, Ashburn W, O'Rourke RA. Serial myocardial (M) imaging with Rubidium-81 after acute myocardial infarction (AMI) [abstract]. Eur J Nucl Med 1976; 1: 99.
5. Jones AG, Abrams MJ, Davison A et al. Biological studies of a new class of technetium complexes: the hexakis (alkylisonitrine) technetium (I) cation. Int J Nucl Med Biol 1984; 11: 225–34.
6. Sia STB, Holman BL, McKusick K et al. The utilization of Tc-99m-TBI as a myocardial perfusion agent in exercise studies: comparison with Tl-201 thallous chloride and examination of its biodistribution in humans. Eur J Nucl Med 1986; 12: 333–6.
7. McKusick K, Holman BL, Jones AG et al. Comparison of 3 Tc99m isonitriles for detection of ischemic heart disease in humans [abstract]. J Nucl Med 1986; 27: 878.
8. Wackers FJ, Berman DS, Maddahi J et al. Technetium-99m hexakis 2-methoxyisobutyl isonitrile: human biodistribution, dosimetry, safety and preliminary comparison to thallium-201 for myocardial perfusion imaging. J Nucl Med 1989; 30: 301–11.
9. Leppo JA, Meerdink DJ. Comparison of the myocardial uptake of a technetium-labeled isonitrile analogue and thallium. Circ Res 1989; 65: 632–9.
10. Sands H, Delano ML, Gallagher BM. Uptake of hexakis-(*t*-butylisonitrile) technetium (I) and hexakis-(isopropyl-isonitrile) technetium (I) by neonatal rat myocytes and human erythrocytes. J Nucl Med 1986; 27: 404–8.
11. Maublant JC, Gachon P, Moins N. Hexakis (2-methoxy isobutylisonitrile) technetium-99m and thallium-201 chloride uptake and release in cultured myocarddial cells. J Nucl Med 1988; 29: 48–54.
12. Fukuda H, Syrota A, Charbonneau P et al. Use of ^{11}C-triphenylmethylphosphonium for the evaluation of membrane potential in the heart by positron-emission tomography. Eur J Nucl Med 1986; 11: 478–83.
13. Chiu ML, Kronauge JF, Piwnica Worms D. Effect of mitochondrial and plasma membrane potentials on accumulation of hexakis (2-methoxyisobutylisonitrile) technetium (I) in cultured mouse fibroblasts. J Nucl Med 1990; 31: 1646–53.
14. Okada RD, Glover D, Gaffney T, Williams S. Myocardial kinetics of technetium-99m-hexakis-2-methoxy-2-methylpropyl-isonitrile. Circulation 1988; 77: 491–8.
15. Glover DK, Okada RD. Myocardial kinetics of Tc-MIBI in canine myocardium after dipyridamole. Circulation 1990; 81: 628–36.
16. Li QS, Frank TL, Franceshi D, Wagner HN Jr, Becker LC. Technetium-99m methoxyisobutyl isonitrile (RP30) for quantification of myocardial ischemia and reperfusion in dogs. J Nucl Med 1988; 29: 1539–48.
17. Li QS, Solot G, Frank TL, Wagner HN Jr, Becker LC. Myocardial redistribution of Technetium-99m-metaboxyisobutyl isonitrile (Sestamibi). J Nucl Med 1990; 31: 1069–76.
18. Camby RC, Silber S, Pohost GM. Relations of the myocardial imaging agents 99mTc-MIBI and 201 Thallium to myocardial blood flow in a canine model of myocardial ischemic insult. Circulation 1990; 81: 289–96.

19. Maddahi J, Kiat H, Van Train KF et al. Myocardial perfusion imaging with technetium-99m sestaMIBI SPECT in the evaluation of coronary artery disease. Am J Cardiol 1990; 66: 55E–62E.

20. Kiat H, Maddahi J, Roy LT et al. Comparison of technetium-99m methoxy isobutyl isonitrile and thallium-201 for evaluation of coronary artery disease by planar and tomographic methods. Am Heart J 1989; 117: 1–11.

21. Larock MP. Apports de la tomographie myocardique d'émission monophotonique et du 99mTc-MIBI dans l'exploration de la maladie coronarienne [dissertation]. Univ of Liège, 1991.

22. Karcher G, Bertrand A, Moretti JL et al. Comparative study by two independent observers of the uptake abnormalities of 201 thallium and Tc-99m MIBI in 81 patients with coronary artery disease [abstract]. J Nucl Med 1988; 29: 793–4.

23. Maddahi J, Merz R, Van Train K, Roy L, Wong C, Berman DS. Tc-99m MIBI (RP30) and Tl-201 myocardial perfusion scintigraphy in patients with coronary artery disease: quantitative comparison of planar and tomographic techniques for perfusion defect intensity and defect reversibility [abstract]. J Nucl Med 1987; 28: 654.

24. Boucher CA. Detection and location of myocardial infarction using technetium-99m sestaMIBI imaging at rest. Am J Cardiol 1990; 66: 32E–5E.

25. Dilsizian V, Rocco TP, Strauss HW, Boucher CA. Technetium-99m isonitrile myocardial uptake at rest. I. Relation to severity of coronary artery stenosis. J Am Coll Cardiol 1989; 14: 1673–7.

26. Verani MS, Jeroudi MO, Mahmarian JJ et al. Quantification of myocardial infarction during coronary occlusion and myocardial salvage after reperfusion using cardiac imaging with technetium-99m hexakis 2-methoxyisobutyl isonitrile. J Am Coll Cardiol 1988; 12: 1573–81.

27. Gibbons RJ, Verani MS, Behrenbeck T et al. Feasibility of tomographic 99mTc-hexakis-2--methoxy-2-methylpropyl-isonitrile imaging for the assessment of myocardial area at risk and the effect of treatment in acute myocardial infarction. Circulation 1989; 80: 1277–86.

28. Bergin JD, Sinusas AJ, Smith WH et al. Quantitative isonitrile imaging for risk area determination following transient coronary occlusion [abstract]. J Nucl Med 1990; 31: 784–5.

29. Prigent F, Maddahi J, Garcia EV, Satoh Y, Van Train K, Berman DS. Quantification of experimental myocardial infarct size by thallium-201 single photon emission computed tomography: experimental validation in the dog. Circulation 1986; 74: 852–61.

30. Grégoire J, Théroux P. Detection and assessment of unstable angina using myocarial perfusion imaging: comparison between technetium-99m Sestamibi SPECT and 12-lead electrocardiogram. Am J Cardiol 1990; 66: 42E–6E.

31. Braat SH, de Swart H, Janssen JH, Brugada P, Rigo P, Wellens HJJ. Use of Technetium-99m Sestamibi to determine the size of the myocardial area perfused by a coronary artery. Am J Cardiol 1990; 66: 85E–90E.

32. Larock MP, Legrand V, Kulbertus H, Rigo P. 99mTc-MIBI to evaluate the extent of myocardial ischemia, the risk area and the results of PTCA. In: 'Radioactive Isotopes in Clinical Medicine and Research', Proceedings of the 19th Bad Gastein Symposium, 1990: 69–73.

33. Faraggi M, Assayag P, Messian O et al. Early isonitrile SPECT in acute myocardial infarction: feasibility and results before and after fibrinolysis. Nucl Med Commun 1989; 10: 539–49.

34. Wackers FJT, Gibbons RJ, Verani MS et al. Serial quantitative planar technetium-99m isonitrile imaging in acute myocardial infarction: efficacy for noninvasive assessment of thrombolytic therapy. J Am Coll Cardiol 1989; 14: 861–73.

35. Borges-Neto S, Coleman RE, Jones RH. Perfusion and function at rest and treadmill exercise using Tc-99m sestaMIBI: comparison of one- and two-day protocols in normal volunteers. J Nucl Med 1990; 31: 1128–32.

36. Larock MP, Cantineau R, Legrand V, Kulbertus H, Rigo P. 99mTc-MIBI (RP-30) to define the extent of myocardial ischemia and evaluate ventricular function. Eur J Nucl Med 1990; 16: 223–30.

37. Najm YC, Timmis AD, Maisey MN et al. The evaluation of ventricular function using gated myocardial imaging with Tc-99m MIBI. Eur Heart J 1989; 10: 142–8.

38. Corbett JR, Henderson EB, Akers MS et al. Gated tomography with technetium-99m RP-30A in patients with myocardial infarcts: assessment of myocardial perfusion and function [abstract]. Circulation 1987; 76 (4 Suppl IV): IV 217.

39. Larock MP, Cantineau R, Van Cutsem JL, Rigo P. Tc-99m MIBI to assess global and regional ventricular function in the acute phase of myocardial infarction. In: Schmidt HAE, Chambron J, editors, Nuclear medicine: quantitative analysis in imaging and function. Stuttgart: Shattauer Verlag 1990: 272–4.

40. Hecht HS, Shaw RE, Bruce TR, Ryan C, Stertzer SH, Myler RK. Usefulness of tomographic thallium-201 imaging for detection of restenosis after percutaneous transluminal coronary angioplasty. Am J Cardiol 1990; 66: 1314–8.

.

7. Is there a specific role for technetium-99m sestaMIBI in the assessment of cardiac arrhythmias?

HANS B.M.R. DE SWART, SIMON H. BRAAT, JOEP SMEETS, PIERRE RIGO and HEIN J.J. WELLENS

Introduction

In a small number of patients, cardiac arrhythmias are treated by transcoronary chemical ablation [1, 2]. Selective intracoronary injection of low amounts of pure ethanol results in permanent damage of the myocardial cells, being the substrate of the arrhythmia. Destroying the substrate can, however, result in deterioration of left ventricular function, especially in patients with ventricular tachycardia after myocardial infarction and a pre-existing low ejection fraction. However, assessment of the presence of viable tissue in and around infarcted areas is very difficult. We have studied the value of selective injections of technetium-99m (Tc-99m) sestaMIBI into main coronary arteries and into small arteries providing blood supply to the substrate of cardiac arrhythmias to detect the flow areas and to estimate the area at risk for chemical ablation. In a previous study [3, 4], we demonstrated that Tc-99m sestaMIBI is able to detect short episodes of ischemia, without the need for studying the patient immediately after injection of the radioactive tracer, which obviously is a prerequisite, when the nuclear agent is administered in the catheterization laboratory. The first part of the study was performed to determine whether intracoronary injection of Tc-99m sestaMIBI could demonstrate the flow area of the myocardium perfused by that artery. In the second part, we studied the value of selective injection of Tc-99m sestaMIBI into the artery providing blood supply to the substrate of the arrhythmia.

Ernst E. van der Wall et al. (eds), What's new in cardiac imaging?, 87–92.
© *1992 Kluwer Academic Publishers. Printed in the Netherlands.*

Patients and methods

Technetium-99m sestaMIBI injection into main coronary arteries

Thirteen patients (group 1) were investigated; nine were male and four female. Age ranged from 31 to 73 years (mean 49 years). Four patients had documented cardiac arrhythmias and nine patients were catheterized for anginal complaints, class II to III according to the classification of the New York Heart Association. All patients had normal resting electrocardiograms, never suffered from myocardial infarction and had a normal left ventricular contraction pattern during cineangiography. Cardiac catheterization was performed using the Judkins technique. Left coronary angiography was performed in 30° and 60° left anterior oblique positions and in 30° right anterior oblique projection. Additional views to demonstrate coronary artery disease were made, when indicated. The right coronary artery was visualized from the 30° right and 60° left anterior oblique position, with additional views, when necessary. One mCi of Tc-99m sestaMIBI was injected into the proximal part of a normal right coronary artery in seven patients, into the left anterior descending coronary artery just after the left main coronary artery in four patients and into the proximal portion of a normal circumflex coronary artery in the remaining two patients. After catheterization patients were brought to the laboratory of nuclear medicine for imaging. For all studies, we used a mobile Technicare gamma camera with an all-purpose parallel hole collimator interfaced to a Technicare 560 mobile computer system (Technicare corporation). Three views were recorded in all patients: 45° left anterior oblique, anterior and lateral using a preset time of 360 seconds. The window was 20% with a photopeak of 140 keV.

Selective technetium-99m sestaMIBI injections

In five male patients (group 2), mean age 63 years, who were candidates for transcoronary chemical ablation, selective injections of Tc-99m sestaMIBI were made into the artery, providing blood supply to the substrate of the arrhythmia. Four patients had an old myocardial infarction with an irreversible defect in the corresponding area during thallium-201 exercise testing; in two of those patients, positron emission tomography did not demonstrate any viable tissue in the infarcted area. One patient was investigated for transcoronary chemical ablation of the atrioventricular node and had a normal contraction pattern of the left ventricle. Blood supply was provided by collateral circulation to the infarcted area in three patients. Collateral circulation originated from the first septal branch of the left anterior descending coronary artery (LAD) to the occluded right coronary artery, from the first septal branch of the occluded LAD to the distal LAD and from the first obtuse marginal branch of the circumflex coronary artery (CX) to the occluded second marginal branch. Anterograde blood supply was present in two patients; one with a reperfused posterolateral branch of the CX and the atrio-ventricular nodal artery in the patient with atrial fibrillation. Cardiac catheterization was performed according to the previously described method. Selective catheterization of the arrhythmia related vessel was performed using a 0.014 inch guide wire and a 2.2 French single lumen catheter. After positioning the single lumen catheter into the artery providing blood supply to the area of interest the radioactive tracer was injected. After the catheterization, nuclear imaging was performed as described above. Finally three patients underwent transcoronary chemical ablation of tachycardia; two patients suffered from medically untreatable ventricular tachycardia and one patient had atrial fibrillation with uncontrollable ventricular rates.

Results

In group 1, coronary angiography revealed that seven patients had normal coronary arteries and six patients had severe coronary artery disease. None of the 13 patients experienced side effects from Tc-99m sestaMIBI. In all patients radioactive uptake was found in the area of the myocardium related to the coronary artery, which was catheterized. The area visualized after nuclear imaging varied with the size of the supplying artery. The target to background ratio was very high because of the absence or minimally present activity outside the flow area of the selectively injected coronary artery. No differences were observed in the absence or presence of coronary artery lesions. The patients in group 2 demonstrated uptake by the myocardial area corresponding to the coronary artery, which was selectively catheterized, although the distribution area was smaller compared to the proximal injection in the patients in group 1. Also, injections of Tc-99m sestaMIBI into the artery providing blood supply to an infarcted area (and an irreversible defect during thallium-201 exercise testing) did show staining by Tc-99m sestaMIBI. The maximal oxalacetic transaminase level in the patients undergoing transcoronary chemical ablation of tachycardia was 202, 109, and 37 units/liter respectively (normal ≤ 40 units/liter). In those patients no new myocardial infarctions could be demonstrated using echocardiography.

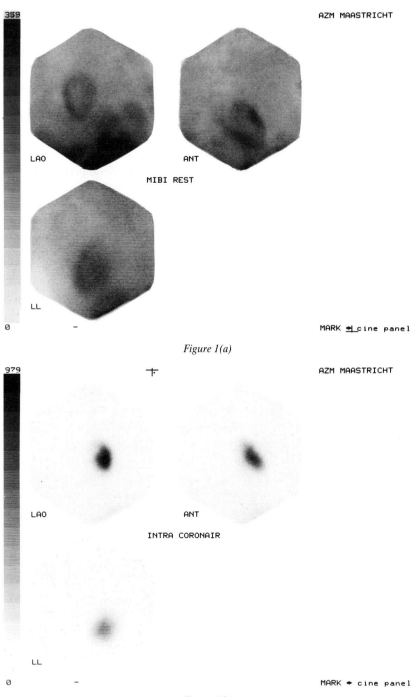

Figure 1(a)

Figure 1(b)

←
Figure 1. (a) Large defect in the posterolateral wall, which remained the same after exercise. Positron emission tomography did not reveal any viable tissue in that area. ANT – anterior view; LAO – left anterior oblique view; LL – left lateral view.
(b) Selective intracoronary injection of Tc-99m sestaMIBI into the first obtuse marginal branch of the circumflex coronary artery, which filled the posterolateral branch colaterally. ANT – anterior view; LAO – left anterior oblique view; LL – left lateral view.

Discussion

In the first part of the study we proved that injection of Tc-99m sestaMIBI into a major coronary artery visualizes the flow-related area. Differences between sizes of coronary arteries and corresponding flow related areas are well visualized by nuclear imaging. The expectation, however, that subselective injections of Tc-99m sestaMIBI are useful in detecting the area at risk for chemical ablation, was not validated. Differentiation between viable and necrotic tissue in the patients in group 2 was impossible, although subselective intracoronary injection of Tc-99m sestaMIBI is still useful to determine the extent of the area of perfusion by the injected coronary artery. The explanation might be the relatively high dosage of radioactive tracer injected into the tachycardia-related artery and still the presence of some viable tissue. Lower dosages of Tc-99m sestaMIBI will probably also cause uptake during nuclear imaging; differences in density will be present, but it is not documented as to what amount of tissue in that area is still viable. This is supported by the results of the positron emission tomography in two of the patients and by the results of the rise in oxalacetic transaminase values after transcoronary chemical ablation in three of our patients. In the latter group of patients, the amount of ethanol injected might be important, however, in general a correlation between enzyme rise after ablation and ethanol dose could not be found. A solution to differentiate between viable and necrotic myocardial tissue might be to compare the exercise and rest nuclear studies with the selective injection studies. If uptake of the nuclear agent is only seen in the area with an irreversible defect in the rest study, we can assume that there is no viable tissue of any importance. Both studies can be superimposed and result in a total nuclear image of the heart, as it is demonstrated in Figures 1(a) and 1(b).

Conclusion

Using intracoronary injections of Tc-99m sestaMIBI the flow area of the coronary artery can be visualized. Visualization is not influenced by lesions in the coronary arteries. Although the number of patients is small, subselective intracoronary injection of Tc-99m sestaMIBI can also be used to determine the size of the area perfused by the tachycardia-related artery, but it does not document what amount of tissue in that area is still viable.

References

1. Brugada P, De Swart H, Smeets JLRM, Wellens HJJ. Transcoronary chemical ablation of ventricular tachycardia. Circulation 1989; 79: 475–82.
2. Brugada P, De Swart H, Smeets JLRM, Wellens HJJ. Transcoronary chemical ablation of atrioventricular conduction. Circulation 1990; 81: 757–61.
3. Braat SH, De Swart H, Janssen JH, Brugada P, Rigo P, Wellens HJJ. Use of technetium-99m sestaMIBI to determine the size of the myocardial area perfused by a coronary artery. Am J Cardiol 1990; 66: 85E–90E.
4. Braat SH, De Swart H, Rigo P, Koppejan L, Heidendal GAK, Wellens HJJ. Value of technetium Mibi to detect short lasting episodes of severe myocardial ischaemia and to estimate the area at risk during coronary angioplasty. Eur Heart J 1991; 12: 30–3.

8. Technetium-99m complexes of functionalized diphosphines for myocardial perfusion imaging in man

BRIAN HIGLEY, AVIJIT LAHIRI and J. DUNCAN KELLY

Introduction

It is almost 15 years since it was suggested that, in the field of myocardial perfusion imaging, the use of a technetium-99m (Tc-99m) based agent could significantly improve image quality as a result of a two-fold increase in resolution and up to four-fold increase in the administered dose compared to the established agent of choice thallous (Tl-201) chloride [1]. In fact, Tc-99m agents that have been developed since those original estimates were made, have even better dosimetry characteristics than predicted. It has, however, taken a considerable amount of effort by numerous research groups to reach the present stage in which several commercially produced Tc-99m myocardial perfusion imaging agents are either already licensed or nearing licence approval.

A key observation, that stimulated much subsequent work, was the finding by Deutsch and co-workers [2] that there is significant uptake of lipophilic Tc-99m cations by cardiac muscle. Following these initial observations, that group [3, 4] and others observed the phenomenon of uptake for a wide range of Tc-99m complex types including the hexakis-isonitriles [5], the bis-arenes [6], and the hexakis-phosphites [7].

Within the various cation series studied, good myocardial uptake can generally be achieved by optimizing lipophilicity. However, there has, until recently, been recurrent failure in man to achieve adequate clearance from nontarget tissues, especially blood and liver and sometimes lung. In recent times, the problem had been adequately addressed for the hexakis-isonitrile complex type, resulting in a series of complexes with significantly improved, though not

93

Ernst E. van der Wall et al. (eds), What's new in cardiac imaging?, 93–109.

necessarily ideal, biodistribution in man. However, a second class of complexes based upon diphosphines has also been the subject of much research. Early studies were restricted to simple alkyl or aryl diphosphines and whilst encouraging in some respects it was clear that these agents were far from ideal. Significant improvements in the biodistribution of diphosphines have been achieved by the introduction of ether functionalities into the molecule.

Simple alkyl and aryl diphosphines

The potential of Tc-99m diphosphine complexes for myocardial perfusion imaging has been extensively explored because of the range of cation cores available with these ligands (L). These core types include: $[TcL_3]^+$, $[TcL_2Cl_2]^+$, $[TcO_2L_2]^+$, $[Tc(NO)L_2Cl]^+$ [8], $[Tc(N)L_2Cl]^+$ [9], $[Tc(NR)L_2Cl]^+$ [10], where R = NMePh, NPh, or $NC_6H_4NO_2$, and $[Tc(CNR)_2L_2]^+$ [11] where R = tBu. Much of the early work was restricted to the first three of these cores. Many different simple alkyl/aryl diphosphines have been synthesized, labeled and the biodistribution studied in animals [12]. However, much of the key research work has been focused upon two of the more readily available simple alkyl diphosphines, 1,2-bis(dimethyl phosphino) ethane (DMPE) and 1,2-bis (diethylphosphino) ethane (DEPE).

The biodistribution of the simple alkyl diphosphine complexes has shown a profound interspecies variability which has been especially well documented in the comprehensive work of Deutsch and co-workers [13, 14]. In all species studied including man, the $[Tc(DMPE)_2O_2]^+$ complex showed extremely poor heart uptake. The remaining biodistribution, however, was quite species dependent especially the relatively slow blood washout in man associated with considerable plasma protein binding. This is in stark contrast to the features displayed by some of the Tc(V) complexes of functionalized diphosphines subsequently developed.

In the early work by the Deutsch group, there was significantly more interesting behaviour exhibited by the Tc(III), $[TcL_2Cl_2]^+$ cations. The study of the $[Tc(DMPE)_2Cl_2]^+$ complex was originally reported in man in 1983 [15, 16]. There was significant heart uptake but slow washout in man which was reasonably well correlated with the behavior of the complex in other animal species. One feature of this Tc(III) complex that was not predictable from animal data was the considerable liver uptake and rather poor clearance seen in man. It was reported that, due to the liver uptake, imaging of the apex of the heart was impaired and that images were significantly worse than achieved with thallium. Despite this, attempts were made to improve the formulation in order to achieve a commercially viable kit [17]. Unfortunately, it did not prove

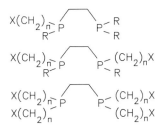

Bridge functions

Figure 1(a) Terminal functionalized diphospines.

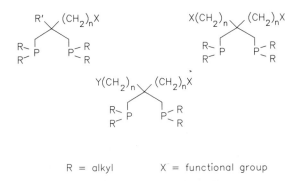

R = alkyl　　　　X = functional group

Figure 1(b) Bridge functionalized diphosphines.

possible to achieve a major improvement in the background clearance with this new formulation.

　Deutsch et al. have indicated that the myocardial washout phenomenon exhibited by $[TcL_2Cl_2]^+$ complexes is linked to the ready reducibility of the Tc(III) species in vivo [18].

　The more lipophilic Tc(III) complex of DEPE has also been studied in man [19, 20] but with even more disappointing results showing either no myocardial uptake or, at best, significantly faster washout than the analogous DMPE complex. Again, it was not possible to predict the failure in man from the available animal biodistribution data. Differences in plasma protein binding between animals and man may, however, begin to shed some light upon the biodistribution differences seen.

　The Tc(I) or 'tris' complexes, $[TcL_3]^+$, have also been widely researched [13, 14, 21]. Once again, there was a significant discrepancy between the biological characteristics of the DMPE complex in man and in animals. There is significant myocardial uptake and excellent retention in all species, including man. However, man is unique in having an extremely long blood clearance time.

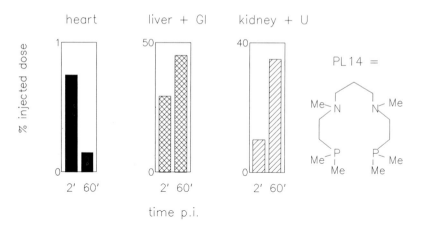

Figure 2. Biodistribution of [Tc-99m(PL14)Cl$_2$]$^+$ in rats.

This resulted in a delay of 10–12 hours being necessary before even rather poor myocardial images could be obtained. This phenomenon is not unique to the DMPE complex but has also been noted for the less lipophilic Tc(I) complex of bis(dimethyl phosphino) methane [22].

The simple alkyl diphosphine complexes pointed the way, indicating that a lipophilic Tc-99m cationic complex could be used for myocardial imaging. However, it seemed clear that there were inherent drawbacks with these very simple systems. Significant progress was made only when a fundamental change was made to the structure of the ligands by introducing new non-chelating functional groups.

The key issues in terms of biodistribution that required improvement were more rapid blood and liver clearance and possible slower myocardial clearance in man.

Development of functionalized diphosphine complexes

(i) Rationale
A limited amount of work has been done to try to overcome one of the recognized drawbacks of the [TcL$_2$Cl$_2$]$^+$ cations, namely the relatively fast myocardial clearance. The objective in this case was to inhibit the reducibility of the Tc(III) complex thought to be the cause of the washout behavior [23].

Additionally, a variety of functional groups has been attached to diphosphine ligands with a view to modifying biological interactions, in particular protein binding, and thus improving clearance from nontarget tissues.

In particular, two different structural types of diphosphine ligand have been

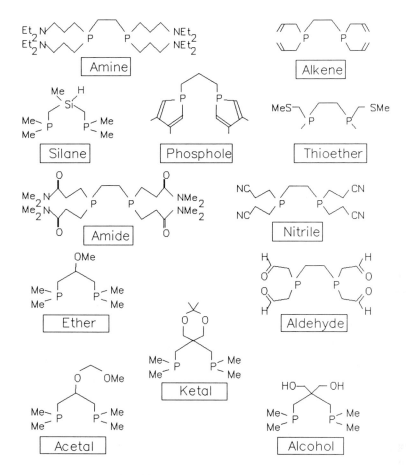

Figure 3. Functionalized diphosphines.

prepared. These involve the attachment of the functional group either via the terminal phosphorus atom or via the hydrocarbon bridge linking the two phosphorus atoms. Functional groups can be added readily two at a time or four at a time (Figure 1a). An alternative approach is to attach the functional group to the hydrocarbon link between the phosphorus atoms. The latter approach is especially favored with propylene-bridged diphosphines, since the introduction of either one or two functions on the central carbon does not give rise to ligand chirality (Figure 1b).

(ii) Choice of functional group
The combination of the TcCl$_2$$^+$ core with mixed phosphine-amine ligands has been examined, as a possible means of counteracting the washout behavior

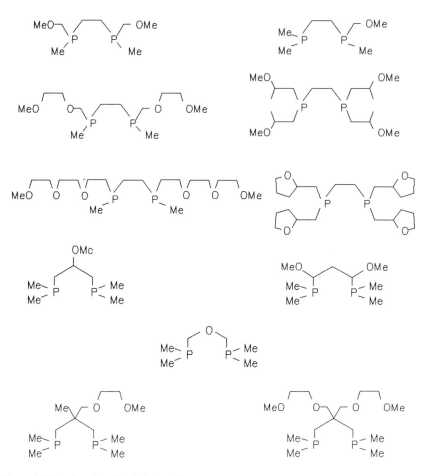

Figure 4. Ether functionalized diphosphines.

exhibited by Tc(III) complexes. For the complex $(TcLCl_2)^+$, where $L =$ PL14 = $Me_2PCH_2CH_2N(Me)CH_2CH_2CH_2N(Me)CH_2CH_2PMe_2$, there was moderate but significant uptake in rat heart at 2 minutes post-injection. By 60 minutes post-injection, however, there was substantial washout (Figure 2). The electrochemistry of the mixed phosphine-amine donor Tc(III) complexes has not yet been evaluated, hence it was not established that the objective of stabilizing the complex to reduction had been achieved. However, the biological results did not provide sufficient justification for pursuing this class of ligand further.

A range of different functional groups has been linked to C2 or C3 bridged diphosphines [23]. Some representative examples are shown in Figure 3.

Technetium-99m complexes have been prepared, employing those core

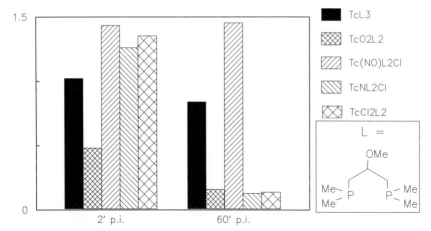

Figure 5. The effect of different Tc-99m core types on the % heart uptake and retention in the rat.

types where the preparative conditions allowed access to the ligand-core combination without significant ligand decomposition. Biodistribution in rats has been evaluated for all preparations yielding lipophilic complexes of adequate radiochemical purity (RCP), the target figure for an initial screen being set at 90% RCP. In parallel with this, studies to determine the binding to human plasma proteins in vitro were performed.

Some of the hydrophilic functional groups had little effect in reducing

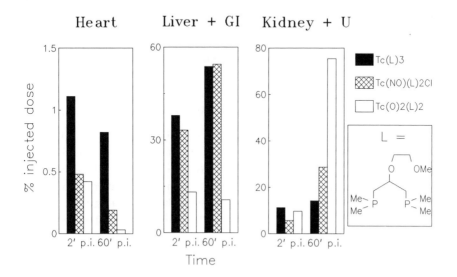

Figure 6. The effect of Tc-99m core type on heart uptake and retention and excretory pattern in the rat.

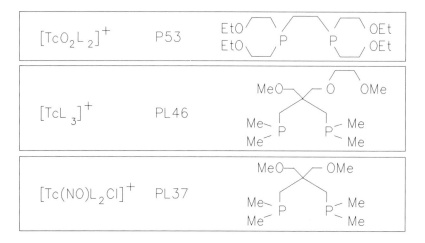

Figure 7. Optimum ligand-core combinations for [TcO₂L₂]⁺, (TcL₃)⁺ and [Tc(NO)L₂Cl]⁺.

plasma protein binding or in improving nontarget clearance, for example alkene, silane, or thio-ether. Amine and nitrile functions gave rise to mixed Tc-99m complexes, presumably because they provide competing ligating moieties. Other functional groups, e.g. alcohol, had too profound an effect in modifying lipophilic behavior; others were too labile to survive any but the mildest labeling conditions, e.g. acetal.

It has been concluded that the ether group presents the best choice of functional group because:

(a) it is quite robust to conditions of ligand synthesis and Tc-99m labeling;
(b) the ether function does not compete with phosphine in binding to Tc-99m and
(c) relatively subtle modification of physicochemical properties can be introduced through modification of the ether function.

(iii) Ligand-core combination

Many ether-functionalized diphosphines have been prepared based on both ethylene and propylene bridged structures. Some examples of the various structural types which have been synthesized are shown in Figure 4.

For the ethylene bridged diphosphines, the main emphasis has been upon symmetrically substituted derivatives.

For the propylene bridged diphosphines, a parallel approach has been taken in combining an alkoxy function with an identical or a different alkoxyalkyl group or with an alkyl function on the central carbon of the propylene bridge.

Combination of phosphino-ethers with the available ligand cores has given

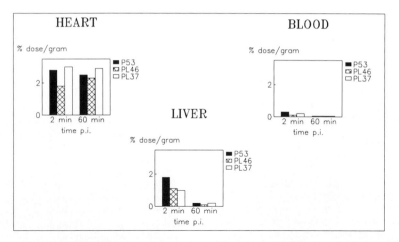

Figure 8(a) Biodistribution of the optimized ligand-core combinations in the rat.

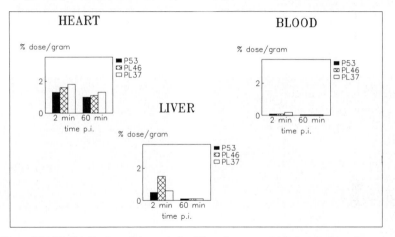

Figure 8(b) Biodistribution of the optimized ligand-core combinations in the guinea pig.

rise to two broad fundamental observations. The first being that the intrinsic properties of the core dominate the uptake and clearance characteristics of the individual complexes. Figure 5 shows the 2 minute and 60 minute biodistribution in rats for the same ligand in combination with five different cores. While the nitrosyl-, nitrido- and dichloro-complexes have all shown similar heart uptake at 2 minutes post-injection, both the nitrido and dichloro complexes show characteristic washout behavior, which is not dissimilar to that displayed by analogous complexes formed with simple alkyl diphosphines. This observation resulted in the limitation of more complex screening programmes to the $[TcL_3]^+$, $[Tc(NO)L_2Cl]^+$, and $[TcO_2L_2]^+$ cores.

The second observation was that, for the three cores studied, the choice of

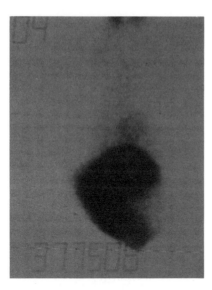

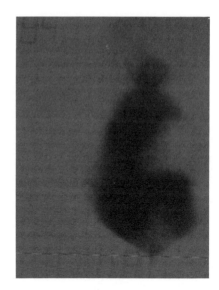

DMPE$_2$Cl$_2$ PL46

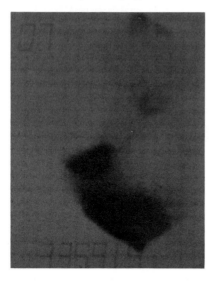

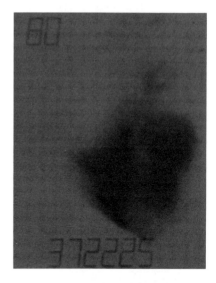

P53   PL37

Figure 9. Biodistribution of four Tc-99m diphosphine complexes in the minipig at 90 minutes post-injection.

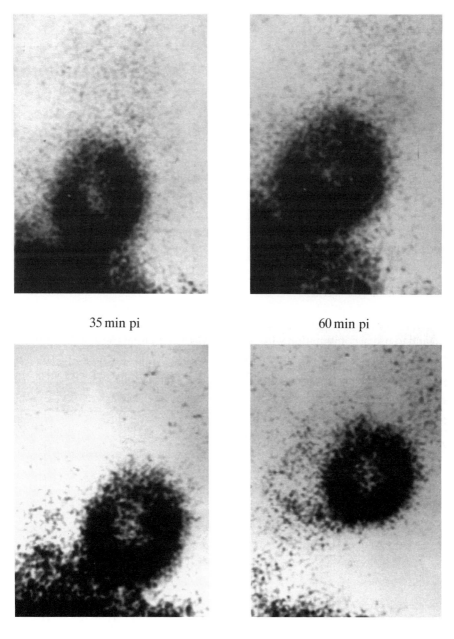

35 min pi   60 min pi

170 min pi   450 min pi

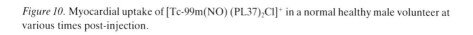

Figure 10. Myocardial uptake of [Tc-99m(NO) (PL37)$_2$Cl]$^+$ in a normal healthy male volunteer at various times post-injection.

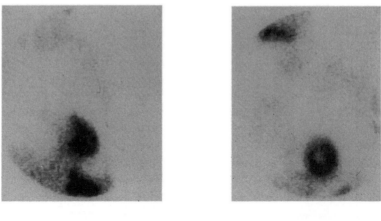

Anterior   LAO

Figure 11. Myocardial uptake of [Tc-99m(P53)₂O₂]⁺ in a normal healthy male volunteer. Anterior and LAO at 3 hr post-injection.

ligand to use in combination with the core was an essential element in optimizing uptake and clearance characteristics (Figure 6). The significantly higher polarity of the dioxo core was apparent from excretion characteristics. In

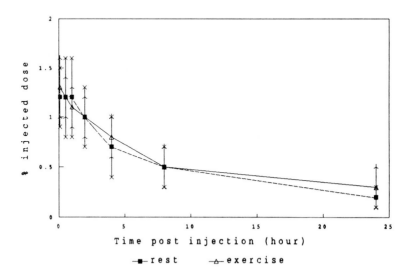

Figure 12. Retention of Tc-99m-P53 formulated as PPN1011 in the heart of normal healthy volunteers.

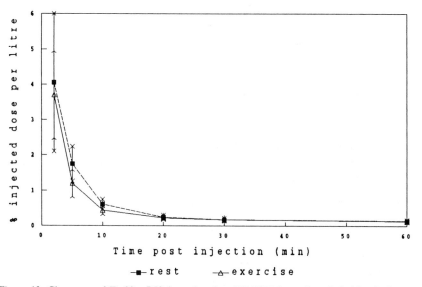

Figure 13. Clearance of Tc-99m-P53 formulated as PPN1011 from the whole blood of normal healthy volunteers.

general, the nitrosyl core, as in this example, gave rise to a less lipophilic complex than the $[TcL_3]^+$ type, though this trend was not universally observed when the size of the functional substituent was increased.

The optimum ligand structure for each of the three core types was sought using a structured screening programme which was developed empirically. The screening programme consisted of a primary screen in rats, a secondary screen in guinea pig, and a tertiary screen in the miniature pig. For each core type, the optimum available ligand has been studied in man. An essential element in the screen was determination in vitro of the interaction of the complex with plasma proteins. The optimal ligands were, respectively, P53 for the dioxo core, PL46 for the Tc(I) core and PL37 for the nitrosyl core (Figure 7).

Rat and guinea pig data are shown for these three complexes in Figure 8. Good heart uptake and retention together with fast blood and liver clearance are seen in all cases. PL46 showed high liver uptake as is typical for a Tc(I) diphosphine complex but rapid liver clearance which is atypical. In the minipig (Figure 9), there was good heart uptake and nontarget clearance for PL37 and P53, but slower liver clearance for PL46. Plasma protein binding of the PL46 complex was significantly different from that exhibited by the other two complexes when tested against both guinea pig and human plasma. These data

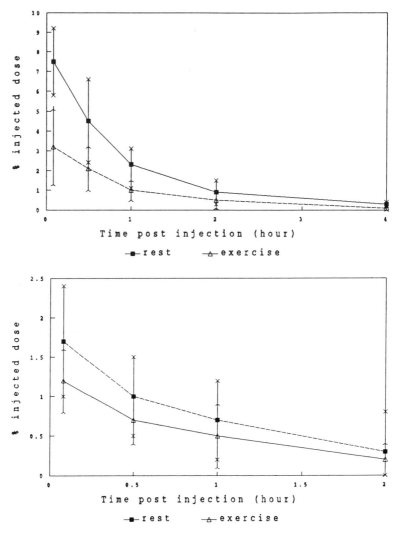

Figure 14. a. Clearance of Tc-99m-P53 formulated as PPN1011 from the liver of normal healthy volunteers.

b. Clearance of Tc-99m-P53 formulated as PPN1011 from the lungs of normal healthy volunteers.

were used to predict significantly poorer performance in both minipig and man.

Studies in man [24] have confirmed very good myocardial uptake and relatively slow clearance for the PL37 and P53 cations (Figures 10 and 11). For these two complexes the background clearance qualities were excellent. As in the minipig, PL46 showed significant heart uptake and retention and there was good background clearance from blood and lung but unsatisfactory clearance from liver. These findings in man were entirely predictable from the data provided by the structured screening programme. One of these ligands, P53, has been developed into a freeze-dried kit (known as PPN1011) and has successfully negotiated both Phase I [25, 26] and Phase II [27, 28] clinical trials.

Data from the Phase I study of this agent were most encouraging. Initial heart uptake (about 1.2%) was well retained for 1 hour followed by a slow fall (Figure 12). Blood activity fell rapidly to less than 0.2%/litre within 30 minutes (Figure 13); lungs and liver largely cleared within the first 4 hours (Figure 14). About 80% of the administered radioactivity was excreted within 48 hours, almost equally via kidneys and gut. After exercise, whole body retention was consistently a few per cent higher than at rest even though some organs cleared more rapidly; this can be explained by increased skeletal muscle uptake after exercise. The highest dose was 3 to 5×10^{-2} mGy/MBq (gall-bladder) followed by doses in the range 1.5 to 3×10^{-2} mGy/MBq (GI tract, urinary bladder) based on a bladder voiding period of 3.5 hours. Effective doses were 8.9×10^{-3} and 7.1×10^{-3} mSv/MBq for the rest and exercise studies respectively. Very good heart to background ratios were rapidly achieved and it has been concluded that diagnostically useful images could be obtained within 30 minutes of injection.

In patient studies it has been reported [27] that a one day imaging protocol involving exercise followed by re-injection at rest within 4 hours is an achievable goal. A comparison of diagnoses, using Tc-99m-P53 and Tl-201 in patients with coronary heart disease, resulted in a high degree of concordance, when the two agents were used in patients having reversible myocardial ischaemia and/or myocardial infarction. It has also been reported [28] that there is no significant difference in diagnosis when data from the same patients are acquired using a one or two day imaging protocol with Tc-99m-P53.

It has been concluded that this new agent P53 has significant potential as a novel Tc-99m labeled myocardial perfusion imaging agent.

References

1. Pitt B, Strauss H. Cardiovascular nuclear medicine. Semin Nucl Med 1977; 7: 3–6.
2. Deutsch E, Glavan KA, Ferguson DL, Lukes SJ, Nishiyama H, Sodd VJ. Development of a Tc-99m myocardial imaging agent to replace Tl-201 [abstract]. J Nucl Med 1980; 21: P56.
3. Deutsch E, Glavan KA, Sodd VJ, Nishiyama H, Ferguson DL, Lukes SJ. Cationic Tc-99m complexes as potential myocardial imaging agents. J Nucl Med 1981; 22: 897–907.
4. Deutsch E, Bushong W, Glavan KA et al. Heart imaging with cationic complexes of technetium. Science 1981; 214: 85–6.
5. Holman BL, Jones AG, Lister-James J et al. A new Tc-99m-labeled myocardial imaging

agent, hexakis(t-butyliso-nitrile)technetium(I) [Tc-99m TBI]: initial experience in the human. J Nucl Med 1984; 25: 1350–5.

6. Dean RT, Wester DW, Nosco DL et al. Progress in the design, evaluation and development of Tc-99m radiopharmaceuticals. In: Nicolini M, Bandoli G, Mazzi U, editors. Technetium in chemistry and nuclear medicine 2. Verona: Raven Press 1986: 147–54.

7. Wester DW, White DH, Miller FW, Dean RT. Synthesis and characterization of a technetium-phosphite complex: hexakis(trimethyl-phosphite)technetium(I) tetraphenylborate. Inorg Chem 1984; 23: 1501–2.

8. Thornback JR, Newman JL, Morgan GF, Nowotnik DP. Novel Tc-99m nitrosyl complexes as potential radiopharmaceuticals [abstract]. Nucl Med Commun 1989; 10: 247.

9. Dilworth JA, Archer CM, Latham IA, Bishop PT, Kelly JD, Higley B. The synthesis of technetium-nitride cations as potential myocardial imaging agents [abstract]. J Nucl Med 1989; 30: 773.

10. Archer CM, Kelly JD, Dilworth JR, Povey DC, Smith GW. The synthesis of technetium-hydrazide complexes. In: Nicolini M, Bandoli G, Mazzi U, editors. Technetium and rhenium in chemistry and nuclear medicine 3. Verona: Raven Press 1990: 159–63.

11. Zanelli GD, Lahiri A, Patel N et al. Animal and human studies of a new Tc-99m labelled phosphine-isocyanide complex with possible applications to radionuclide ventriculography. Eur J Nucl Med 1987; 13: 12–7.

12. Glavan KA, Kronauge JF, Blaubaugh E, Neirinckx RD, Eakins MN, Loberg MD. Synthesis, characterization and electrochemistry of trans dihalo technetium phosphine complexes: potential myocardial imaging agents. J Label Compounds Radiopharm 1982; 19: 1609–11.

13. Ketring AR, Deutsch E, Libson K et al. The Noah's Ark experiment. A search for a suitable animal model for the evaluation of cationic Tc-99m myocardial imaging agents [abstract]. J Nucl Med 1983; 24: P9.

14. Deutsch E, Ketring AR, Libson K, Vanderheyden JL, Hirth WW. The Noah's Ark experiment: species dependent biodistributions of cationic Tc-99m complexes. Int J Rad Appl Instrum 1989; 16: 191–232.

15. Gerson MC, Deutsch EA, Nishiyama H et al. Myocardial perfusion imaging with Tc-99m-DMPE in man. Eur J Nucl Med 1983; 8: 371–4.

16. Dudczak R, Angelberger P, Homan R, Kletter K, Schmoliner R, Frischauf H. Evaluation of Tc-99m-dichloro bis(1,2-dimethylphosphino)ethane (Tc-99m-DMPE) for myocardial scintigraphy in man. Eur J Nucl Med 1983; 8: 513–5.

17. Mohnike W, Schmidt J, Uhlich F, Seifert S, Syhre R, Munze R. Clinical results on myocardial perfusion diagnostics using Tc-99m-DPO – a preparation from ROTOP-MYOSPECT. Nuc Compact 1987; 18: 184–8.

18. Nishiyama H, Deutsch E, Adolph RJ et al. Basal kinetic studies of Tc-99m DMPE as a myocardial imaging agent in the dog. J Nucl Med 1982; 23: 1093–101.

19. Thakur ML, Park CH, Fazio F et al. Preparation and evaluation of [Tc-99m]DEPE as a cardiac perfusion agent. Int J Appl Radiat Isot 1984; 35: 507–15.

20. Zanelli GD, Cook N, Lahiri A, Ellison D, Webbon P, Woolley G. Protein binding studies of technetium-99m-labeled phosphine and isocyanide cationic complexes. J Nucl Med 1988; 29: 62–7.

21. Gerson MC, Deutsch EA, Libson KF et al. Myocardial scintigraphy with Tc-99m-tris-DMPE in man. Eur J Nucl Med 1984; 9: 403–7.

22. Chui KW, Higley B, Latham IA, Lahiri A, Kelly JD. Unpublished data.

23. Kelly JD, Higley B, Archer CM et al. Technetium-99m complexes of functionalised diphosphines for myocardial imaging. In: Nicolini M, Bandoli G, Mazzi U, editors. Technetium and rhenium chemistry and nuclear medicine 3. Verona: Raven Press, 1990: 405–12.

24. Lahiri A, Higley B, Smith T et al. Myocardial perfusion imaging in man using new Tc-99m-labelled diphosphine complexes [abstract]. Nucl Med Commun 1989; 10: 245.
25. Smith FW, Smith T, Gemmell H et al. Phase I study of Tc-99m diphosphine (P53) for myocardial imaging [abstract]. J Nucl Med 1991; 32: 967.
26. Smith T, Lahiri A, Gemmell HG et al. Dosimetry of Tc-99m-P53, a new myocardial perfusion imaging agent. Proceedings of Oak Ridge Radiation Dosimetry Symposium, (in press).
27. Sridhara BS, Braat S, Itti R, Rigo P, Cload P, Lahiri A. Early and late myocardial imaging with a new technetium-99m diphosphine (PPN1011) in coronary artery disease [abstract]. J Am Coll Cardiol 1992 (in press).
28. Rigo P, Braat S, Itti R et al. Myocardial imaging with technetium P53. Comparison with thallium in suspected coronary artery disease [abstract]. J Am Coll Cardiol 1992 (in press).

9. Myocardial perfusion imaging with technetium-99m teboroxime

ROBERT C. HENDEL

Introduction

Myocardial perfusion imaging at rest and following stress is an extensively utilized and widely accepted method for the detection and evaluation of coronary artery disease. Perfusion imaging, in conjunction with exercise or pharmacologic hyperemia, provides physiologic information regarding coronary blood flow reserve and is often complementary to the anatomic data obtained through coronary angiography. Although thallium-201 has been used in clinical practice for more than 15 years and has demonstrated both diagnostic and prognostic value, its availability, as it is a cyclotron-produced product, may be limited. Furthermore, its photon energy is not well suited for an Anger camera and its prolonged half-life limit the dosimetry which results in less photon flux.

Recently, several technetium-based myocardial perfusion tracers (teboroxime and sestamibi) have become available and more are under development. The higher energy (140 keV) of these technetium-99m agents is well suited to gamma camera imaging and the shorter half-life (6 hours) allows for higher doses resulting in improved count statistics. Furthermore, as technetium-99m may be eluted from an on-site generator, technetium compounds are readily available.

Physical properties and transport characteristics

Technetium-99m teboroxime (CDO-MEB; SQ30217; CardioTec, Squibb Di-

111

Ernst E. van der Wall et al. (eds), What's new in cardiac imaging?, 111–126.
© *1992 Kluwer Academic Publishers. Printed in the Netherlands.*

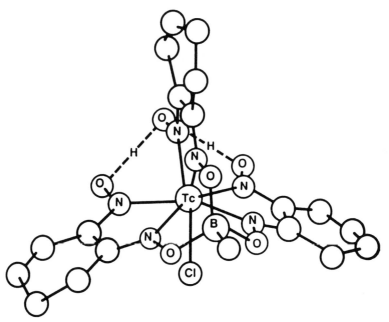

Figure 1. The molecular structure of Tc-99m teboroxime (reprinted with permission from W.B. Saunders Company from Johnson LL. Clinical Experience with Technetium 99m Teboroxime. Seminars in Nuclear Medicine 1991; 23: 183).

agnostics) is a new radiopharmaceutical formed by template synthesis when technetium 99m (Tc-99m) is added to a vial of vicinal dioxime and boronic acid. This results in the formation of a member of a new class of compounds, known as boronic acid adducts of technetium dioxime or BATO compounds (Figure 1). These neutral, lipophilic compounds diffuse quickly into cell membranes, most likely due to passive transport. It is unclear whether teboroxime enters the cytosol of the myocyte or binds only to the cell membrane. The preparation of Tc-99m teboroxime is outlined in Table 1. The Tc-99m teborox-

Table 1. Preparation and quality control.

1. Add 100 mCi of Tc-99m in 1 cc of saline
2. Heat for 15 minutes at 100° C
3. Cool and inspect visually
4. Quality control (paper chromatography)
   Spot two strips of Whatman 31 ET-Chrom paper strips
   Develop-mobile phase solvent fronts of saline, acetone : saline
   Measure activity in well counter or dosimeter
   Calculate % noncomplexed and reduced hydrolyzed Tc-99m

Refer to product package insert for details of preparation and quality control.

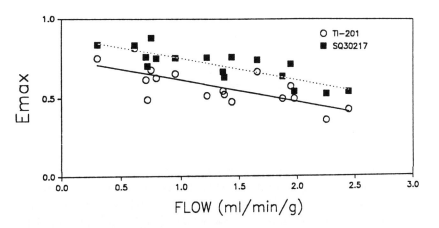

Figure 2. Comparative extraction, E_{max}, for thallium (closed squares) and SQ30217 or teboroxime (open circles). (Adapted and reprinted with permission from the Society of Nuclear Medicine from reference [9].)

ime complex is stable for approximately 6 hours [1] and each vial provides 1–2 doses.

Teboroxime demonstrates good correlation with blood flow as assessed with microspheres, and unlike thallium, this linear relationship is preserved with all levels of coronary perfusion including those obtained with pharmacologic hyperemia [2–6]. Teboroxime does appear to underestimate true levels of flow however, especially at high coronary flow rates and when beyond the early post injection period [5, 6]. Other tracers currently used, thallium and sestamibi, demonstrate a diffusion limitation with increasing coronary blood flows, which potentially limits the accurate assessment of coronary perfusion in high flow states [7].

The clearance of teboroxime from the blood in humans is rapid and biexponential, with a first half-life of 0.79 minutes (88%) [8]. Two minutes after teboroxime injection in dogs, only 8% of the peak blood activity remains [2]. Experimental work has demonstrated that the myocardial extraction of teboroxime is also high. The cardiac uptake of teboroxime is 3.44% of the injected dose at 1 minute post-injection in rats, substantially higher than with thallium, suggesting a high myocardial extraction [1]. In an isolated blood perfused rabbit heart model, the peak first-pass extraction, E_{max}, for teboroxime was significantly higher than thallium (0.72 vs 0.57) [9], and was inversely related to blood flow (Figure 2). In another model, using intracoronary injections of teboroxime in open-chest dogs, the initial myocardial retention of teboroxime was also high (> 90%) [2]. Additionally, the capillary permeation (PS_{cap}) of teboroxime, a measure of solute exchange, is higher than thallium and has a direct linear relationship to flow [9]. The net extraction (E_{net}) of teboroxime in this rabbit heart model is greater than thallium but the difference is relatively small compared to E_{max}. This observation suggests rapid back diffusion of the tracer, since E_{net} represents the retention of the perfusion agent over time (3–5 minutes) [9]. Therefore, despite initially rapid extraction and high capillary permeation, this experimental model suggests that rapid teboroxime myocardial washout occurs.

A biexponential myocardial clearance curve is noted for teboroxime in both animals [1, 2] and humans [8], with about 70% of the clearance occurring within the first 5 minutes [2]. In the canine, the first two thirds of the activity is cleared for the heart in 2.3–3.6 minutes [1, 2]. Initial myocardial clearance data revealed that the effective first half-time in humans is 5.2 minutes with the second effective half-life of teboroxime washout being 3.8 hours [8]. Therefore, the first half-life for the myocardium in humans of approximately 11 minutes. Subsequent research acquiring rapid sequential images using a multi-detector tomographic (SPECT) system suggests that the washout of teboroxime may be even more rapid, with a half-time of myocardial washout of 2.8 minutes for the first phase and 58 minutes for the second [10]. The explanation for the rapid clearance of teboroxime is not entirely known. The relatively small volume of distribution in the myocyte plays some part in the retention but the arterial input function may also be reduced. The amount of teboroxime available for myocardial extraction is reduced as time progresses, as has been shown in rats [11] and following incubation with bovine erythrocytes [12].

The half-time of the early rapid component of myocardial clearance is markedly decreased following dipyridamole infusion [2, 4], similar to that seen following exercise [14], which suggests flow-dependent kinetics of Tc-99m teboroxime. Delayed myocardial clearance has been noted in regions of reduced coronary perfusion and has been described both experimentally [6, 14–16] and clinically [17, 18]. Ischemic, hypoperfused zones have a prolonged cardiac half-time as compared with normal issue. These flow related differences in teboroxime clearance may allow the improved detection of ischemic but viable myocardium and permit the detection of mild to moderate coronary stenoses [16]. The effect of metabolic influence on teboroxime uptake and retention is not well defined. It appears that thallium may be more sensitive to hypoxia and reperfusion injury than is teboroxime, however there is certainly some metabolic influence on teboroxime kinetics [19, 20].

Technetium-99m teboroxime is excreted by the hepatobiliary route, with peak liver activity noted between 4.5 and 7 minutes. The major target organ for dosimetry is the upper large intestine, receiving approximately 6.15 rads following a 50 mCi dose of teboroxime. The mean effective dose equivalent (International Committee on Radiation Protection) is 1.78 rem/30 mCi of

Tc-99m teboroxime, approximately 50% higher than for 3 mCi of thallium-201.

Imaging protocols

The physical and transport properties of Tc-99m teboroxime mandate a different approach to clinical imaging than do other perfusion agents. The prompt blood pool clearance and rapid myocardial washout necessitate rapid data acquisition. Initial studies with teboroxime used protocols in which imaging was performed up to 10 minutes post-injection. It is now evident that expeditious data acquisition is required for optimal image quality. Furthermore, the accurate assessment of ischemia depends on the rapid collection of data in order to minimize the effect of differential myocardial clearance, which is reliant on the level of coronary blood flow. Therefore, the exercise area (with treadmill or bicycle) and camera system need to be in close proximity to one another, to allow for the initiation of data collection with 2 minutes post Tc-99m teboroxime injection.

The exact protocols for teboroxime imaging are still undergoing revisions for optimal results. The dose of teboroxime was approximately 15 mCi per dose in initial reports, however additional clinical experience now demonstrates that 20–25 mCi is the preferred dosage, with a total not to exceed 50 mCi per patient study. Unlike sestaMIBI [21], there does not appear to be a significant difference regarding the results of teboroxime scanning with respect to the order of imaging, i.e. stress followed by rest or vice versa. In patients without known ischemic heart disease, it may be preferable to perform the stress scintigram first, so that if it appears normal, no additional isotope need be given and the study would be completed within minutes of the stress procedure. However, if the detection of viable, ischemic myocardium is the key question, then the resting imaging is acquired first, eliminating the potential influence by background activity. The time between the first and second studies has also not been fully defined. One to two hours separated the image acquisitions in most of the early studies [8, 13, 17, 22, 23], however it may be feasible to begin the second study as early as 20 minutes after the first (DS Berman, personal communication). The temporal sequence of events for Tc-99m teboroxime is displayed in Figure 3.

Planar imaging should be completed within 5 minutes of teboroxime administration, with the acquisition started after the disappearance of blood pool activity. If a dynamic mode is used (Figure 4) 20–30 second frames of information are collected continuously, and later 2–4 frames are summated for each projection. Static collection of 45–60 seconds per view is optimal, provid-

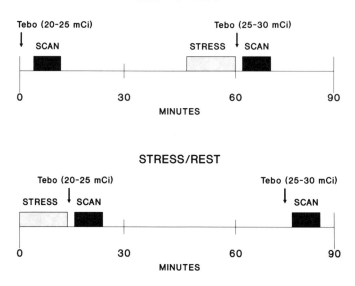

Figure 3. Timing of events for teboroxime imaging (Tebo = teboroxime injection). It may be feasible to reduce the time between scans to 20 minutes. The preference for the stress/rest or rest/stress sequence is discussed in the text.

ed the camera system can reset for each projection within a brief period of time. Imaging vertically, with the patient standing or seated, allows for maximum myocardial-hepatic separation. This also permits the camera to remain stationary while the patient is pivoted in front of the collimator, thereby minimizing the time required for patient/camera positioning. Obtaining the left lateral view first may reduce hepatic interference which may be noted in this projection. Suggestions for planar teboroxime methodology are outlined in Table 2.

SPECT teboroxime scintigraphy has been performed successfully, again with an emphasis on rapid acquisition methods [22–24]. Rehearsing the transfer of the patient to the camera gantry allows for rapid and accurate patient and camera positioning following the teboroxime injection. Following exercise, image acquisition should begin as soon as possible. As the scintigraphic procedure begins immediately after exercise, imaging artifacts may be present due to changes in chamber size, respiratory motion and cardiac 'creep' [25]. However, these artifacts may not be problematic, due to the very short imaging times. Many different acquisition parameters have been attempted with a variety of SPECT systems. The choice of collimators will depend on the system, however a low-energy, all-purpose collimator may provide the best

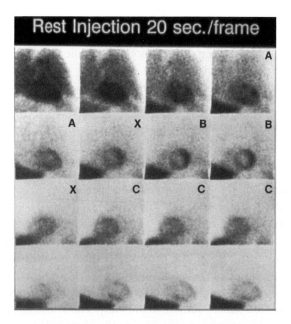

Figure 4. An example of dynamic planar imaging with Tc-99m teboroxime. Each frame represents 20 second. The letters 'A', 'B', 'C' indicate the anterior, 45° LAO and left lateral projections, respectively. The frames labeled with 'X' are frames during which motion artifacts are present due to patient repositioning. Note the rapid and intense appearance of hepatic activity and the virtual disappearance of tracer activity within 5 minutes (reprinted courtesy of Dr Jeffrey Leppo).

sensitivity/resolution relationship. In order to minimize hepatic interference, starting the acquisition in the 45° left posterior oblique projection may be worthwhile. For a single detector SPECT, a continuous acquisition is ideal but limited to certain systems. Reconstruction limits should be as close to the myocardium as possible to eliminate hepatic influence, but without cutting off

Table 2. Planar acquisition parameters.

Camera	Large field of view
Collimator	Low energy, all purpose
Data matrix	128×128 $(64 \times 64)^*$
Mode	Dynamic (20 sec/frame) or static
Projection	LLAT (70° LAO), ANT, 45° LAO
Time per view	40–90 seconds
Total acquisition time	2.5–4.0 minutes
Background subtraction	None
Quantitation	Not available

Items in parentheses and with an asterisk indicate alternative methods.

the inferior wall which may produce an artifactual defect. Multidetector SPECT cameras not only have the advantage of only requiring a 120° rotation, but are also designed for rapid continuous data collection [10, 26, 27]. Serial scanning can be performed with both planar and multi-SPECT cameras to examine regional differences in myocardial washout. A summary of many of the technical aspects of SPECT teboroxime scintigraphy is depicted in Table 3.

Clinical trials

The early clinical experience with teboroxime perfusion imaging was obtained as part of a multicenter trial in which the results of Tc-99m teboroxime scintigraphy were compared to the 'clinical impression' of the presence of coronary artery disease based on coronary angiography and/or thallium scanning in 155 patients [28, 29]. The results of clinical laboratory tests failed to demonstrate any significant changes attributable to teboroxime administration and no serious adverse effects have been described in over 300 patients [13, 29; unpublished data, Squibb Diagnostics]. The sensitivity and specificity for the detection of coronary artery disease was 82 and 91%, respectively, and the concordance between thallium and teboroxime was 90% [28, 29]. As part of this multicenter study, Seldin et al. performed planar teboroxime perfusion imaging in conjunction with bicycle ergometry in 30 subjects [13]. In this initial report of the clinical utility of Tc-99m teboroxime, the imaging was completed approximately 17 minutes after tracer injection. When compared with thallium scintigraphy, teboroxime scintigraphy was equally sensitive for detecting angiographically documented coronary artery disease (thallium = 80% vs teboroxime = 85%; p = NS). The recent Canadian Multicenter Trial has also demonstrated that similar sensitivities exist for thallium and teboroxime for

Table 3. Tomographic acquisition parameters.

	Single detector	Multiple detectors
Collimator	LEAP (high resolution)*	High resolution
Data matrix	64 × 64	128 × 128 (64 × 64)*
Orbit	180° circular	120° elliptical
Mode	Step-shoot (continuous)*	Continuous
Time per stop	32 stops, 5–10 sec/stop	–
Time per scan	4–8 min (2.5–3.5 min)*	1–2.5 min
Total scan time	4–8 min (2.5–3.5 min)*	4–10 min

Items in parentheses and with an asterisk indicate alternative methods.

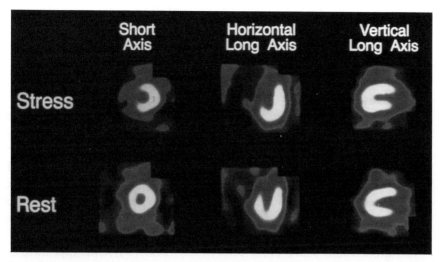

Figure 5. An example of a SPECT teboroxime scan, demonstrating a completely reversible septal defect, consistent with ischemia in the left anterior descending territory (reprinted courtesy of Dr Raye Bellinger).

the angiographic presence of coronary artery disease (thallium = 85% vs teboroxime = 83%; p = NS) [30].

Investigators at the University of Massachusetts Medical Center also examined 30 patients with Tc-99m teboroxime using a rapid planar imaging protocol [17]. The total imaging time was approximately 4 minutes for each study, with approximately 90 minutes separating the stress and rest examinations. Diagnostic agreement was present in 28 of 30 studies. When teboroxime was compared with thallium for the detection of transient (ischemic) and persistent (infarction) defects, the concordance was 89 and 86%, respectively. Due to the significant hepatic uptake of teboroxime and its possible interference with the detection of inferior wall abnormalities, the data was also analyzed on the basis of vascular distributions. The major coronary artery territories were concordant between thallium and teboroxime in 82–85% of these regions, suggesting that the diagnostic accuracy for a particular vascular region is not reduced [31].

The ability to detect coronary artery disease with teboroxime using SPECT was questioned in the early trials due to the rapid myocardial clearance of this perfusion agent from the myocardium. However, minor modifications in SPECT methodology has demonstrated that this technique is feasible. Using SPECT, teboroxime and thallium are in agreement for the detection of coronary artery disease in 73–80% of myocardial segments [22, 32, 33] and a per-patient diagnostic correlation of 88–100% [23, 32]. Fleming et al. have also demonstrated that concordance of perfusion regions and quantitative arteriographic data was 76% for teboroxime and 73% for thallium (p = NS; 22). Therefore, it appears that that Tc-99m-teboroxime SPECT imaging is comparable to tomographic thallium scintigraphy for the detection of coronary artery disease (Figure 5).

A continuous acquisition is an optimal way for a single detector SPECT to decrease camera acquisition time by the removal of camera dead time. Furthermore, the loss of 15–25% of available activity would be eliminated. Utilizing a 3-minute continuous acquisition, Burns and Wright have demonstrated 78% segmental concordance for normal, reversible or fixed defects when teboroxime was compared with thallium [24]. This type of rapid SPECT imaging may minimize the effects of differential washout and improve the scintigraphic detection of viable myocardium. While this methodology has significant benefits for teboroxime imaging, this technology is not available on all camera systems.

The initial results with multidetector SPECT camera systems appears to be very encouraging, with a similar efficacy for the detection of coronary artery disease [10, 26]. As cardiac imaging optimally uses 180° rotations, an ideal camera system may be with two detectors in an orthogonal arrangement. These rapid sequential images with multidetector cameras also allow for the collection of myocardial washout data [27], which may enhance the detection of coronary artery disease and allow for the rapid detection of viable myocardium.

The use of Tc-99m teboroxime combined with pharmacologic vasodilation may be an ideal way to use this perfusion agent. Technetium-99m teboroxime uptake and early clearance has a uniquely linear relationship to flow, as compared with other myocardial perfusion agents, even at the high levels of coronary blood flow associated with pharmacologic hyperemia [3, 5]. Additionally, patients may be prepositioned prior to the initiation of the stress state and scan acquisition may be initiated easily within the recommended 2 minutes post-injection. Preliminary reports using both adenosine [34] and dipyridamole [35] have been very favorable, as segmental concordance with thallium studies is 82–85%. As the washout of teboroxime is rapid and flow-related, most investigators have attempted to delay the Tc-99m washout by reversing the coronary hyperemia of dipyridamole with aminophylline or by discontinuing the adenosine infusion.

Differential washout and myocardial viability

Regional differences in the myocardial washout of Tc-99m teboroxime have been demonstrated clinically, as well as in animal models [6, 14–16]. The

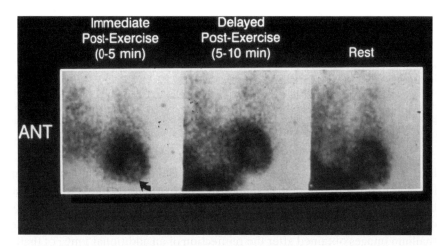

Figure 6. An example of rapid differential washout in the anterior (ANT) view. Note the inferoapical region (arrow) has significant improvement on the delayed (5–10 minute post-exercise scan) as compared with the immediate post-stress study (reprinted with permission from the American College of Cardiology from reference [17]).

well-described dependence of teboroxime clearance on flow was felt to lead to the early 'redistribution' of a perfusion defect [2]. Differential washout was noted on serial planar scanning and in 9 of 11 patients on delayed, post-exercise images (5–10 minutes after tracer injection) correlated better with the resting image than with the immediate, post exercise (0–5 minutes) study [17] (Figure 6). Ischemic zone to normal zone ratios (IZ : NZ) have quantitatively confirmed this effect, with the IZ : NZ ratios diminishing on delayed stress views in 65% of patient studies [18]. Rapid changes in teboroxime perfusion defects have also been noted using multidetector SPECT systems [10, 27]. Drane and co-workers have reported that by using 10 two-minute acquisitions, the 'redistribution' observed by other investigators, with the rapid normalization of images is due to differential washout with delayed clearance of teboroxime in regions with stenotic coronary arteries [27]. As these initial defects may decrease in severity with time, this method may allow the rapid determination of hypoperfused, viable cardiac tissue following a single tracer injection [7, 17, 18, 27] and may obviate the need for true rest images in some patients.

The detection of coronary artery disease is no longer sufficient for clinical cardiology. Many therapeutic decisions rest on the assessment of ischemic, viable myocardium. Several reports have noted that more persistent defects are present with Tc-99m teboroxime than with thallium imaging and that teboroxime may be less sensitive in detecting ischemia [8, 13, 22, 26]. Our laboratory, however, has noted more transient perfusion abnormalities and

→

Figure 7. Planar exercise thallium (A) and teboroxime (B) scans in a patient with known coronary artery disease. The left, center and right columns represent the anterior, 45° LAO, and left lateral projections respectively. The top rows are the immediate post-stress scans. The bottom row of the teboroxime study is the rest scan. On the thallium scan, the middle row is the redistribution images and the bottom is the reinjection study. The thallium images demonstrate partially reversible anterior and septal defects, which following thallium reinjection reveals almost complete reversibility. The teboroxime images also demonstrate the finding of anterior wall and septal ischemia, in corcordance with the thallium reinjection images (reprinted courtesy of Dr Jeffrey Leppo).

less fixed defects with Tc-99m teboroxime as compared to thallium imaging [17, 36]. In order to more fully evaluate the relative abilities of teboroxime and thallium to detect viable myocardium, teboroxime scans were compared not only to the routine stress and redistribution thallium images, but also to thallium images obtained after the reinjection of an additional 1 mCi of thallium. This reinjection method has been shown to enhance detection of ischemic but viable myocardium [37]. The preliminary results with teboroxime are quite promising, as persistent perfusion defects are similar in number with teboroxime and thallium reinjection studies, in contrast to routine thallium imaging [36] (Figure 7).

Newer applications

As teboroxime has its initial distribution in the blood pool, it is possible to obtain functional information by means of first-pass radionuclide ventriculography. Johnson, Seldin, and colleagues, using a small, high count rate multicrystal scintillation camera (SIM-400, Scinticor), have developed a protocol to obtain both first pass ventriculograms and perfusion images [8]. Motion correction is accomplished by dual isotope imaging of a point source (americium-241) and the technetium agent [38]. Thus, an ejection fraction and regional wall motion assessment may be obtained, as well as myocardial perfusion data. The image quality of the perfusion scan is limited, however, due to the reduced resolution of the multicrystal camera.

Future applications may include the delineation of flow in acute coronary syndromes. As sestamibi has shown utility in the diagnosis and prognosis of acute myocardial infarction, research is presently underway using teboroxime in a similar fashion. Additionally, there is optimism that reperfusion after thrombolytic therapy may be accurately assessed by Tc-99m teboroxime as has been shown with sestamibi [39]. This new agent may also be of use in delineating vascular territories prior to percutaneous transluminal coronary angioplasty and may be of value in the detection of early restenosis after angioplasty.

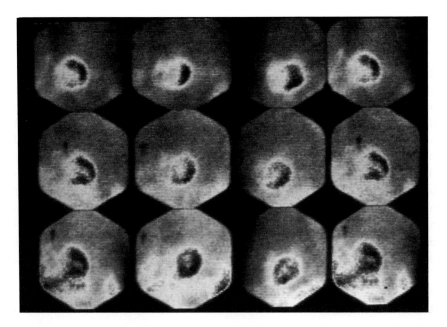

(A)

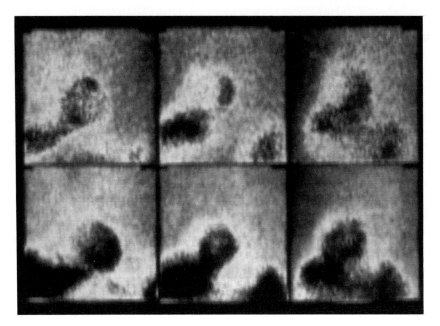

(B)

Conclusion

In conclusion, Tc-99m teboroxime is a unique myocardial perfusion agent with documented safety and efficacy. The kinetics of this tracer are ideally suited to imaging in conjunction with pharmacologic stress and/or multidetector SPECT camera systems. However, diagnostic quality information may be obtained following exercise or with planar or SPECT imaging. Teboroxime has a clear advantage over existing perfusion agents with regards to time until study completion, which impacts both on patient acceptance and laboratory throughput. Other theoretical benefits, such as the improved relationship between activity and flow, as well as improved ischemia detection have not been fully realized at this time. Although possibly more demanding on personnel and equipment, Tc-99m teboroxime is a valuable agent in one's armamentarium of techniques for the noninvasive assessment of ischemic heart disease.

Acknowledgements

The author wishes to acknowledge the continued support from Dr Jeffrey Leppo, whose thoughtful comments on this manuscript were most appreciated. The assistance of Squibb Diagnostics is also acknowledged.

References

1. Narra RK, Nunn AD, Kuczynski BL, Feld T, Wedeking P, Eckelman WC. A neutral technetium-99m complex for myocardial imaging. J Nucl Med 1989; 30: 1830–7.
2. Stewart RE, Schwaiger M, Hutchins GD et al. Myocardial clearance kinetics of technetium-99m-SQ30217: a marker of regional myocardial blood flow. J Nucl Med 1990; 31: 1183–90.
3. Coleman RE, Maturi M, Nunn AD, Eckelman WC, Cobb FR. Myocardial perfusion: comparison of SQ 30217, thallium-201 and microspheres in dogs [abstract]. J Nucl Med 1987; 28 suppl: 1080.
4. Li QS, Solot G, Frank TL, Wagner HN Jr, Becker LC. Serial rest and dipyridamole tomographic myocardial perfusion studies with the rapidly clearing Tc-99m agent SQ 30217 [abstract]. J Nucl Med 1988; 29 Suppl: 938.
5. Beanlands R, Muzik O, Nguyen N, Schwaiger M. Comparison of the myocardial retention of technetium-99m-teboroxime and thallium-201 [abstract]. J Am Coll Cardiol 1991; (2 Suppl A): 252A.
6. Beanlands R, Muzik O, Nguyen N, Petry N, Schwaiger M. The relationship of technetium-99m teboroxime retention and myocardial blood flow [abstract]. J Nucl Med 1991; 32 Suppl: 947.

7. Mousa SA, Williams SJ, Sands H. Characterization of in vivo chemistry of cations in the heart. J Nucl Med 1987; 28: 1351–7.

8. Johnson LL, Seldin DW. Clinical experience with technetium-99m teboroxime, a neutral, lipophilic myocardial perfusion agent. Am J Cardiol 1990; 66: 63E–67E.

9. Leppo JA, Meerdink DJ. Comparative myocardial extraction of two technetium-labeled BATO derivatives (SQ30217, SQ32014) and thallium. J Nucl Med 1990; 31: 67–74.

10. Nakajima K, Taki J, Bunko H et al. Dynamic acquisition with a three-headed SPECT system; application to technetium 99m-SQ30217 myocardial imaging. J Nucl Med 1991; 32: 1273–7.

11. Rumsey WL, Rosenspire K, Nunn AD. Extraction and metabolism of teboroxime in the isolated perfused rat heart [abstract]. J Nucl Med 1991; 32 Suppl: 948.

12. Dahlberg ST, Gilmore MP, Siwko R, Leppo JA. Incubation with red blood cells reduces the extraction of technetium-99m teboroxime in the isolated rabbit heart [abstract]. J Nucl Med 1991; 32 Suppl: 910.

13. Seldin DW, Johnson LJ, Blood DK et al. Myocardial perfusion imaging with technetium-99m SQ30217: comparison with thallium-201 and coronary anatomy. J Nucl Med 1989; 30: 312–9.

14. Gray W, Gewirtz H. Evidence of differential washout of Tc-99m teboroxime from normal and ischemic myocardium [abstract]. J Am Coll Cardiol 1991; 17 (2 Suppl A): 286A.

15. Glover DK. Okada RD, Hebert CB. Tc-99m-teboroxime (SQ30217 Cardiotec) kinetics in normal and ischemic canine myocardium [abstract]. Circulation 1990; 82 (4 Suppl III): III486.

16. Johnson G3d, Okada RD, Hebert CB. Myocardial kinetics of technetium-99m teboroxime in a canine stenosis model following dipyridamole [abstract]. J Nucl Med 1991; 32 Suppl: 948.

17. Hendel RC, McSherry B, Karimeddini M, Leppo JA. Diagnostic value of a new myocardial perfusion agent, teboroxime (SQ 30217), utilizing a rapid planar imaging protocol: preliminary results. J Am Coll Cardiol 1990; 16: 855–61.

18. Levine D, Gewirtz H. Evidence of differential technetium-99m teboroxime washout in myocardial images of patients with known or suspected ischemic heart disease [abstract]. J Nucl Med 1991; 32 Suppl: 930.

19. Dahlberg ST, Gilmore M, Meerdink DJ, Leppo JA. Effect of global cardiac ischemia and reperfusion on the extraction of thallium-201 and technetium-teboroxime in the isolated rabbit heart [abstract]. J Am Coll Cardiol 1991; 17 (2 Suppl A): 286A.

20. Okada RD, Johnson G3d, Glover DK, Hebert CB. Myocardial Tc-99m-teboroxime (Cardiotec, SQ30217) clearance is reduced in ischemic myocardium due to a combination of hypoxic and low flow factors [abstract]. J Am Coll Cardiol 1991; 17 (2 Suppl A): 286A.

21. Taillefer R, Gagnon A, Laflamme L, Gregoire J, Leveille J, Phaneuf DC. Same day injections of Tc-99m methoxy isobutyl isonitrile (hexamibi) for myocardial tomographic imaging: comparison between rest-stress and stress-rest injection sequences. Eur J Nucl Med 1989; 15: 113–7.

22. Fleming RM, Kirkeeide RL, Taegtmeyer H, Adyanthaya A, Cassidy DB, Goldstein RA. Comparison of technetium-99m teboroxime tomography with automated quantitative coronary arteriography and thallium-201 tomographic imaging. J Am Coll Cardiol 1991; 17: 1297–302.

23. Iskandrian AS, Heo J, Nguyen T, Mercuro J. Myocardial imaging with Tc-99m teboroxime: technique and initial results. Am Heart J 1991; 121: 889–94.

24. Burns RJ, Wright L. Three-minute acquisition of exercise Tc-99m-teboroxime cardiac SPECT with a single-head detector [abstract]. J Nucl Med 1991; 32 Suppl: 929.

25. Friedman J, Van Train K, Maddahi J. 'Upward creep' of the heart: a frequent source of false-positive reversible defects during thallium-201 stress-redistribution SPECT. J Nucl Med 1989; 30: 1718–22.

26. Kim AS, Quaife RA, Akers MS, Faber TL, Corbett JR. Sequential tomographic myocardial

perfusion imaging with Tc-99m teboroxime in patients: comparison with thallium-201 and arteriography [abstract]. J Nucl Med 1991; 32 Suppl: 919.

27. Drane WE, Decker M, Strickland P, Tineo A, Zmuda S. Measurement of regional myocardial perfusion using Tc-99m teboroxime (Cardiotec) and dynamic SPECT [abstract]. J Nucl Med 1989; 30: 1744.

28. Zielonka JS, Bellinger R, Coleman RE et al. Multicenter clinical trial of 99m-Tc teboroxime (SQ30217; Cardiotec) as a myocardial perfusion agent [abstract]. J Nucl Med 1989; 30: 1745.

29. Zielonka JS, Cannon P, Johnson L et al. Multicenter trial of Tc-99m teboroxime (Cardiotec): a new myocardial perfusion agent [abstract]. J Nucl Med 1990; 31 Suppl: 827.

30. Taillefer R, Freeman M, Greenberg D et al. Detection of coronary artery disease: comparison between 99m-Tc-teboroxime and 201-thallium planar myocardial perfusion imaging (Canadian multicenter clinical trial) [abstract]. J Nucl Med 1991; 32 Suppl: 919.

31. Hendel RC, Dahlberg ST, McSherry BA, Leppo JA. Diagnostic correlation between rapid planar teboroxime imaging and thallium scintigraphy: general concordance and a comparison by vascular territory [abstract]. J Nucl Med 1990; 31 Suppl: 827–8.

32. Serafini AN, Friden A, Topchik S et al. Tomographic SPECT myocardial imaging – A comparative study between Tc-99m-teboroxime (teboroxime) and 201 thallium [abstract]. J Nucl Med 1991; 32 Suppl: 920.

33. Burns RJ, Fung A, Iles S, Daigneault L, Lalonde L, Hong Tai Eng F. Exercise Tc-99m-teboroxime cardiac SPECT: results of a Canadian multicenter trial [abstract]. J Nucl Med 1991; 32 Suppl: 919.

34. Nguyen T, Heo J, Beer S, Cassel D, Cave V, Iskandrian AS. SPECT teboroxime imaging during adenosine-induced coronary hyperemia [abstract]. J Nucl Med 1991; 32 Suppl: 1036.

35. Labonte C, Taillefer R, Lambert R et al. Comparison between Tc-99m-teboroxime and 201-thallium dipyridamole imaging in detection of coronary artery disease [abstract]. J Nucl Med 1991; 32 Suppl: 919–20.

36. Hendel RC, McSherry BA, Leppo JA. Teboroxime and thallium (with reinjection) scintigraphy for the detection of myocardial ischemia and infarction [abstract]. Circulation 1990; 82 (4 Suppl III): III320.

37. Dilsizian V, Rocco TP, Freedman NM, Leon MB, Bonow RO. Enhanced detection of ischemic but viable myocardium by the reinjection of thallium after stress-redistribution imaging. N Engl J Med 1990; 323: 141–6.

38. Port S, Gal S, Grenier R, Acharya K, Shen Y, Skrade B. First-pass radionuclide angiography during treadmill exercise: evaluation of patient motion and a method for motion correction [abstract]. J Nucl Med 1989: 30 Suppl: 770.

39. Wackers FJ, Gibbons RJ, Verani MS et al. Serial quantitative planar technetium-99m isonitrile imaging in acute myocardial infarction: efficacy for noninvasive assessment of thrombolytic therapy. J Am Coll Cardiol 1989; 14: 861–73.

10. Clinical applications of rubidium-82 for myocardial perfusion imaging

KIM A. WILLIAMS

Introduction

The many recent advances in the fields of diagnostic and interventional cardiology have placed growing importance on the noninvasive approaches to myocardial perfusion imaging. The goals of such imaging has been to determine the extent of coronary artery disease, its impact on myocardial blood flow under varied physiologic and pathophysiologic states, the presence, location and extent of myocardial infarction, and residual myocardial segmental viability. Recently, new myocardial perfusion imaging tracers have been developed which are capable of addressing these important clinical issues. This article aims to review the application of one of these tracers, rubidium-82 (Rb-82). The clinical potential of this tracer will be highlighted by a review of the fundamentals and history of myocardial perfusion imaging.

Nuclear imaging of myocardial perfusion

Radionuclide imaging of myocardial perfusion requires injection, usually intravenously, of an isotope which undergoes radioactive decay. This process results in the emission of a 'photon' or energy packet, which can then be detected by imaging devices or 'cameras'. The emissions that come from the nucleus of an isotope (as it changes to a more stable and lower energy state) are called 'gamma (γ) rays'. The rearrangement of an isotope's electron configuration (again, changing to a lower energy state) results in the emission of a 'characteristic x-ray'. Proton-rich isotopes may also undergo a transformation

127

Ernst E. van der Wall et al. (eds), What's new in cardiac imaging?, 127–141.
© *1992 Kluwer Academic Publishers. Printed in the Netherlands.*

by 'positron emission', in which a proton is converted to a neutron, resulting in the release of a positron and a neutrino. The positron, (or β^+-particle) is the antimatter of the electron (β^--particle). A positron will travel a few millimeters before it collides with an electron. Their interaction results in annihilation of both particles and the emission of two oppositely directed relatively high energy (511 keV) photons, called coincidence photons. Thus, the radiation produced by these three radioactive decay processes, gamma emission, x-ray emission, and positron annihilation photons, varies in photon energy.

Most radiation imaging devices, i.e. gamma cameras, employ an energy sensitive crystal of sodium iodide mixed with a small amount of thallium, abbreviated Na-I(Tl). This crystal is a scintillator which produces visible light when struck by radiation photons. The intensity of this visible light is proportional to the energy of the incident photon. The visible light is then amplified and converted to electrical current by an array of photomultiplier tubes which are connected to the crystal by light pipes. Thus, a photon of radiation is converted into a voltage pulse which identifies its energy and spatial location. Modern camera systems record these voltage pulses, or 'counts', in digital computer memory for storage and processing. The positioning of events in the image to correspond spatially with the imaged object is enhanced by photon focusing, or 'collimation'. The collimators used for this purpose employ a heavy metal (such as lead or tungsten) with long holes (usually parallel to each other) in order to exclude tangential photons, while allowing only those photons which are directed perpendicularly from the organ toward the crystal surface to comprise an image. Long exposure images obtained from a few angles (usually three views) is called planar imaging. Many camera systems have rotational capabilities, for single photon emission computed tomography (SPECT). SPECT images are obtained by taking brief exposure images from multiple stops (usually 32 or 60) along a rotation of 180 or 360 degrees. These images are then back projected and filtered into a three-dimensional reconstruction of the organ.

An alternative approach to imaging positrons, called positron emission tomography (PET), relies on coincidence-counting circuitry [1]. To detect the coincident oppositely directed 511 keV positron annihilation photons, radiation detectors are placed facing one another. One 'count' occurs when each detector is simultaneously struck by one of an annihilation photon pair. Decays striking only one detector are not counted. Thus, PET cameras are electronically 'collimated', ignoring stray single photons. Several banks of rings of hundreds of coincidence detectors encircle the patient in modern PET cameras. Back projection of this circle of images (similar in principle to SPECT imaging or CT scanning) gives three-dimensional tomographic images. As with SPECT imaging, the three-dimensional information can be displayed in multiple two-dimensional slices, polar maps (also called 'bullseye' plots), or in rotating three-dimensional topographic displays. Attenuation correction information is obtained from transmission scanning by placing a positron-emitting ring source (usually gallium-68) between the patient and the detector prior to injection of a radionuclide for emission scanning. Thus, PET has the combination of intrinsic tomographic spatial and contrast resolution, quantitation and attenuation correction which are currently unobtainable with single photon gamma cameras.

Myocardial perfusion imaging: a historical perspective

Myocardial perfusion scintigraphy has progressed over the past two decades from the early-use monovalent cationic radioactive isotopes of potassium, potassium analogs (rubidium, cesium, and thallium) and nitrogen-13 ammonia [1], to the more recent introduction of technetium-99m complexes, including the monovalent cation methoxyisobutylisonitrile (MIBI) [2] and the neutral lipophilic boronic acid adduct of technetium dioxime (BATO) [3].

The clinical impact of noninvasive determination of relative regional myocardial perfusion has been very large in the diagnosis and management of coronary heart disease over the past two decades. Diagnosis of inducible ischemia, evaluation of therapy, detection and sizing of myocardial infarction, and determination of myocardial viability are among the many current indications for perfusion scintigraphy. The current standards, thallium-201 (Tl-201) and the new technetium-labeled agents, are imaged with either planar or SPECT techniques. While planar imaging is technically less demanding, rotational tomographic imaging provides three-dimensional images and superior perfusion defect definition.

Although each of the aforementioned perfusion tracers has been imaged with single photon techniques, the development of positron emission tomography (PET) imaging [4] has provided two major advantages: quantitation of myocardial perfusion and intrinsic correction for attenuation. These factors have made PET imaging superior to the single photon technique for both clinical and research applications. However, the expense of PET has precluded its widespread use. Over the past decade it has been primarily as a research technique at major university medical centers. Although a cogent case can be made that PET is indeed cost-effective [5], the relatively large initial investment has made it unattractive to most medical centers at this time.

Thallium-201 imaging

Thallium-201 has been the perfusion imaging standard for the past 15 years [6]. However, the physical characteristics of Tl-201 are not optimal for myocardial perfusion imaging. It has a long physical half-life (73 hours), resulting in difficulty in performing serial studies. The long half-life also results in significant radiation doses to the target organ, the kidney (1.2 rads/millicurie), when serial studies are undertaken [7]. Thallium-201 produces low-energy photons (primarily 68 to 83 keV mercury characteristic x-rays) which are below the optimal range for gamma camera imaging. These photons are easily attenuated by body tissues, often resulting in apparent perfusion defects which are due to breast, chest wall, or diaphragmatic attenuation [8]. Moreover, Tl-201 is cyclotron produced. This results in the need for frequent deliveries from an off-site manufacturer.

Technetium-labeled compounds

Since technetium-99m (Tc-99m) has the best physical imaging properties for gamma cameras, Tc-99m-labeled compounds have been actively sought for myocardial perfusion imaging. At this time, the most promising agents are Tc-99m-labeled MIBI and BATO. The myocardial uptake of these agents are similar to those of Tl-201; BATO has a slightly higher myocardial extraction at high blood flows, while MIBI has a slightly lower extraction under these conditions. However, myocardial retention of MIBI is extremely high, while myocardial washout of BATO is very rapid. Thus, delayed imaging to examine myocardial redistribution is not feasible for MIBI [9] and has not yet been shown to be clinically practical for BATO. As a result, two injections are needed to detail differences between resting and exercise or pharmacological stress perfusion patterns. A major advantage of compound labeling to Tc-99m is its lower radiation dosimetry, allowing higher doses of tracer to be administered (10 to 50 millicuries Tc-99m total,versus 3 to 5 millicuries for Tl-201). This should result in better count density in the images. Also, these tracers can be bolus-injected for first-pass studies of ventricular function, followed by perfusion imaging of the same injection [10]. The combination of perfusion and ventricular function imaging with one tracer injection may provide risk stratifying information not currently available from other clinical and laboratory indicators [11] in patients with coronary artery disease. Serial imaging with these tracers requires either split dosing (e.g. 7 to 10 millicuries at rest followed by 20 to 30 millicuries with stress), or imaging with full doses on separate days. As with Tl-201, despite the somewhat higher photon energy of Tc-99m (140 keV), the lack of tissue attenuation corrections impedes the accuracy of these studies. Without appropriate mathematical modeling for SPECT, absolute quantitation of perfusion is not possible.

Positron-emitting perfusion tracers

The difficulty with serial imaging, caused by the relatively long physical half-lives of Tc-99m (6 hours) and Tl-201 (73 hours), can be eliminated by the use of short-lived perfusion tracers, such as Rb-82 and nitrogen-13 (N-13) ammonia. Both of these tracers are positron-emitting isotopes with myocardial uptake characteristics similar to Tl-201.

Positron-emitting isotopes are generally imaged using PET imaging. However, a planar imaging technique has been described which allows application of these tracers in the coronary care unit with a mobile gamma camera [12, 13]. The original description of N-13 ammonia for myocardial perfusion imaging was with a planar gamma camera at the University of Chicago [12]. Images were obtained with a mobile Pho-Gamma IV camera (Searle Radiographics) fitted with lead shielding and a rotating tungsten collimator. This collimator was designed for high energy (511 keV) photons of positron-emitting isotopes. It rotates circumferentially, resulting in the absence of the septation and hole pattern from the image without loss of spatial resolution [14]. The gamma camera was mounted on a truck-driven mechanism, so that imaging could be performed either in the coronary care unit or nuclear imaging laboratory.

Rubidium-82 for myocardial perfusion imaging

Advantages of Rubidium-82

Isotopes of the alkali metal rubidium (Rb) including Rb-81, Rb-82, and Rb-86, are potassium analogs and have been used for myocardial perfusion imaging for nearly two decades [1]. Rubidium-82 is a positron-emitting isotope with a physical half-life of 75 seconds, which is now commercially available. It is eluted from an on-site generator that can be used for up to six weeks [15]. The parent radionuclide is accelerator produced strontium-82 (Sr-82), which is housed in a lead shielded generator column and has a physical half-life of 25 days. This column has negligible Sr-82 breakthrough due to the secure binding of strontium to its stannic oxide adsorbent. Elution of Rb-82 is performed with isotonic saline, similar to the technique of the molybdenum-99-technetium-99m generator. The generator is contained in an infusion system (Figure 1) which is on a mobile cart. The infusion system is self-monitored for radiation delivery, with dial-in settings for the dose of Rb-82 (in millicuries), dose rate,

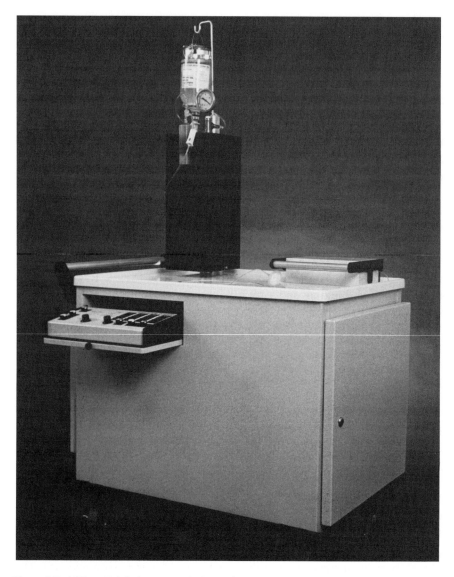

Figure 1. Rubidium-82 infusion system is shown (courtesy of ER Squibb, Inc).

and volume to be delivered to the patient. After each elution, the infusion system is regenerated to full capacity within 10 minutes, since the half-life of Rb-82 is far shorter than that of Sr-82 (secular equilibrium).

The major advantages of rubidium-82 over other perfusion tracers are its very short physical half-life and immediate availability without the need for frequent deliveries or kit preparation. The short half-life allows the performance of serial studies, with a relatively low radiation dose. Each 40 millicurie dose results in only 0.78 rad to the kidneys (the target organ), 0.30 rad to the heart walls, and a 0.06 rad estimated whole body radiation absorbed dose [16]. The half-life is also helpful for imaging rest/stress studies and for rapidly evolving clinical situations, such as pre- and post-thrombolytic therapy or coronary angioplasty in the setting of acute myocardial infarction or observing transient ischemic phenomenon. Serial images can be obtained within a few minutes of one another in these circumstances without contamination of the second image with counts from a previous dose. In comparison with the positron-emitting perfusion tracer N-13 ammonia (10 minute half-life), Rb-82 has several advantages. It does not require an on site cyclotron, has inherently shorter acquisition times, and does not show increased uptake in the lungs of patients who smoke cigarettes.

Clinical uses of rubidium-82

Quantitation of myocardial perfusion

Early PET studies demonstrated that Rb-82 could be used as a quantitative marker of myocardial perfusion [17, 18]. Utilizing arterial input curves to estimate tracer delivery to the myocardium, flow-dependent tracer uptake can be directly related to myocardial blood flow. It has been shown that myocardial uptake of Rb-82 correlates linearly with myocardial blood-flow measurements obtained with microspheres over a wide range of experimental flow rates during both pharmacologic and metabolic interventions [18]. Similar to Tl-201 and potassium isotopes, Rb-82 is rapidly and efficiently concentrated in the myocardium, with the first-pass extraction fraction in the range of 60% at rest and 30% at high levels of coronary blood flow [17–19]. During myocardial ischemia, there is a relative Rb-82 deficiency in the regions of reduced blood flow which may be due to a reduction in sodium-potassium-ATPase mediated myocardial cellular cation transport [20].

Detection of coronary artery disease

Since coronary artery disease is the leading cause of mortality in the industrialized western world, improved methods of early detection are needed. Provocative testing with exercise or pharmacological stress and rest or redistribution myocardial perfusion imaging has become commonplace. However, traditional methods have had limitations in diagnostic accuracy, and are very time-consuming for patients and laboratory personnel. Using Rb-82 and PET, rapid patient throughput high diagnostic accuracy have been attained. A complete rest and stress study can be performed in less than one hour (Plates 10.1 and 10.2).

Imaging with vasodilators

Although exercise is possible in combination with Rb-82 imaging, most investigators have opted for pharmacological stress using dipyridamole or adenosine. Dipyridamole is an inhibitor of cellular uptake and metabolism of adenosine, a potent vasodilator which produces maximal coronary flow more reliably than exercise [21]. Similarly, some investigators have used direct acting intravenous adenosine infusion as an adjunct to myocardial perfusion imaging [22]. Invasive studies have utilized intracoronary papaverine for this purpose. Using these agents, resistance arterioles are dilated, resulting in a 3 to 6 fold increase in the flow through normal coronary beds. The ratio between maximal and resting flow has been termed 'absolute coronary flow reserve' [23]. Another index, 'relative coronary flow reserve' is defined as the ratio of the maximal myocardial blood flow in a given segment to the maximal myocardial blood flow in the segment with the highest level of flow in the heart [4]. These indices appear to be complementary in clinical application. The often-cited but rarely observed 'balanced' three-vessel disease could potentially result in a falsely normal relative flow reserve measurement. However, the absolute flow reserve would show a reduced increment in global myocardial flow with vasodilation. Conversely, the relationship between resting and maximal coronary flow can be altered by ventricular hypertrophy [24], loading conditions, heart rate, and cardiac workload [25], adversely affecting the usefulness of the measurement of absolute coronary flow reserve. Using these concepts, diagnostic accuracy of PET studies can be optimized for the detection of even mild coronary artery stenoses.

It has been shown that measures of coronary flow reserve are superior to visually interpreted coronary arteriograms in the assessment of the physiologic impact of coronary stenoses [26]. This fact makes suspect the value of the myriad of studies which describe the 'diagnostic accuracy' of noninvasive tests for ischemic heart disease which have been compared with coronary arteriography. Thus, any discussion of test severity and specificity obtained in such a manner has serious limitations. Quantitative coronary angiography, employing objective computer derived videodensitometric measurement of coronary stenosis sensitity, has been validated as a better measure of coronary flow reserve [27].

Accuracy of PET for coronary artery disease

Using quantitative angiography, PET perfusion imaging with Rb-82 or N-13 ammonia and dipyridamole has been shown to have sensitivities and specificities ranging from 94 to 100% [28–30]. Reviews of the accuracy of SPECT Tl-201 imaging would suggest that it has far less sensitivity and specificity than PET [4, 31, 32], estimated at 65 to 75%. However, the studies comprising these reviews were reported from visually analyzed coronary arteriograms, and are therefore suspect. Little data comparing thallium scintigraphy and quantitative angiographic measures of coronary arterial stenoses are available, but one study suggests that excellent correlation exists in patients with single-vessel disease [33]. One direct comparison between SPECT and PET in patients with severe ischemic disease found no significant difference between the two [34], while other studies suggest that PET is far superior [4, 28, 35]. The exact degree to which the accuracy of PET exceeds that of SPECT remains to be determined, using a truer gold standard in a large series of patients.

Evaluation of patients with known disease

Importantly, PET perfusion indices are useful in the delineation of the extent and severity of myocardial perfusion deficits and, thus, provide a measure of coronary disease extent and severity [4]. This is of demonstrated value in the assessment of revascularization procedures, such as coronary angioplasty [36] and bypass surgery [37]. Under the influence of pharmacologic vasodilators, especially when combined with hand-grip exercise to increase coronary tone, a fall in measured coronary blood flow may occur in collateral flow-dependent myocardial segments. This phenomenon has been termed 'coronary steal' and can be identified by PET perfusion imaging [38] as a fall in absolute Rb-82 or N-13 ammonia content in the myocardium after dipyridamole administration.

Detection of acute infarction with planar imaging

Despite the elegance of the information obtained from PET studies, the immobility of PET technology hinders its wide spread application in the coronary care unit. Rb-82 myocardial perfusion imaging has also been performed in the coronary care unit utilizing the planar mobile gamma camera described earlier. In one study [13] which included 22 patients with myocardial infarction, planar rubidium-82 images were compared with resting planar Tl-201 images (Figure 2). Myocardial perfusion defect detection and severity scoring were found to have good correlation between the two tracers. Both

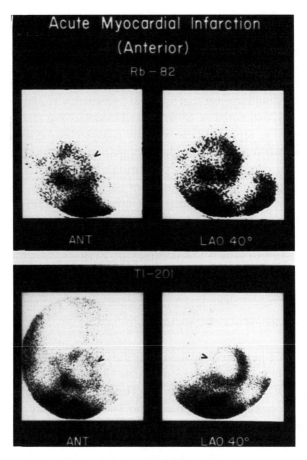

Figure 2. Planar rubidium-82 (Rb-82) and thallium-201 (Tl-201) images obtained in a patient with occlusion of the left anterior descending coronary artery and an acute anteroseptal myocardial infarction are shown. Images were obtained at rest in the coronary care unit. Perfusion defects in the anterolateral (ANT projection) and anteroseptal segments (LAO 40° projection) are demonstrated (arrows). [ANT = anterior, LAO = left anterior oblique]

perfusion techniques had diagnostic accuracies similar to regional wall motion for identification of the infarct-related artery.

Detection of silent ischemia

Most, if not all, patients with ischemic heart disease experience intermittent episodes of silent (asymptomatic) ischemia. There appears to be little difference in prognosis for patients with inducible ischemia, whether symptomatic or silent. Many noninvasive diagnostic techniques have enabled the detection of episodes of myocardial ischemia which would have otherwise been unapparent. Exercise electrocardiography and ambulatory ECG Holter monitoring have been frequently used for this purpose [39, 40]. However, myocardial perfusion and ventricular function studies are even better suited for ischemia detection than the ECG, since perfusion disparities and segmental dysfunction are pathophysiologically earlier events in the ischemic cascade [41, 42]. Indeed, PET studies have been critical in removing much of the diagnosis of silent ischemia, demonstrating that the ischemic ST-segment depression is associated with transient reduction of regional myocardial blood flow, as reflected by reversible Rb-82 perfusion defects [43].

Several studies have shown that PET imaging of Rb-82 is an extremely useful tool for the detection of silent myocardial ischemia in patients with coronary artery disease. Silent ischemia has been documented in these patients using Rb-82 PET during cold provocation, mental stress, mastication, after cigarette smoking, and spontaneously [37, 44–50].

Assessment of myocardial viability

In addition to myocardial perfusion, PET facilities have examined segmental myocardial ischemia and viability using metabolic markers such as fluorine-18-deoxyglucose and carbon-11-palmitate. During exercise or post-myocardial infarction, much diagnostic and prognostic information has been obtained using the combination of metabolic and perfusion imaging [51–53]. Some myocardial segments with severely reduced blood flow may have contractile dysfunction and nonreversible perfusion defects, but have enough flow to maintain cell-membrane integrity, substrate metabolism, and viability. Such segments may improve in contractile performance with time, especially if revascularization is undertaken. These segments can be identified as viable tissue by imaging substrate metabolism [52, 53]. Furthermore, myocardial segments without preserved metabolism have been shown to be unlikely to improve [53]. Thus, metabolic imaging can guide the clinician to a decision about revascularization procedures in a given patient. In segments with Tl-201 perfusion defects after exercise, myocardial viability has been assessed with delayed redistribution imaging and, more recently, with Tl-201 reinjection [54]. However, segments without improvement with delayed imaging or reinjection may still have metabolic evidence for viability [55, 56].

There is recent evidence that examination of myocardial membrane integrity with resting Rb-82 PET perfusion imaging may play a role in the assessment of myocardial viability [57]. With newer 'fast' PET camera technology, list mode acquisition of PET data allows reformatting of the Rb-82 perfusion data into two high-count images, begun 80 seconds after injection. The first image consists of data from 15 to 110 seconds, while the second image is comprised of the data from 120 to 360 seconds. The difference between the early and late images represents tracer washout and/or tracer trapping. Failure to trap Rb-82 is reflected by a new or worsening defect on the second image, and presumably represents necrotic myocardium. A defect on the initial scan which improves on the second set of images suggests the presence of membrane integrity and tracer trapping, and therefore regional myocardial viability. Although large-scale multicenter experience remains to be accumulated with resting Rb-82 imaging for the assessment of myocardial viability, this technique appears promising for speed and simplicity, relative to other PET technology.

Conclusion

Rubidium-82 is a generator produced positron-emitting potassium analog with a very short half-life of 75 seconds. This tracer has been utilized for the assessment of myocardial perfusion in a variety of clinical settings. These include planar imaging for detection and localization of myocardial infarction in the CCU, and qualitative or quantitative perfusion imaging with positron emission tomography (PET) for diagnosis and assessment of coronary artery disease.

The short half-life of Rb-82 allows serial perfusion studies under varied physiologic conditions, such as drug or exercise-induced hyperemic flow, within 10 minutes of each other. Its production in the strontium-82 generator provides convenient tracer availability at the bedside in the coronary care unit, or in the clinical or PET imaging laboratory. Newer PET techniques may provide accurate quantitation of absolute myocardial blood flow and indices of regional myocardial viability after myocardial infarction.

Acknowledgements

I gratefully acknowledge the expert editorial assistance of Ms Mary D. Spainhour and the kind help of Mr Kevin Brooks of Squibb Diagnostics. This work was supported in part by a National Institute of Health training grant, HL-7381.

References

1. Budinger TF. Physiology and physics of nuclear cardiology. Cardiovasc Clin 1979; 10: 9–78.
2. Machac J: Technetium-99m isonitrile: a perfusion or a viability agent? [editorial]. J Am Coll Cardiol 1989; 14: 1685–8.
3. Johnson LL, Seldin DW. Clinical experience with technetium-99m teboroxime, a neutral, lipophilic myocardial perfusion imaging agent. Am J Cardiol 1990; 66: 63E–67E.
4. Gould KL. PET perfusion imaging and nuclear cardiology. J Nucl Med 1991; 32: 579–606.
5. Gould KL, Goldstein RA, Mullani NA. Economic analysis of clinical positron emission tomography of the heart with rubidium-82. J Nucl Med 1989; 30: 707–17.
6. Berman DS, Garcia EV, Maddahi J et al. Thallium-201 myocardial perfusion scintigraphy. In: Freeman LM, editor. Freeman and Johnson's clinical radionuclide imaging. 3rd ed. Orlando: Grune & Stratton, 1984: 485.
7. Thallous Chloride Tl-201 (product insert). North Billerica, Mass.: New England Nuclear Medical Products, May, 1984.
8. Gordon DG, Pfisterer M, Williams R, Walaski S, Ashburn W. The effect of diaphragmatic attenuation on Tl-201 images. Clin Nucl Med 1979; 4: 150–1.
9. Okada RD, Glover D, Gaffney T, Williams S. Myocardial kinetics of technetium-99m-hexakis-2-methoxy-2-methylpropyl-isonitrile. Circulation 1988; 77: 491–8.
10. Sporn V, Perez Balino N, Holman BL et al. Simultaneous measurement of ventricular function and myocardial perfusion using the technetium-99m isonitriles. Clin Nucl Med 1988; 13: 77–81.
11. Perez-Gonzalez J, Botvinick EH, Dunn R et al. The late prognostic value of acute scintigraphic measurement of myocardial infarction size. Circulation 1982; 66: 960–71.
12. Walsh WF, Fill HR, Harper PV. Nitrogen-13-labeled ammonia for myocardial imaging. Semin Nucl Med 1977; 7: 59–66.
13. Williams KA, Ryan JW, Resnekov L et al. Planar positron imaging of rubidium-82 for myocardial infarction: a comparison with thallium-201 and regional wall motion. Am Heart J 1989; 118: 601–10.
14. Brunsden B, Harper PV, Beck RN. Elimination of collimator-hole pattern by double displacement of a hexagonal array [abstract]. J Nucl Med 1975; 16 Suppl: 517.
15. Neirinckx RD, Kronauge JF, Gennaro GP, Loberg MD. Evaluation of inorganic adsorbents for the rubidium-82 generator. I. Hydrous SnO_2. J Nucl Med 1982; 23: 245–9.
16. Ryan JW, Harper PV, Stark VS et al. Radiation absorbed dose estimate for rubidium-82 determined from in vivo measurements in human subjects. In: Schlafke-Stelson AT, Watson EE, editors. Fourth international radiopharmaceutical dosimetry symposium: proceedings of a conference held at Oak Ridge, Tennessee; November 5–8, 1985. Oak Ridge: Oak Ridge Associated Universities Publishers, 1986; 346–58.
17. Mullani NA, Gould KL. First-pass measurements of regional blood flow with external detectors. J Nucl Med 1983; 24: 577–81.
18. Mullani NA, Goldstein RA, Gould KL et al. Myocardial perfusion with rubidium-82. I. Measurement of extraction fraction and flow with external detectors. J Nucl Med 1983; 24: 898–906.
19. Goldstein RA, Mullani NA, Marani SK, Fisher DJ, Gould KL, O'Brien HA Jr. Myocardial perfusion with rubidium-82. II. Effects of metabolic and pharmacologic interventions. J Nucl Med 1983; 24: 907–15.
20. Selwyn AP, Allan RM, L'Abbate A et al. Relation between regional myocardial uptake of

rubidium-82 and perfusion: absolute reduction of cation uptake in ischemia. Am J Cardiol 1982; 50: 112–21.

21. Leppo JA. Dipyridamole-thallium imaging: the lazy man's stress test. J Nucl Med 1989; 30: 281–7.

22. Verani MS, Maharian JJ, Hixson JB, Boyce TM, Staudacher RA. Diagnosis of coronary artery disease by controlled coronary vasodilation with adenosine and thallium-201 scintigraphy in patients unable to exercise. Circulation 1990; 82: 80–7.

23. Gould KL, Lipscomb K. Effects of coronary stenosis on coronary flow reserve and resistance. Am J Cardiol 1974; 34: 48–55.

24. Goldstein RA, Haynie M. Limited myocardial perfusion reserve in patients with left ventricular hypertrophy. J Nucl Med 1990; 31: 255–8.

25. Gould KL, Kirkeeide Rl, Buchi. Coronary flow reserve as a physiologic measure of stenosis severity. J Am Coll Cardiol 1990; 15: 459–74.

26. White CW, Wright CB, Doty DB. Does visual interpretation of the coronary arteriogram predict the physiologic importance of a coronary stenosis? N Engl J Med 1984; 310: 819–24.

27. Goldstein RA, Kirkeeide RL, Demer LL et al. Relations between geometric dimensions of coronary artery stenoses and myocardial perfusion reserve in man. J Clin Invest 1987; 79: 1473–8.

28. Gould KL, Goldstein RA, Mullani NA et al. Noninvasive assessment of coronary stenoses by myocardial perfusion imaging during pharmacologic coronary vasodilation. VIII. Clinical feasibility of positron cardiac imaging without a cyclotron using generator-produced rubidium-82. J Am Coll Cardiol 1986; 7: 775–89.

29. Demer L, Gould KL, Goldstein RA. Assessment of coronary artery disease severity by positron emission tomography. Comparison with quantitative arteriography in 193 patients. Circulation 1989; 79: 825–35.

30. Yonekura Y, Tamaki N, Senda M, Nohara R, Kambara H, Konishi Y et al. Detection of coronary artery disease with 13N-ammonia and high-resolution positron-emission computed tomography. Am Heart J 1987; 113: 645–54.

31. Gould KL. How accurate is thallium exercise testing for the diagnosis of coronary artery disease [editorial]. J Am Coll Cardiol 1989; 14: 1487–90.

32. Diamond GA. How accurate is SPECT thallium scintigraphy? [editorial]. J Am Coll Cardiol 1990; 16: 1017–21.

33. Zijlstra F, Fioretti P, Reiber JH, Serruys PW. Which cineangiographically assessed anatomic variable correlates best with functional measurements of stenosis severity? A comparison of quantitative analysis of the coronary cineangiogram with measured coronary flow reserve and exercise/redistribution thallium-201 scintigraphy. J Am Coll Cardiol 1988; 12: 686–91.

34. Tamaki N, Yonekura Y, Senda M et al. Value and limitation of stress thallium-201 single photon emission computed tomography: comparison with nitrogen-13 ammonia positron tomography. J Nucl Med 1988; 29: 1181–8.

35. Go RT, Marwick TH, MacIntyre WJ et al. A prospective comparison of rubidium-82 PET and thallium-201 SPECT myocardial perfusion imaging utilizing a single dipyridamole stress in the diagnosis of coronary artery disease. J Nucl Med 1990; 31: 1899–1905.

36. Goldstein RA, Kirkeeide RL, Smalling RW. Changes in myocardial perfusion reserve after PTCA: noninvasive assessment with positron tomography. J Nucl Med 1987; 28: 1262–7.

37. Ribeiro P, Shea M, Deanfield JE. Different mechanisms for the relief of angina after coronary bypass surgery. Physiological versus anatomical assessment. Br Heart J 1984; 52: 502–9.

38. Demer LL, Gould KL, Goldstein RA, Kirkeeide RL. Noninvasive assessment of coronary collaterals in man by PET perfusion imaging. J Nucl Med 1990; 31: 259–70.

39. Conti CR. Silent myocardial ischemia: prognostic significance and therapeutic implications. Clin Cardiol 1988; 11: 807–11.
40. Gottlieb SO. Association between silent myocardial ischemia and prognosis: insensitivity of angina pectoris as a marker of coronary artery disease activity. Am J Cardiol 1987; 60: 33J–38J.
41. Nesto RW, Kowalchuk GJ. The ischemic cascade: temporal sequence of hemodynamic, electrocardiographic and symptomatic expressions of ischemia. Am J Cardiol 1987; 59: 23C–30C.
42. Beller GA. Myocardial perfusion imaging for detection of silent myocardial ischemia. Am J Cardiol 1988; 61: 22F–28F.
43. Nabel EG, Rocco MB, Selwyn AB. Characteristics and significance of ischemia detected by ambulatory electrocardiographic monitoring. Circulation 1987; 75 (6 Suppl): V74–83.
44. Deanfield JE, Shea MJ, Wilson RA, Horlock P, deLandsheere CM, Selwyn AP. Direct effects of smoking on the heart: silent ischemic disturbances of coronary flow. Am J Cardiol 1986; 57: 1005–9.
45. Deanfield JE, Shea MJ, Selwyn AP. Clinical evaluation of transient myocardial ischemia during daily life. Am J Med 1985; 79: 18–24.
46. Selwyn AP, Shea MJ, Deanfield JE, Wilson RA, DeLandsheere C. Jones T. Clinical problems in coronary disease are caused by wide variety of ischemic episodes that affect patients out of hospital. Am J Med 1985; 79: 12–7.
47. Deanfield JE, Shea M, Kensett M et al. Silent myocardial ischaemia due to mental stress. Lancet 1984; 2: 1001–5.
48. Shea MJ, Deanfield JE, Wilson RA, deLandsheere C, Selwyn AP. Silent myocardial ischemia during mastication. Am J Med 1987; 82: 357–60.
50. Shea MJ, Deanfield JE, deLandsheere CM, Wilson RA, Kensett M, Selwyn AP. Asymptomatic myocardial ischemia following cold provocation. Am Heart J 1987; 114: 469–76.
51. Camici P, Araujo LI, Spinks T et al. Increased uptake of 18F-fluorodeoxyglucose in postischemic myocardium of patients with exercise-induced angina. Circulation 1986; 74: 81–8.
52. Sobel BE, Geltman EM, Tiefenbrunn AJ et al. Improvement of regional myocardial metabolism after coronary thrombolysis induced with tissue-type plasminogen activator or streptokinase. Circulation 1984; 69: 983–90.
53. Schwaiger M, Brunken R, Grover-McKay M. Regional myocardial metabolism in patients with acute myocardial infarction assessed by positron emission tomography. J Am Coll Cardiol 1986; 8: 800–8.
54. Dilsizian V, Rocco TP, Freedman NM, Leon MB, Bonow RO. Enhanced detection of ischemic but viable myocardium by the reinjection of thallium after stress-redistribution imaging. N Engl J Med 1990; 323: 141–6.
55. Brunken R, Schwaiger M, Grover-McKay M. Positron emission tomography detects tissue metabolic activity in myocardial segments with persistent thallium perfusion defects. J Am Coll Cardiol 1987; 10: 557–67.
56. Tamaki N, Ohtani H, Yamashita K. Metabolic activity in the areas of new fill-in after thallium-201 reinjection: comparison with positron emission tomography using fluorine-18-deoxyglucose. J Nucl Med 1991; 32: 673–8.
57. Gould KL, Yoshida K, Hess MJ, Haynie M, Mullani NA, Smalling RW. Myocardial metabolism of fluorodexoglucose compared to cell membrane integrity for the potassium analog Rubidium-82 for assessing infarct size in man by PET. J Nucl Med 1991; 32: 1–9.

11. Nitrogen-13 ammonia perfusion imaging

MENCO G. NIEMEYER, AAF F.M. KUIJPER,
EDUARD G.M. D'HAENE and ERNST E. VAN DER WALL

Summary

Positron emission tomography (PET) provides an advanced imaging technology that permits the accurate definition of regional tracer distribution. In
combination with nitrogen-13 (N-13) ammonia, PET allows for the sensitive
and specific detection of coronary artery disease. Several studies indicate the
superiority of this approach in comparison to standard thallium-201 (Tl-201)
tomographic (SPECT) imaging. In addition, regional blood flow can be accurately measured using N-13 ammonia PET, and this approach can be employed
in conjunction with pharmacologic stress imaging to quantify regional flow
reserve. In combination with metabolic markers, N-13 ammonia is capable of
assessing myocardial viability. Furthermore, the N-13 ammonia PET approach may differentiate between various forms of cardiomyopathy. More
studies are needed to define the cost-benefit ratio of the N-13 ammonia PET
technique for the management of patients with coronary artery disease or
cardiomyopathy.

Introduction

The conventional imaging techniques provide a quite clear evaluation of the
anatomy and function of the heart. However, these methods show limitations
in answering questions of physiologic significance of given anatomy or of
myocardial viability. Whereas planar and SPECT imaging have major practical advantages and can be applied in almost any hospital with current commer-

Ernst E. van der Wall et al. (eds), What's new in cardiac imaging?, 143–156.
© *1992 Kluwer Academic Publishers. Printed in the Netherlands.*

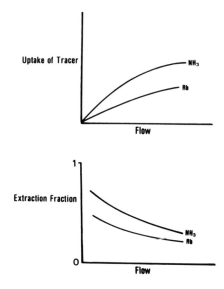

Figure 1. Uptake and extraction fraction of two partially extracted tracers, N-13 ammonia and rubidium-82, are shown as a function of flow. Extraction of these and similar tracers falls off at higher flows because shortened residence time in the capillary bed reduces uptake across capillary membranes. From Gould KL, Mullani N, Wong W, Goldstein RA. Positron emission tomography. In: Collins SE, Skorton DJ (eds) Cardiac imaging and image processing, pp 330–60, 1986. (Reproduced with permission.)

cially available nuclear medicine equipment and radiopharmaceuticals, PET theoretically offers major advantages in its ability to quantitatively study regional myocardial metabolism and blood flow. PET measures local tissue concentrations of radioisotopes in the body and differs from tomographic imaging with techniques such as computed tomography or magnetic resonance imaging in that it provides functional information [1]. In cardiac studies, PET can be used for the detection of myocardial ischemia, identification of tissue viability, and pathophysiologic assessment of various myocardial diseases, such as coronary artery disease and hypertrophic cardiomyopathy [2, 3]. With diffusible tracers such as N-13 and rubidium-82 (Rb-82) it is possible to measure the myocardial blood flow with PET (Figure 1). The application of N-13 as a marker for myocardial blood flow was supported by animal studies in which it was shown that myocardial blood flow deficits could be measured over a wide flow range [4, 5]. In addition to its ability to measure myocardial perfusion, PET is currently the only available technique that can assess cardiac metabolism in patients. To study metabolism of myocardial tissue with PET, two different types of metabolic compounds are available: fluorine-18 (F-18) labeled fluorodeoxyglucose (FDG) and carbon-11 labeled palmitic acid. The evaluation of cardiac metabolism and perfusion enables detection of viable myocardium, which is crucial for determination of appropriate therapy. Also, gated cardiac PET images may enable determination of myocardial function, perfusion, and metabolism at the same time [6].

Local tissue perfusion, blood volume, glucose and oxygen consumption, and fractional extractions of various metabolites and substances have all been quantitated and imaged with accuracy [7]. In this, the use of a positron emitting isotope as a tracer is crucial. The background of the PET technique is addressed in Chapter 10.

Positron emitting agents

Radioactive forms of oxygen, nitrogen, and carbon can be made and sub-stituted for the same stable elements in the molecules to be studied, thus avoiding alterations of the normal metabolic rate after introduction into the body that may result from the use of 'foreign' isotopes such as iodine or technetium. The activity passing through a volume of scanned tissue can then be measured. Although some radiopharmaceuticals can be used as they are produced by the cyclotron such as oxygen-15 (O-15) and N-13, or generator-produced (e.g. Rb-82), whereas others require radiosynthesis such as F-18 FDG. The variety of functions that can be assessed and imaged is limited by the availability of tracers that can be rapidly labeled chemically with the isotopes, which have extremely short half-lives. For example, the half-life of O-15 is 2.07 minutes and that of N-13 9.96 minutes. Measuring the amount of labeled molecule in the tissue depends on several chemical, physical, and biological factors, any of which may be the focus of primary, clinical, or biological interest. Because of the short half-lives of the positron-emitting radionuclides, the synthesis must be performed expeditiously. Work is pro-gressing to automate and make routine the synthesis of PET radiopharmaceut-icals. The short half-lives permit serial studies at short time intervals. Three positron-emitting tracers have shown to have clinical value as markers of myocardial perfusion: Rb-82 (Chapter 10), O-15 labeled water (Chapter 12), and N-13 ammonia. In this chapter, the clinical value of N-13 ammonia is discussed.

Measurement of regional myocardial blood flow by N-13 ammonia

Tracers of blood flow may be classified as extractable particles and extractable diffusion indicators. Labeled albumin microspheres are the most widely used

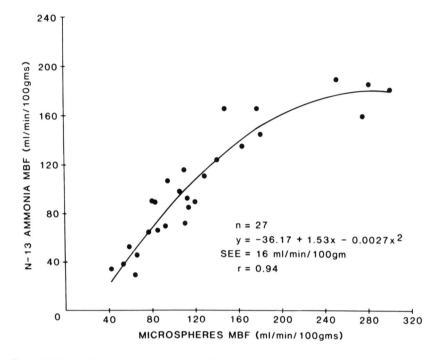

Figure 2. Relation between regional myocardial blood flow (MBF) determined with the microspheres technique and with nitrogen-13 labeled-positron emmission tomography in 27 dog experiments. From Ref. [8] Shah A et al. J Am Coll Cardiol 1985; 5: 92–100. (Reprinted with permission from the American College of Cardiology.)

agents in the first group. Since they are extracted almost 100% during a single capillary transit, the local deposited activity reflects local capillary blood flow. Nitrogen-13 ammonia is a flow tracer which also mimics microspheres after intravenous injection due to its high clearance from the blood. Nitrogen-13 ammonia as an indicator of myocardial blood flow appears to diffuse across capillary and cellular membranes and becomes metabolically trapped in the myocardium.

Excellent correlation between this method and the microsphere technique has been demonstrated in animal models, although at high rates, flow will be underestimated by N-13 ammonia [8] (Figure 2). This method has extensively been studied in humans [9, 10]. The advantages of N-13 ammonia include rapid clearance from blood and high myocardial extraction (80–90%) and retention (82%), which results in high contrast myocardial images [11]. A linear relationship was observed between microspheres and N-13 ammonia for myocardial blood flow. Potential disadvantages of N-13 ammonia are that it is probably retained in the myocardium by metabolic trapping mainly by the glutamic

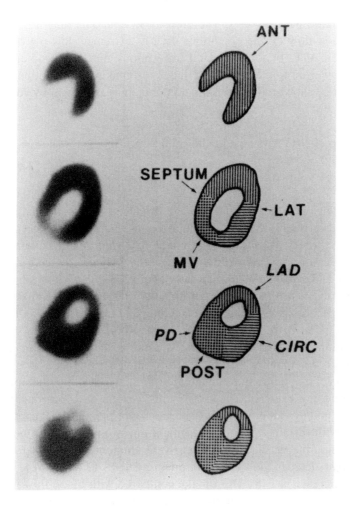

Figure 3. Contiguous cross-sectional images of the heart obtained after intravenous administration of 13-N ammonia in a normal volunteer. The cross-sections of the left ventricular myocardium are displayed as if viewed from below. The cross-section on the top is through the high anterior wall, whereas the image at the bottom is at an oblique angle through the posterior and inferior wall of the left ventricle. The schematic representation of the cross-sectional images on the right indicates the intraventricular septum and the anterior (ANT), lateral (LAT), and posterior (POST) walls of the left ventricle and mitral valve (MV). The distributions of the left anterior descending (LAD), left circumflex (CIRC), and posterior descending (PD) coronary arteries are indicated by the different shades of gray. From Ref. [15] Schelbert et al. Am J Cardiol 1982; 49: 1197–207. (Reproduced with permission.)

acid-glutamine pathway [12]. Therefore N-13 ammonia may not accurately reflect blood flow during conditions such as extremely low pH or reduced intracellular ATP. In addition, after intravenous injection, N-13 ammonia is rapidly converted to metabolic intermediates, making quantitation problematic. Figure 3 shows a normal N-13 ammonia image in a healthy volunteer.

Indications of N-13 ammonia in clinical practice

A. Coronary artery disease

PET imaging of the heart with cyclotron-produced N-13 ammonia, preferably in conjunction with F-18 FDG is optimal for (1) accurate noninvasive diagnosis of coronary artery disease in symptomatic or asymptomatic patients [13–17], for (2) assessing physiologic stenosis severity [18], (3) imaging myocardial infarction and determining myocardial viability [19–23], (4) assessing effects of interventions such as thombolysis on metabolism [24], PTCA on coronary flow reserve [25], and bypass surgery on function and metabolism [26], (5) following progression or regression of coronary artery disease during risk factor modification, and (6) noninvasively evaluating collateral function [27].

Accurate detection of coronary artery disease using PET is possible by evaluation of blood flow at rest compared with images after either intravenous dipyridamole or exercise. The assessment of extent of myocardial infarction, ischemia, and/or viability by PET seems promising in clinical cardiology. In patients with sustained myocardial infarction, two patterns can be observed when comparing cardiac PET using N-13 ammonia and F-18 FDG: (1) a concordant decrease in N-13 ammonia and F-18 FDG uptake, and (2) a relative increase in F18 FDG uptake compared with blood flow (Figure 4). This latter pattern is predominantly observed with patients with persistent symptoms and signs of ischemia and is thought to represent viable myocardial tissue that is still able to metabolize glucose anaerobically [28]. In the presence of injured or ischemic but viable myocardial cells, myocardial metabolism is shifted toward anaerobic glycolysis. Fluorine-18 FDG uptake then increases relative to the rest of the myocardium, thereby identifying ischemic, viable tissue, since necrotic myocardium does not extract FDG. In patients with chronic coronary artery disease and acute myocardial infarction, myocardial areas with a N-13 ammonia rest perfusion defect and normal F-18 FDG uptake after oral glucose loading (flow-metabolism mismatch) are hypothesized to be viable and may demonstrate improved left ventricular function after revascularization [26].

Studies have further suggested that the blood flow-metabolism mismatch

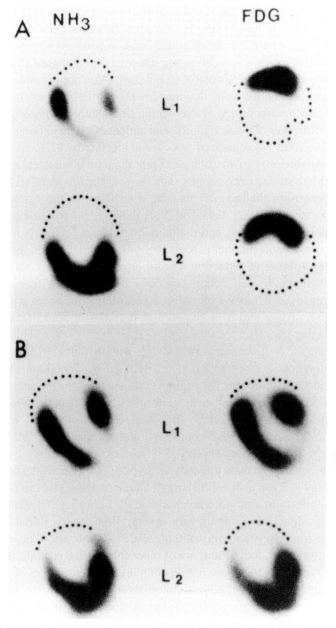

Figure 4. Cross-sectional N-13 ammonia (NH$_3$) and F-18-fluorodeoxyglucose (FDG) images at two levels (L) obtained 48 hours (A) and 6 weeks (B) after the onset of acute symptoms. In the study, there is a mismatch of FDG and NH$_3$ uptake, suggesting viable tissue in the segments with decreased flow. On the study at 6 weeks (B), the patient's infarct was complete, suggesting salvage of myocardium after restoration of blood flow. From Schwaiger M et al. Metabolism and flow in acute myocardial infarction. J Am Coll Cardiol 1986; 8: 806. (Reprinted with permission from the American College of Cardiology.)

may reflect different states of ischemia such as 'stunned myocardium' (reperfusion ischemia) and 'hibernating myocardium' (low-flow ischemia) [29].

The wider use of PET viability studies may depend on whether this approach provides incremental diagnostic information compared with less expensive and more routinely available techniques. More importantly, comparison with results obtained using thallium-201 myocardial imaging is required. The presence of redistribution of stress-induced thallium-201 defects is widely accepted as a marker of tissue viability, and patients with these findings are not usually referred for assessment of myocardial viability by PET.

The clinical dilemma arises when persistent thallium-201 defects are present 3–4 hours after stress, since reports indicate that the standard technique of stress-redistribution thallium-201 imaging overestimates the extent of non-viable myocardium [30–32]. Based on PET, thallium-201 redistribution imaging at 24 hours after stress, and thallium-201 findings following revascularization, a considerable number of segments with fixed defects on thallium-201 images after 4 hours of redistribution did have evidence of viability. Most recently, thallium-201 reinjection has been proposed as a technique that provides improved detection of viable myocardium compared with 4 hour redistribution images and is more practical than the 24 hour delayed thallium-201 imaging [33, 34].

Comparing the N-13 ammonia PET images with thallium-201 SPECT images, the differences are not apparent, as outlined by Tamaki et al. [35]. A limitation in their study was the high prevalence of coronary artery disease (94%) and the use of treadmill exercise instead of dipyridamole, which gives a higher increase of coronary flow. In a subsequent study, they found that rest-stress N-13 ammonia PET could accurately predict reversible ischemia and asynergy after coronary surgery [36]. It could even identify irreversible areas more accurately than the commonly performed stress-delayed thallium-201 imaging. Even using reinjection thallium imaging, the extent of tissue viability is underestimated when compared to PET imaging [37]. PET viability studies are valuable in patients with severely impaired regional or global function, with coronary anatomy suitable for revascularization regions of wall motion abnormality, and the absence of reversible perfusion abnormalities on thallium-201 imaging following reinjection [38]. The advantages of advanced PET technology are best observed for intermediate disease prevalence ($<60\%$ of the study population) and/or moderate to less severe coronary artery disease, in which the question of medical or mechanical intervention is unclear and thallium stress testing is least accurate [14].

B. Dilated cardiomyopathy

This condition is unrelated to coronary artery disease and may also be diagnosed by positron imaging as an enlarged, poorly functioning heart with no resting or stress perfusion defects typical of ischemic cardiomyopathy due to coronary artery disease [6]. In cases of dilated congestive cardiomyopathy, PET has been found to accurately distinguish between idiopathic and ischemic types of cardiomyopathy [39, 40]. Idiopathic dilated cardiomyopathy characteristically exhibits homogeneous blood flow, homogeneous glucose utilization, and diffusely heterogeneous fatty acid uptake and metabolism. In contrast, ischemic types of dilated cardiomyopathy characteristically exhibit large discrete reductions in regional myocardial blood flow, corresponding to well-defined vascular territories. Relative increases in glucose utilization in such segments identify myocardium as viable and predict a potential functional improvement after interventional revascularization. Loss of metabolic activity, on the other hand, defines such hypoperfused regions as irreversibly injured without the potential for functional recovery [29].

Duchenne's muscular dystrophy has been shown to selectively involve the posterolateral wall of the left ventricle as the initial and primary site of myocardial dystrophy [41]. Electrocardiographic changes in this patient population suggest myocardial damage in corresponding ventricular segments. Perloff et al. [42] investigated 15 patients with Duchenne's muscular dystrophy and reported decreased N-13 ammonia uptake but maintained or increased F-18 FDG uptake in the posterolateral wall.

C. Hypertrophic cardiomyopathy

Patients with classic hypertrophic cardiomyopathy have been studied with N-13 ammonia PET [43–45]. By gating the positron-emission tomograms with the electrocardiogram, left ventricular function and wall thickening may be assessed regionally in three dimensions [46]. Grover-McKay et al. [3] found a reduced N-13 ammonia concentration in the septum compared with the free wall of wall of the left ventricle in patients with hypertrophic cardiomyopathy studied at rest (Figure 5). Camici et al. [45] showed, in a study of patients with hypertrophic cardiomyopathy, using N-13 ammonia PET, that coronary vasodilatory reserve is abnormal not only in the hypertrophied interventricular septum, but also in the nonhypertrophied-free wall of the left ventricle, suggesting that the reduction in coronary flow reserve is not necessarily due to myocardial hypertrophy, but may be a primary defect.

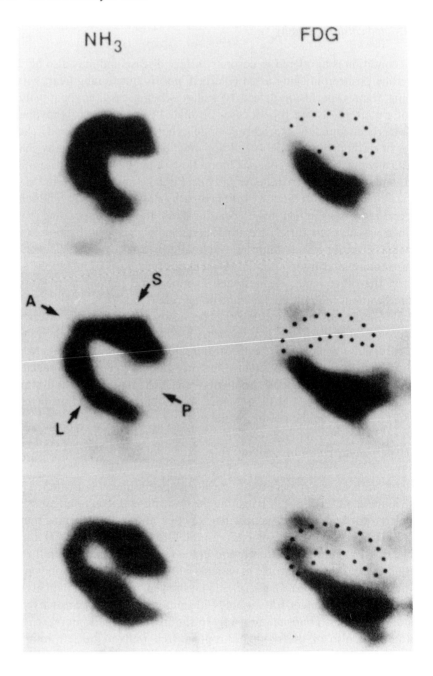

←

Figure 5. Transverse tomographic reconstructions acquired after the intravenous administration of N-13 ammonia ($^{12}NH_3$) (*left*) and ^{18}F-2-deoxyglucose (^{18}FDG) (*right*), acquired in the fasting state in a patient with hypertrophic cardiomyopathy. Three levels of the heart are shown; L-1 is the most basal and L-3 the most apical. The distribution of $^{13}NH_3$ is relatively homogeneous, but there is markedly depressed accumulation of ^{18}FDG in the interventricular septum. The location of the septum is indicated by the dotted lines. From Ref. [3], Grover-McKay M et al. J Am Coll Cardiol 1989; 13: 317–24. (Reprinted with permission from the American College of Cardiology.)

Conclusion

Serial imaging with the perfusion-marker N-13 ammonia PET shows promise as a noninvasive technique for accurately assessing myocardial perfusion both at rest and with stress. This method can now be applied to the study of patients to obtain more precise information relating to diagnostic and prognostic value of this technique in a variety of cardiac diseases. In patients with coronary artery disease, it should permit more accurate characterization of the severity of their coronary artery disease both by the accurate assessment of perfusion alone and in combination with F-18 FDG, which assists in the assessment of myocardial viability [9]. The cost of providing PET imaging in a medical center is, however, expensive. Such facilities require an investment for a cyclotron and a PET imaging device and also the services of both well-trained radiochemists and physicists for maintenance and operation.

References

1. Phelps ME, Mazziotta JC, Schelbert HR. Positron emission tomography and autoradiography: principles and applications for the brain and heart. New York: Raven Press, 1986.
2. Yamashita K, Tamaki N, Yonekura Y et al. Regional wall thickening of left ventricle evaluatied by gated positron emission tomography in relation to myocardial perfusion and glucose metabolism. J Nucl Med 1991; 32: 679–85.
3. Grover-McKay M, Schwaiger M, Krivokapich J, Perloff JK, Phelps ME, Schelbert HR. Regional myocardial blood flow and metabolism at rest in mildly symptomatic patients with hypertrophic cardiomyopathy. J Am Coll Cardiol 1989; 13: 317–24.
4. Schelbert HR. Blood flow and substrate use in normal and diseased myocardium. Ann Intern Med 1983; 98: 339–59.
5. Nienaber CA, Ratib O, Gambhir SS et al. A quantitative index of regional blood flow in canine myocardium derived noninvasively with N-13 ammonia and dynamic positron emission tomography. J Am Coll Cardiol 1991; 17: 260–9.
6. Hoffman EJ, Phelps ME, Wisenberg G, Schelbert HR, Kuhl DE. Electrographic gating in positron emission computed tomography. J Comput Assist Tomogr 1979; 3: 733–9.
7. Gould KL. PET perfusion imaging and nuclear cardiology. J Nucl Med 1991; 32: 579–606.
8. Shah A, Shelbert HR, Schwaiger M et al. Measurement of regional myocardial blood flow

with N-13 ammonia and positron emission tomography in intact dogs. J Am Coll Cardiol 1985; 5: 92–100.

9. Krivokapich J, Smith GT, Huang SC et al. 13-N ammonia myocardial imaging at rest and exercise in normal volunteers. Quantification of absolute myocardial perfusion with dynamic positron emission tomography. Circulation 1989; 80: 1328–37.

10. Hutchins GD, Schwaiger M, Rosenspire KC, Krivokapich J, Schelbert HR, Kuhl DE. Noninvasive quantification of regional blood flow in the human heart using N-13 ammonia and dynamic positron emission tomographic imaging. J Am Coll Cardiol 1990; 15: 1032–42.

11. Schelbert HR, Phelps ME, Huang SC et al. N-13 ammonia as an indicator of myocardial blood flow. Circulation 1981; 63: 1259–72.

12. Rauch B, Helus F, Grunze M et al. Kinetics of 13-N ammonia uptake in myocardial single cells indicating potential limitations in its applicability as a marker of myocardial blood flow. Circulation 1985; 71: 387–93.

13. Kambara H, Fudo T, Hashimoto T et al. Silent myocardial ischemia in patients with myocardial infarction: evaluation with positron emission computed tomography. Jpn Circ J 1989; 53: 1437–43.

14. Gould KL. Clinical cardiac positron emission tomography: state of the art. Circulation 1991; 84 (3 Suppl I): I23–I36.

15. Schelbert HR, Wisenberg G, Phelps ME et al. Noninvasive assessment of coronary stenosis by myocardial imaging during pharmacologic coronary vasodilation. VI. Detection of coronary artery disease in man with intravenous N-13 ammonia and positron computed tomography. Am J Cardiol 1982; 49: 1197–207.

16. Yonekura Y, Tamaki N, Senda M et al. Detection of coronary artery disease with 13-N ammonia and high resolution positron emission computed tomography. Am Heart J 1987; 113: 645–54.

17. Zimmermann R, Tillmanns H, Knapp WH et al. Regional myocardial nitrogen-13 glutamate uptake in patients with coronary artery disease: inverse post-stress relation to thallium-201 uptake in ischemia. J Am Coll Cardiol 1988; 11: 549–56.

18. Gould KL. Percent coronary stenosis: battered gold standard pernicious relic, or clinical practicality? J Am Coll Cardiol 1988; 11: 886–8.

19. Schwaiger M, Brunken RC, Krivokapich J et al. Beneficial effect of residual anterograde flow on tissue viability as assessed by positron emission tomography in patients with myocardial infarction. Eur Heart J 1987; 8: 981–8.

20. Brunken K, Schwaiger M, Grover-McKay M, Phelps M, Tillisch J, Schelbert HR. Positron emission tomography detects tissue metabolic activity in myocardial segments with persistent thallium perfusion defects. J Am Coll Cardiol 1987; 10: 557–67.

21. Marshall RC, Tillisch JH, Phelps ME et al. Identification and differentiation of resting myocardial ischemia and infarction in man with positron computed tomography. ^{18}F-labeled fluorodeoxyglucose and N-13 ammonia. Circulation 1983; 67: 766–78.

22. Williams BR. Positron emission tomography for the assessment of ischemia and myocardial viability. J Myocardial Ischemia 1990; 2: 33–64.

23. Bonow RO, Dilsizian V, Cuocolo A, Bacharach SL. Identification of viable myocardium in patients with chronic coronary artery disease and left ventricular dysfunction. Comparison of thallium scintigraphy with reinjection and PET imaging with 18-F-fluorodeoxyglucose. Circulation 1991; 83: 26–37.

24. Sobel BE, Geltman EM, Tiefenbrunn AJ et al. Improvement of regional myocardial metabolism after coronary thrombolysis induced with tissue-type plasminogen activator or streptokinase. Circulation 1984; 69: 983–90.

25. Goldstein RA, Kirkeeide R, Smalling RW et al. Changes in myocardial perfusion reserve after PTCA: noninvasive assessment with positron tomography. J Nucl Med 1987; 28: 1262–7.
26. Tillisch J, Brunken R, Marschall R et al. Reversibility of cardial wall-motion abnormalities predicted by positron tomography. N Engl J Med 1986; 314: 884–8.
27. Demer LL, Gould KL, Goldstein R, Kirkeeide L. Noninvasive assessment of coronary collaterals in man by PET perfusion imaging. J Nucl Med 1990; 31: 259–70.
28. Brunken K, Kottou S, Nienaber CA et al. PET detection of viable tissue in myocardial segments with persistent defects at Tl-201 SPECT. Radiology 1989; 172: 65–73.
29. Schelbert HR. Positron emission tomography for the assessment of myocardial viability. Circulation 1991; 84 (Suppl I): I122–I131.
30. Liu P, Kiess MC, Okada RD et al. The persistent defect on exercise thallium imaging and its fate after myocardial revascularization: does it represent scar or ischemia? Am Heart J 1985; 110: 996–1001.
31. Kiat H, Berman DS, Maddahi J et al. Late reversibility of tomographic myocardial thallium-201 defects: an accurate marker of myocardial viability. J Am Coll Cardiol 1988; 12: 1456–63.
32. Dilsizian V, Rocco TP, Freedman NMT, Leon MB, Bonow RO. Enhanced detection of ischemic but viable myocardium by reinjection of thallium after stress-redistribution imaging. N Engl J Med 1990; 323: 141–6.
33. Ohtani H, Tamaki N, Yonekura Y et al. Value of thallium-201 reinjection after delayed SPECT imaging for predicting reversible ischemia after coronary artery bypass grafting. Am J Cardiol 1990; 66: 394–9.
34. Dilsizian V, Smeltzer WR, Freedman NMT, Dextras R, Bonow RO. Thallium reinjection after stress-redistribution imaging. Does 24-hour delayed imaging after reinjection enhance detection of viable myocardium? Circulation 1991; 83: 1247–55.
35. Tamaki N, Yonekura Y, Senda M et al. Value and limitation of stress thallium-201 single photon emission computed tomography: comparison with nitrogen-13 ammonia positron tomography. J Nucl Med 1988; 29: 1181–8.
36. Tamaki N, Yonekura Y, Yamashita K et al. Value of rest-stress myocardial positron tomography using nitrogen-13 ammonia for preoperative prediction of reversible asynergy. J Nucl Med 1989; 30: 1302–10.
37. Tamaki N, Ohtani H, Yamashita K et al. Metabolic activity in the areas of new fill-in after thallium-201 reinjection: comparison with positron emission tomography using fluorine-18-deoxyglucose. J Nucl Med 1991; 32: 673–8.
38. Schwaiger M, Hicks R. The clinical role of metabolic imaging of the heart by positron emission tomography. J Nucl Med 1991; 32: 565–78.
39. Vaghaiwalla-Mody FV, Brunken RC, Warner Stevenson L, Nienaber CA, Phelps ME, Schelbert HR. Differentiating cardiomyopathy of coronary artery disease from nonischemic dilated cardiomyopathy utilizing positron tomography. J Am Coll Cardiol 1991; 17: 373–83.
40. Geldman EM, Smith JL, Beecker D, Ludbrook PA, Ter-Pogossian MM, Sobel BE. Altered regional myocardial metabolism in congestive cardiomyopathy detected by positron tomography. Am J Med 1983; 4: 773–85.
41. Perloff JK, Roberts WC, Deleon ACJ, O'Doherty D. The distinctive electrocardiogram of Duchenne's progressive muscular dystrophy. An electrocardiographic pathologic correlative study. Am J Med 1967; 42: 179–88.
42. Perloff JK, Henze E, Schelbert HR. Alterations in regional myocardial metabolism perfusion, and wall motion in Duchenne's muscular dystrophy studied by radionuclide imaging. Circulation 1984; 69: 33–42.

43. Endo M, Yoshida K, Iinuma TA et al. Noninvasive quantification of regional myocardial blood flow and ammonia extraction fraction using nitrogen-13 ammonia and positron emission tomography. Ann Nucl Med 1987; 1: 1–6.
44. Yoshida K, Endo M, Himi T et al. Measurement of regional myocardial blood flow in hypertrophic cardiomyopathy: application of the first-pass flow model using 13-N ammonia and PET. Am J Physiol Imaging 1989; 4: 97–104.
45. Camici P, Chiriatti G, Lorenzoni R et al. Coronary vasodilatation is impaired in both hypertrophied and nonhypertrophied myocardium of patients with hypertrophic cardiomyopathy: a study with nitrogen-13 ammonia and positron emission tomography. J Am Coll Cardiol 1991; 17: 879–86.
46. Kehtarnavaz N, Defigueiredo RJP. A novel surface reconstruction and display method for cardiac PET imaging. IEEE Trans Med Imaging 1984; 3: 108–15.

12. Quantification of myocardial perfusion with oxygen-15 water

PILAR HERRERO and STEVEN R. BERGMANN

Introduction

Assessment of regional myocardial perfusion at rest or in response to exercise or pharmacologic interventions, is crucial in the diagnosis of coronary artery disease and in the evaluation of the efficacy of therapies designed to restore nutritive perfusion. In some instances, such as in the diagnosis of high-grade, single-vessel coronary artery disease, qualitative assessment of myocardial perfusion with conventional nuclear medicine techniques may suffice. However, quantitative estimates (e.g., ml/g/min) are necessary for the objective evaluation of myocardial perfusion reserve (the ability of the vasculature to increase perfusion maximally in response to a hyperemic stimulus) and may be important for the evaluation of patients in whom myocardial uptake of flow tracers may be homogeneous (without regional disparities), such as those with chest pain but angiographically normal coronary arteries, those who have undergone cardiac transplantation, those with cardiomyopathy, and those with balanced lesions or multivessel coronary artery disease.

Advantages of positron-emission tomography

Conventional nuclear medicine procedures such as thallium-201 scintigraphy provide only qualitative information regarding myocardial blood flow because of the nonphysiologic nature of the tracers used and because absolute tracer concentration in the myocardium cannot be measured accurately with gamma cameras that cannot correct for photon attenuation, superimposition of radioactivity, effects of scatter, and depth-dependent resolution [1]. Single-photon

157

Ernst E. van der Wall et al. (eds), What's new in cardiac imaging?, 157–164.
© *1992 Kluwer Academic Publishers. Printed in the Netherlands.*

emission computed tomography (SPECT) has been developed to improve the physical limitations of planar gamma scintigraphy, but its usefulness also is limited by problems associated with attenuation correction of gamma emissions and the nonphysiologic nature of single photon-emitting tracers.

Positron-emission tomography (PET) overcomes many of the limitations inherent to conventional single-photon imaging because of its ability to measure the distribution of positron-emitting tracers within the body and it is therefore an attractive tool for the noninvasive quantification of myocardial perfusion. The short half-life positron-emitting isotopes such as oxygen-15 (^{15}O), nitrogen-13 (^{13}N), rubidium-82 (^{82}Rb), potassium-38 (^{38}K), and copper-62 (^{62}Cu) can be used to label tracers of myocardial perfusion. With the use of appropriate mathematical models to describe the kinetic behavior of radiotracers in blood and myocardial tissue over time, quantitative estimates of regional myocardial perfusion can be made.

Classes of perfusion tracers

Two classes of tracers are presently used for estimates of myocardial perfusion with PET: those that are partially extracted and retained by the myocardium, such as ^{13}N-ammonia, ^{38}K-chloride, ^{82}Rb-chloride, and ^{62}Cu-pyruvaldehyde bis-N^4-methylthiosemicarbazone, and those that are freely diffusible in myocardium, such as ^{15}O-water. ^{15}O-water has a major advantage over partially extracted tracers because its kinetics are solely related to flow and are not altered by changes in metabolism [2–4]. Furthermore, its short half-life ($t_{1/2} = $ 2.1 min) allows for rapid sequential measurements of flow with modest radiation exposure.

Basis of the kinetic model used in estimating myocardial perfusion with ^{15}O-water

The approach currently used for quantification of myocardial perfusion with ^{15}O-water is based on the work of Kety [5], who developed mathematical relationships incorporating principles governing the exchange of inert gas between blood and tissue. With the development of PET instruments with rapid data acquisition capabilities, in vivo application of the Kety approach became feasible [6, 7]. For estimation of myocardial perfusion, the approach uses a one-compartment kinetic model. The operational equation derived from the model defines myocardial tissue activity over time as a function of myocardial perfusion and tracer activity in arterial blood. Myocardial perfusion can be estimated based on the measurement of arterial and tissue concentration of tracer and knowledge of the tissue/blood partition coefficient.

Bergmann et al. [2] and Tripp et al. [8] have shown that myocardial perfusion can be measured accurately in dogs with the use of radiolabeled water and this model when the arterial input function and tissue radioactivity are measured directly after a bolus injection of labeled water. However, accurate measurements of the concentration of tracer within the heart with PET is complicated by cardiac motion and by the limited spatial resolution of available tomographic systems (8–12 mm full-width half-maximum) in relation to the dimensions of the myocardial wall imaged, in addition to factors such as inaccurate random and photon attenuation corrections and the path length of the positrons in tissue before annihilation [1, 9–11]. Interrogation of regions smaller than two times the full-width half-maximum resolution of the tomograph results in partial volume effects (underestimation of true radiotracer concentration) and spillover (contamination of activity in one region with that from an adjacent region) [9]. These effects contaminate the measure of myocardial tissue activity obtained noninvasively with PET. Thus, to estimate myocardial perfusion accurately with this technique, tissue activity must be corrected for these effects. Correction methods using independent estimations of partial volume and spillover factors have been proposed [12, 13], but they are not in general use because of the complexity of their implementation and practical problems such as the need to measure the dimensions of the cardiac tissue with independent modalities such as echocardiography, gated x-ray computed tomography, or nuclear magnetic resonance imaging. The routine use of dual-modality imaging makes this approach impractical. Recently developed techniques entail estimation of the recovery coefficient and the spillover fraction along with myocardial perfusion by including in the operational equation the mathematical relationship between observed PET tissue activity and true tissue activity [4, 14–16]. Estimation of these parameters along with myocardial perfusion not only obviates the need for a dual imaging modality, making the approach more useful in the clinical setting, but also allows for more accurate correction for the effects of the parameters on tissue activity: the estimates give information about the effects of both limited resolution and linear cardiac and respiratory motion. The use of this mathematical technique to estimate myocardial perfusion noninvasively with PET has been validated in a number of studies in intact dogs over a wide range of physiologic flows and interventions [4, 15, 16] (Figure 1).

Clinical applications

The use of ^{15}O-labeled water and PET in the measurement of regional myocardial perfusion in human subjects has been validated in a number of studies. In a study by Bergmann et al. [4], myocardial perfusion in normal subjects studied

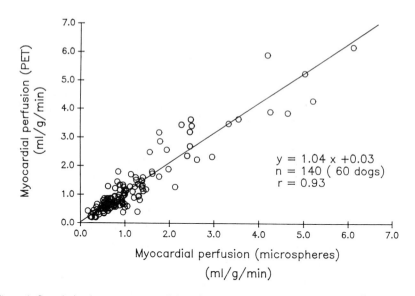

Figure 1. Correlation between myocardial perfusion estimated noninvasively with ^{15}O-water and PET and that obtained with radiolabeled microspheres in 140 observations in 60 dogs over the flow range of 0.2 to 6.2 ml/g/min. The excellent agreement between the results validates the use of ^{15}O-water and PET for the noninvasive quantification of myocardial perfusion. (Reproduced, with permission, from Bergmann [22].)

at rest averaged 0.90 ± 0.22 ml/g/min, and increased to 3.55 ± 1.15 ml/g/min after intravenous administration of dipyridamole. Myocardial perfusion reserve averaged 4.1 ± 1.3, comparable to values for coronary flow reserve reported by others using invasive techniques. Similar results have recently been reported by Araujo et al. [16]. With increasing life expectancy due to advances in medical technology and improved habits regarding health and fitness, a better understanding of the effects of aging on the cardiovascular system is needed. Senneff et al. studied 15 older adults with a mean age of 55 years and a low likelihood of coronary artery disease and demonstrated that myocardial perfusion at rest was similar to that observed in younger subjects but that peak myocardial perfusion was blunted in these older, healthy subjects (3.12 ml/g/min compared with 4.25 ± 1.54 ml/g/min in younger adults [17]).

   The approach developed has been used to identify patients with coronary artery disease. Iida et al. [14] showed diminished flow in patients with coronary artery disease with the use of PET. Araujo et al. [16] quantified blood flow in eight patients with chronic stable angina and single-vessel disease. In these patients, myocardial perfusion reserve assessed after intravenous dipyridamole was diminished in areas supplied by the stenotic vessel when compared

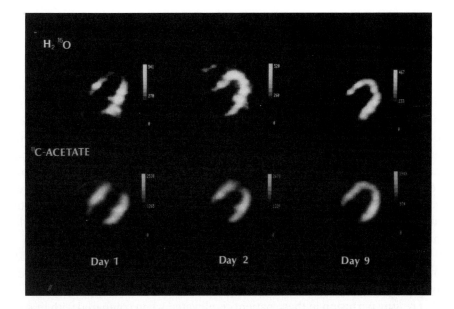

Figure 2. Sequential midventricular PET reconstructions of perfusion, assessed with ^{15}O-water (top), and of oxidative metabolism, assessed with ^{11}C-acetate (bottom), from a patient with anterior myocardial infarction after thrombolysis with tissue-type plasminogen activator (*t*-PA). The top of each image corresponds to the anterior wall, while the septum is to the left and lateral wall to the right. Both perfusion and metabolism images show decreased activity in the anterior region indicative of impaired perfusion and metabolism on day 1. By day 2, perfusion is restored to normal levels in the anterior wall while oxygen consumption is still impaired. By day 9 both perfusion and oxygen consumption are restored to nearly normal levels, indicative of the beneficial effects of successful thrombolysis. (Reproduced, with permission, from Henes et al. [19].)

with that in areas supplied by normal vessels, whereas no disparities in resting myocardial perfusion were observed between normal and abnormal areas.

To evaluate effects of coronary angioplasty on myocardial perfusion at rest and in response to dipyridamole, Walsh et al. [18] evaluated 13 patients before and again after single-vessel coronary angioplasty. Myocardial perfusion reserve in regions distal to stenosis was impaired before angioplasty, but normalized after a successful procedure, demonstrating the utility of ^{15}O-water and PET for quantitative delineation of the effects of coronary angioplasty on nutritive perfusion and perfusion reserve.

To elucidate the extent to which thrombolytic therapy early after the onset of acute myocardial infarction can restore nutritive perfusion and myocardial metabolic function in patients, Henes et al. [20] studied eight patients with coronary occlusion after thrombolysis with tissue-type plasminogen activator and demonstrated that pharmacologic recanalization promptly improves nutritive perfusion in jeopardized, ischemic zones to nearly normal levels. In contrast, restoration of oxidative metabolism was markedly slower than restoration of perfusion (Figure 2).

Between 10 and 30% of patients with chest pain who undergo cardiac catheterization are found to have normal coronary arteries. To assess the value of PET and ^{15}O-labeled water in the determination of whether angina in these patients is attributable to abnormalities of perfusion at rest or after pharmacologic stress, Geltman et al. [20] evaluated 17 patients with chest pain but angiographically normal coronary arteries. Approximately 50% of patients had high blood flow at rest (average of 1.61 ml/g/min) and impaired flow reserve in response to intravenous dipyridamole (myocardial perfusion reserve averaged 1.4). Myocardial perfusion in these patients was homogeneous at rest and after dipyridamole (Plate 12.1), so that qualitative imaging would have revealed no flow perturbation.

One of the areas in which quantification of myocardial perfusion with PET might be valuable is in the early diagnosis of coronary artery disease in cardiac transplant recipients. In a preliminary report, Senneff et al. [21] have shown that resting perfusion in these patients is elevated when compared with that in normal volunteers (but is appropriate for the increased work performed by the allograft) and that perfusion reserve is moderately blunted.

Limitation of the approach

Although results obtained with ^{15}O-water are promising and are helping to answer clinically important questions, quantification of perfusion with this tracer has some limitations. Since ^{15}O is cyclotron produced, centers must have a cyclotron on site. After intravenous administration, ^{15}O-water is distributed in the tissue as well as the vascular volume. Thus, for visualization of the myocardium, ^{15}O-water images need to be corrected for activity in the vascular compartment. This typically requires labeling the vascular volume with a second tracer such as ^{15}O-carbon monoxide [4, 14, 16]. Because of the dynamic model used, data acquisition at high temporal rates is necessary with a rapidity that exceeds the capabilities of many of the currently commercially available tomographic units. A slow and continuous delivery of the tracer as $C^{15}O_2$ gas, which is transformed into $H_2^{15}O$, has been shown to be a potential alternative method of delivery [16]. Quantification of myocardial perfusion in very low-flow regions may be limited by the low count rates observed in damaged regions due partially to the thinning of the myocardial wall. This limitation, however, applies to all tracers of perfusion. Improved instrumentation with enhanced spatial resolution and sensitivity and new mathematical approaches to correct for count spillover from adjacent, normal regions may enhance the ability to quantitate flow in severely ischemic regions.

Conclusions

PET with ^{15}O-water is currently the most promising noninvasive approach for quantification of myocardial perfusion. It allows accurate estimation of myocardial perfusion and perfusion reserve, and its utility has been demonstrated in patients with cardiac disease of diverse causes, permitting an enhanced understanding of the regulation of myocardial perfusion and its perturbation with disease, and in the objective assessment of the effects of pharmacologic and surgical interventions designed to enhance nutritive myocardial perfusion.

Acknowledgement

The authors thank Elizabeth Engeszer for editorial review and Becky Leonard for preparation of the manuscript.

References

1. Bergmann SR, Fox KA, Geltman EM, Sobel BE. Positron emission tomography of the heart. Prog Cardiovasc Dis 1985; 28: 165–94.
2. Bergmann SR, Fox KA, Rand AL et al. Quantification of regional myocardial blood flow in vivo with $H_2^{15}O$. Circulation 1984; 70: 724–33.
3. Knabb RM, Fox KA, Sobel BE, Bergmann SR. Characterization of the functional significance of subcritical coronary stenoses with $H_2^{15}O$ and positron emission tomography. Circulation 1985; 71: 1271–8.
4. Bergmann SR, Herrero P, Markham J, Weinheimer CJ, Walsh MN. Noninvasive quantitation of myocardial blood flow in human subjects with oxygen-15-labeled water and positron emission tomography. J Am Coll Cardiol 1989; 14: 639–52.
5. Kety S. Theory and applications of exchange of inert gas at lungs and tissues. Pharmacol Rev 1951; 3: 1–41.
6. Herscovitch P, Markham J, Raichle ME. Brain blood flow measured with intravenous $H_2^{15}O$. I. Theory and error analysis. J Nucl Med 1983; 24: 782–9.
7. Raichle ME, Martin WR, Herscovitch P, Mintun MA, Markham J. Brain blood flow measured with intravenous $H_2^{15}O$. II. Implementation and validation. J Nucl Med 1983; 24: 790–8.
8. Tripp MR, Meyer MW, Einzig S, Leonard JJ, Swayze CR, Fox IJ. Simultaneous regional myocardial blood flows by tritiated water and microspheres. Am J Physiol 1977; 232: H173–90

 9   Hoffman EJ, Huang SC, Phelps ME. Quantitation in positron emission computed tomography: 1. Effect of object size. J Comput Assist Tomogr 1979; 3: 299–308

10. Huang S-C, Hoffman EJ, Phelps ME, Kuhl DE. Quantitation in positron emission computed tomography: 2. Effects of inaccurate attenuation correction. J Comput Assist Tomogr 1979; 3: 804–14.

11. Hoffman EJ, Huang SC, Phelps ME, Kuhl DE. Quantitation in positron emission computed tomography: 4. Effect of accidental coincidences. J Comput Assist Tomogr 1981; 5: 391–400.

12. Henze E, Huang SC, Ratib O, Hoffman E, Phelps ME, Schelbert HR. Measurements of regional tissue and blood-pool radiotracer concentrations from serial tomographic images of the heart. J Nucl Med 1983; 24: 987–96.

13. Herrero P, Markham J, Myears DW, Weinheimer CJ, Bergmann SR. Measurement of myocardial blood flow with positron emission tomography: correction for count spillover and partial volume effects. Math Comput Modelling 1988; 11: 807–12.

14. Iida H, Kanno I, Takahashi A. et al. Measurement of absolute myocardial blood flow with $H_2^{15}O$ and dynamic positron-emission tomography. Strategy for quantification in relation to the partial-volume effect. Circulation 1988; 78: 104–15.

15. Herrero P, Markham J, Bergmann SR. Quantitation of myocardial blood flow with $H_2^{15}O$ and positron emission tomography: assessment and error analysis of a mathematical approach. J Comput Assist Tomogr 1989; 13: 862–73.

16. Araujo LI, Lammertsma AA, Rhodes CG et al. Noninvasive quantification of regional myocardial blood flow in coronary artery disease with oxygen-15-labeled carbon dioxide inhalation and positron emission tomography. Circulation 1991; 83: 875–85.

17. Senneff MJ, Geltman EM, Bergmann SR. Noninvasive delineation of the effects of moderate aging on myocardial perfusion. J Nucl Med 1991; 32: 2037–42.

18. Walsh MN, Geltman EM, Steel RL et al. Augmented myocardial perfusion reserve after coronary angioplasty quantified by positron emission tomography with $H_2^{15}O$. J Am Coll Cardiol 1990; 15: 119–27.

19. Henes CG, Bergmann SR, Perez JE, Sobel BE, Geltman EM. The time course of restoration of nutritive perfusion, myocardial oxygen-consumption, and regional function after coronary thrombolysis. Coronary Artery Dis 1990; 1: 687–96.

20. Geltman EM, Henes CG, Senneff MJ, Sobel BE, Bergmann SR. Increased myocardial perfusion at rest and diminished perfusion reserve in patients with angina and angiographically normal coronary arteries. J Am Coll Cardiol 1990; 16: 586–95.

21. Senneff MJ, Genton RE, Kenzora JL et al. Perfusion abnormalities in cardiac allografts demonstrable with positron emission tomography (PET) [abstract]. J Nucl Med 1990; 31 Suppl: 841.

22. Bergmann SR. Assessment of myocardial perfusion with PET. In: Bergmann SR, Sobel BE, editors. Positron emission tomography of the heart. New York: Futura Publishing (in press).

13. Myocardial perfusion imaging with copper-62 labeled Cu-PTSM

MARK A. GREEN

Introduction

The value of positron emission tomography (PET) in the study of myocardial physiology and the clinical diagnosis of cardiac disease is widely recognized. The short-lived radionuclides most commonly used as labels for PET radiopharmaceuticals are ^{15}O, ^{13}N, ^{11}C, and ^{18}F. These have proven particularly useful because they allow natural biochemical substrates to be labeled by isotopic substitution for tracer studies of a diversity of discrete physiological processes. Unfortunately, the short half-lives of these radionuclides (2, 10, 20, and 110 minutes, respectively) pose problems with regard to isotope production and delivery. Hospitals that employ ^{15}O, ^{13}N, ^{11}C, and ^{18}F radiopharmaceuticals will generally find it necessary to operate an in-house cyclotron facility for radionuclide production, since only ^{18}F is sufficiently long-lived to allow remote production for distribution via a regional delivery system. For many hospitals, the expense of operating a cyclotron for radionuclide production presents a barrier to the use of PET in clinical diagnosis.

The need for an in-house cyclotron to support PET activities could be reduced or eliminated through the use of positron-emitting isotopes that are available from parent/daughter radionuclide generator systems (e.g. ^{62}Cu, ^{82}Rb, ^{68}Ga). With a parent/daughter generator system, the short-lived 'daughter' radionuclide that is to be used as a radiopharmaceutical label is produced by the decay of a long-lived 'parent' radionuclide. If the parent nuclide is irreversibly adsorbed onto a solid chromatography matrix from which the daughter nuclide can be selectively and efficiently eluted, then the parent/daughter pair effectively becomes a long-lived source or 'generator' of the

Ernst E. van der Wall et al. (eds), What's new in cardiac imaging?, 165–177.

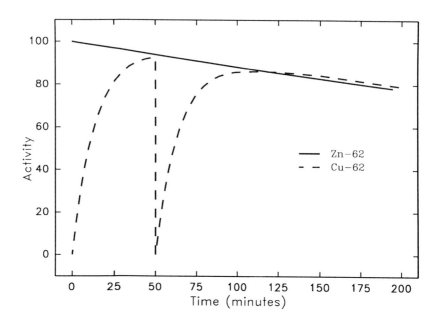

Figure 1. Graphic illustration of the relationship between parent and daughter radioactivity levels on the column of the ^{62}Zn/^{62}Cu generator with one ^{62}Cu elution at $t = 50$ minutes.

short-lived daughter (Figure 1). While several radioisotopes of copper decay by positron emission (Table 1), copper-62 is of the greatest clinical interest due to its availability from such a parent/daughter (^{62}Zn/^{62}Cu) generator system.

The ^{62}Zn/^{62}Cu generator

The 9.7 minute half-life of ^{62}Cu makes this nuclide an attractive generator-produced label for PET radiopharmaceuticals. This short half-life would allow multiple imaging studies at reasonably brief time intervals, without interference of background activity from a previous dose. However, the ^{62}Cu half-life remains sufficiently long to permit the rapid synthesis of a variety of radiopharmaceuticals. The 9.7 minute half-life is well-suited to the time frame of PET perfusion imaging, particularly if long (10–20 minute) image acquisition periods can be used to improve counting statistics.

An inherent disadvantage of the ^{62}Zn/^{62}Cu generator is the rather short (9.26 hour) half-life of the zinc-62 parent. This problem is somewhat offset by the ease with which ^{62}Zn can be produced with a medium energy (>20 MeV) cyclotron via the ^{63}Cu(p,2n)^{62}Zn nuclear reaction [4, 5]. Cyclotrons capable of producing large quantities of ^{62}Zn currently exist at a number of commercial facilities for the production of routinely used medical radionuclides, as well as at several clinical PET centers. Nevertheless, a continuously operating PET facility relying on ^{62}Cu would require ^{62}Zn/^{62}Cu generator replacement at 1–2 day intervals [4]. While the overnight delivery services routinely employed for shipment of medical radionuclides could deliver ^{62}Zn/^{62}Cu generators over great distances, reliance on a regional cyclotron facility for ^{62}Zn production may be more attractive, especially if that facility could also supply ^{18}F-fluoro-deoxyglucose for metabolic studies that would not be feasible with ^{62}Cu.

A number of ^{62}Zn/^{62}Cu generator systems are described in the literature. One of the simplest and best characterized systems separates the ^{62}Cu-daughter from the ^{62}Zn-parent by column chromatography, employing a Dowex 1 × 8 anion exchange resin that avidly retains Zn(II) and allows the Cu^{2+} ion to be eluted with aqueous HCl [4–6]. The best Zn(II)/Cu(II) separations with this system occur using 2N HCl as the eluent [7]. Such a system employing a 0.7 cm diameter × 4.0 cm column gives excellent parent/daughter separations and high ^{62}Cu elution yields [5]. High-level (> 300 mCi) generators with this configuration provide consistent performance with ^{62}Zn breakthrough at less than 2×10^{-3}% eluted ^{62}Cu activity [5]. Alternatively, Fujibayashi et al. [8] have described a generator employing a strong cation exchange resin ad-

Table 1. Properties of copper radioisotopes [1].

Isotope	Half-life	Radiation	Average energy per β disintegration (keV)	Production
Cu-62	9.74 min	β$^+$ (97%)	1280	Daughter of ^{62}Zn ($t_{1/2}$ = 9.26 hours)
Cu-60	23.3 min	β$^+$ (92%) 826 keV (22%) 1332 keV (88%) 1792 keV (45%)	894	^{60}Ni$(p,n)^{60}$Cu ^{60}Ni$(d,2n)^{60}$Cu
Cu-61	3.41 hour	β$^+$ (61%) 283 keV (12%) 656 keV (11%)	306	^{60}Ni$(d,n)^{61}$Cu ^{59}Co$(\alpha,2n)^{61}$Cu
Cu-64	12.7 hour	β$^+$ (18%) β$^-$ (37%)	49.8 71	^{63}Cu$(n,\gamma)^{64}$Cu ^{64}Zn$(n,p)^{64}$Cu[a] ^{64}Ni$(d,2n)^{64}$Cu[b]
Cu-67	2.58 day	β$^-$ (100%) 91 keV (7%) 93 keV (16%) 184 keV (49%)	142	^{67}Zn$(n,p)^{67}$Cu ^{64}Ni$(\alpha,p)^{67}$Cu

[a] Reference [2]; [b] Reference [3].

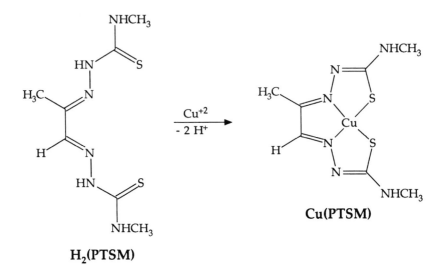

Figure 2. Synthesis and structural formula of Cu-PTSM. The Cu^{II}-PTSM complex is quite stable, with a formation constant $K = 10^{17.9}$ at physiological pH [9].

sorbent (CG-120, Amberlite) that allows the ^{62}Cu daughter to be eluted in 0.2 M glycine. A potential advantage of this latter system is the suitability of its eluate for direct intravenous injection; however, the performance of the 0.2 M glycine generator at high activity levels has not yet been reported.

Pyruvaldehyde bis(N⁴-methylthiosemicarbazonato)copper(II), Cu-PTSM

Pyruvaldehyde bis(N⁴-methylthiosemicarbazone) (H$_2$PTSM) reacts with the copper(II) ion to form a highly-stable Cu^{II}-PTSM complex in which the metal is coordinated in a square-planar geometry by two 'imino' nitrogen atoms and two sulfur atoms of the doubly deprotonated PTSM^{2-} ligand (Figure 2). Since the organic backbone of the PTSM^{2-} ligand is a conjugated π-system, the entire Cu-PTSM molecule is essentially planar [10]. This uncharged Cu-PTSM complex is quite lipophilic, exhibiting an octanol/water partition coefficient $P = 100$ [11–13].

Animal testing has been done to determine the acute toxicity of Cu-PTSM administered by intravenous injection [14]. In the rat Cu-PTSM has an i.v. LD$_{50}$ of 26 mg/kg, while in the rabbit the LD$_{50}$ was found to be 2 mg/kg. In a separate rabbit study, i.v. administration of Cu-PTSM at 2.16 μg/kg/day, 5 days per week for 2 weeks, resulted in no changes in histopathology, hematology, or clinical chemistry parameters. In this latter treatment protocol, each *daily* dose of Cu-PTSM is at least 80 times greater than the dose of Cu-PTSM that would be administered in a single injection to a 70 kg man, based on the reported performance of the Dowex 1 × 8/2N HCl generator and [62]Cu-PTSM remote synthetic apparatus [5, 15].

The radiolabeled Cu-PTSM complex has been synthesized with most of the copper nuclides shown in Table 1 for various chemical and biological studies [2, 3, 11–13, 16–19]. Although the 10 minute half-life of [62]Cu is quite attractive from the standpoint of PET perfusion imaging, it is inconveniently short for laboratory studies. Consequently, longer-lived [67]Cu and ^{64}Cu have been extensively used in research to screen and evaluate potential [62]Cu-labeled radiopharmaceuticals [2, 3, 11–13, 16, 17].

Synthesis of [62]Cu-PTSM

The synthesis of [62]Cu-labeled Cu-PTSM is straightforward and can be accomplished in high radiochemical yield in a time frame compatible with the 9.7 minute half-life of the nuclide using the eluate from the Dowex 1 × 8/2N HCl generator system [5, 15]. The procedure requires buffering the acidic generator eluate by addition of 2 equivalents of sodium acetate prior to mixing with an ethanol solution of the H_2(PTSM) ligand (1.5 μg H_2PTSM in 0.10 mL ethanol). After allowing 2–3 minutes for the chelation reaction to take place, the lipophilic [62]Cu-PTSM product is isolated from this hypertonic solution by adsorption onto a C_{18}-Sep-Pak® solid phase extraction cartridge. The [62]Cu-PTSM radiopharmaceutical is then recovered from the C_{18}-Sep-Pak® cartridge by washing with 0.1–0.2 mL absolute ethanol. Finally this ethanol solution is diluted with sterile saline to a 5% alcohol concentration and filtered through a sterile 0.2 μm fluorocarbon polymer membrane to provide a radiopharmaceutical product suitable for intravenous injection. Radiochemical purity of the product is verified by thin layer chromatography on silica gel eluted with either ethyl acetate or ethanol [5, 15]. The short half-life of the product will almost always require that TLC be a *retrospective* quality control procedure.

A remote system has been described that allows this entire synthetic procedure to be conducted in a shielded apparatus minimizing radiation exposure to the operator [15]. Using this remote system the [62]Cu-PTSM radiopharmaceutical can be reproducibly obtained with > 98% radiochemical purity in ca 40% end-of-synthesis radiochemical yield (yield based on [62]Cu activity available at end of generator elution, without decay correction). Use of the remote system results in a synthesis time of 7–8 minutes, which is somewhat longer than a 'hands-on' synthesis but judged acceptable in view of the stringent need for worker radiation protection in the routine repetitive preparation of [62]Cu-PTSM.

The specific activity of the ^{62}Cu-PTSM radiopharmaceutical will be determined by the purity of the Dowex 1 × 8 ion exchange resin, the HCl eluent, and the reagents used in the radiopharmaceutical synthesis. (The specific activity of *carrier-free* ^{62}Cu is $1.89 × 10^{10}$ Ci/mole.) To minimize the introduction of non-radioactive carrier copper or other metals into the radiopharmaceutical preparation, only ultrapure reagents are employed in the radiopharmaceutical synthesis. The copper content of the final ^{62}Cu-PTSM radiopharmaceutical preparation has been found to be < 0.1 μg using the synthetic techniques just described [5, 15], an amount dwarfed by the normal 1.4–2.1 mg/kg copper content of the human body [20].

The synthesis of ^{62}Cu-PTSM has also been reported using the CG-120/0.2 M glycine generator system [8]. An advantage of this approach is the formation of the ^{62}Cu-PTSM radiopharmaceutical in a solution suitable for direct intravenous administration, although the stability of the Cu^{II}-glycine complex may require slightly higher H$_2$PTSM concentrations than those employed with the Dowex 1 × 8/2N HCl generator. Time is saved in ^{62}Cu-PTSM synthesis with the glycine-based eluate by elimination of the C$_{18}$-Sep-Pak® purification procedure that is required to separate ^{62}Cu-PTSM from the hypertonic reaction mixture obtained when using the Dowex 1 × 8/2N HCl generator. However, in comparing the two synthetic methods, consideration must also be given to two additional benefits of employing the C$_{18}$-Sep-Pak® chromatographic procedure. This purification step in the synthesis not only desalts the product, but also serves as a *prospective* radiochemical quality control procedure verifying that the desired lipophilic ^{62}Cu complex is indeed present [5, 15]. In addition, the C$_{18}$-Sep-Pak® procedure has been found to remove $> 99.97\%$ of the ^{62}Zn-breakthrough present in the initial generator eluate from the final ^{62}Cu-PTSM radiopharmaceutical [5, 15]. Thus, although the level of ^{62}Zn breakthrough in the Dowex 1 × 8/2N HCl generator is acceptably low, the C$_{18}$-Sep-Pak® procedure insures an even greater margin of safety.

Cu-PTSM biodistribution and pharmacokinetics

The tissue distribution and pharmacokinetics of copper-labeled Cu-PTSM following intravenous injection makes the ^{62}Cu-radiopharmaceutical attractive for PET studies to image the brain, heart, and kidneys [2, 5, 11–13, 16, 17]. The rat biodistribution data presented in Table 2 illustrates that ^{67}Cu-PTSM is rapidly cleared from the blood following intravenous administration. In addition, at one minute post-injection relatively high tracer uptake is seen in the brain, heart, and kidney, followed by prolonged 'microsphere-like' tissue retention of the copper radiolabel.

The relatively high uptake of Cu-PTSM in the major organs suggests that it is behaving as a highly-diffusible tracer; thus a correlation should exist between its regional deposition and regional rates of cerebral and myocardial perfusion. In addition, Cu-PTSM is attractive as a radiopharmaceutical because the efficient tissue trapping of the copper radiolabel would allow imaging over a time frame limited only by the physical half-life of the copper radionuclide.

To better define the potential of ^{62}Cu-PTSM as a PET perfusion tracer, a number of studies have been conducted in order to (i) establish the chemical mechanism for Cu-PTSM trapping in tissue [12, 13]; (ii) directly compare regional Cu-PTSM uptake to that of validated perfusion tracers [2, 5, 12, 16, 17, 21]; and (iii) to establish that the tissue uptake of Cu-PTSM is related only to the rate of regional perfusion and not dependent upon other physiological or biochemical processes [2, 16, 17].

Molecular basis for the tissue trapping of ^{62}Cu-PTSM

Bis(thiosemicarbazone) derivatives of α-ketoaldehydes and their copper(II) complexes have been extensively investigated in biological systems, due to observations that some derivatives exhibit antineoplastic and antitrichomonal activity [9, 22, 23]. These studies have provided a wealth of information regarding the intracellular fate of copper(II) bis(thiosemicarbazone) complexes and allow the tissue trapping of copper-labeled Cu-PTSM to be understood at the molecular level [12, 13].

The uncharged lipophilic Cu$^{(II)}$-PTSM complex has been shown to readily diffuse across tumor cell membranes (Figure 3), whereupon it is quite susceptible to reductive decomposition by reaction with ubiquitous intracellular thiols such as glutathione [9, 22, 23]. Electron transfer from R-S$^-$ produces the

Table 2. Biodistribution of ^{67}Cu-PTSM in the rat following intravenous injection [13].

Organ	% Injected dose per organ			
	1 min	5 min	15 min	2 hours
Blood	9.3 ± 1.3	8.0 ± 1.7	6.6 ± 1.7	6.5 ± 2.5
Heart	2.7 ± 0.3	3.4 ± 1.2	2.5 ± 0.2	3.3 ± 0.9
Kidney (1)	3.7 ± 0.7	3.1 ± 0.1	3.1 ± 0.9	4.3 ± 0.4
Brain	3.0 ± 0.7	3.0 ± 0.6	2.7 ± 0.6	3.2 ± 0.4
Heart/blood	5.9 ± 1.0	9.7 ± 2.9	8.9 ± 1.2	10.7 ± 3.8

Values shown represent the mean (± standard deviation) of four rats, 195–225 grams.

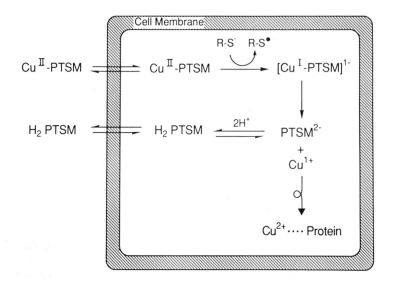

Figure 3. Schematic diagram illustrating the thiol-mediated intracellular reductive decomposition of Cu^{II}-PTSM that is believed to account for the 'microsphere-like' tissue retention of the ^{62}Cu-radiolabel.

unstable Cu$^{(I)}$-PTSM complex, which decomposes by the dissociation of the PTSM^{2-} ligand. This leads to an effectively irreversible deposition of ionic copper throughout the cell (bound to macromolecules), while the re-protonated ligand can diffuse back through the cell membrane into the extracellular space [9, 22, 23].

Such a mechanism appears to account for the non-specific tissue trapping of the copper radiolabel following i.v. administration of tracer Cu-PTSM [2, 11–13, 16]. Fortunately, while glutathione occurs intracellularly in millimolar concentrations, it exists in only micromolar concentrations in plasma [24]. Thus, the Cu-PTSM radiopharmaceutical does not encounter high glutathione concentrations until it reaches the target tissues where trapping is desired.

Cu-PTSM in isolated perfused hearts

To better define the myocardial kinetics of Cu-PTSM, the extraction and retention of ^{67}Cu-PTSM have been studied in an isolated perfused rabbit heart preparation in which variables of tracer delivery, myocardial perfusion, and perfusate oxygenation were carefully controlled [16]. In this model the single-pass extraction of Cu-PTSM was > 40% and invariate over a range of conditions including normal physiologic flow, hyperemia, ischemia, and hypoxia

(Table 3). The extraction of Cu-PTSM at 1.5 mL · min^{-1} · g^{-1} (control flow condition) is similar to that observed for ^{13}NH$_3$ [25] (Table 3). However, ^{13}NH$_3$ extraction is more sensitive to the physiologic status of the heart, with 48% extraction under ischemic conditions but only 18% extraction during hypoxia [25]. Other cationic tracers for estimation of flow, such as ^{201}Tl$^+$, also exhibit a dependence of extraction and clearance on the metabolic status of the heart [26].

Once extracted, the ^{67}Cu label used in these Cu-PTSM isolated heart studies showed essentially irreversible retention under all experimental conditions, with a biological clearance half-time of greater than 3600 minutes [16]. The fastest ^{67}Cu clearance observed was sufficiently long that it would not influence flow estimates over the 20 minute image acquisition period that would be feasible with ^{62}Cu.

PET imaging with ^{62}Cu-PTSM

The ^{62}Cu-PTSM radiopharmaceutical has been investigated as a tracer for both myocardial and cerebral perfusion in PET studies employing animal models and human subjects [5, 17, 27–29]. In the dog and baboon, as well as in a limited number of human studies, ^{62}Cu-PTSM has been found to provide high-quality images of the heart in which regional myocardial perfusion is accurately delineated [5, 27]. In a normal human subject studied with ^{62}Cu-

Table 3. Comparison of myocardial perfusion tracers in isolated rabbit hearts perfused with erythrocyte-enriched modified Krebs-Henseleit buffer.

Tracer	Flow (mL · min^{-1} · g^{-1})	Residual fraction (%)	Clearance half-time
Cu-PTSM[a]	1.5	45 ± 7	> 60 hours
	3.0	43 ± 8	> 60 hours
	0.15	45 ± 20	> 60 hours
	1.5[b]	49 ± 8	> 60 hours
^{13}NH$_3$[c]	1.4	55 ± 2	41 ± 6 min
	0.7	48 ± 5	46 ± 7 min
	0.3	58 ± 4	35 ± 10 min
	1.2[b]	18 ± 1	15 ± 3 min
^{201}Tl^{+}[d]	1.4	81 ± 7	22 ± 2 min
	0.6	94 ± 4	44 ± 17 min
	2.3	68 ± 6	15 ± 5 min

[a] From reference [16]. [b] Hypoxic buffer perfusate. [c] From reference [25]. [d] From reference [26].

PTSM (Plate 13.1) the distribution of ^{62}Cu in the heart was found to correlate closely to the distribution of ^{15}O-water, a validated PET tracer for quantitation of regional myocardial perfusion [5]. As predicted from animal studies, the ^{62}Cu label was effectively trapped in human myocardium, allowing a 10–20 minute image acquisition time.

In dogs studied with ^{64}Cu and ^{67}Cu-labeled Cu-PTSM at rest, after ischemia, and after coronary hyperemia induced by intravenous dipyridamole, myocardial tracer levels were found to increase proportionately with blood flow over a 0.0–6.0 mL $\cdot$ min^{-1} $\cdot$ g^{-1} flow range (measured concomitantly with radiolabeled microspheres) [17]. The increase in copper radioactivity was linear up to a flow of 2.5 mL $\cdot$ min^{-1} $\cdot$ g^{-1} and then increased more gradually at higher flows. Over the entire flow range studied, the data best fit a second order polynomial.

To complement the information available with ^{62}Cu-PTSM, ventricular blood volume images can be obtained with ^{62}Cu by employing a bifunctional chelate to label human serum albumin (HSA) [27]. The ^{62}Cu-benzyl-TETA-HSA complex has been shown to provide myocardial blood-pool images identical to those produced with ^{15}O-carboxyhemoglobin [27]. These ^{62}Cu-images of the ventricular blood volume were used for blood-pool subtraction of ^{62}Cu-PTSM images of the myocardium [27], although high quality images of the myocardium are obtained with ^{62}Cu-PTSM even without blood-pool correction. Blood pool subtraction from ^{62}Cu-PTSM myocardial images does facilitate their comparison with blood-pool subtracted ^{15}O-water myocardial perfusion images, however, by removing any contribution from blood-bound ^{62}Cu and by indirectly compensating for some of the effects of the higher β^+-energy of the ^{62}Cu radionuclide. (The average β^+ energies for ^{15}O, ^{82}Rb, and ^{62}Cu are 0.74 MeV, 1.41 MeV, and 1.28 MeV, respectively [1].) Myocardial image quality with ^{62}Cu-PTSM is expected to be better than that observed with generator-produced ^{82}Rb$^+$, due to problems with counting statistics imposed by the ultra-short 76 second half-life of rubidium-82 [5].

The results from animal and human studies with ^{62}Cu-PTSM to date suggest that this radiopharmaceutical should be particularly useful in hospitals that wish to employ PET to diagnose coronary artery disease in the absence of an 'in-house' cyclotron [5]. The availability of such a generator-produced flow tracer should enable the study of patients with acute cardiac disorders, such as acute ischemia, 24 hours per day. In addition, ^{62}Cu-PTSM should allow assessment of the adequacy of reperfusion after interventions such as thrombolytic therapy or balloon angioplasty [5]. Recent efforts to model the myocardial ^{62}Cu-PTSM kinetics suggest that flow quantitation may be possible with this tracer, if modeling includes correction of the input function for the fraction of ^{62}Cu in arterial blood that is no longer ^{62}Cu-PTSM [30].

In addition to its use to study myocardial perfusion, ^{62}Cu-PTSM has also been shown in both animal models and human subjects to be a useful tracer for PET studies of regional cerebral blood flow [2, 5]. In sequential baseline/ activation PET imaging studies, ^{62}Cu-PTSM is sufficiently sensitive as a tracer of cerebral blood flow to allow detection of focal areas of increased cerebral perfusion that result from neurological stimulation [5, 29]. In addition, ^{62}Cu-PTSM appears suitable as a tracer for evaluation of regional blood flow in the kidney [17, 21]. Thus, hospitals employing ^{62}Cu-PTSM might not need to rely entirely on their cardiac case load to support the costs of ^{62}Zn/^{62}Cu generator purchase and PET camera operation.

Acknowledgements

Financial support for this work was provided by a grant from the National Cancer Institute of the U.S. Public Health Service (RO1-CA46909). The author also wishes to thank Professors Michael J. Welch, Steven R. Bergmann, Marcus E. Raichle, Joel S. Perlmutter and their colleagues at Washington University for the substantial contributions they have made as collaborators in the investigation of ^{62}Cu-PTSM as a PET radiopharmaceutical.

References

1. Browne E, Firestone RB. Table of radioactive isotopes. New York: John Wiley, 1986.
2. Mathias CJ, Welch MJ, Raichle ME et al. Evaluation of a potential generator-produced PET tracer for cerebral perfusion imaging: single-pass cerebral extraction measurements and imaging with radiolabeled Cu-PTSM. J Nucl Med 1990; 31: 351–9.
3. Zweit J, Smith AM, Downey S, Sharma HL. Excitation functions for deuteron induced reactions in natural nickel: production of no-carrier-added ^{64}Cu from enriched ^{64}Ni targets for positron emission tomography. Appl Radiat Isot 1991; 42: 193–8.
4. Robinson GD Jr, Zielinski FW, Lee AW. The zinc-62/copper-62 generator: a convenient source of copper-62 for radiopharmaceuticals. Int J Appl Radiat Isot 1980; 31: 111–6.
5. Green MA, Mathias CJ, Welch MJ et al. Copper-62 labeled pyruvaldehyde bis(N^4-methylthiosemicarbazonato)copper(II): synthesis and evaluation as a positron emission tomography tracer for cerebral and myocardial perfusion. J Nucl Med 1990; 31: 1989–96.
6. Yagi M, Kondo K. A ^{62}Cu generator. Int J Appl Radiat Isot 1979; 30: 569–70.
7. Kraus KA, Moore GE. Anion exchange studies. VI. The divalent transition elements manganese to zinc in hydrochloric acid. J Am Chem Soc 1953; 75: 1460–2.
8. Fujibayashi Y, Matsumoto K, Yonekura Y, Konishi J, Yokoyama A. A new zinc-62/copper-62 generator as a copper-62 source for PET radiopharmaceuticals. J Nucl Med 1989; 30: 1838–42.
9. Winkelmann DA, Bermke Y, Petering DH. Comparative properties of the anti-neoplastic

agent 3-ethoxy-2-oxobutyraldehyde bis(thiosemicarbazone) copper(II) and related chelates: linear free energy correlations. Bioinorg Chem 1974; 3: 261–77.

10. John E, Fanwick PE, McKenzie AT, Stowell JG, Green MA. Structural characterization of a metal-based perfusion tracer: copper(II) pyruvaldehyde bis(N^4-methylthiosemicarbazone). Int J Rad Appl Instrum [B] 1989; 16: 791–7.

11. Green MA. A potential copper radiopharmaceutical for imaging the heart and brain: copper-labeled pyruvaldehyde bis(N^4-methylthiosemicarbazone). Int J Rad Appl Instrum [B] 1987; 14: 59–61.

12. Green MA, Klippenstein DL, Tennison JR. Copper(II) bis(thiosemicarbazone) complexes as potential tracers for evaluation of cerebral and myocardial blood flow with PET. J Nucl Med 1988; 29: 1549–57.

13. John EK, Green MA. Structure-activity relationships for metal-labeled blood flow tracers: comparison of keto aldehyde bis(thiosemicarbazonato)-copper(II) derivatives. J Med Chem 1990; 33: 1764–70.

14. Kostyniak PJ, Nakeeb SM et al. Acute toxicity and mutagenicity of the copper complex of pyruvaldehyde-bis(N^4-methylthiosemicarbazone), Cu-PTSM. J Appl Toxicol 1990; 10: 417–21.

15. Mathias CJ, Margenau WH, Brodack JW, Welch MJ, Green MA. A remote system for the synthesis of copper-62 labeled Cu(PTSM). Appl Radiat Isot 1991; 42: 317–20.

16. Shelton ME, Green MA, Mathias CJ, Welch MJ, Bergmann SR. Kinetics of copper-PTSM in isolated hearts: a novel tracer for measuring blood flow with positron emission tomography. J Nucl Med 1989; 30: 1843–7.

17. Shelton ME, Green MA, Mathias CJ, Welch MJ, Bergmann SR. Assessment of regional myocardial and renal blood flow with copper-PTSM and positron emission tomography. Circulation 1990; 82: 990–7.

18. Stone CK, Martin CC, Mueller B, Pyzalski RA, Perlman SB, Nickles RI. Comparison of myocardial uptake of copper pyruvaldehyde thiosemicarbazone with N-13 ammonia in humans by PET [abstract]. J Nucl Med 1991; 32 Suppl: 999.

19. Martin CC, Oakes TR, Nickles RJ. Small cyclotron production of [Cu-60] Cu-PTSM for PET blood flow measurements [abstract]. J Nucl Med 1990; 31 Suppl: 815.

20. Howard-Lock HE, Lock CJL. Uses in therapy. In: Wilkinson G (ed). Comprehensive coordination chemistry: the synthesis, reactions, properties and applications of coordination compounds: volume 6: applications. Oxford: Pergamon Press 1987: 765.

21. Barnhart AJ, Voorhees WD, Green MA. Correlation of Cu(PTSM) localization with regional blood flow in the heart and kidney. Int J Rad Appl Instrum [B] 1989; 16: 747–8.

22. Petering DH. Carcinostatic copper complexes. In: Sigel H (ed) Metal complexes as anticancer agents. New York: Marcel Dekker, 1980: 197–229.

23. Minkel DT, Saryan LA, Petering DH. Structure-function correlations in the reaction of bis(thiosemicarbazone) copper(II) complexes with Ehrlich acites tumor cells. Cancer Res 1978; 38: 124–9.

24. Meister A, Anderson ME. Glutathione. Annu Rev Biochem 1983; 52: 711–60.

25. Bergmann SR, Hack S, Tewson T, Welch MJ, Sobel BE. The dependence of accumulation of $^{13}NH_3$ by myocardium on metabolic factors and its implications for quantitative assessment of perfusion. Circulation 1980; 61: 34–43.

26. Bergmann SR, Hack SN, Sobel BE. Redistribution of myocardial thallium-201 without reperfusion: implications regarding absolute quantification of perfusion. Am J Cardiol 1982; 49: 1691–8.

27. Mathias CJ, Welch MJ, Green MA et al. In vivo comparison of copper blood-pool agents: potential radiopharmaceuticals for use with copper-62. J Nucl Med 1991; 32: 475–80.

28. Beanlands R, Muzik O, Lee K et al. Evaluation of copper-62 PTSM as a myocardial flow tracer [abstract]. J Nucl Med 1991; 32 Suppl: 1028.

29. Lee KS, Mangner TJ, Petry NA, Moskwa JJ, Mintun MA. Evaluation of Cu-62 PTSM in the detection of neural activation foci [abstract]. J Nucl Med 1991; 32 Suppl: 1072.

30. Herrero P, Markham J, Weinheimer J, Green MA, Welch MJ, Bergmann SR. Quantification of myocardial perfusion with Cu-62 PTSM and positron emission tomography [abstract]. J Nucl Med 1991; 32 Suppl: 937.

14. Application of contrast agents in magnetic resonance imaging: additional value for detection of myocardial ischemia?

CHRISTOPHER L. WOLFE

Summary

Magnetic resonance imaging (MRI) is a useful technique for assessing cardiac anatomy, function, and the identification of infarcted myocardium. However, the assessment of ischemic and infarcted myocardium can be further enhanced with the use of paramagnetic to contrast agents. This chapter discusses the advantages of using contrast enhanced MRI for the study of ischemic and infarcted myocardium.

Identifying myocardial infarction by noncontrast enhanced MRI

Many investigators have reported that noncontrast enhanced MRI can be used to identify myocardial infarction in animal models [1–5], and in patients [6]. Previous studies by Higgins [1], Wesby [5], Pflugfelder [3], and co-workers have shown that, in the canine model, areas of increased signal intensity in T2-weighted images signify the presence of infarcted myocardium. The increased signal intensity within the infarcted region corresponded with an increase in tissue T2 value secondary to the presence of tissue edema which can occur as early as three hours following coronary artery occlusion [1, 3–5]. Furthermore, Tscholakoff et al. [4] have reported that the difference in signal intensity between infarcted and normal myocardium in nonenhanced T2-weighted images was similar to that seen in contrast enhanced images with gadolinium-diethylene triamine pentaacetic acid (Gd-DTPA).

Other investigators [2, 7–9] have noted that noncontrast MR images may be

179

Ernst E. van der Wall et al. (eds), What's new in cardiac imaging?, 179–199.

suboptimal for identifying infarcted myocardium within the first one to two days after infarction. Rehr and co-workers [9] noted difficulty in visualizing the infarcted region within the first 40 hours of occlusion using non-contrast T2-weighted images in the canine model of infarction. In a study by Checkley et al. [8], serial MRI studies performed on nine mini-pigs with acute myocardial infarction failed to detect acute myocardial infarction at 30 hours in all cases. They were able to identify only one of six infarcts by noncontrast enhanced MRI after 3 days following fixed coronary artery occlusion. However, at 10 days, nine of nine documented infarcts were successfully identified by areas of increased signal intensity on MR images. The investigators hypothesized that, due to the relative paucity of coronary collaterals in the pig heart compared to that in the canine heart, the onset of tissue edema within the infarcted region may have been significantly delayed, making the identification of myocardial infarction difficult with noncontrast MRI.

In studies involving patients, several investigators have noted that noncontrast MRI lacks specificity for the identification of acute myocardial infarction. Filipchuk and colleagues [10] reported that although increased signal intensity was seen within the myocardium in a high percentage of patients with acute myocardial infarction, this finding was frequently present in normal volunteers. They noted that increased myocardial signal intensity detected acute myocardial infarction with an 88% sensitivity but only a 17% specificity. The most reliable indicator of acute myocardial infarction on MRI was regional wall thinning within the area of infarction. This finding was present in 68% of patients with acute myocardial infarction and only 11% of normal volunteers (88% specificity).

The problem in detecting acute myocardial infarction with noncontrast enhanced MRI results from the fact that tissue edema may not occur within the first several hours after coronary artery occlusion. The increased signal intensity within the infarct zone is due to two factors resulting from the development of edema within the infarcted tissue: there is an increase in the proton density within the infarcted region resulting in an increase in signal intensity on spin-echo images; and the edema within the infarcted tissue also increases the T2 relaxation time which also increases signal intensity. It is important to note that because the T1 is also increased within the infarcted zone, which tends to reduce signal intensity. Paramagnetic contrast agents are helpful in increasing the contrast between the infarcted and normally perfused myocardium by accentuating differences in the T1 and T2 relaxation times between the normally perfused and ischemic and/or infarcted regions.

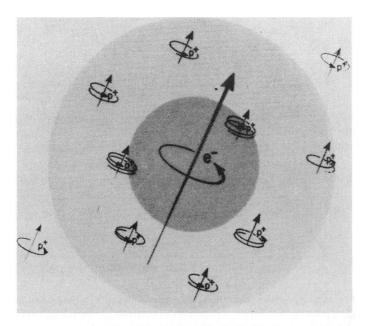

Figure 1. Schematic diagram of a paramagnetic molecule with a spinning unpaired electron (large arrow) in close proximity with nearby hydrogen nuclei with unpaired electrons (small arrows). The paramagnetic molecule causes proton relaxation of nearby hydrogen nuclei resulting in a decrease in T1 and T2 values. This phenomenon, known as proton relaxation enhancement, is one means of increasing contrast differences on MR images. (From Brasch RC. Work in progress: methods of contrast enhancement of NMR imaging and potential applications. Radiology 1983; 147: 781–788, with permission.)

Principles of MRI signal intensity

Three intrinsic signal characteristics determine the signal intensity in conventional spin-echo MRI images: (1) hydrogen concentration within the tissue, (2) T1, and (3) T2 relaxation values of the tissue. These factors determine the signal intensity on spin-echo images according to the following equation:

$$I = H\, f(v) \times [1 - e^{(-TR/T1)}]e^{(-TE/T2)},$$

where I is the signal intensity, H is the local concentration of hydrogen ion, $F(v)$ is a function of proton velocity, TE is the echo time, TR is the repetition time, and T1 and T2 are the proton relaxation times for the tissue [11]. Therefore, the signal intensity on MRI spin-echo images increases when there is an increase in hydrogen ion concentration (H), an increase in the tissue T2 value, or a decrease in the T1 value [12]. Furthermore, by adjusting the TE and

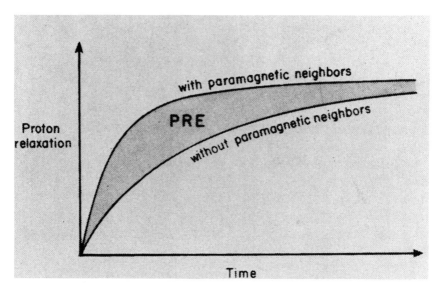

Figure 2. The degree of proton relaxation enhancement plotted as a function of time after a radiofrequency pulse. In the presence of paramagnetic molecules, proton relaxation enhancement is increased, regardless of the echo delay. This effect is increased with shorter echo times. (From Brasch RC. Work in progress: methods of contrast enhancement for NMR imaging and potential applications. Radiology 1983; 147: 781–788, with permission.)

TR, tissues with relatively low T1 values can be enhanced using T1-weighted spin-echo pulse sequences (using relatively short TE and TR) or by using an inversion recovery pulse sequence [13]. Similarly, tissues with relatively long T2 can be further enhanced using the T2-weighted spin-echo sequence (using a relatively long TE and TR). In cardiac imaging, the TR is usually the R-R cycle length or a multiple of this interval as determined by a gated EKG signal.

Paramagnetic contrast agents

A variety of compounds and elements possess unpaired electrons that generate local magnetic fields and shorten the magnetic relaxation time of surrounding hydrogen nuclei (Figure 1). This proton relaxation effect is roughly proportional to the concentration of the paramagnetic agent and results in an increase in the signal intensity on MRI by decreasing the tissue T1 value (Figure 2) [11]. This results in increased signal intensity that is most prominent with a T1-weighted sequence that has a relatively short echo time (TE). Thus, if a paramagnetic agent is infused within an organ with regional differences in blood flow, differences in the T1 relaxation time between normally perfused

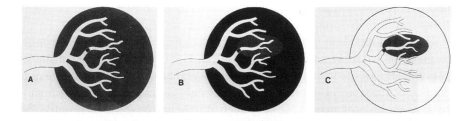

Figure 3. The influence of paramagnetic (T1-enhancing) and magnetic susceptibility contrast media on acutely ischemic myocardium. (A) In the absence of magnetic resonance contrast media, there is no difference in signal intensity between normal and ischemic regions. (B) In the presence of a paramagnetic (T1-enhancing) contrast media there is an increased signal intensity of the normal myocardium due to increased proton relaxation (resulting in a corresponding decrease in T1 value) in the tissue perfused by the contrast agent. This results in the ischemic region being demarcated as a 'cold spot'. (C) Magnetic susceptibility contrast agent causes a decrease in the signal intensity of normal myocardium due to alterations in the local magnetic field within the perfused region. Since the signal intensity of the ischemic region has unaltered magnetic suscepti-bility, this appears as a 'hot spot'. (From Higgins CB, Saeed M, Wendland M. MRI in ischemic heart disease: expansion of the current capabilities with MR contrast. Am J Card Imag 1991; 5: 38–50, with permission.)

Table 1. Paramagnetic substances with unbalanced electron spins.

Unpaired electrons
Nitric oxide (NO)
Nitrogen dioxide (NO_2)
Paired electrons with parallel spins
   Molecular oxygen (O_2)
Ions containing unpaired electrons
   Transition metal series
      Mn^{2+}, Mn^{3+}
      Fe^{2+}, Fe^{3+}
      Ni^{2+}
      Cr^{2+}
      Cu^{2+}
   Lanthanide series
      Gd^{3+}
      Eu^{2+}
   Actinide series
      Pa^{4+}
   Stable fee radicals
      Nitroxides
      Triphenylmethyl

From Brash RC. Work in progress: methods of contrast enhancement for NMR imaging and potential applications. Radiology 1983; 147: 781–788, with permission.

and hypoperfused regions can enhance differences in MRI signal intensity between normally reperfused and ischemic regions (Figure 3A, B).

Transition metals in the lanthanide series have received the most attention as potential paramagnetic contrast agents to date (Table 1). The manganese cation (Mn^{2+}) is taken up by viably myocytes and has proved to be useful as a cardiac contrast agent in animals [14]. Because the manganese ion is highly toxic, complexes of manganese have been utilized and have shown promise for the identification of ischemic and nonischemic myocardium [14–17, 51]. The metal complex that has shown the most potential as an MRI contrast agent is Gd-DTPA [12, 15, 18–31]. Again, because free gadolinium is potentially toxic, this cation has been complexed with various ligands such as DTPA to limit toxicity. This agent and other Gd complexes have shown promise for identifying myocardial ischemia, myocardial infarction, and myocardial salvage following reperfusion.

Recently, magnetic susceptibility contrast media have been utilized to identify ischemic regions within the heart [37]. These agents induce changes in the local magnetic field within the tissue, creating a marked decrease in signal intensity within the region perfused by the contrast agent. Since the ischemic region is not perfused by the susceptibility agent (Figure 3C), the signal intensity of ischemic tissue is unchanged, giving it the appearance of a 'hot spot' on T2-weighted images.

Detection of acute myocardial ischemia

A number of investigators have demonstrated that contrast enhanced MRI using either manganese chloride [14], Gd-DTPA [22, 23, 32, 35], manganese-ethyl diamine tetraphosphonate [33] or albumin Gd-DTPA [28, 30, 34–36] is useful in identifying acutely ischemic myocardium in animal models of ischemia. Brady and co-workers [14] demonstrated that normal and perfused myocardium was significantly enhanced compared to the ischemic zone after administration of manganese chloride in 12 dogs who had undergone left circumflex coronary artery occlusion. Similarly, Johnston et al. [22], showed that signal intensity was increased in normally perfused myocardium compared to ischemic myocardium after infusion of Gd-DTPA (Figure 4). Similar findings were noted by McNamara and co-workers [23] as early as two minutes after coronary artery occlusion.

Although Gd-DTPA has shown utility for the delineation of ischemic myocardium, the fact that it enters the extra vascular space and is rapidly cleared from normal myocardium potentially limits its usefulness in this role. Macromolecular paramagnetic contrast agents stay within the intravascular compart-

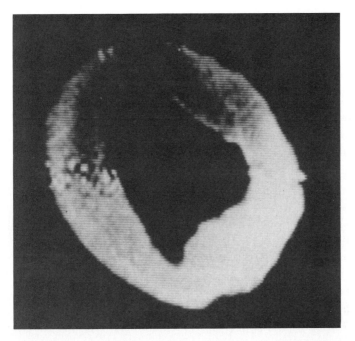

Figure 4. The magnetic resonance image of an excised heart after occlusion of the left anterior descending coronary artery and following infusion of Gd-DTPA. There is marked signal enhancement in the normally perfused posterior and lateral wall compared to the non-enhanced ischemic region in the anterior wall. (From Johnston DL, Liu P, Lauffer RB et al. Use of gadolinium-DTPA as a myocardial perfusion agent: potential applications and limitations for magnetic resonance imaging. J Nucl Med 1987; 28: 871–877, with permission.)

ment and, therefore, enhance normally perfused myocardium for prolonged periods of time. Manganese-ethyl diamine tetraphosphonate (Mn-TP) was used to delineate ischemic from non-ischemic myocardium in vivo in the rat model of myocardial ischemia by Pflugfelder et al. [33]. They found that normally perfused myocardium was markedly enhanced compared to ischemic myocardium, a pattern that had persisted for 60 minutes after the administration of MN-TP infusion. Albumin-(Gd-DTPA) (molecular weight = 92K Da) is another agent that remains in the intravascular space for prolonged periods of time resulting in persistent enhancement of vascular tissues such as heart and liver. Schmiedl et al. [34–36], and Wolfe et al. [30], have demonstrated that normal myocardium is enhanced significantly over ischemic myocardium following administration of albumin-(Gd-DTPA). This pattern of myocardial enhancement persisted for up to 90 minutes of myocardial ischemia.

As mentioned above, magnetic susceptibility contrast agents can be utilized to identify ischemic regions as well [37]. Because these agents create local

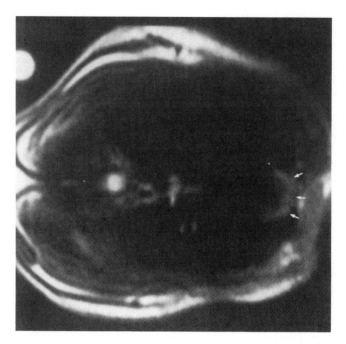

Figure 5. MR images acquired after the administration of dysprosium-DTPA-MBA, a magnetic susceptibility contrast agent in a rat with acute ischemia in the anterior wall of the left ventricle. Note that after infusion of the magnetic susceptibility contrast agent, the non-ischemic regions exhibit a marked decrease in signal intensity yet the ischemic anterior wall maintains relatively unchanged signal intensity resulting in the appearance of a 'hot spot' in the ischemic region (arrows). (From Saeed M, Wendland MF, Tomei E et al. Demarcation of myocardial ischemia: magnetic susceptibility effect of contrast medium in MR imaging. Radiology 1989; 173: 763–767, with permission.)

magnetic field gradients within the tissues they perfuse, they markedly decrease the signal intensity within normally perfused regions of the heart. This leaves the signal intensity of the ischemic tissue relatively unchanged, giving it the appearance of a 'hot spot' on T2-weighted MR images (Figure 3C). One potential disadvantage of the use of magnetic susceptibility contrast agents is that, although they readily identify ischemic regions of the heart, there is considerable loss of information about the anatomy of the normally perfused areas of the heart (Figure 5).

Assessment of acute myocardial infarction

Although many investigators reported that noncontrast MRI has the potential to identify acute myocardial infarction [1, 2, 4–6, 38, 39], others have reported that this technique lacks specificity, especially in the early phase after acute myocardial infarction [2, 7–10]. In this regard, contrast enhanced MRI may be helpful in the early identification of acute myocardial infarction. McNamara and co-workers [24] and Rehr and co-workers [9] reported that in the canine model of acute myocardial infarction, the use of Gd-DTPA significantly enhanced the contrast between infarcted and noninfarcted regions. Rehr et al. [9] studied 10 dogs with acute myocardial infarction between 1 and 5 days following ligation of the left anterior descending coronary artery. They found that administration of Gd-DTPA improved the visualization of the infarcted segment in three of four dogs at 2 days post-infarction and six of six dogs between 4 and 5 days post-infarction. The signal intensity ratio between infarcted and noninfarcted tissue was significantly greater after the infusion of Gd-DTPA. The ratio of infarcted to normal myocardium was 1.4 in non-contrast MR images at 24 to 48 hours post-occlusion and increased to 1.7 following Gd-DTPA administration. Similarly, the intensity ratio of infarcted to noninfarcted tissue in noncontrast images was 1.5 at 4 to 5 days post-occlusion and increased to 1.8 after infusion of Gd-DTPA.

De Roos and co-workers [21] showed that Gd-DTPA improved the signal contrast of infarcted and noninfarcted tissue in patients as well. They obtained MRI on five patients between 2 and 17 days following acute myocardial infarction and showed that the intensity ratio between the infarcted and normal tissue in noncontrast MR images was 1.1 using a T1-weighted sequence (TE = 30 msec) and 1.4 using a T2-weighted sequence (TE = 60 msec). After infusion of Gd-DTPA, the signal intensity of the infarcted region increased to 1.6 times that of normal tissue, significantly greater than in nonenhanced images.

Contrast enhanced MRI is also useful for the quantitation of infarct size in both animal models as well as in patients. Goldman and co-workers [40] measured the infarct size in six canine hearts with contrast enhance MRI using magnesium chloride, 24 hours after circumflex coronary artery occlusion (Figure 6). They found that the area of nonenhanced (infarcted) myocardium on MR images corresponded well with the infarct size determined by triphe-nyltetrazolium chloride (TTC) staining. Potential for contrast enhanced MRI to quantitate infarct size in patients was demonstrated by De Roos and co-workers [41]. They studied 21 patients with acute myocardial infarction from 2 to 8 days following Gd-DTPA administration with the area of increased signal intensity on noncontrast T2-weighted MR images. They noted a good correlation between the Gd-DTPA enhanced area and the area of high signal intensity on T2-weighted images. Furthermore, they noted that infarct size measured by contrast enhanced MRI was significantly smaller in patients who

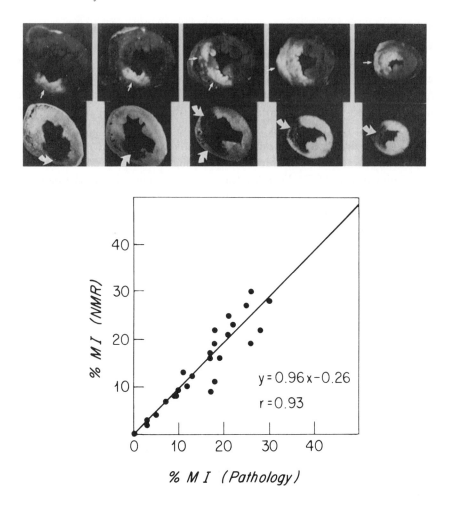

Figure 6. The use of contrast enhanced MRI for infarct sizing. (A) top, sections of a canine heart that was stained with triphenyltetrazolium chloride (TTC) after 24 hours of left circumflex coronary artery occlusion. Note the area of infarcted myocardium within the circumflex distribution (white, small arrows). Bottom, magnetic resonance images of the corresponding levels of the unsliced heart. Note that the normally perfused myocardium is markedly enhanced leaving the nonenhanced infarcted myocardium (curved arrows) appearing as a 'cold spot'. This nonenhanced infarcted region on MRI corresponds well with the area that is infarcted by TTC staining. (B) infarct size determined by MR imaging compared to infarct size determined by TTC staining from 26 myocardial sections obtained from six dog hearts. (From Goldman MR, Brady TJ, Pykett IL et al. Quantification of experimental myocardial infarction using nuclear magnetic imaging and paramagnetic ion contrast enhancement in excised canine hearts. Circulation 1982; 66: 1012–1016, with permission.)

had received reperfusion therapy compared to those that were not reperfused (8% ± 5% vs 15% ± 4% respectively, $p = 0.001$).

Other investigators have shown that infarct size can be reliably estimated by MRI using noncontrast T2-weighted images as well. Ryan and co-workers [42] performed noncontrast MRI and two-dimensional contrast enhanced echocardiography in 16 canines after coronary artery occlusion and reperfusion. They noted that the area of increased signal intensity on MRI correlated well with infarct size although MRI appeared to overestimate infarct size somewhat. Using a similar technique, Johns et al. [43] noted a good correlation between the infarct volume on T2-weighted images and the area of hypokinesis on left ventriculography in patients. Others have noted good correlation between infarct size and the area of increased signal intensity on T2-weighted images in both ischemic [44, 45] and reperfused [46] infarcts where the imaging was performed ex vivo on the excised heart. Further work is necessary to fully evaluate the potential role of both contrast enhanced and noncontrast MRI for infarct sizing in vivo in both animal models of acute myocardial infarction and in patients.

Assessment of reperfusion and myocardial salvage

With the current potential of thrombolytic therapy to decrease infarct size and improve survival in patients with acute myocardial infarction, it is important that noninvasive techniques be developed to evaluate the presence or absence of successful coronary reperfusion and to assess the degree of myocardial salvage. Although several ex vivo studies have shown significant increases in T2 values and increased signal intensity in reperfused infarcts compared to ischemic infarcts [37, 47], noncontrast enhanced MRI has not been reliable in distinguishing between reperfused and nonreperfused infarcts [7]. Because T2 values increase in nonreperfused infarcts due to the development of tissue edema through collateral circulation, changes in T2 are not always sufficient to permit the early assessment of reperfusion. Several investigators have demonstrated that contrast enhanced MRI is useful for identifying the presence of reperfusion after acute myocardial ischemia [30, 36] and after myocardial infarction [25, 27, 30, 39, 48].

In the rat model of coronary occlusion and reperfusion, Schmiedl and co-workers [36] and Wolfe and co-workers [30] demonstrated that, with T1-weighted contrast enhanced MRI using albumin-(Gd-DTPA), normal myocardium was significantly enhanced compared to ischemic myocardium during coronary artery occlusion (Figure 7). After reperfusion, there was a

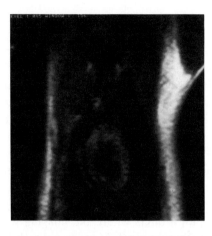

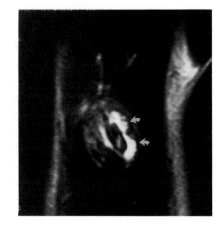

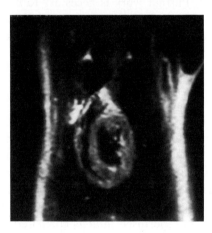

Figure 7. T1-weighted MR images of a rat heart subjected to 30 minutes of ischemia followed by reperfusion.
(A) Baseline image prior to ischemia and prior to administration of contrast agent.
(B) Following occlusion of the left coronary artery and after administration of albumin-(Gd-DTPA). Note the area of nonenhanced ischemic myocardium (curved arrows) and the highly enhanced signal from intercavitary blood adjacent to the ischemic myocardium.
(C) After 15 minutes of reflow. Note there is uniform enhancement of the previously ischemic zone and the non-ischemic zone. Histopathologic examination revealed no evidence of myocardial necrosis.
(From Wolfe CL, Moseley ME, Wikstrom MG et al. Assessment of myocardial salvage after ischemia and reperfusion using magnetic resonance imaging and spectroscopy. Circulation 1989; 80: 969–982, with permission.)

normalization of this enhancement pattern such that the ischemic myocardium appeared homogeneous with nonischemic regions of the heart.

Others have shown that contrast enhanced MRI is useful in differentiating reperfused from ischemic infarcts [25, 27, 30, 39, 48]. Peshock et al. demonstrated that in the canine model, there was significant contrast enhancement between normal and ischemic myocardium after the administration of Gd-DTPA that was further augmented following reperfusion [25]. This enhancement was best demonstrated using inversion recovery pulse sequences following reperfusion. Schaeffer and co-workers [27] showed that, in 28 dogs with coronary artery occlusion and reperfusion, there was marked enhancement of

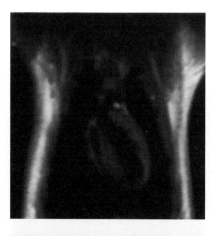

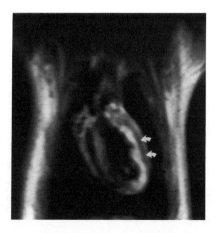

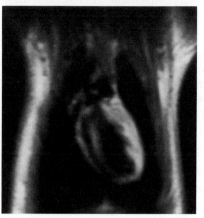

Figure 8. T1-weighted MR images of a rat heart subjected to 90 minutes of ischemia followed by reperfusion.

(A) Baseline image before ischemia and before administration of contrast agent.

(B) After occlusion of left coronary artery and administration of albumin-(Gd-DTPA), the ischemic myocardium remains non-enhanced (arrows) and the signal from the left ventricular cavity adjacent to the ischemic zone is markedly enhanced, likely secondary to stasis of blood adjacent to this region.

(C) Following 90 minutes of ischemia and reperfusion, there was marked enhancement of the reperfused zone. Histopathologic examination revealed contraction band necrosis and evidence of intramyocardial hemorrhage signifying a loss of vascular integrity within this region. (From Wolfe CL, Moseley ME, Wickstrom MG et al. Assessment of myocardial salvage after ischemia and reperfusion using magnetic resonance imaging and spectroscopy. Circulation 1989; 80: 969–982, with permission.)

the ischemic and reperfused region following administration of Gd-DTPA. Furthermore, the area of enhanced myocardium corresponded with the anatomic area of risk.

Contrast enhanced MRI has also shown potential for identifying myocardial salvage after reperfusion [16, 30]. In the canine model of ischemia and reperfusion, McNamara and co-workers [16] found that irreversibly injured myocardium demonstrated a marked increase in signal intensity following Gd-DTPA administration. However, dogs with reversible injury showed no difference in signal intensity between normal and perfused and ischemic myocardium fol-

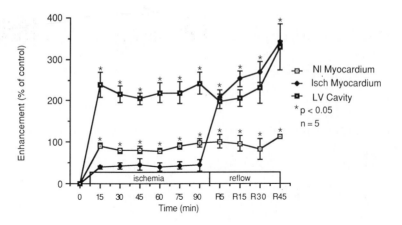

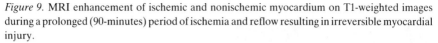

Figure 9. MRI enhancement of ischemic and nonischemic myocardium on T1-weighted images during a prolonged (90-minutes) period of ischemia and reflow resulting in irreversible myocardial injury.

(A) Albumin-(Gd-DTPA) was administered immediately after the onset of ischemia. The normally perfused zone showed significant enhancement compared to baseline, and the ischemic zone showed no significant enhancement during the period of left coronary occlusion. There was marked enhancement of the intracavitary blood immediately adjacent to the ischemic zone. After reperfusion, the ischemic zone became markedly enhanced. Histopathologic examination revealed evidence or contraction and necrosis, and leakage of red blood cells into the extravascular space signifying loss of vascular integrity within the reperfused and necrotic region.

lowing reperfusion. In the rat model of ischemia and reperfusion, Wolfe and co-workers [30] demonstrated that contrast enhanced MRI with albumin-(Gd-DTPA), a macro-molecular paramagnetic contrast agent was helpful in distinguishing between reversible and irreversible injury following reperfusion. Reversible myocardial injury was characterized by uniform enhancement of both normal and ischemic regions after reperfusion (Figure 7). Irreversible ischemic injury was characterized by marked transmural enhancement of the reperfused region on contrast enhanced MRI (Figures 8, 9). This finding correlated with presence of infarcted myocardium by TTC staining and the presence of myocardial hemorrhage on histologic examination. Similar findings have been noted by Saeed and co-workers [49] using a non-ionic Gd chelate (Gd-DTPA bismethylamide).

Although contrast enhanced MRI has shown potential for detecting reperfusion in animal models of acute myocardial infarction, current studies with contrast enhanced MRI in patients have been unable to detect differences between reperfused and nonreperfused infarcts. Van der Wall and co-workers [48] studied 27 patients with acute myocardial infarction with contrast enhanced MRI and was unable to demonstrate differences in the intensity ratios

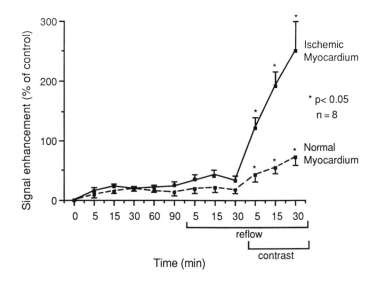

Figure 9. (B) Albumin-(Gd-DTPA) was not given until 30 minutes after reperfusion. No significant enhancement of the ischemic or non-ischemic regions was noted during coronary artery occlusion or reperfusion prior to the administration of albumin-(Gd-DTPA). Following the intravenous administration of the contrast agent, the reperfused zone became markedly enhanced compared to the nonischemic zone. Histopathologic examination again revealed evidence of contraction band necrosis and evidence of intra-myocardial hemorrhage within the area of ischemia. (From Wolfe CL, Moseley ME, Wickstrom MG et al. Assessment of myocardial salvage after ischemia and reperfusion using magnetic resonance imaging and spectroscopy. Circulation 1989; 80: 969–982, with permission.)

between 19 patients who had undergone successful reperfusion compared to eight patients who were not reperfused. De Roos and co-workers [50] performed contrast enhanced MRI with Gd-DTPA in 45 patients with acute myocardial infarction and again were unable to demonstrate differences in infarct enhancement between reperfused and nonreperfused infarcts. However, it should be noted that these patients underwent MRI imaging from 37 to 240 hours after acute presentation. After such a long delay, one would expect that even nonreperfused infarcts could have developed significant collateral blood flow to the ischemic region, potentially allowing the delivery of Gd-DTPA into the infarcted region despite persistent coronary artery occlusion. Further work is necessary to determine if contrast enhanced MRI is necessary to determine if contrast enhanced MRI is useful in identifying reperfusion in the first several hours of reperfusion.

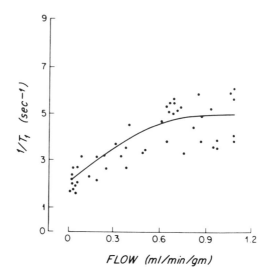

Figure 10. Relationship between 1/T1 and myocardial blood flow in ischemic canine myocardium after a bolus infusion of Gd-DTPA. There is good correlation between blood flow and 1/T1 where resting flow values are less than or equal to 0.5 ml per minute per g. (From Johnston DL, Liu P, Lauffer RB et al. Use of gadolinium-DTPA as a myocardial perfusion agent: Potential applications and limitations for magnetic resonance imaging. J Nucl Med 1987; 28: 871–877, with permission.)

The assessment of myocardial perfusion during ischemia

Although many previous studies have emphasized the qualitative differences between ischemic and non-ischemic myocardium with enhanced and non-enhanced MRI, several studies have shown the potential for MRI to assess the degree of myocardial ischemia quantitatively. Ratner and co-workers [26] demonstrated a significant inverse relationship between T1 and T2 relaxation values and myocardial blood flow within the ischemic endocardium in a canine model of coronary artery occlusion. After reflow, there is a direct relationship between myocardial blood flow in both T1 and T2 relaxation values in the previously ischemic zone. In an ex-vivo study, Johnston and co-workers [43] noted an inverse nonlinear mono-exponential relationship between increasing T1 and T2 values and decreasing myocardial blood flow in an ischemic canine model. Although these studies demonstrate the feasibility of assessing myocardial blood flow with noncontrast enhanced MRI, it should be noted that the changes in T1 and T2 during ischemia were relatively small. Any error in the measurement of these values would therefore, result in a significant error in the quantitative estimation of tissue blood flow.

Several investigators have demonstrated the potential feasibility for con-

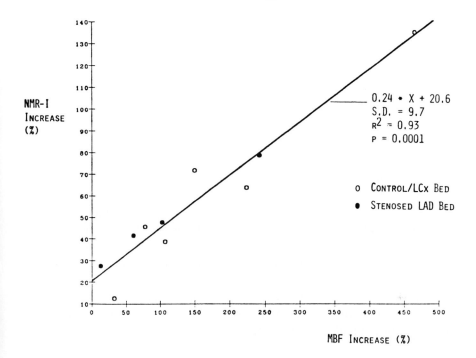

Figure 11. The relationship between the relative increase in myocardial blood flow vs the increase in MR signal intensity in contrast enhanced MR images after infusion of dipyridamole in four dogs with left anterior descending coronary artery stenosis and two control dogs. There is a significant correlation between changes in the hyperemic coronary blood flow reserve after dipyridamole administration and the increase in MR signal intensity. (From Miller DD, Holmvan G, Gill JB et al. Magnetic resonance imaging for detection of coronary artery stenosis by continuous gadolinium-DTPA paramagnetic contrast infusion during dipyridamole-induced hyperemia. Magn Reson Med 1989; 10: 246–255, with permission.)

trast enhanced MRI to quantitate regional myocardial blood flow. In an in vivo canine study, Johnston et al. [2], demonstrated that there was significant relationship between $1/T1$ and myocardial blood flow during ischemia after a bolus infusion of Gd-DTPA (Figure 10). This correlation existed primarily when the blood flow was less than or equal to 0.5 cc/min/gram of tissue. There was no significant relationship between $1/T1$ and myocardial blood flow when the flow was greater than 1 cc/min/gram tissue (Figure 10). Schaefer and co-workers [51] have shown that manganese gluconate may be useful for quantitatively assessing myocardial perfusion, as well. These investigators found a linear relationship between myocardial blood flow and myocardial manganese concentration in a canine model of myocardial ischemia. They did not correlate changes in T1 and T2 or MRI signal intensity with myocardial perfusion, however.

During pharmacologic stress with dipyridamole infusion, Miller and co-workers [52] demonstrated that changes in MRI signal intensity on contrast enhanced MR images (using a constant infusion of Gd-DTPA) correlated with changes in myocardial blood flow in the canine model of coronary artery stenosis. They showed a direct linear correlation between the increase in signal intensity and the increase in myocardial blood flow during infusion of dipyridamole (Figure 11). Vexler and co-workers [53] demonstrated that by using the macromolecular contrast agent, albumin-(Gd-DTPA), there were significant increases in signal intensity within the heart during adenosine infusion, another potent coronary vasodilator. In a preliminary study by Galjee et al. [54], less contrast enhancement was noted in regions supplied by stenotic coronary arteries in patients after infusion of Gd-DTPA and dipyridamole. These studies, however, demonstrate the potential for contrast enhanced MRI for quantitative assessment of myocardial perfusion. Furthermore, contrast enhanced MRI in conjunction with pharmacologic coronary vasodilators may potentially allow for the detection of significant, but nonocclusive coronary artery stenosis in patients in the future.

Conclusions

Contrast enhanced MRI is helpful in identifying and quantitating ischemic and infarcted myocardium with increased specificity over noncontrast enhanced MRI. Preliminary studies in animal models of ischemia and reperfusion suggests that contrast enhanced MRI is useful for identifying reperfusion and assessing myocardial salvage following reperfusion in a setting of acute myocardial infarction. Contrast enhanced MRI in conjunction with the infusion of pharmacologic coronary vasodilators may potentially enable detection of significant but nonocclusive coronary artery stenosis in the future.

Acknowledgement

We wish to thank Richard Aleguas for his help in preparing this manuscript. This work was supported in part by the NHLBI (Grant # HL-01972-05) and the California Affiliate of the American Heart Association (Grant # 88-N135).

References

1. Higgins CB, Herfkens R, Lipton MJ et al. Nuclear magnetic resonance imaging of acute myocardial infarction in dogs: alterations in magnetic relaxation times. Am J Cardiol 1983; 52: 184–8.
2. Johnston DL, Thompson RC, Liu P et al. Magnetic resonance imaging during acute myocardial infarction. Am J Cardiol 1986; 57: 1059–65.
3. Pflugfelder PW, Wisenberg G, Prato FS, Carroll SE, Turner KL. Early detection of canine myocardial infarction by magnetic resonance imaging in vivo. Circulation 1985; 71: 587–94.
4. Tscholakoff D, Higgins CB, McNamara MT, Derugin N. Early-phase myocardial infarction: evaluation by MR imaging. Radiology 1986; 159: 667–72.
5. Wesbey G, Higgins CB, Lanzer P, Botvinick E, Lipton MJ. Imaging and characterization of acute myocardial infarction in vivo by gated nuclear magnetic resonance. Circulation 1984; 69: 125–30.
6. Higgins CB, Lanzer P, Stark D. Imaging by nuclear magnetic resonance in patients with chronic ischemic heart disease. Circulation 1984; 69: 523–31.
7. Aisen AM, Buda AJ, Zotz RJ, Buckwalter KA. Visualization of myocardial infarction and subsequent coronary reperfusion with MRI using a dog model. Magn Reson Imaging 1987; 5: 399–404.
8. Checkley D, Loveday BE, Waterton JC, Zhu XP, Isherwood I. Detection of myocardial infarction in the mini-pig using NMR imaging. Magn Reson Med 1987; 5: 201–16.
9. Rehr RB, Peshock RM, Mallow CR et al. Improved in vivo magnetic resonance imaging of acute myocardial infarction after intravenous paramagnetic contrast agent administration. Am J Cardiol 1986; 57: 864–8.
10. Checkley D, Loveday BE, Waterton JC, Zhu XP, Isherwood I. Detection of myocardial infarction in the minipig using NMR imaging. Magn Reson Med 1987; 5: 201–16.
11. Brasch RC. Work in progress: methods of contrast enhancement for NMR imaging and potential applications. Radiology 1983; 147: 781–8.
12. Johnston DL, Liu P. Evaluation of myocardial ischemia and infarction by nuclear magnetic resonance techniques. Can J Cardiol 1988; 4: 116–29.
13. Wolf GL, Joseph PM, Goldstein EJ. Optimal pulsing sequences for MR contrast agents. AJR Am J Roentgenol 1986; 147: 367–71.
14. Brady TJ, Goldman MR, Pykett IL et al. Proton nuclear magnetic resonance imaging of regionally ischemic canine hearts: effect of paramagnetic proton signal enhancement. Radiology 1982; 144: 343–7.
15. Boudreau RJ, Burbidge S, Sirr S, Loken MK. Comparison of the biodistribution of manganese-54 DTPA and gadolinium-153 DTPA in dogs. J Nucl Med 1987; 28: 349–53.
16. Kang YS, Gore JC. Studies of tissue NMR relaxation enhancement by manganese. Dose and time dependences. Invest Radiol 1984; 19: 399–407.
17. Wolf GL, Baum L. Cardiovascular toxicity and tissue proton T1 response to manganese injection in the dog and rabbit. AJR Am J Roentgenol 1983; 141: 193–7.
18. Boudreau RJ, Frick MP, Levey RM, Lund G, Sirr SA, Loken MK. The preliminary evaluation of Mn DTPA as a potential contrast agent for nuclear magnetic resonance imaging. Am J Physiol Imaging 1986; 1: 19–25.
19. Brasch RC, Weinmann HJ, Wesbey GE. Contrast-enhanced NMR imaging: animal studies using gadolinium-DTPA complex. AJR Am J Roentgenol 1984; 142: 625–30.
20. Brown JJ, Higgins CB. Myocardial paramagnetic contrast agents for MR imaging. AJR Am J Roentgenol 1988; 151: 865–71.

21. de Roos A, Doornbos J, van der Wall EE, van Voorthuisen AE. MR imaging of acute myocardial infarction: value of Gd-DTPA. AJR Am J Roentgenol 1988; 150: 531–4.

22. Johnston DL, Liu P, Lauffer RB et al. Use of gadolinium-DTPA as a myocardial perfusion agent: potential applications and limitations for magnetic resonance imaging. J Nucl Med 1987; 28: 871–7.

23. McNamara MT, Higgins CB, Ehman RL, Revel D, Sievers R, Brasch RC. Acute myocardial ischemia: magnetic resonance contrast enhancement with gadolinium-DTPA. Radiology 1984; 153: 157–63.

24. McNamara MT, Tscholakoff D, Revel D et al. Differentiation of reversible and irreversible myocardial injury by MR imaging with and without gadolinium-DTPA. Radiology 1986; 158: 765–9.

25. Peshock RM, Malloy CR, Buja M, Nunnally RL, Parkey RW, Willerson JT. Magnetic resonance imaging of acute myocardial infarction: gadolinium diethylenetriamine pentaacetic acid as a marker of reperfusion. Circulation 1986; 74: 1434–40.

26. Ratner AV, Okada RD, Newell JB, Pohost GM. The relationship between proton nuclear magnetic resonance relaxation parameters and myocardial perfusion with acute coronary arterial occlusion and reperfusion. Circulation 1985; 71: 823–8.

27. Schaefer S, Malloy CR, Katz J et al. Gadolinium-DTPA-enhanced nuclear magnetic resonance imaging of reperfused myocardium: identification of the myocardial bed at risk. J Am Coll Cardiol 1988; 12: 1064–72.

28. Schmiedl U, Ogan MD, Paajanen H et al. Albumin labeled with Gd-DTPA as an intravascular, blood pool-enhancing agent for MR imaging: biodistribution and imaging studies. Radiology 1987; 162: 205–10.

29. Wesbey GE, Higgins CB, McNamara MT et al. Effect of gadolinium-DTPA on the magnetic relaxation times of normal and infarcted myocardium. Radiology 1984; 153: 165–9.

30. Wolfe CL, Moseley ME, Wikstrom MG et al. Assessment of myocardial salvage after ischemia and reperfusion using magnetic resonance imaging and spectroscopy. Circulation 1989; 80: 969–82.

31. Wolfe CL. Assessment of myocardial ischemia and infarction by contrast enhanced magnetic resonance imaging. Cardiol Clin 1989; 7: 685–96.

32. Runge VM, Clanton JA, Wehr CJ, Pautain CL, James AE Jr. Gated magnetic resonance imaging of acute myocardial ischemia in dogs: application of multiecho techniques and contrast enhancement with Gd-DTPA. Magn Reson Imaging 1985; 3: 255–66.

33. Pflugfelder PW, Wendland MR, Holt WW et al. Acute myocardial ischemia: MR imaging with Mn-TP. Radiology 1988; 167: 129–33.

34. Schmiedl U, Moseley ME, Ogan MD, Chen WM, Brasch RC. Comparison of initial biodistribution patterns of Gd-DTPA and albumin-(Gd-DTPA) using rapid spin echo MR imaging. J Comput Assist Tomogr 1987; 11: 306–13.

35. Schmiedl U, Moseley ME, Sievers R et al. Magnetic resonance imaging of myocardial infarction using albumin-(Gd-DTPA), a macromolecular blood-volume contrast agent in a rat model. Invest Radiol 1987; 22: 713–21.

36. Schmiedl U, Sievers R, Brasch RC et al. Acute myocardial ischemia and reperfusion: MR imaging with albumin-Gd-DTPA. Radiology 1989; 170: 351–6.

37. Saeed M, Wendland MF, Tomei E et al. Demarcation of myocardial ischemia: magnetic susceptibility effect of contrast medium in MR imaging. Radiology 1989; 173: 763–7.

38. McNamara MT, Higgins CB, Schechtmann N et al. Detection and characterization of acute myocardial infarction in man with use of gated magnetic resonance. Circulation 1985; 71: 717–24.

39. Tscholakoff D, Higgins CB, Sechtem U, McNamara MT. Occlusive and reperfused myocardial infarcts: effect of Gd-DTPA on ECG-gated MR imaging. Radiology 1986; 160: 515–9.

40. Goldman MR, Brady TJ, Pykett IL et al. Quantification of experimental myocardial infarction using nuclear magnetic resonance imaging and paramagnetic ion contrast enhancement in excised canine hearts. Circulation 1982; 66: 1012–6.

41. de Roos A, Matheijssen NA, Doornbos J et al. Myocardial infarct size after reperfusion therapy: assessment with Gd-DTPA-enhanced MR imaging. Radiology 1990; 176: 517–21.

42. Ryan TS, Tarver RD, Duerk JL, Sawada SG, Hollenkamp NC. Distinguishing viable from infarcted myocardium after experimental ischemia and reperfusion by using nuclear magnetic resonance imaging. J Am Coll Cardiol 1990; 15: 1355–64.

43. Johns JA, Leavitt MB, Newell JB et al. Quantitation of acute myocardial infarct size by nuclear magnetic resonance imaging. J Am Coll Cardiol 1990; 15: 143–9.

44. Caputo GR, Sechtem U, Tscholakoff D, Higgins CB. Measurement of myocardial infarct size at early and late intervals using MR imaging: an experimental study in dogs. AJR Am J Roentgenol 1987; 149: 237–43.

45. Rokey R, Verani MS, Bolli R et al. Myocardial infarct size quantification by MR imaging early after coronary artery occlusion in dogs. Radiology 1986; 158: 771–4.

46. Buda AJ, Aisen AM, Juni JE, Gallagher KP, Zotz RJ. Detection and sizing of myocardial ischemia and infarction by nuclear magnetic resonance imaging in the canine heart. Am Heart J 1985; 110: 1284–90.

47. Johnston DL, Brady TJ, Ratner AV et al. Assessment of myocardial ischemia with proton magnetic resonance: effects of a three hour coronary occlusion with and without reperfusion. Circulation 1985; 71: 595–601.

48. van der Wall EE, van Dijkman PR, De Roos A et al. Diagnostic significance of gadolinium-DTPA (diethylenetriamine penta-acetic acid) enhanced magnetic resonance imaging in thrombolytic treatment for acute myocardial infarction: its potential in assessing reperfusion. Br Heart J 1990; 63: 12–7.

49. Saeed M, Wendland MF, Takehara Y, Higgins CB. Reversible and irreversible injury in the reperfused myocardium: differentiation with contrast material-enhanced MR imaging. Radiology 1990; 175: 633–7.

50. de Roos A, van Rossum AC, van der Wall E et al. Reperfused and nonreperfused myocardial infarction: diagnostic potential of Gd-DTPA-enhanced MR imaging. Radiology 1989; 172: 717–20.

51. Schaefer S, Lange RA, Gutekunst DP, Parkey RW, Willerson JT, Peshock RM. Contrast-enhanced magnetic resonance imaging of reperfused myocardium. Invest Radiol 1991; 26: 551–6.

52. Miller DD, Holmvang G, Gill JB et al. MRI detection of myocardial perfusion changes by gadolinium-DTPA infusion during dipyridamole hyperemia. Magn Reson Med 1989; 10: 246–55.

53. Vexler VS, Berthezene Y, Wolfe CL et al. MRI demonstration of pharmacologically induced myocardial vasodilation using a macromolecular contrast agent [Abstract]. In: Society of magnetic resonance in medicine: tenth annual scientific meeting and exhibition; August 10–16, 1991; San Francisco, California, USA: book of abstracts. Berkeley: Society of Magnetic Resonance in Medicine, 1991: 239.

54. Galjee MA, van Rossum AC, Visser FC, Valk J, Roos JP. Magnetic resonance imaging of myocardial ischemia using continuous infusion of gadolinium-DTPA after dipyridamole [Abstract]. In: Society of magnetic resonance in medicine: tenth annual scientific meeting and exhibition; August 10–16, 1991; San Francisco, California, USA: book of abstracts. Berkeley: Society of Magnetic Resonance in Medicine, 1991: 241.

15. Magnetic resonance imaging using paramagnetic contrast agents in the clinical evaluation of myocardial infarction

PAUL R.M. VAN DIJKMAN and ERNST E. VAN DER WALL

Summary

Magnetic resonance imaging (MRI) is a noninvasive and specific method for production of high resolution tomographic images in blocks of three-dimensional information. Apart from scintigraphic techniques and computed tomography for the evaluation of myocardial ischemia and infarcts, MRI has emerged as a new diagnostic technique to study the extent of anatomical and functional abnormalities in patients with coronary artery disease. Conventional noncontrast MRI can identify acutely infarcted myocardial areas, although the difficulty in identifying myocardial ischemia and infarcts with noncontrast MRI suggests a potential role for contrast enhanced MRI. The use of the paramagnetic contrast agent gadolinium (Gd)-diethylene triamine pentaacetic acid (DTPA) improves depiction of infarcted myocardium on T1-weighted spin-echo MR images that are obtained soon after acute myocardial infarction. This is of particular interest for the estimation of myocardial infarct size. Furthermore, ultrafast subsecond imaging, in combination with Gd-DTPA, offers the potential to analyze cardiac first pass and myocardial perfusion. The development of nontoxic paramagnetic contrast agents which are selectively taken up by viable myocardium would be helpful in assessing the presence of ischemic/infarcted myocardium and myocardial salvage by MRI following reperfusion.

Ernst E. van der Wall et al. (eds), What's new in cardiac imaging?, 201–220.
© *1992 Kluwer Academic Publishers. Printed in the Netherlands.*

Introduction

With the advent of nuclear magnetic resonance imaging (MRI) in cardiology, an important diagnostic tool to the currently available diagnostic arsenal is added for the evaluation of patients with heart disease. Proton nuclear MRI has been applied clinically to many areas of the body. It is noninvasive, gives excellent anatomic resolution, provides inherent contrast between tissues and flowing blood, is intrinsically three-dimensional, and can often distinguish between normal and abnormal tissue based on tissue relaxation properties.

The identification of ischemic and infarcted myocardial tissue by MRI has been greatly aided by the use of gadolinium containing paramagnetic contrast agents. Rather than aiming at competing with established imaging techniques, MRI techniques in cardiology are to be used in those conditions for which they are uniquely suited: (1) myocardial tissue characterization, (2) regional myocardial blood flow distribution with contrast agents, (3) noninvasive angiography, (4) flow imaging of the great vessels, and (5) in vivo myocardial biochemistry (MR spectroscopy). These applications are typically for MRI and MR spectroscopy and cannot be simply duplicated by other imaging technique.

This chapter discusses the current knowledge of the application of paramagnetic MRI contrast agents in ischemic heart disease. Most emphasis has been laid on our own experimental results and on clinical results in patients with myocardial infarction; the general experimental findings are predominantly discussed in Chapter 14.

Unenhanced cardiac MRI

The detection of acute myocardial ischemia and infarction is based on alterations in tissue relaxation times T1 and T2 with resultant changes in image intensity.

Experimental findings

First experimental studies in dog hearts showed that the relaxation times T1 and particularly T2 are usually prolonged in disease states which are characterized by edematous changes that occur in regions with acute myocardial ischemia or infarction [1–7]. The magnitude of increase in T1 and T2 was proportional to the magnitude of changes in blood flow [2]. Changes in T1 and T2 can be detected in vivo 3–6 hours after coronary occlusion in infarcted areas, whereas reperfused areas showed these changes already by 30 minutes after reperfusion [4]. MRI also allows the assessment of infarct size based on different T2-relaxation times between infarcted and normal tissue, although unenhanced MRI may not be suitable for early detection of infarct size [6]. Serial MRI measurements of left ventricular infarct size 3 and 21 days after coronary artery ligation using T2 measurements correlated well with histopathologically assessed infarct size [7].

Clinical results

Clinical studies in patients with documented myocardial infarction have also shown T1 and T2 alterations in infarcted myocardium. McNamara et al. [8] studied nine patients with acute myocardial infarction 5–12 days after the acute onset and showed that the infarcted areas were characterized by increased signal intensity of the infarcted region and prolonged T2 relaxation time. Distinction between normal and infarcted myocardium was sufficient to estimate infarct size. Johnston et al. [9] studied 34 patients 3 to 30 days after myocardial infarction and showed that regional increase of signal intensity in the patients was consistent with the electrocardiographic location of the infarction and with the presence of hypokinetic segments on the left ventriculogram. Fisher et al. [10] showed in 29 patients, 3 to 17 days after myocardial infarction, prolonged T2 relaxation times in infarcted myocardial regions. On the other hand, they observed that increased signal intensity on T2-weighted images may be very difficult to distinguish from slowly moving intraventricular blood flow. In addition, Ahmad et al. [11] showed that T2 prolongation may not be a specific marker for acute myocardial infarction but can also be observed in abnormally perfused myocardial segments of patients with unstable angina. Been et al. [12] demonstrated in 10 of 13 patients with recent myocardial infarction a 40% increase of T1 values in the infarcted areas. In a subsequent study, Been et al. [13] showed in 41 patients with acute myocardial infarction that maximum T1 values were observed at 2 weeks after the acute onset, suggesting that the increase of T1 reflects cellular infiltration as much or more than tissue edema. No differences in T1 values were observed between the patients with or without reperfusion, indicating that alterations of T1 are complex and may bear no relationship to specific histological findings. Infarcted myocardial areas are not only detectable by changes in T1 and T2 relaxation times, but can also be seen by MRI using morphological features like increased signal intensity, ventricular cavitary signal and regional wall thinning. Filipchuk et al. [14] showed increased myocardial signal intensity in 88%, cavitary signal in 74% and regional wall thinning in 67% of 27 patients with acute myocardial infarction. However, in 18 asymptomatic volunteers increased myocardial signal intensity was also observed in 83%, cavitary signal in 94%, and wall thinning in 11% of cases. These findings imply that increased signal both from myocardial tissue and from the cavity are sensitive but not specific for myocardial infarction. Of the three features therefore, wall thinning was the most predictive and specific for acute myocardial infarction. Krauss et al. [15] showed in 20 patients with acute myocardial infarction who underwent MRI with a mean of 8 days after the acute event, that regional T2 abnormalities in 82% of patients correlated with the presence and location of thallium perfusion defects, thereby emphasizing the value of MRI tissue characterization in flow-deprived injured myocardial tissue. In a subsequent study, Krauss et al. [16] showed in 20 patients 7–14 days after acute myocardial infarction that MRI provided an accurate means of assessing infarct size and left ventricular function. Also Wisenberg et al. [17] demonstrated in 66 patients 3 weeks after acute infarction that infarct size could be determined very well by MRI. They also demonstrated that, in the 41 patients who had received acute streptokinase therapy, a significant reduction in MRI measured infarct size was observed compared to the patients without thrombolytic therapy. White et al. [18] showed in patients with a recent myocardial infarction a good comparison between MRI and two-dimensional echocardiography for demonstrating regional wall motion abnormalities. Moreover, they observed that the extent of regional wall thinning by MRI can be used to measure infarct size.

MRI is also capable for detecting long-term sequelae of myocardial infarction. Segmental wall thinning can be clearly defined and is indicative of a sustained myocardial infarction. The site of an old myocardial infarction may be recognized as a region with decreased signal intensity, suggesting that MRI can identify replacement of myocardial tissue by fibrous scar. Also complications of acute myocardial infarction including thrombo-embolism, ventricular aneurysm, ventricular septum perforation, and mitral regurgitation can be readily demonstrated by MRI. Early detection of complications by MRI is very important for guiding proper patient management.

Contrast agents

An intravenous contrast agent may improve the sensitivity and specificity of MRI and provide more direct and precise information concerning the state of myocardial perfusion. The objectives for a myocardial contrast agent for MRI are (1) to provide a method for assessing myocardial perfusion, (2) to delineate the area at risk for infarction after acute coronary artery occlusion, (3) to show more accurately the site and extent of an acute or chronic infarction by improving contrast between normal and infarcted myocardium, and (4) to distinguish between occlusive and reperfused myocardial infarctions [19].

The use of MRI contrast agents is based on the attempt to influence the tissue relaxation parameters T1 and T2 [20]. Certain substances enhance tissue relaxation because they can be induced by an external magnetic field to produce an additive magnetic field. The ratio of induced magnetization to that of the external magnetic field is termed the magnetic susceptibility of the substance. Paramagnetic contrast agents have positive magnetic susceptibilities because their induced magnetic fields are additive to that of the applied magnetic field. A compound that has negative magnetic susceptibility is termed a diamagnetic agent. Positive magnetic susceptibility causes increased magnetic flux in the vicinity of the compound and thus produces increased relaxation in the surrounding tissue. Paramagnetic substances have magnetic moments only in the presence of an external magnetic field. The magnitude of relaxation enhancement depends on the proximity of the paramagnetic agent to the nuclear spin. Paramagnetic agents are capable of realigning the bulk magnetic moment and therefore increasing T1 relaxation rates. They also produce local magnetic inhomogeneities and thus shorten T2 relaxation times as well.

The paramagnetic agents that have received the most attention are the paramagnetic lanthanide complexes, transition metals, and organic free radicals. In the lanthanide series, gadolinium and europium have the highest spin quantum numbers, and in the transition-metal group, manganese, chromium, and ferrum are the most potent relaxation agents. Because of toxicity, both the lanthanides and transition metals have been complexed with chelates.

The degree to which myocardial signal intensity reflects myocardial perfusion after intravenous administration of a paramagnetic contrast agent depends on multiple factors, including the affinity of the agent for myocardial cells, the rate of elimination of the agent from the blood stream, the degree of diffusion of the agent through the capillaries, and the volume of the interstitial space. Therefore, the accumulation of a contrast agent in myocardial tissue before and during the acquisition of MR images is affected not only by the rate of myocardial perfusion, but by additional factors. Further development of MRI techniques may allow rapid-sequence scanning in the future [21]. However, use of paramagnetic contrast agents for quantitative measurement of perfusion still may not be feasible because of problems in relating tissue MR signal intensity to precise tissue concentrations of the contrast agent. Therefore, most of the research into myocardial contrast agents for MRI has been directed towards a qualitative measure of relative tissue perfusion sufficient to distinguish ischemic from nonischemic myocardium.

Metal ions

The bivalent transition metal cation manganese was the first paramagnetic pharmaceutical studied as a potential myocardial contrast agent [22]. Manganese is actively taken up by viable myocardial cells and has a short half-life in the blood pool, resulting in a high myocardial-to-blood ratio. It is strongly paramagnetic by virtue of its five unpaired electrons, resulting in dramatic T1 shortening in normal myocardial tissue. Ischemic myocardial areas are well delineated as areas of low signal intensity relative to the brightly enhancing normal myocardium.

As with manganese, the free gadolinium ion (Gd^{3+}) is limited by serious toxicity [23]. However, the complexing of these cations with a variety of ligands greatly reduces their toxicity while significant paramagnetic, proton-relaxation, enhancement properties are retained. Toxic effects from a metal complex can arise from, (1) free metal ion, released by dissociation; (2) free ligand, which also arises from dissociation; and (3) the intact metal complex. The available toxicological data [24] point to the importance of metal complex dissociation as an important source of toxicity. Both metal ions and free ligands tend to be more toxic than metal chelates. The degree of toxicity of a metal chelate is related to its degree of dissociation in vivo before excretion. The coordination of ions to oxygen, nitrogen, or sulfur heteroatoms in macromolecules and membranes alters the dynamic equilibria necessary to sustain life. Gd^{3+}, for example, can bind to calcium (Ca^{2+}) binding sites, often with higher affinity owing to its greater charge/radius ratio. The toxicity of free ligands, which is less understood, can stem from the sequestration of essential metal ions such as Ca^{2+} in addition to 'organic' toxicity. The toxicity of intact metal complexes can stem from a wide variety of specific and nonspecific effects. A difference in osmolality between intracellular and extracellular compartments is established after injection of large quantities of the ionic complexes and appropriate counter ions. Water is drawn out of the cells as a result of the osmotic gradient, causing cellular and circulatory damage. Other possible mechanisms of chelate toxicity include enzyme inhibition, nonspecific protein conformational effects, or alteration of membrane potentials.

Gadolinium-DTPA

Gd^{3+}, gadolinium, a rare-earth element, possesses as a Gd^{3+} ion seven unpaired electrons and has powerful effects on T1 and T2. When administered as free ion it is toxic for the liver, spleen and bone marrow. Because no covalent bonds are formed with organic molecules, complexing with diethylene tria-

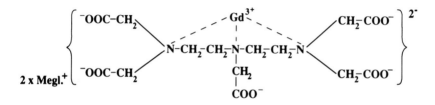

Figure 1. Structural formula of Gd-DTPA/Dimeglumine.

mine pentaacetic acid (DTPA) (Figure 1) is performed for detoxification [25]. The effectivity as a contrast agent depends on the properties of the DTPA molecule. The molecular weight is 600 daltons. In vitro, the signal shows a maximum at about 1.5 mmol/l in aqueous solution and at 0.6–0.7 mmol/l plasma, but these concentrations depend on the employed pulse sequence. Gd-DTPA has been applied intravenously (0.1–0.2 mmol/kg body weight) to enhance lesions within the heart, brain, liver, urinary tract, breast, etc. As with contrast-enhanced computed tomography, the effect of an extracellular contrast agent such as Gd-DTPA is not critically time-dependent for cerebral lesions. For other organs such as the heart, one should be aware of the pharmacokinetic behavior of the contrast agent. In dogs, following rapid intravenous injection (0.1 mmol/kg body weight in 10 ml within 1 minute) only minor hemodynamic effects of short duration have been noted. If the period taken for administration is 15 minutes, no effect is seen at all [26]. Using a rat model, the following data have been obtained [27]. Optimal dose for contrast is 0.1–0.5 mmol/kg body weight and the LD_{50} (interpolated dose at which 50% of the animals would die) is 10 mmol/kg body weight. In vivo the Gd-DTPA complex does not dissociate. Five minutes after intravenous administration, only 10% of the dose is still intravascularly located, which indicates a rapid spread, probably exclusively into the extracellular compartment. The intact blood-brain barrier is not passed. A fast renal excretion results in a 20 minutes half-life of the plasma concentration. After 3 hours the renal excretion amounts to more than 85% of the administrated dose. About 7.5% of the dose is lost with the faeces. One week after administration 0.3% of the dose is still present in the body, mainly in liver and renal tissue. In the rabbit, 5 minutes after administration the distribution is governed by organ perfusion, as shown by Strich et al. [28], using radioactive labeled Gd-DTPA.

In a review by Niendorf et al. [29] the tolerance and safety of Gd-DTPA at 0.1 and at 0.2 mmol/kg body weight in more than 13,000 patients appeared to be excellent. The overall incidence of adverse drug reactions after intravenous injection of Gd-DTPA was in the order of magnitude of 1% as determined in clinical trials in Europe and Japan. At a dose of 0.1 mmol/kg body weight slight, transient increases of serum levels of iron within normal range were seen in 20% to 30% of patients at 4 hours post-injection. Serum levels were back to baseline range at 24 hours post-injection. No clinical relevance is attributed to this side effect. Urticaria was reported in 0.14% and focal convulsion in 0.11%. The latter was found only in patients with respective history. Only recently one severe anaphylactoid reaction to Gd-DTPA was reported [30].

Detection of myocardial perfusion

A number of investigators has evaluated the utility of Gd-DTPA in detecting acute myocardial ischemia and infarction.

Experimental findings

Holman et al. [31] showed the potential of Gd-DTPA enhanced T1-weighted MRI to assess the presence and absence of myocardial perfusion after varying periods of ischemia with and without reperfusion in isolated, perfused rat hearts. After induction of ischemia unperfused subendocardial areas were detected on both MR images and Evans Blue stained slices. After reperfusion, the unperfused areas dissolved on both MR images and Evans Blue stained slices depending on duration and severity of ischemia. McNamara et al. [32] showed that Gd-DTPA enhanced MRI detected ischemia as early as 2 minutes after coronary artery occlusion. Six dogs were injected with Gd-DTPA immediately after left anterior descending occlusion. Images of the excised hearts revealed increased signal intensity in the ischemic myocardium compared to normally perfused zone due to the presence of the contrast media. This was most prominent in the relatively T2-weighted second spin-echo images (TE = 56 msec). Three dogs that were injected with normal saline showed no difference in signal intensity between normally perfused and ischemic myocardium. A study by Johnson et al. [33] showed that T1-weighted images (TE = 15 msec) acquired after coronary artery occlusion and infusion with Gd-DTPA demonstrated increased signal intensity in the normally perfused myocardium compared to the ischemic region. This was due to decreased tissue T1 in normally perfused tissue due to the presence of Gd-DTPA. They showed that there was a significant relationship between 1/T1 and regional myocardial flow when resting blood flow was less than or equal to 0.5 ml per minute per gram tissue. There was no significant relationship between tissue perfusion and 1/T1 when the myocardial flow was greater than 1 ml/min/g tissue. In a study by Miller et al. [34] in dogs, changes in myocardial flow following dipyridamole

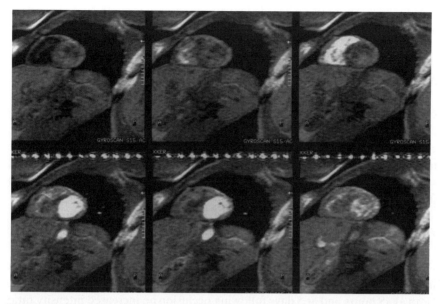

Figure 2. Series of six sequential short-axis images obtained by ultrafast magnetic resonance imaging. Following the baseline MRI scan (upper left panel), note the signal enhancement after administration of Gd-DTPA in the right ventricular cavity (upper middle and upper right panel), the pulmonary vasculature (lower left panel), the left ventricular cavity (lower left and lower middle panel), the aorta (lower left and lower middle panel), and the left ventricular myocardial wall (lower right panel). (Image provided by courtesy of F.P. van Rugge, Ref. [35].)

infusion were noted to correlate with changes in MRI signal intensity with contrast enhanced MRI using Gd-DTPA. A direct linear correlation between the increase in MRI signal intensity and the increase in myocardial blood flow as assessed by radioactive microspheres was shown with an r^2 value of 0.93.

Clinical results

Recently, ultrafast imaging sequences have been developed, requiring a fraction of a second for acquisition (subsecond imaging). In combination with rapid bolus injection of Gd-DTPA, this technique offers the potential to analyze cardiac first-pass and myocardial perfusion. In a study by Van Rugge et al. [35] progressively increasing signal intensities were observed in the right ventricular cavity, the left ventricular cavity and in the myocardial wall in seven normal subjects after bolus administration of Gd-DTPA (0.05 mmol/kg body weight). Gd-DTPA enhanced subsecond MRI offers temporal information of the first transit in the cardiac chambers and may provide useful clinical data for assessment of myocardial perfusion in patients with coronary artery disease (Figure 2).

Assessment of acute myocardial infarction

Conventional noncontrast MRI can identify acute myocardial infarction in the canine model and in humans, although investigators have reported difficulties, especially in the early phase of infarction. The difficulty in identifying acute myocardial infarction early after coronary occlusion with noncontrast MRI suggests a potential role for contrast enhanced MRI for diagnosing myocardial infarction with greater specificity.

Experimental findings

Rehr et al. [36] found in dog hearts that MRI using Gd-DTPA significant improved the visualization of infarcted tissue compared to nonenhanced MRI. Both at 48 hours and at 5 days following occlusion an increased intensity ratio (infarcted/noninfarcted myocardium) was observed in favor of Gd-DTPA.

Clinical results

Only few clinical studies with Gd-DTPA have been performed. Matheijssen et al. [37] compared the use of T2-weighted and T1-weighted Gd-DTPA enhanced MRI for the detection of acute myocardial infarction. It appeared that the detectability of acutely infarcted myocardial areas was similar at TE = 60 ms and at Gd-DTPA enhanced short TE (30 ms) MRI. However, image quality proved to be superior using the Gd-DTPA enhanced short TE technique. Eichstaedt et al. [38] showed in 26 patients with acute myocardial infarction that the 11 patients who were studied with Gd-DTPA 5–10 days after the acute event had a 70% average increase of signal intensity within zones of infarcted myocardium, while only a 20% increase of signal intensity in normal myocardial tissue was observed. The other 15 patients were imaged later in the course of infarction and did not show differences in intensity ratio between infarcted and normal tissue. Therefore, administration of Gd-DTPA resulted in significantly improved contrast between acutely infarcted and normal myocardium because of accumulation of Gd-DTPA in injured tissue. In a study by De Roos et al. [39] patients underwent MRI using Gd-DTPA 2–17 days after myocardial infarction. The signal intensity ratio of infarcted versus normal myocardium was significantly greater after Gd-DTPA administration than before Gd-DTPA, both by visual and computer-assessed analysis

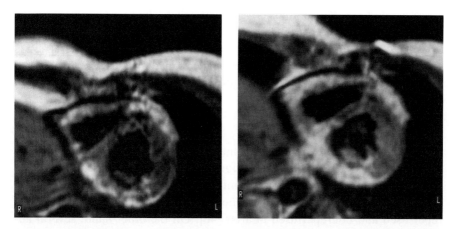

Figure 3. Cardiac MR images of a short-axis, midventricular section of a patient with transmural inferior wall infarction obtained 1 week after acute myocardial infarction, before (left) and 20 minutes after (right) administration of intravenous Gd-DTPA. Increased signal intensity of the inferior wall is visible after gadolinium enhancement. From Van Dijkman PRM, Van der Wall EE, De Roos A et al. Radiology 1991; 180: 147–51, reproduced by permission.

(Figure 3). This study was extended to 20 patients with acute myocardial infarction by Van Dijkman et al. [40] and showed maximal contrast 20–25 minutes after administration of Gd-DTPA. Moreover, a good correlation between electrocardiographic infarct site and local increase of signal intensity based on region of interest analysis was observed. In 27 patients, of whom 10 were studied within 72 hours after myocardial infarction, Van der Wall et al. [41] showed that signal intensity of Gd-DTPA was significantly increased in the infarcted areas of the 17 patients who were studied more than 72 hours after the acute onset, indicating increased accumulation of Gd-DTPA in a more advanced stage of the disease process. Nishimura et al. [42] studied 17 patients with gadolinium-enhanced MRI at an average of 5, 12, 30, and 90 days after acute myocardial infarction. At these four points in time, the percentage of patients with increased signal intensity increased to 94% (day 12) and then gradually decreased to 38%. We also assessed the value of gadolinium enhancement to enable detection of infarcted myocardium at longer time intervals after acute myocardial infarction in 84 patients [43]. After Gd-DTPA administration the signal intensity ratio of infarcted and normal myocardium was abnormally increased in 82% of MR examinations of patients imaged within 1 week, in 62% of patients imaged between 1 and 3 weeks, in 58% in patients imaged between 3 and 6 weeks and only in 12% of patients imaged more than 6 weeks after the acute event.

Assessment of reperfused infarcts and myocardial salvage

With the current efforts to decrease infarct size with thrombolytic therapy, it is important that noninvasive techniques be developed to assess the presence of coronary reperfusion in myocardial salvage.

Experimental findings

MRI has shown promise in this role and several ex vivo studies have shown an increase in T2 values and increased signal intensity in reperfused myocardial infarcts compared to nonreperfused infarcts [44, 45]. However, in an in vivo canine study, unenhanced MRI was not able to reliably distinguish between reperfused and nonreperfused infarcts [46]. On the other hand, several authors [45, 47] demonstrated that intravenous administration of Gd-DTPA significant improved the contrast between infarcted and normal myocardium in dogs that had undergone 1 hour [45] or 2 hours [47] of coronary occlusion followed by reperfusion. Schaefer et al. [48] showed in dogs that the area of enhanced myocardium after ischemia and reperfusion following Gd-DTPA administration correlated with the area of jeopardized myocardium. All animals given Gd-DTPA demonstrated increased signal intensity in reperfused regions. The extent of the enhanced region on MRI corresponded well with the bed at risk determined anatomically using a dye perfusion technique. McNamara et al. [49] found that irreversible injury in a canine model of ischemia and reperfusion resulted in marked contrast enhancement following Gd-DTPA, but in dogs with reversible injury no difference in signal intensity or in relaxation times between normally perfused and ischemic myocardium following reperfusion was observed.

Clinical results

On the basis of differences in signal intensity ratios the gadolinium-enhanced MR images do not enable sufficient distinction between patients treated with and those treated without streptokinase [41, 43]. However, Van Rossum et al. [50] studied the early dynamics of contrast enhancement using Gd-DTPA in 18 patients with acute myocardial infarction and they observed a significant difference in signal intensity ratio between patients with occluded infarct-related coronary arteries without collateral filling and patients with reperfused infarct vessels or occluded vessels with collateral supply on MR images obtained early (within 6–8 minutes) after injection of Gd-DTPA (1.14 ± 0.05 versus 1.29 ± 0.10, $p < 0.02$). Furthermore, it has been observed that the morphological appearance of contrast enhancement by Gd-DTPA may provide some clues as to the presence or absence of reperfusion; reperfusion goes along with a homogeneous aspect, while lack of reperfusion may be visualized as a heterogeneous enhancement of contrast [41, 51]. More recently, we assessed acute myocardial infarct size after thrombolytic therapy using Gd-DTPA enhanced MRI in 23 patients [52]. The extent of areas with enhanced signal intensity was measured by planimetry in each slice, and summed for all eight slices. The total area with contrast enhancement was expressed as percentage of the total left ventricular muscle. At 1 week after infarction patients treated with streptokinase had an infarct size of $9.8 \pm 5.5\%$, while the patients without streptokinase treatment had an infarct size of $14.5 \pm 4.2\%$ ($p = 0.052$). This favorable trend in the streptokinase-treated group was a fortiori present in the patients who underwent MRI studies at 4 weeks after the acute event. Infarct size was $9.6 \pm 3.1\%$ in the treated group versus $14.7 \pm 4.9\%$ in the patients without streptokinase treatment ($p < 0.03$) [53].

Other potential contrast agents

Several contrast agents with more prolonged intravascular retention show promise for myocardial imaging. Gd-DTPA has been covalently bound to albumin to produce an agent that remains largely confined within the intravascular space during the time required for MRI. The large size of this molecule (molecular weight 92,000 daltons) slows the rate of molecular rotation resulting in a correlation time that more closely approximates the Larmor frequency. This results in a marked increase in the effectiveness of proton relaxation per gadolinium group [54]. Schmiedl et al. [55] investigated the use of albumin-(Gd-DTPA) in a rat model in which MRI was performed at 6–8 hours after coronary artery occlusion. They demonstrated significantly increased contrast between normal and infarcted myocardium on T1-weighted images, which persisted without change from 5 to 60 minutes after administration. These findings indicate an accumulation of albumin-(Gd-DTPA) in the infarct zone by 6–8 hours after coronary occlusion, suggesting delivery of the contrast agent to the infarcted area via collateral vessels in this experimental model. The accumulation of this contrast medium reflects blood volume in the tissue rather than blood flow; the greater enhancement of infarcted compared with normal myocardium is hypothesized to be due to microvascular vasodilatation and capillary leakage of contrast agent within the infarcted area [55]. Another macromolecular intravascular contrast agent, Gd-DTPA poly-lysine, has recently been developed. The Gd-DTPA polylysine complex is composed of amino group 312 and gadolinium 60 per molecule, with a molecular weight of 4,000–5,000 daltons. Saeed et al. [56] evaluated Gd-DTPA

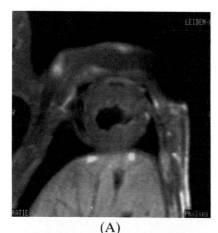

(A)

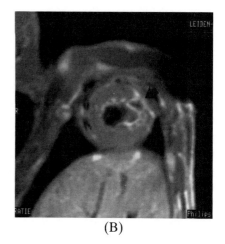

(B)

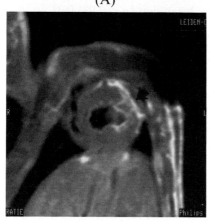

(C)

Figure 4. In vivo cardiac MR images of a short-axis section of a pig with occlusion of a diagonal branch, obtained 1 week after surgery, before (A), 5 minutes after (B) and 30 minutes after (C) administration of intravenous Gd-DTPA. Only after gadolinium enhancement, infarcted myocardium is clearly demarcated (arrow in (B): dark area surrounded by rim with high signal intensity; arrow in (C): enhanced intensity of the core surrounded by rim with high signal intensity).

polylysine in acute, subacute and chronic myocardial infarctions in rats. In acute and subacute infarctions, Gd-DTPA polylysine produced greater enhancement (over 60 minutes) in the peri-infarction zone than in the normal or infarcted myocardium. In chronic infarction, Gd-DTPA polylysine had no discernible effect on the signal intensity of the central infarction zone. The same pattern of early infarct delineation was otherwise observed by Van Dijkman et al. [57] after administration of Gd-DTPA in pigs with acute myocardial infarction (Figures 4–6). No studies of the metabolism, toxicity, and elimination of albumin-(Gd-DTPA) and Gd-DTPA polylysine have been published.

Additional paramagnetic agents are being developed and tested that are designed to have some degree of specificity for myocardial cells [19]. Gadolini-

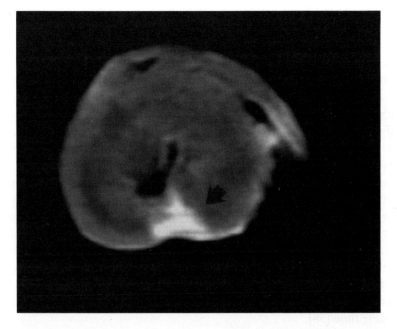

Figure 5. T2-weighted MRI scan of the excised heart of the same animal of Figure 4. The infarcted area is visible as an area with enhanced signal intensity (arrow).

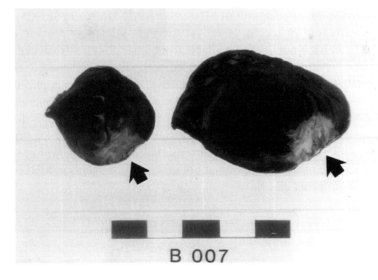

Figure 6. Two short axis slices of the heart of the same animal of Figure 4 stained with Nitroblue tetrazolium with occlusion of a diagonal branch. The infarcted myocardium is unstained (arrow).

um has been complexed with various phosphonates and related compounds for the purpose of creating an agent with an affinity for myocardium.

Another approach to differential enhancement of normal and ischemic myocardium is to highlight the ischemic region by using magnetic susceptibility to diminish or eliminate signal intensity of the normal myocardial region. The MR contrast agent dysprosium DTPA, causes such a differential magnetic susceptibility effect, and this effect persists for nearly 60 minutes. After acute coronary occlusion, the dysprosium DTPA erases the signal intensity of the normally perfused myocardium and shows the ischemic area as a region of high signal intensity [19].

The costs of the development of new paramagnetic contrast agents are relatively high but there appear to be major opportunities to increase value. Even without providing the equivalent of coronary angiography, a single contrast-enhanced MR examination that quantitatively evaluated cardiac anatomy, function and myocardial perfusion would be cost-effective. Such an examination would reduce the use of ultrasound, radionuclide scanning and cine-computed tomography and could relegate coronary angiography to a setting where an interventional procedure was also likely to be performed at the same time [58].

Conclusion

The cardiovascular applications of MRI in coronary artery disease have considerably increased in recent years. At present, MRI may provide useful information which is not readily available from other noninvasive conventional modalities. Although MRI can be used without contrast media, the information it generates in coronary artery disease is increased by application of paramagnetic contrast agents. Most clinical experience has been obtained with Gd-DTPA, which can be safely used in patients with ischemic heart disease. Future technical developments including faster imaging sequences, automatic quantitation algorithms, and three-dimensional angiography, will automatically expand the use and development of new contrast agents in MRI for the investigation of heart disease.

References

1. Tscholakoff D, Higgins CB, McNamara MT, Derugin N. Early-phase myocardial infarction: evaluation by MR imaging. Radiology 1986; 159: 667–2.
2. Ratner AV, Okada RD, Newell JB, Pohost GM. The relationship between proton nuclear

magnetic resonance relaxation parameters and myocardial perfusion with acute coronary arterial occlusion and reperfusion. Circulation 1985; 71: 823–8.

3. Pflugfelder PW, Wisenberg G, Prato FS, Carroll SE, Turner KL. Early detection of canine myocardial infarction by magnetic resonance imaging in vivo. Circulation 1985; 71: 587–94.

4. Tscholakoff D, Higgins CB, Sechtem U, Caputo G, Derugin N. MRI of reperfused myocardial infarct in dogs. AJR Am J Roentgenol 1986; 146: 925–30.

5. Bouchard A, Reeves RC, Cranney G, Bishop SO, Pohost GM, Bischoff P. Assessment of myocardial infarct size by means of T2-weighted ^{1}H nuclear magnetic resonance imaging. Am Heart J 1989; 117: 281–9.

6. Wisenberg G, Prato FS, Carroll SE, Turner KL, Marshall T. Serial nuclear magnetic resonance imaging of acute myocardial infarction with and without reperfusion. Am Heart J 1988; 115: 510–8.

7. Caputo GR, Sechtem U, Tscholakoff D, Higgins CB. Measurements of myocardial infarct size at early and late time intervals using MR imaging: an experimental study in dogs. AJR Am J Roentgenol 1987; 149: 237–43.

8. McNamara MT, Higgins CB, Schechtmann N et al. Detection and characterization of acute myocardial infarction in man with the use of gated magnetic resonance. Circulation 1985; 71: 717–24.

9. Johnston DL, Thompson RC, Liu P et al. Magnetic resonance imaging during acute myocardial infarction. Am J Cardiol 1986; 57: 1059–65.

10. Fisher MR, McNamara MT, Higgins CB. Acute myocardial infarction: MR evaluation in 29 patients. AJR Am J Roentgenol 1987; 148: 247–51.

11. Ahmad M, Johnson RF Jr, Fawcett HD, Schreibert MH. Magnetic resonance imaging in patients with unstable angina: comparison with acute myocardial infarction and normals. Magn Reson Imaging 1988; 6: 527–34.

12. Been M, Smith MA, Ridgeway JP et al. Characterisation of acute myocardial infarction by gated magnetic resonance imaging. Lancet 1985; 2: 348–50.

13. Been M, Smith MA, Ridgeway JP et al. Serial changes in the T1 magnetic relaxation parameter after myocardial inafarction in man. Br Heart J 1988; 59: 1–8.

14. Filipchuk NG, Peshock RM, Malloy GR et al. Detection and localization of recent myocardial infarction by magnetic resonance imaging. Am J Cardiol 1986; 58: 214–9.

15. Krauss XH, Van der Wall EE, Doornbos J et al. The value of nuclear magnetic resonance imaging in patients with a recent myocardial infarction: comparison with planar thallium-201 scintigraphy. Cardiovasc Intervent Radiol 1989; 12: 119–24.

16. Krauss XH, Van der Wall EE, Van der Laarse A et al. Follow-up of regional myocardial T2 relaxation times in patients with myocardial infarction evaluated with magnetic resonance imaging. Eur J Radiol 1990; 11: 110–9.

17. Wisenberg G, Finnie KJ, Jablonsky G, Kostuk WJ, Marshall T. Nuclear magnetic resonance and radionuclide angiographic assessment of acute myocardial infarction in a randomized trial of intravenous streptokinase. Am J Cardiol 1988; 62: 1011–6.

18. White RD, Cassidy MM, Melvin MD et al. Segmental evaluation of left ventricular wall motion after myocardial infarction: magnetic resonance imaging versus echocardiography. Am Heart J 1988; 115: 166–75.

19. Brown JJ, Higgins CB. Myocardial paramagnetic contrast agents for MR imaging. AJR Am J Roentgenol 1988; 151: 865–72.

20. Young SW. Magnetic resonance imaging: basic principles. 2nd ed. New York: Raven Press, 1988: 98–100.

21. Atkinson DJ, Burstein D, Edelman RR. First-pass cardiac perfusion: evaluation with ultra-fast MR imaging. Radiology 1990; 174: 757–62.

22. Goldman MR, Brady TJ, Pykett IL et al. Quantification of experimental myocardial infarction using nuclear magnetic resonance imaging and paramagnetic ion contrast enhancement in excised canine hearts. Circulation 1982; 66: 1012–6.
23. Arvelo P. Toxicity of rare-earths. Prog Pharmacol 1979; 2: 262–8.
24. Lauffer RB. Magnetic resonance contrast media: principles and progress. Magn Reson Q 1990; 6: 65–84.
25. Engelstad BL, Wolf GL. Contrast agents. In: Stark DD, Bradley WG Jr, editors. Magnetic resonance imaging. St. Louis: Mosby, 1988: 161–81.
26. Slutsky RA, Peterson T, Strich G, Brown JJ. Hemodynamic effects of rapid and slow infusions of manganese chloride and gadolinium-DTPA in dogs. Radiology 1985; 154: 733–5.
27. Brasch RC, Weinmann HJ, Wesbey GE. Contrast-enhanced NMR imaging: animal studies using gadolinium-DTPA complex. AJR Am J Roentgenol 1984; 142: 625–30.
28. Strich G, Hagan PL, Gerber KH, Slutsky RA. Tissue distribution and magnetic resonance spin lattice relaxation effects of gadolinium-DTPA. Radiology 1985; 154: 723–6.
29. Niendorf HP, Dinger JC, Haustein J, Cornelius I, Alhassan A, Clauss W. Tolerance data of Gd-DTPA: a review. Eur J Radiol 1991; 13: 15–20.
30. Weiss KL, Jhaveri HS. Severe anaphylactoid reaction after IV Gd-DTPA [abstract]. Magn Reson Imaging 1990; 8 suppl 1: 81.
31. Holman ER, Van Dijkman PRM, Van der Wall EE et al. Assessment of myocardial perfusion during ischemia and reperfusion in isolated rat hearts using Gadolinium-DTPA enhanced magnetic resonance imaging. Coronary Artery Dis 1991; 2: 789–98.
32. McNamara MT, Higgins CB, Ehman RL, Revel D, Sievers R, Brasch RC. Acute myocardial ischemia: magnetic resonance contrast enhancement with gadolinium-DTPA. Radiology 1984; 153: 157–63.
33. Johnston DL, Liu P, Lauffer RB et al. Use of gadolinium-DTPA as a myocardial perfusion agent: potential applications and limitations for magnetic resonance imaging. J Nucl Med 1987; 28: 871–7.
34. Miller DD, Holmvang G, Gill JB et al. MRI detection of myocardial perfusion changes by gadolinium-DTPA infusion during dipyridamole hyperemia. Magn Reson Med 1989; 10: 246–55.
35. Van Rugge FP, Boreel JJ, Van der Wall EE et al. Assessment of cardiac first-pass and myocardial perfusion in normal subjects using Gadolinium-DTPA enhanced subsecond magnetic resonance imaging. J Comput Assist Tomogr 1991; 15: 959–65.
36. Rehr RB, Peshock RM, Malloy CR et al. Improved in vivo magnetic resonance imaging of acute myocardial infarction after intravenous paramagnetic contrast agent administration. Am J Cardiol 1986; 57: 864–8.
37. Matheijssen NAA, De Roos A, Van der Wall EE et al. Acute myocardial infarction: comparison of T2-weighted and T1-weighted gadolinium-DTPA enhanced MR imaging. Magn Reson Med 1991; 17: 460–9.
38. Eichstaedt HW, Felix R, Dougherty FC, Langer M, Rusch W, Schmutzler H. Magnetic resonance imaging (MRI) in different stages of myocardial infarction using the contrast agent gadolinium-DTPA. Clin Cardiol 1986; 9: 527–35.
39. De Roos A, Doornbos J, Van der Wall EE, Van Voorthuisen AE. MR imaging of acute myocardial infarction: value of Gd-DTPA. AJR Am J Roentgenol 1988; 150: 531–4.
40. Van Dijkman PRM, Doornbos J, De Roos A et al. Improved detection of acute myocardial infarction by magnetic resonance imaging using gadolinium-DTPA. Int J Card Imaging 1989; 5: 1–8.
41. Van der Wall EE, Van Dijkman PRM, De Roos A et al. Diagnostic significance of gadolini-

um-DTPA (diethylenetriamine penta-acetic acid) enhanced magnetic resonance imaging in thrombolytic therapy for acute myocardial infarction: its potential in assessing reperfusion. Br Heart J 1990; 63: 12–7.

42. Nishimura T, Kobayashi H, Ohara Y et al. Serial assessment of myocardial infarction by using gated MR imaging and Gd-DTPA. AJR Am J Roentgenol 1989; 153: 715–20.

43. Van Dijkman PRM, Van der Wall EE, De Roos A et al. Acute, subacute and chronic myocardial infarction: quantitative analysis of gadolinium-enhanced MR images. Radiology 1991; 180: 147–51.

44. Johnston DL, Brady TJ, Ratner AV et al. Assessment of myocardial ischemia with proton magnetic resonance: effects of three hour coronary occlusion with and without reperfusion. Circulation 1985; 71: 595–601.

45. Tscholakoff D, Higgins CB, Sechtem U, McNamara MT. Occlusive and reperfused myocardial infarcts: effect of Gd-DTPA on ECG-gated MR imaging. Radiology 1986; 160: 515–9.

46. Aisen AM, Buda AJ, Zotz RJ, Buckwalter KA. Visualization of myocardial infarction and subsequent coronary reperfusion with MRI using a dog model. Magn Reson Imaging 1987; 5: 399–404.

47. Peshock RM, Malloy CR, Buja LM, Nunnally RL, Parkey RW, Willerson JT. Magnetic resonance imaging of acute myocardial infarction: gadolinium diethylenetriamine pentaacetic acid as a marker of reperfusion. Circulation 1986; 74: 1434–40.

48. Schaefer S, Malloy CR, Katz J et al. Gadolinium-DTPA enhanced nuclear magnetic resonance imaging of reperfused myocardium: identification of the myocardial bed at risk. J Am Coll Cardiol 1988; 12: 1064–72.

49. McNamara MT, Tscholakoff D, Revel D et al. Differentiation of reversible and irreversible myocardial injury by MR imaging with and without gadolinium-DTPA. Radiology 1986; 158: 765–9.

50. Van Rossum AC, Visser FC, Van Eenige MJ et al. Value of gadolinium-diethylene-triamine pentaacetic acid dynamics in magnetic resonance imaging of acute myocardial infarction with occluded and reperfused coronary arteries after thrombolysis. Am J Cardiol 1990; 65: 845–51.

51. De Roos A, Van Rossum AC, Van der Wall EE et al. Reperfused and nonreperfused myocardial infarction: diagnostic potential of Gd-DTPA-enhanced MR imaging. Radiology 1989; 172: 717–20.

52. De Roos A, Matheijssen NAA, Doornbos J, Van Dijkman PRM, Van Voorthuisen AE, Van der Wall EE. Myocardial infarct size after reperfusion therapy: assessment with Gd-DTPA-enhanced MR imaging. Radiology 1990; 176: 517–21.

53. Van Dijkman PRM, De Roos A, Van der Wall EE et al. Reduction of infarct size after thrombolytic therapy by Gadolinium-DTPA enhanced magnetic resonance imaging. In: Schmidt HA, Van der Schoot JB, editors. Nuclear medicine: the state of the art of nuclear medicine in Europe. Stuttgart: Schattauer, 1991: 68–70.

54. Schmiedl U, Ogan MD, Moseley ME, Brasch RC. Comparison of the contrast-enhancing properties of albumin-(Gd-DTPA) and Gd-DTPA at 2.0 T: an experimental study in rats. AJR Am J Roentgenol 1986; 147: 1263–70.

55. Schmiedl U, Moseley ME, Sievers R et al. Magnetic resonance imaging of myocardial infarction using albumin-(Gd-DTPA), a macromolecular blood-volume contrast agent in a rat model. Invest Radiol 1987; 22: 713–21.

56. Saeed M, Wendland MF, Masui T et al. Myocardial infarction: assessment with an intravascular MR contrast medium. Radiology 1991; 180: 153–60.

57. Van Dijkman PRM, Höld KM, Van der Laarse A et al. Sequential analysis of infarcted and

normal myocardium in pigs using in vivo Gadolinium-DTPA enhanced magnetic resonance imaging. Magn Reson Imaging (In press).

58. Wolf GL. Role of magnetic resonance contrast agents in cardiac imaging. Am J Cardiol 1990; 66: 59F–62F.

SECTION TWO

Metabolism

16. Assessment of myocardial metabolism in vivo: a biochemist's view

ARNOUD VAN DER LAARSE

Summary

Due to extensive biochemical investigations on myocardial tissue during the last 50 years and the recent development of techniques (positron emission tomography, magnetic resonance imaging, magnetic resonance spectroscopy, single photon emission computed tomography) to visualize and/or quantify biochemical parameters in the human heart in vivo, the era of metabolic imaging has begun. In addition to imaging of metabolic substrates and intermediates (palmitate, glucose, ATP, phosphocreatine) future contributions regarding receptor-effector-second messenger functions will augment our understanding of normal myocardial metabolism and its regulation, but particularly of their abnormalities in cardiac diseases.

Introduction

In clinical cardiology, diagnostic investigation of *cardiac contractile function* is performed routinely, providing detailed temporal and regional information about wall motion. Functional assessment using contrast angiography, M-mode and two-dimensional echocardiography, and radionuclide blood pool scanning has been, since the mid seventees, supplemented with *regional perfusion imaging*. First with thallium-201, and later with technetium-99 m labeled hexakis 2-methoxyisobutyl isonitrile and related radiolabeled perfusion markers, abnormalities considering regional myocardial perfusion are visualized. Especially with single photon emission computed tomography,

Ernst E. van der Wall et al. (eds), What's new in cardiac imaging?, 223–228.
© *1992 Kluwer Academic Publishers. Printed in the Netherlands.*

great spatial resolution is achieved. Recently, also magnetic resonance imaging with paramagnetic contrast agents like gadolinium-DTPA, ultrafast computed tomography, and positron emission tomography using rubidium-82, nitrogen-13 labeled ammonia and oxygen-15 labeled water provide facilities to quantify regional myocardial blood flow.

As cardiac function is driven by energy from metabolic processes, and perfusion is essential to maintain adequate intensity of metabolism, metabolic information is crucial in the understanding of several pathological conditions of the heart, present either globally or regionally. Now that great technical achievements have made possible the construction of equipment to 'image' certain aspects of cardiac metabolism, *metabolic imaging* is receiving tremendous interest.

Rationale for metabolic imaging

The question 'What biochemical product or process can we measure' is dealt with in detail in the following chapters about scintigraphy with radiolabeled fatty acids, and about positron emission tomography using radiolabeled palmitate, acetate, and glucose.

From the standpoint of a biochemist, another question can be raised: 'What do we want to know as myocardial biochemistry is concerned in relation to cardiac pathophysiology'. Before I address that question, I would like to distinguish four major issues in myocardial biochemistry:

(1) *Energy production and conservation.* Energy liberated from metabolic pathways is invested in the phosphorylation of ADP to ATP. Normally, $>95\%$ of energy production and conservation takes place in the mitochondria of the myocyte.

(2) *Sarcomere shortening.* Shortening of sarcomeres includes actin-myosin interaction, requiring ATP and Ca^{2+}-ions.

(3) *Membranes and membrane processes.* These are pertinent to ionic homeostasis (particularly Na^+-, K^+-, and Ca^{2+}-ions), excitation-contraction coupling, and receptor-effector-second messenger actions.

(4) *Synthesis and degradation of proteins.* Protein synthesis takes place at the ribosomes in the cytoplasm, directed by substances (mRNA) produced in the nucleus, and protein degradation takes place in the lysosomes. Soon after birth myocyte proliferation comes to a stop and each myocyte has to last for a lifetime. Due to a sustained process of protein turnover, the myocyte renews itself continuously.

In a biochemical investigation of a heart with a certain pathologic abnormality, the metabolic product or process to be measured should be chosen such that the particular abnormality is addressed specifically, either by localizing it or by quantifying it.

In an arbitrarily chosen number of cardiac diseases, a discussion on the 'metabolic marker of choice' is presented below, which is sometimes more theoretical than practical.

Coronary artery disease

Three important issues concerning coronary heart disease have attracted much attention lately: *stunning* which is encountered during reperfusion after ischemia, remaining *viable myocytes* in acutely or recently infarcted segments, and *hibernation* which is a state of atrophic survival of myocytes in scarred myocardium.

Stunned myocardium

The process of stunning myocardial tissue is, by definition, visualized by time-dependent improvement of regional wall motion after reperfusion following a period of ischemia. To date, no deficiencies have been reported with respect to the ATP-generating capacity of the stunned myocardium, nor to the ATP and phosphocreatine levels themselves [1]. One of the key features of stunned myocardium disclosed so far is the ability to perform (almost) normally if positive inotropic stimuli are applied [2]. Therefore, metabolic imaging should be directed at visualization of cytoplasmic Ca^{2+}-ion concentration, revealing information of the aberrant action of actin-myosin interaction (diminished affinity to Ca^{2+}) or of the aberrant sarcoplasmic reticulum function, with and without a positive inotropic intervention. In isolated cells and in isolated hearts, two methodologies are currently used to measure intracellular Ca^{2+}-ion concentration, fluorimetry using fluorescent calcium indicators, such as Fura-2 and Indo-1 [3], and magnetic resonance spectroscopy using fluorine-19 labeled calciumchelators, such as BAPTA [4].

Remaining viable tissue in acutely infarcted segments

Assessment of the presence and quantity of viable tissue in acutely or recently infarcted segments is important in predicting the benefit of revascularization procedures. Especially, fluorine-18 labeled 2-deoxyglucose imaging with positron emission tomography has been shown to be extremely valuable in this respect, as surviving myocytes reveal increased glycolytic flux and decreased β-oxidation rates [5]. Therefore, lactate imaging is also advocated, although only animal studies have been reported [6]. As it is expected that surviving myocytes have an increased intracellular Na$^+$-ion concentration, sodium imaging may be of value. The use of shift reagents, such as dysprosium complexed to a carrier (bis-tripolyphosphate, TTHA or DOTP) enables discrimination between extracellular and intracellular Na$^+$ pools. Another approach is the use of multiple quantum filter techniques which have resulted in sodium images of dog hearts before and after a period of ischemia [7].

Hibernating myocytes

Recent studies have shown that the morphological hallmark of hibernating myocytes surrounded by scar tissue is dystrophy characterized by loss of sarcomeres, loss of mitochondria, and accumulation of glycogen [8]. It is expected that these myocytes are completely dependent on glucose utilization and that cellular oxygen consumption is low. Until the characterization of hibernating myocytes is described in more detail, imaging of glucose uptake seems the only biochemical way to visualize these cells.

Cardiomyopathies

Of the different forms of cardiomyopathies known, the hypertrophic cardiomyopathy and the dilated cardiomyopathy are regularly seen in clinical cardiology. The metabolic derangement(s) is (are) unknown, but from a number of studies, several suggestions as to what to measure can be given.

Hypertrophic cardiomyopathy

Experimental and clinical evidence has made clear that hypertrophied hearts have a diminished tolerance to ischemia. One of the responsible factors is a diminished coronary reserve, particularly in the subendocardial regions of the left ventricle [9]. Biochemical studies have revealed an increased glycolytic capacity [10], a diminished β-oxidation [11], and a weakened coupling between ATP consumption and ATP production [12]. Therefore, metabolic imaging of these hearts should include glucose imaging in combination with fatty acid (e.g. palmitate) imaging, pH imaging, and measurement of phosphocreatine to βATP ratios, especially during a stress test, for instance before, during, and after dobutamine infusion.

Since cardiac hypertrophy in experimental animals was associated with an increased rate of myocardial protein synthesis [13], it would be interesting to investigate the uptake of labeled amino acids by the hearts of patients with different types of cardiac hypertrophy, such as hypertrophic cardiomyopathy.

Dilated cardiomyopathy

If left ventricular wall thickness does not adequately compensate for increased wall stress, myocardial oxygen consumption increases and thereby produces exhaustion of reserve capacities of the myocardium. Whether coronary heart disease or an idiopathic origin is the underlying cause of the heart failure, myocardial ischemia is present or nearby in the majority of the patients presenting with dilated cardiomyopathy in the failing stage. Myocardial phosphocreatine to βATP ratios will therefore be depressed. Due to the 'stressed' nature of this disease, abnormalities as to the adrenoceptor density and/or affinity is expected. Imaging with radiolabeled metaiodobenzylguanidine (MIBG) has already shown myocardial adrenergic nervous system disintegrity in patients with idiopathic dilated cardiomyopathy [14].

Conclusion

Due to extensive biochemical investigations on myocardial tissue during the last 50 years and the recent development of techniques (positron emission tomography, magnetic resonance imaging, magnetic resonance spectroscopy, single photon emission computed tomography) to visualize and/or quantify biochemical parameters in the human heart in vivo, the era of metabolic imaging has begun. This interesting extension of diagnostic modalities will gain tremendous impact, especially if temporal (time-dependent processes) and/or spatial (well-defined regions) resolution are improved even more.

Finally, in addition to imaging of metabolic substrates and intermediates (palmitate, glucose, ATP, phosphocreatine), future contributions regarding receptor-effector-second messenger functions will augment our understanding of normal myocardial metabolism and its regulation, but particularly of their abnormalities in cardiac diseases.

References

1. Bolli R. Mechanism of myocardial 'stunning'. Circulation 1990; 82: 723–38.
2. Ito BR, Tate H, Kobayashi M, Schaper W. Reversibly injured, postischemic canine myocardium retains normal contractile reserve. Circ Res 1987; 61: 834–46.

3. Moore EDW, Becker PL, Fogarty KE, Williams DA, Fay FS. Ca^{2+} imaging in single living cells: theoretical and practical issues. Cell Calcium 1990; 11: 157–79.

4. Kusuoka H, Koretsune Y, Chacko VP, Weisfeldt ML, Marban E. Excitation-contraction coupling in postischemic myocardium. Does failure of activator Ca^{2+} transients underlie stunning? Circ Res 1990; 66: 1268–76.

5. Schelbert HR, Buxton D. Insights into coronary artery disease from metabolic imaging. Circulation 1988; 78: 496–505.

6. Keller AM, Sorce DJ, Sciacca RR, Barr ML, Cannon PJ. Very rapid lactate measurement in ischemic perfused hearts using ^1H MRS continuous negative echo acquisition during steady-state frequency selective excitation. Magn Reson Med 1988; 7: 65–78.

7. Cannon PJ, Maudsley AA, Hilal SK, Simon HE, Cassidy F. Sodium nuclear magnetic resonance imaging of myocardial tissue of dogs after coronary artery occlusion and reperfusion. J Am Coll Cardiol 1986; 7: 573–9.

8. Borgers M. Morphology of human hibernating myocardium [abstract]. J Mol Cell Cardiol 1991; 23 (suppl V): S12.

9. Vatner SF, Shannon R, Hittinger L. Reduced subendocardial coronary reserve. A potential mechanism for impaired diastolic function in the hypertrophied and failing heart. Circulation 1990; 81 (suppl III): III-8–III-14.

10. Anderson PG, Allard MF, Thomas GD, Bishop SP, Digerness SB. Increased ischemic injury but decreased hypoxic injury in hypertrophied rat hearts. Circ Res 1990; 67: 948–59.

11. Kagaya Y, Kanno Y, Takeyama D et al. Effects of long-term pressure overload on regional myocardial glucose and free fatty acid uptake in rats. A quantitative autoradiographic study. Circulation 1990; 81: 1353–61.

12. Miller DD, Walsh RA. In vivo phosphorus-31 NMR spectroscopy of abnormal myocardial high-energy phosphate metabolism during cardiac stress in hypertensive-hypertrophied non-human primates. Int J Card Imag 1990/91; 6: 57–70.

13. Parmacek MS, Magid LM, Lesch M, Decker RS, Samarel AM. Cardiac protein synthesis and degradation during thyroxine-induced left ventricular hypertrophy. Am J Physiol 1986; 251: C727–36.

14. Schofer J, Spielmann R, Schuchert A et al. Iodine-123 metaiodobenzylguanidine scintigraphy. A noninvasive method to demonstrate myocardial adrenergic nervous system disintegrity in patients with idiopathic dilated cardiomyopathy. J Am Coll Cardiol 1988; 12: 1252–8.

17. Myocardial metabolic imaging with iodine-123 fatty acids

FRANS C. VISSER, GERRIT W. SLOOF and FURN F. KNAPP

Introduction

The maintainance of a normal metabolism is most important for the heart because it forms the basis for contractile function. Although the clinician is accustomed to evaluating symptoms and derangement of pump function during manifestations of disease, often an appreciation is lacking that abnormalities in metabolism precede functional derangements. For example, one of the first problems in ischemia is the rapid depletion of high-energy phosphates, which are necessary to maintain contraction. On the other hand, chronic increased demand, which occurs with hypertrophy, may lead to metabolic changes. These considerations indicate that it is important to study myocardial metabolism in patients with cardiac disease.

Of all the possible cardiac nutrients, free fatty acids contribute most under physiological conditions to the energy production of the heart. In contrast, during ischemia, oxidation of fatty acids is reduced or stopped. Therefore, fatty acids radiolabeled with an appropriate radioisotope can be used to study a major aspect of cardiac metabolism.

For patient studies, free fatty acids radiolabeled with carbon-11 (C-11) and iodine-123 (I-123) have been developed. Carbon-11-labeled fatty acids in conjunction with positron emission tomography (PET) are discussed in Chapter 18.

The advantage of using radioiodinated fatty acids in comparison to the positron emitters, is that radioiodide can be traced with conventional Anger cameras, and it is therefore potentially applicable in routine nuclear medicine. Iodine-123 decays with the emission of a photon peak with an energy of 159

Ernst E. van der Wall et al. (eds), What's new in cardiac imaging?, 229–247.
© *1992 Kluwer Academic Publishers. Printed in the Netherlands.*

keV which is almost optimal for gamma camera detection. The disadvantage of limited in-depth resolution in planar fatty acid imaging can be partially overcome using single photon emission computerized tomographic (SPECT imaging.

To be applicable in clinical cardiology as a metabolic tracer, the radio-iodinated fatty acids require the following profile:

(1) The modified fatty acid must be recognized by the myocardium as a natural long-chain fatty acid. Therefore, uptake, oxidation, and incorporation should be, to some extent, similar to the natural fatty acids.

(2) Because the biochemistry of fatty acids is extremely complex, involving numerous enzymatic steps and various metabolic pathways for different fatty acid molecules, the scintigraphic data should clearly provide information on a discrete part of the metabolic process.

(2) The parameters obtained by scintigraphy can be used as a diagnostic test, yielding information which cannot be obtained by other tests (e.g. abnormal fatty acid metabolism) or should provide at least the same diagnostic information and preferably more than the conventional cardiac diagnostic agents (e.g. improved detection of coronary artery disease).

(3) The I-123-labeled fatty acid analogues should be relatively inexpensive. At the present time, fatty acid imaging is still relatively expensive because of I-123 production and labeling. However, if the I-123-labeled fatty acids were accepted as useful clinical tools and there was a widespread demand for their availability, one could envision that the costs would approach that of conventional imaging agents like thallium-201 (T1-201).

In this chapter, the biochemical and scintigraphic characteristics of the radio-iodinated fatty acids and the results of clinical patient studies are reviewed.

Metabolic and scintigraphic characteristics of the radioiodinated fatty acids

Although a large number of radioiodinated fatty acid analogues have been developed, a limited number has been used in patient studies and include the following (Figure 1):

(1) *Iodoalkyl fatty acids:* 17–I–heptadecanoic acid (IHDA) and 17–I–hexadecenoic acid (IHA),

(2) *Terminal iodophenyl fatty acids:* 15-(p-I-phenyl)-pentadecanoic acid (pIPPA) and 15-(o-I-phenyl)pentadecanoic acid (oIPPA),

(3) *Methyl branched fatty acids:* 15-(p-I-phenyl)-3-R,S-methylpentadecanoic acid (3-BMIPPA), 15-(p-I-phenyl)-9-R,S-methylpentadecanoic acid (9-BMIPPA) and 14-(p-I-phenyl)-3-R,S-methyltetradecanoic acid (IPBMTA).

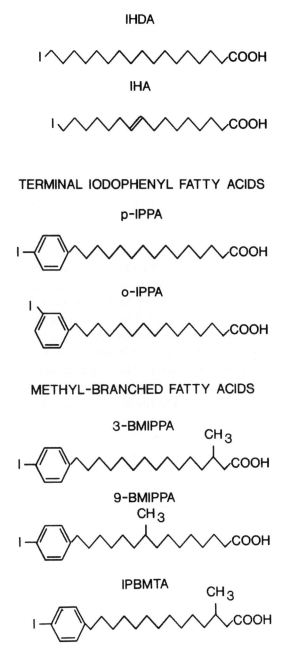

IODOALKYL FATTY ACIDS

IHDA

IHA

TERMINAL IODOPHENYL FATTY ACIDS

p-IPPA

o-IPPA

METHYL-BRANCHED FATTY ACIDS

3-BMIPPA

9-BMIPPA

IPBMTA

Figure 1. Structure of the radioiodinated free fatty acids.

(1) *17-I-123-heptadecanoic acid and 17-I-123-hexadecanoic acid.* These fatty acids are efficiently extracted by the myocardium, with extraction fractions in the range of natural fatty acids. After uptake, a major part of the fatty acids is immediately oxidized, splitting off the radiolabel. This radioiodide probably leaves the cell by simple diffusion and enters the circulation, giving rise to background activity. A minor part is stored into lipids, mainly phospholipids (Figure 2a).

Scintigraphic evaluation of regional uptake and regional clearance of radioactivity following intravenous administration of I-123 labeled fatty acids involves acquisition of serial planar images of the myocardium followed by generation of time-activity curves of defined regions of interest. In this manner, clearance kinetics from 'normal' regions can be readily compared to different clearance kinetics from impaired regions.

With IHDA, two parameters can be obtained from an analysis of the scintigram. They are the uptake of the tracer and the washout or clearance of radioactivity. The time-activity curve can be described as either a (bi)-exponential or as mono-exponential plus constant. Correction for free iodide has been used but the need for this background subtraction is debatable. Although the structures of the IHA and IHDA fatty acid analogues are slightly different and they are catabolized differently, the curves obtained from an analysis of the serial planar scintigram are similar. Due to the relatively rapid disappearance of the tracer from the myocardium under normal conditions (the half-time value T1/2 in patients varies between 18 and 33 minutes), SPECT imaging is not possible. However, after exercise [1, 2] or after lactate loading [3], the clearance of the tracer is delayed, which allows SPECT acquisition. Plate 17.1 shows a IHDA scintigram of a patient with a myocardial infarction in the posterior wall. The region of the myocardial infarction is clearly detected by the tracer defect. Figures 3a and 3b show the time-activity curves of the anteroseptal and posterior wall in this patient. The uptake in the septal area is higher than in the posterior wall and the exponential part of the time-activity curve shows a normal clearance rate with a T1/2 of 22 minutes. The mono-exponential fitted time-activity curve of the posterior wall is clearly abnormal with a T1/2 of 65 minutes.

(2) *15-(p-I-Phenyl)pentadecanoic acid and 15-(o-I-Phenyl)pentadecanoic acid.* Because of the high background activity of IHDA and IHA, Machulla et al. [4] proposed terminal phenyl-substitution of fatty acids and developed 15-(p-I-phenyl)pentadecanoic acid (*p*-IPPA). The *p*-IPPA analog is catabolized to para-iodobenzoic acid (*p*-IBA) rather than free iodide, and is either directly excreted or transformed in the liver to para-iodohippuric acid and then excreted by the kidneys [5]. Rapid excretion would lower levels of radioactivity in the

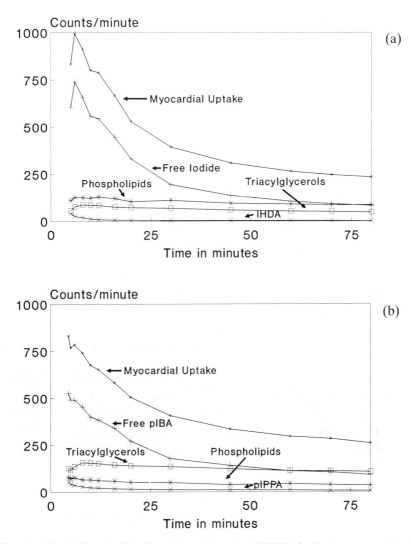

Figure 2a. Metabolism of radioiodinated heptadecanoic acid (IHDA): after intravenous injection at *t* = 0 minutes, multiple biopsy specimens are taken from normal canine myocardium in an assay period of 80 minutes and the fractional distribution of the samples is analyzed. A major part of IHDA is immediately oxidized, liberating the radioiodide (free iodide). Free iodide leaves the cell probably by simple diffusion. The remainder is incorporated into complex lipids, mainly phospholipids and triacylglycerols. Thus, the time-activity curve as obtained by a gamma camera is composed of an exponential part with a fast elimination of the radioactivity (free iodide) and an exponential with a slow elimination being constant or exponential (lipids) [69].

Figure 2b. Metabolism of radioiodinated paraiodo-phenylpentadecanoic acid (*p*-IPPA). See Figure 2a. Oxidation leads to formation of paraiodobenzoic acid, which leaves the cell probably by simple diffusion.

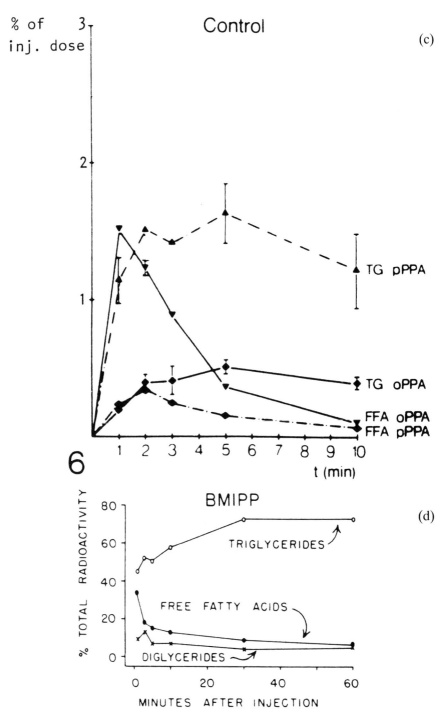

←

Figure 2c. Incorporation into lipids of *o*-IPPA compared to *p*-IPPA in rat hearts. Free *o*-IPPA was high and incorporation into triacylglycerols was low compared to *p*-IPPA. (From Beckurts et al. [7] with permission.)

Figure 2d. Distribution of radioactivity in lipid pools of rat hearts following intravenous administration of BMIPPA. The majority of radioactivity at all assay times was found in the triacylglycerol fraction.

blood, resulting in more favorable heart to blood ratios. Uptake of *p*-IPPA is similar to that of IHDA and for a major part, although less than IHDA, oxidized (Figure 2b). The *p*-IPPA isomer is, to a greater degree than IHDA, incorporated into triacylglycerols, and less into phospholipids. In addition, *p*-IPPA clearance from the myocardium is slightly slower (T1/2 higher) than of IHDA. From the scintigraphic data, the uptake, clearance, and fatty acid extraction can be obtained. The fatty acid extraction can be measured when the radioiodinated fatty acid is administered simultaneously with Tl-201 [6].

Although only the position of the radiolabel in the phenyl ring of *o*-IPPA is different from *p*-IPPA, the metabolism is quite different. In animal experiments, *o*-IPPA is rapidly oxidized accompanied by a very low rate of incorporation into triacylglycerols [7] (Figure 2c). In contrast, in humans, *o*-IPPA is well retained with elimination half times longer than 200 minutes [8], allowing measurement of uptake differences between normal and diseased myocardium.

The differences between myocardial uptake and retention of radioiodinated *o*-IPPA in comparison with *p*-IPPA are quite striking and totally unexpected, since the *o*-IPPA analogue shows washout kinetics in animal studies similar to *p*-IPPA, while in humans, *o*-IPPA shows nearly irreversible retention. Extensive earlier structure-activity studies by several groups [9, 10] demonstrated that many structural alterations on the terminus of long-chain fatty acids can be tolerated without drastically affecting the myocardial clearance kinetics. The behavior of *o*-IPPA represents a unique example of a fatty acid where behavior in lower animals is completely different than in humans. Thus, animal data cannot be used as a prelude to predict the expected behavior in humans or used for absorbed radiation dose estimates.

(3) Methyl-branched iodinated fatty acids. The methyl-branched fatty acids have been designed to overcome the problem of rapid clearance of radioactivity of the 'straight-chain' fatty acids, due to oxidation. Although the position of the methyl group differs in the three radioiodinated fatty acid analogues which have been used in clinical studies, the global effect is that oxidation is apparently prevented or changed by the introduction of the methyl group. This results in a prolonged myocardial retention. In animal experi-

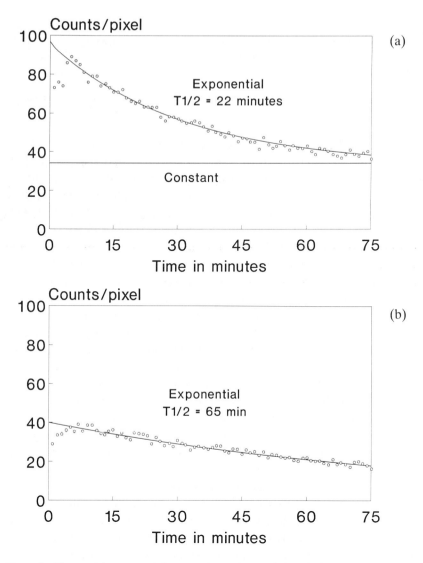

Figure 3a. Time-activity curve of the normal septal area of the scintigram of Plate 17.1. The time-activity curve is fitted with a monoexponential plus constant.

Figure 3b. Time-activity curve of the abnormal posterior area of the scintigram of Plate 17.1. The peak activity is reduced compared to Figure 3a and the time-activity curve is fitted with a monoexponential.

ments, it was demonstrated that 3-BMIPPA was mainly incorporated into triacylglycerols and, to a lesser extent, into diacylglycerols and phospholipids [11–13]. Unmetabolized radioiodinated free fatty acids also remained rela-

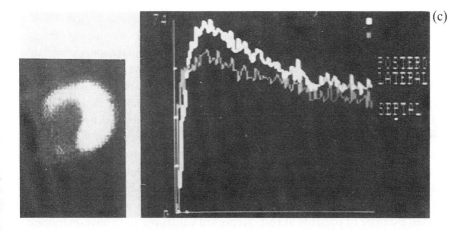

Figure 3c. Left: example of a 9-BMIPPA scintigram (view: LAO 45 degrees) of a patient with a septal infarction. Left: an area of diminished tracer uptake is seen in the septum. Right: time-activity curves of the normal posterolateral wall and the abnormal septal area in this patient. Elimination of the radioactivity from the normal myocardium is slow, allowing SPECT imaging. (From Knapp et al. [14] with permission.)

tively high (Figure 2d, [14]). The long myocardial retention allows the determination of uptake differences between normal and diseased myocardium. Figure 3c shows the 9-BMIPPA scintigram of a patient with an anteroseptal infarction. The time-activity curve of the normal myocardium demonstrates a slow clearance of the radioactivity over a study period of 100 minutes.

The following clinical topics have been studied with radioiodinated free fatty acids:
(1) Diagnosis of coronary artery disease,
(2) changes in fatty acid metabolism in coronary artery disease,
(3) infarct sizing and tissue viability/prognosis after infarction,
(4) bypass surgery/coronary angioplasty (PTCA),
(5) hypertrophy, cardiomyopathy and congestive heart failure,
(6) heart transplantation,
(7) valvular disease.

Changes in fatty acid metabolism during ischemia and diagnosis of coronary artery disease

During ischemic conditions, both uptake and oxidation of natural fatty acids is diminished and a greater portion of the extracted fatty acids is stored in lipids.

The altered oxidation and storage of radioiodinated fatty acids during ischemia has also been demonstrated in animal studies [15–18]. A number of studies with patients at rest using various radioiodinated fatty acids demonstrated that the normal scintigraphic pattern of uptake, distribution, and turnover was disturbed in patients with coronary artery disease. The most striking results were decreased uptake and extraction [19–21] of the straight-chain radioiodinated fatty acids in those areas of the myocardium supplied by a stenosed coronary artery. The clearance of radioactivity in these areas was also decreased [5, 20, 22–26], and a decrease in the relative oxidation size of the exponential curve [24] or component ratio [27] was observed. The same pattern of reduced uptake was observed with the methyl-branched fatty acids, [14, 28]. The abnormal regional fatty acid metabolism was found in a substantial number of patients at rest. Reported values for the above-mentioned studies ranged from 37 to 100%. One may speculate that the altered metabolic handling can be regarded as a metabolic variety of silent ischemia. However, the clinical relevance of this form of silent ischemia in terms of therapeutic management and prognosis still has to be resolved. Much attention has been focused on the diagnostic ability of radioiodinated fatty acid scintigraphy after exercise to detect coronary artery disease (CAD). Metabolic imaging may be more sensitive than other modalities to detect CAD, because the fatty acid oxidation strongly depends on oxygen supply. Thus, even in conditions where a relative lack in aerobic oxidation is completely compensated by anaerobic glycolysis, fatty acid metabolism may be 'visibly' disturbed. Using uptake, extraction, and clearance criteria, both *o*-IPPA [29] and *p*-IPPA [6, 30–33] and 9-BMIPPA [34] have demonstrated a high sensitivity to detect CAD. Hansen et al. [30] and Chouraqui et al. [34] compared the diagnostic ability of radioiodinated fatty acid imaging with Tl-201 perfusion imaging and concluded that fatty acid imaging is at least as sensitive as the Tl-201 perfusion data.

With IHDA, more conflicting results have been published. Van der Wall et al. [35] described patient studies after exercise and found slower clearance rates of IHDA in patients compared to volunteers. Hoeck et al. [36] and Stoddart et al. [37] described a reduced uptake of IHDA in patients with coronary artery disease. In contrast, Stoddart et al. [37] found nonsignificant slower clearance rates in patients having CAD with a large range of values. The contrasting results are probably due to methodological problems in the studies with heptadecanoic acid. These problems are related with the short acquisition period, the curve fitting and the background correction procedures [38–40].

Infarct imaging and tissue viability/prognosis after infarction

Myocardial infarctions are easily identified by a reduced tracer uptake with the straight-chain as well as with the methyl-branched fatty acids. In this context, initial uptake (extraction) is directly correlated with flow. Studies report similar distribution and image quality compared to the Tl-201 studies in the same group of patients [10, 41, 42]. However, infarct detection and localization can also be easily performed with other readily available clinical tools such as ECG, cardiac enzyme determination, and echocardiography. Thus, radioiodinated fatty acids do not represent a unique or cost-effective tool for this application.

Tissue viability and prognosis are clinically much less easy to ascertain. Tissue viability is currently a very important issue because of the widespread use of thrombolytic agents which limit infarct size and improve prognosis. At this moment, the only diagnostic tool which might readily assess tissue viability is PET imaging with Fluorine-18 2-fluorodeoxyglucose (FDG). However, PET imaging is costly, complex, and time-consuming and would not be expected to be routinely available in the near future for use in the majority of patients treated with thrombolytic agents.

Studies with radioiodinated fatty acids have focused on the relation between the clearance of radioactivity and tissue viability. Van der Wall et al. [43] reported that increased elimination compared to controls was associated with infarcted tissue and decreased elimination with ischemia. A similar finding was reported in patients intracoronary treated with thrombolytic therapy. Patients with decreased clearance had better preserved ventricular function than patients with increased clearance [44]. However, increase in elimination is also found in patients with coronary artery disease without infarction [45]. Stoddart et al. [46] found a weak relation between clearance rates and improvement in ventricular ejection fraction, however the variable response reduced the ability to predict individual improvement. Similar results were reported by Roesler et al. [47, 48], demonstrating that ischemic lesions did not lead to improvement of the ejection fraction. Only a slight reduction in end-diastolic volume was observed in the ischemic lesions. The problem with these types of studies is that, apart from the earlier-mentioned methology, direct evidence for tissue viability in patients is difficult to obtain. Studies, as reported by Tillisch et al. [49], which demonstrate that tissue with increased FDG uptake improve in contractile function after revascularization, have not been published so far. On the other hand, Chappuis et al. [50] showed in a canine occlusion-reperfusion model, that HDA uptake was found to be the single-most important predictor of viability, whereas Tl-201 was only of limited importance [50]. Recently, Henrich et al. [51] published a comparison between SPECT *o*-IPPA uptake and PET FDG uptake in myocardial infarction patients with persistent Tl-201 defects. Twenty-two percent of the patients had both normal *o*-IPPA and FDG uptake in the Tl-201 defects. Also, a significant correlation of *o*-IPPA and FDG uptake was found in the persistent Tl-201 defects [51], suggesting that viability may well be demonstrated with radioiodinated fatty acids.

Studies with Tl-201 have demonstrated that ischemic changes in and outside the infarct area have prognostic value for patients after a myocardial infarction [52]. Prognostic studies with radioiodinated fatty acids are not yet available which demonstrate differences in survival or major cardiac events in patients with and without abnormal metabolism of radioiodinated fatty acid.

Bypass surgery/PTCA

Relatively few metabolic studies have focused on the effects of bypass surgery/ PTCA on fatty acid metabolism in patients. Fridrich et al. [53] reported normalization of tracer elimination despite the fact that ventricular function could remain impaired. Interestingly, there seems to be a dissociation between restoration of flow and metabolism after revascularization, since the uptake of fatty acids normalizes only in some of the patients [37, 54, 55] and decreased metabolism may not return to normal [55, 56]. The significance of this finding is not clear, but may indicate restenosis, incomplete revascularization, cellular ischemia, or focal necrosis. Furthermore, it may have significance for the long-term patency of bypass grafts. Similar studies with Tl-201 after bypass surgery indicate that reversible defects may not completely disappear. An example is reported by Fioretti et al. where the number of reversible segments decreased after bypass grafting only with 60% [57].

Hypertrophy, cardiomyopathy and congestive heart failure

From the early studies with radioiodinated fatty acids, attention has been paid to the uncommon but interesting cardiac diseases: the cardiomyopathies. Metabolic studies in patients with congestive cardiomyopathy and heart failure indicate that regional uptake/extraction of fatty acids is inhomogeneously reduced and clearance of the radioactivity from the myocardium is delayed [23, 25, 27, 41, 58–60]. Ugolini et al. [61] reported increased elimination of the radioactivity. In contrast, the study of Rabinovitch et al. [62] showed abnormal uptake and turnover in only 2 out of 16 patients with cardiomyopathy of different etiology.

In patients with hypertrophy and hypertrophic cardiomyopathy [59, 63, 64], a decrease in uptake and extraction was noted and the latter was related with degree of hypertrophy [65].

It is obvious from these studies that accurate discrimination between the different etiologies of the cardiomyopathies cannot be expected from metabolic studies. Possibly, metabolic imaging can discriminate better than other noninvasive tools, discriminate between ischemic and idiopathic congestive cardiomyopathy. Likewise, metabolic imaging can possibly discriminate between physiological and pathological hypertrophy of the myocardium. Moreover, progression of the disease in all types of cardiomyopathies, assessment of prognosis, and the influence of therapy may be assessed by metabolic studies [66].

Heart transplantation

Fridrich et al. [67] published the preliminary results of fatty acid imaging in patients with heart transplantation. In his small group of patients, histological evidence of rejection was not correlated with abnormalities in fatty acid turnover, but depression of metabolism was related with an inadequate ventricular ejection fraction response during exercise. This inadequate exercise response was thought to be an early sign of functional derangement in chronic rejection.

At this moment, histology of biopsies is the golden standard for the diagnosis of rejection. Because of the necessity to frequently repeat the procedure, it poses an increasing burden on patients and catheterization laboratories. The role of metabolic imaging still needs careful evaluation.

Valvular heart disease

Only one study has reported fatty acid imaging in valvular disease. Voth et al. [68] investigated the relation with perfusion imaging in mitral valve prolapses and concluded that the Tl-201 abnormalities were similar to the metabolic abnormalities. The diagnosis and assessment of the severity of valvular heart disease can be routinely determined with noninvasive techniques such as Doppler echocardiography. The timing of valvular replacement can still form a problem because too early replacement exposes patients to the operation and reimplantation risk and sometimes long-life anticoagulants. Too late replacement may lead to persistent damage of the ventricles. Metabolic studies may play a role in this respect, hypothesizing that functional changes of the myocardium may be preceded by metabolic changes.

Future perspectives

Further advances and a renewed interest in the use of straight-chain iodine-123-labeled fatty acids such as *p*-IPPA and IHDA, may be on the horizon with the availability of new three-headed SPECT systems such as the Triad® camera, which will now, for the first time, allow rapid tomographic acquisitions. The methyl-branched fatty acids such as 3-BMIPPA were originally developed by Knapp et al. and others as a strategy to facilitate SPECT imaging because of the significantly longer myocardial retention in comparison with the straight-chain analogues. The relative rapid clearance of IHDA and *p*-IPPA coupled with the long acquisition times required for traditional SPECT with a single-headed camera (e.g. 15–20 minutes) often make SPECT imaging not possible. Since maximal physiologic information could be expected to be obtained from an evaluation of both the regional uptake and clearance kinetics, SPECT imaging with an evaluation of clearance kinetics would be an important capability. The new three-headed camera would be expected to offer this opportunity, since rapid SPECT acquisition times of, for example, 5 minutes, are possible. Thus, one should be able to construct regional time-activity curves from tomographic data, in a fashion similar to the well-established approaches developed for PET. Because of the inherently improved opportunity to evaluate target tissue uptake with SPECT with a significant reduction of the contribution of nontarget tissue radioactivity in the field of view, this approach should offer a new important oppertunity to evaluate radioiodinated fatty acid metabolism by 'serial SPECT'.

In summary, a variety of radioiodinated fatty acids with specific metabolic behavior have been developed and have been applied in different cardiac diseases. Because metabolism is a 'condition sine qua non' for maintaining cellular integrity and cardiac contraction, the major advantage of using radioiodinated fatty acids is that they provide a specific insight into metabolic abnormalities which can be obtained with widely available gamma cameras. Although metabolic studies have not yet established diagnostic tools like the perfusion agents, the potential is such that, in the near future, radioiodinated fatty acids will have their own clinical application.

References

1. Visser FC, Van Eenige MJ, Duwel CM, Van Lingen A, Roos JP. Radioiodinated fatty acid scintigraphy of the normal human myocardium during exercise testing: a new interpretation. Nuc Compact 1990; 21: 236–40.
2. Kuikka JT, Mustonen JN, Uusitupa MI et al. Demonstration of disturbed free fatty acid metabolism of myocardium in patients with non-insulin-dependent diabetes mellitus as measured with iodine-123-heptadecanoic acid. Eur J Nucl Med 1991; 18: 475–81.
3. Duwel CM, Visser FC, Van Eenige MJ, Den Hollander W, Roos JP. The fate of 131I-17-iodoheptadecanoid acid during lactate loading: its oxidation is strongly inhibited in favor to its esterification. A radiochemical study in the canine heart. Nuklearmedizin 1990; 29: 24–7.
4. Machulla HJ, Marsmann M, Dutchka K. Biochemical concept and synthesis of a radioiodinated phenylfatty acid for in vivo metabolic studies of the myocardium. Eur J Nucl Med 1980; 5: 171–3.
5. Dudczak R, Schmolinger R, Kletter K, Frischauf H, Angelberger P. Clinical evaluation of 123I-labeled-*p*-phenylpentadecanoic acid (*p*-IPPA) for myocardial scintigraphy. J Nucl Med Allied Sci 1983; 27: 267–79.
6. Vyska K, Machulla HJ, Stremmel W et al. Regional myocardial free fatty acid extraction in normal and ischemic myocardium. Circulation 1988; 78: 1218–33.
7. Beckurts TE, Shreeve WW, Schieren R, Feinendegen LE. Kinetics of different 123I- and 14C-labelled fatty acids in normal and diabetic rat myocardium in vivo. Nucl Med Commun 1985; 6: 415–24.
8. Antar MA, Spohr G, Herzog HH et al. 15-(ortho-123I-phenyl)-pentadecanoic acid, a new myocardial imaging agent for clinical use. Nucl Med Commun 1986; 7: 683–96.
9. Westera G, Visser FC. Myocardial uptake of radioactively labelled free fatty acids. Eur Heart J 1985; 6 Suppl B: 3–12.
10. Fischman AJ, Saito T, Dilsizian V et al. Myocardial fatty acid imaging: rationale, comparison of (11)C- and (123)I-labeled fatty acids, and potential clinical utility. Am J Card Imaging 1989; 3: 288–96.
11. Ambrose KR, Owen BA, Callahan AP, Goodman MM, Knapp FF Jr. Effects of fasting on the myocardial subcellular distribution and lipid distribution of terminal p-iodophenyl-substituted fatty acids in rats. Int J Rat Appl Instrum [B] 1988; 15: 695–700.
12. Ambrose KR, Rice DE, Goodman MM, Knapp FF. Effect of 3-methyl-branching on the metabolism in rat hearts of radioiodinated iodovinyl long chain fatty acids. Eur J Nucl Med 1987; 13: 374–9.
13. Ambrose KR, Owen BA, Goodman MM, Knapp FF Jr. Evaluation of the metabolism in rat hearts of two new radioiodinated 3-methyl-branched fatty acid myocardial imaging agents. Eur J Nucl Med 1987; 12: 486–91.
14. Knapp FF Jr, Goodman MM, Ambrose KR et al. The development of radioiodinated 3-methylbranched fatty acids for evaluation of myocardial disease by single photon techniques. In: van der Wall EE, editor. Noninvasive imaging of cardiac metabolism: single photon scintigraphy, positron emission tomography and nuclear magnetic resonance. Dordrecht: Martinus Nijhoff, 1987: 159–261.
15. Hudon MP, Lyster DM, Jamieson WR, Qayumi AK, Sartori C, Dougan H. The metabolism of 15-*p*-[123I]-iodophenylpentadecanoic acid in a surgically induces canine model of regional ischemia. Eur J Nucl Med 1990; 16: 199–204.
16. Visser FC, Westera G. Radioiodinated free fatty acids: a clue to myocardial metabolism? In: van der Wall EE, editor. Noninvasive imaging of cardiac metabolism: single photon scintigra-

phy, positron emission tomography and nuclear magnetic resonance. Dordrecht: Martinus Nijhoff, 1987: 127–38.

17. Visser FC, Sloof GW, Comans E, van Eenige MJ, Knapp FF. Metabolism of radioiodinated 17-iodo heptadecanoic acid in the normal and ischemic dog heart. Eur Heart J 1990; 11 Suppl: 137.

18. Rellas JR, Corbett JR, Kulkarni PV et al. Iodine-123 phenylpentadecanoic acid: detection of acute myocardial infarction and injury in dogs using an iodinated fatty acid and single-photon emission tomography. Am J Cardiol 1983; 52: 1326–32.

19. Reske SN. 123I-phenylpentadecanoic acid as a tracer of cardiac free fatty acid metabolism. Experimental and clinical results. Eur Heart J 1985; 6 Suppl B: 39–47.

20. Reske SN, Koischwitz D, Reichmann K et al. Cardiac metabolism of 15 (*p*-I-123 phenyl-) pentadecanoic acid after intracoronary tracer application. Eur J Radiol 1984; 4: 144–9.

21. Railton R, Rodger JC, Small DR, Harrower AD. Myocardial scintigraphy with I-123 heptadecanoic acid as a test for coronary heart disease. Eur J Nucl Med 1987; 13: 63–6.

22. Dudczak R, Kletter K, Frischauf H, Losert U, Angelberger P, Schmoliner R. The use of 123I-labeled heptadecanoic acid (HDA) as metabolic tracer: preliminary report. Eur J Nucl Med 1984; 9: 81–5.

23. Dudczak R, Schmoliner R, Angelberger P, Kletter K, Losert U, Frischauf H. Myocardial perfusion and metabolism as assessed by Tl-201 and I-123 heptadecanoic acid scintigraphy. Nuklearmedizin 1982; 21 Suppl 19: 540–4.

24. Van Eenige MJ, Visser FC, Duwel CM, Roos JP. Clinical value of studies with radioiodinated heptadecanoic acid in patients with coronary artery disease. Eur Heart J 1990; 11: 258–68.

25. Freundlieb C, Hock A, Vyska K, Feinendegen LE, Machulla HJ, Stoklin G. Myocardial imaging and metabolic studies with [17-123I]iodoheptadecanoic acid. J Nucl Med 1980; 21: 1043–50.

26. Visser FC, Van Eenige MJ, Van der Wall EE et al. The elimination rate of 123I-heptadecanoic acid after intracoronary and intravenous administration. Eur J Nucl Med 1985; 11: 114–9.

27. Fridrich L, Pichler M, Gassner A, Vagner M, Mostbeck G, Eghbalian F. Tracer elimination in I-123-heptadecanoic acid: half-life, component ratio and circumferential profiles in patients with cardiac disease. Eur Heart J 1985; 6 Suppl B: 61–70.

28. Dudczak R, Schmoliner R, Angelberger P, Knapp FF, Goodman MM. Structurally modified fatty acids: clinical potential as tracers of metabolism. Eur J Nucl Med 1986; 12 Suppl: 545–8.

29. Kaiser KP, Vester E, Grossmann K, Geuting B, Loesse B, Feinendegen LE. 15-(ortho-I-123-phenyl)pentadecanoic acid (OPPA) in the human myocardium: clinical applications. Nuc Compact 1990; 21: 213–5.

30. Hansen CL, Corbett JR, Pippin JJ et al. Iodine-123 phenylpentadecanoic acid and single photon emission computed tomography in identifying left ventricular regional metabolic abnormalities in patients with coronary heart disease: comparison with thallium-201 myocardial tomography. J Am Coll Cardiol 1988; 12: 78–87.

31. Kennedy PL, Corbett JR, Kulkarni PV et al. Iodine 123-phenylpentadecanoic acid myocardial scintigraphy: usefulness in the identification of myocardial ischemia. Circulation 1986; 74: 1007–15.

32. Schad N, Wagner RK, Hallermeier J, Daus HJ, Vattimo A, Bertelli P. Regional rates of myocardial fatty acid metabolism: comparison with coronary angiography and ventriculography. Eur J Nucl Med 1990; 16: 205–12.

33. Reske SN, Nitsch J, Von der Lohe E, Simon HJ, Bardos P. Eingeschrankte myokardiale Feltsaure-Utilisation bei koronarer Herzerkrankung nach symptomlimitierter ergometrischer Belastung. Nachweis pathologischer Stoffwechselmuster mit Hilfe von Iod-123-Phenyl-pentadekansaure und sequentieller SPECT, Bull U. Z Kardiol 1989; 78: 262–70.

34. Chouraqui P, Maddahi J, Henkin R, Karesh SM, Galie E, Berman DS. Comparison of myocardial imaging with iodine-123-iodophenyl-9-methyl pentadecanoic acid and thallium-201-chloride for assessment of patients with exercise-induced myocardial ischemia. J Nucl Med 1991; 32: 447–52.

35. Van der Wall EE, Heidendal GA, Den Hollander W, Westera G, Roos JP. Metabolic myocardial imaging with 123I-labeled heptadecanoic acid in patients with angina pectoris. Eur J Nucl Med 1981; 6: 391–6.

36. Hoeck A, Freundlieb C, Vyska K, Feinendegen LE, Rost R, Schuerch PM et al. The influence of rehabilitation training on fatty acid metabolism in patients after myocardial infarction. In: Faivre G, Bertrand A, Cherrier F, Amor M, Neiman JL, editors. Noninvasive methods in ischemic heart disease. Nancy: Specia, 1982: 300–3.

37. Stoddart PG, Papouchado M, Vann Jones J, Wilde P. Practical and technical problems of myocardial imaging with 17-(123-iodo)-heptadecanoic acid. Nuc Compact 1990; 21: 244–7.

38. Van Eenige MJ, Visser FC, Duwel CM, Bezemer PD, Karreman AJ, Roos JP. Analysis of myocardial time-activity curves of 123I-heptadecanoic acid I. Curve fitting. Nuklearmedizin 1987; 26: 241–7.

39. Van Eenige MJ, Visser FC, Karreman AJ, Duwel CM, Bezemer PD, Roos JP. Analysis of myocardial time-activity curves of 123I-heptadecanoic acid II. The acquisition time. Nuklearmedizin 1987; 26: 248–52.

40. Van Eenige MJ, Visser FC, Karreman AJ, Bezemer PD, Westera G, Van Lingen A et al. Analysis of time-activity curves related to myocardial metabolism. The case of 123I-heptadecanoic acid. Nucl Med Commun 1991; 12: 115–25.

41. Abdullah AZ, Hawkins LA, Britton KE, Elliot AT, Stephens JD. I-123-labelled heptadecanoic acid as myocardial imaging agent: comparison with thallium-201 and first-pass nuclear ventriculography. Nucl Med Commun 1981; 2: 268–77.

42. Van der Wall EE, Heidendal GA, Den Hollander W, Westera G, Roos JP. I-123 labeled hexadecenoic acid in comparison with thallium-201 for myocardial imaging in coronary heart disease: a preliminary study. Eur J Nucl Med 1980; 5: 401–5.

43. Van der Wall EE, Den Hollander W, Heidendal GA, Westera G, Majid PA, Roos JP. Dynamic myocardial scintigraphy with 123I-labeled free fatty acids in patients with myocardial infarction. Eur J Nucl Med 1981; 6: 383–9.

44. Visser FC, Westera G, Van Eenige MJ, Van der Wall EE, Heidendal GA, Roos JP. Free fatty acid scintigraphy in patients with successful thrombolysis after acute myocardial infarction. Clin Nucl Med 1985; 10: 35–9.

45. Reske SN. Cardiac metabolism of I-123 phenylpentadecanoic acid. In: Van der Wall EE, editor. Noninvasive imaging of cardiac metabolism: single photon scintigraphy, positron emission tomography, and nuclear magnetic resonance. Dordrecht: Martinus Nijhoff, 1987: 139–58.

46. Stoddart PG, Papouchado M, Wilde P. Prognostic value of 123-iodo-heptadecanoic acid imaging in patients with acute myocardial infarction. Eur J Nucl Med 1987; 12: 525–8.

47. Roesler H, Hess T, Weiss M et al. Tomographic assessment of myocardial metabolic heterogenity. J Nucl Med 1983; 24: 285–96.

48. Rosler H, Noelpp U, Toth T, Schubiger PA, Hunziker HR. On the prognostic potential of the sequential 123-I-HDA-tomoscintigram after the first MI. Eur Heart J 1985; 6 Suppl B: 49–55.

49. Tillisch J, Brunken R, Marchall R et al. Reversibility of cardiac wall-motion abnormalities predicted by positron tomography. N Engl J Med 1986; 314: 884–8.

50. Chappuis F, Meier B, Belenger J, Blauenstein P, Lerch R. Early assessment of tissue viability with radioiodinated heptadecanoic acid in reperfused canine myocardium: comparison with thallium-201. Am Heart J 1990; 119: 833–41.

51. Henrich MM, Vester E, Von der Lohe E et al. The comparison of 2-F 18-deoxyglycose and 15-(ortho-123-I-phenyl)-pentadecanoic acid uptake in persisting defects on Thallium-201 tomography in myocardial infarction. J Nucl Med 1991; 32: 1353–7.

52. Gibson RS, Watson DD, Craddock GB et al. Prediction of cardiac events after uncomplicated myocardial infarction: a prospective study comparing predischarge exercise thallium-201 scintigraphy and coronary angiography. Circulation 1983; 68: 321–36.

53. Fridrich L, Gassner A, Sommer G et al. Dynamic 123I-HDA myocardial scintigraphy after aortocoronary bypass grafting. Eur J Nucl Med 1986; 12 Suppl: 524–6.

54. Stoddart PG, Papouchado M, Jones JV, Wilde P. Assessment of percutaneous transluminal coronary angioplasty with 123IODO-heptadecanoic acid. Eur J Nucl Med 1987; 12: 605–8.

55. Kropp J, Koehler U, Nitch J, Likungu J, Biersack HJ, Knapp FF. Imaging of myocardial metabolism before and after revascularisation. Nuc Compact 1990; 21: 219–22.

56. Kropp J, Likungu J, Kirchhoff PG et al. Single photon emission tomography imaging of myocardial oxidative metabolism with 15-(p-[123I]iodophenyl) pentadecanoic acid in patients with coronary artery disease and aorto-coronary bypass graft surgery. Eur J Nucl Med 1991; 18: 467–74.

57. Fioretti P, Reijs AE, Neumann D et al. Improvement in transient and 'persistent' perfusion defects on early and late post-exercise thallium-201 tomograms after coronary artery bypass grafting. Eur Heart J 1988; 9: 1332–8.

58. Hock A, Freundlieb C, Vyska K, Losse B, Erbel R, Feinendegen LE. Myocardial imaging and metabolic studies with [17-123I]-iodoheptadecanoic acid in patients with idiopathic congestive cardiomyopathy. J Nucl Med 1983; 24: 22–8.

59. Knapp WH, Vyska K, Machulla HJ et al. Double-nuclide study of the myocardium using 201Tl and 123I-labeled fatty acids in non-ischemic myocardial diseases. Nuklearmedizin 1988; 27: 72–8.

60. Schad N, Daus HJ, Ciavolella M, Maccio A. Noninvasive functional imaging of regional rate of myocardial fatty acids metabolism. Cardiologia 1987; 32: 239–47.

61. Ugolini V, Hansen CL, Kulkarni PV, Jansen DE, Akers MS, Corbett JR. Abnormal myocardial fatty acid metabolism in dilated cardiomyopathy detected by iodine-123 phenyl-pentadecanoic acid and tomographic imaging. Am J Cardiol 1988; 62: 923–8.

62. Rabinovitch MA, Kalff V, Allen R et al. ω-123I-hexadecanoic acid metabolic probe of cardiomyopathy. Eur J Nucl Med 1985; 10: 222–7.

63. Livni E, Elmaleh DR, Barlai-Kovach MM, Goodman MM, Knapp FF Jr, Strauss HW. Radioiodinated beta-methyl phenyl fatty acids as potential tracers for myocardial imaging and metabolism. Eur Heart J 1985; 6 Suppl B: 85–9.

64. Notohamiprodjo G, Vyska K, Knapp WH et al. Fatty acid extraction in hypertrophied myocardium in hypertensive heart disease. Nuc Compact 1990; 21: 241–3.

65. Wolfe CL, Kennedy PL, Kulkarni PV, Jansen DE, Gabliani GI, Corbett JR. Iodine-123 phenylpentadecanoic acid myocardial scintigraphy in patients with left ventricular hypertrophy: alterations in left ventricular distribution and utilization. Am Heart J 1990; 119: 1338–47.

66. Som P, Oster ZH, Kubota K et al. Studies of a new fatty acid analog (DMIVN) in hypertensive rats and the effect of verapamil using ARG microimaging. Int J Rad Appl Instrum [B] 1989; 16: 483–90.

67. Fridrich L, Havel M, Horvat R, Wollenek G, Laczkovics A. Myocardial fatty acid metabolism in patients after orthotopic heart transplantation. Nuc Compact 1990; 21: 216–8.

68. Voth E, Schicha H, Tebbe U, Neumann P, Emrich D. Fatty acid metabolism in symptomatic patients with mitral valve prolapse but without coronary artery disease-comparison with 201Tl myocardial perfusion scintigraphy. Nuklearmedizin 1987; 26: 172–6.

69. Van Eenige MJ, Visser FC, Duwel CM, Karreman AJ, Van Lingen A, Roos JP. Comparison of 17-iodine-131 heptadecanoic acid kinetics from externally measured time-activity curves and from serial myocardial biopsies in an open-chest canine model. J Nucl Med 1988; 29: 1934–42.

18. Assessment of myocardial fatty acid metabolism with carbon-11 palmitate

RENÉ LERCH

Introduction

The positron emitting radionuclide carbon-11 allows the labeling of fatty acids without alteration to their molecular structure. Accordingly, the labeled fatty acid is taken up by the myocardium and metabolized in proportion to the unlabeled circulating counterpart. The availability of a true tracer of fatty acid metabolism combined with the quantitative capabilities positron imaging represent the framework for the noninvasive assessment of regional fatty acid metabolism with positron emission tomography (PET) [1–3]. Furthermore, the short half-life of carbon-11 (half-life 20.4 minutes) enables sequential evaluation of metabolism which is important if the method is used to study transient metabolic alterations or to monitor the effect of a therapeutic intervention on regional metabolism. These advantages of PET over the approaches using single photon emitting radioiodinated fatty acids have to be weighed against the higher costs involved in both the logistics required for on-site cyclotron-production of short-lived isotopes and the ensuing radiochemistry.

For the study of myocardial fatty acid metabolism with PET, palmitate, a saturated fatty acid with 16 carbon atoms, has been labeled with carbon-11 in the first position, the carboxyl group [4, 5]. Strictly speaking, metabolic studies with (1-^{11}C)-palmitate apply only to metabolism of this particular fatty acid. However, because circulating fatty acids with a chain length of 16 or 18 atoms are metabolized in a similar fashion [6], and because these fatty acids account for more than 85% of myocardial fatty acid uptake [7], observations with

Ernst E. van der Wall et al. (eds), What's new in cardiac imaging?, 249–261.
© *1992 Kluwer Academic Publishers. Printed in the Netherlands.*

(1-^{11}C)-palmitate can be considered as representative for myocardial fatty acid utilization.

Despite the intrinsically favourable properties of (1-^{11}C)-palmitate for metabolic studies, interpretation of tomographic observations is complicated by the multiple metabolic fate of the label [1–3, 8, 9]. Fatty acids are transported in the plasma bound to albumin. The precise mechanism of transfer of fatty acids from the intracapillary to the myocytoplasmic compartment has yet to be determined, but it is known to require a concentration gradient. This gradient is maintained both by the steady supply of fatty acids from the coronary circulation and by intracellular metabolism. After having crossed the sarcolemma, fatty acids may diffuse back [10]. However, in normoxic myocardium, most of extracted fatty acid is thioesterified with coenzyme A (CoA) which prevents back-diffusion [8, 9]. There are two main pathways for further metabolism of acyl-CoA. The first pathway is transport into the mitochondrial matrix by a carnitine-dependent transfer system, followed by β-oxidation to acetyl-CoA and further catabolism to CO_2 in the Krebs cycle. The second main pathway is incorporation into triacylglycerols or phospholipids and subsequent hydrolysis [8, 9]. Studies have been conducted in experimental animals to characterize the interrelations between myocardial fatty acid metabolism and externally detectable myocardial kinetics of (1-^{11}C)-palmitate.

This chapter is intended to provide both a review of the experimental results relevant to the understanding of the myocardial kinetics of (1-^{11}C)-palmitate and a survey of clinical studies performed with this tracer.

Myocardial kinetics of (1-^{11}C)-palmitate

After intravenous administration in dogs, (1-^{11}C)-palmitate is avidly taken up by the myocardium and disappears rapidly from blood with a half-time of 2 minutes, permitting clear delineation of the left ventricular myocardium on tomographic images initiated 5 minutes after tracer injection [11]. Subsequently, radioactivity is cleared from the myocardium in a multiexponential fashion [11–13]. For the discussion of myocardial kinetics of (1-^{11}C)-palmitate, it is convenient to deal separately with the initial myocardial tracer uptake and clearance of myocardial activity.

Myocardial uptake of (1-^{11}C)-palmitate

In normal canine hearts, the initial distribution of (1-^{11}C)-palmitate radioactivity is homogeneous throughout the left ventricular myocardium [11]. In contrast, in animals with experimental coronary occlusion [4] or severe coronary stenosis and atrial pacing [14], an uptake defect is readily visible in the critically supplied region. In hearts with regional ischemia, initial uptake of (1-^{11}C)-palmitate correlated roughly with myocardial perfusion [14, 15]. However, unlike a flow tracer (1-^{11}C)-palmitate exhibits a variable single-pass extraction fraction [4, 10, 13]. Characteristic of a diffusion-limited tracer the extraction fraction of (1-^{11}C)-palmitate is inversely related to myocardial blood flow, provided the metabolic demand of the myocardium and arterial substrate concentrations are kept constant [13]. Furthermore, at a given level of myocardial perfusion, the extraction fraction of (1-^{11}C)-palmitate my alter with variation in intracellular metabolism. For example, the extraction fraction of (1-^{11}C)-palmitate decreased both in isolated rabbit hearts subjected to prolonged low-flow ischemia [4] and in canine myocardium perfused in vivo with hypoxic blood at normal flow [10, 12].

Since oxidation is not the only possible intracellular fate of extracted (1-^{11}C)-palmitate [1, 8, 9], the single-pass extraction fraction is not directly related to the rate of β-oxidation. In dog experiments, myocardial regions with impaired fatty acid oxidation continue to extract substantial amounts of (1-^{11}C)-palmitate from the blood [10, 12]. The importance of nonoxidative pathways for myocardial extraction of (1-^{11}C)-palmitate has recently been demonstrated by Wyns et al. [16]. In their study in dogs, pharmacological inhibition of mitochondrial fatty acid transfer elicited a marked reduction of myocardial (1-^{11}C)-palmitate extraction. However, the baseline extraction fraction was restored when glucose was administered concomitantly with the inhibitor of fatty acid oxidation, presumably reflecting stimulation of the synthesis of triacylglycerol by glycolytic production of the precursor glycerol-3-phosphate [17]. Thus, initial accumulation of (1-^{11}C)-palmitate reflects regional fatty acid uptake, which is influenced by numerous factors including arterial supply, transfer from the plasma to the myocytoplasma and intracellular metabolism.

PET with (1-^{11}C)-palmitate has been used to noninvasively measure infarct size. Weiss et al. [18] observed in dogs that, 48 hours after coronary occlusion, the size of the region with less than 50% of peak left ventricular radioactivity on PET images obtained after injection of (1-^{11}C)-palmitate, correlated closely with infarct size as delineated postmortem using morphological criteria.

Furthermore, in myocardial samples taken from the region at risk, the reduction of tracer uptake compared to normal myocardium correlated closely with myocardial loss of creatine kinase. Thus, in hearts with completed myocardial infarction, PET with (1-^{11}C)-palmitate permitted accurate delineation of viable myocardium.

(1-^{11}C)-palmitate may be useful for the characterization of metabolic recovery after postischemic reperfusion. In dogs with experimental coronary thrombosis, the size of the (1-^{11}C)-palmitate uptake defect measured after coronary

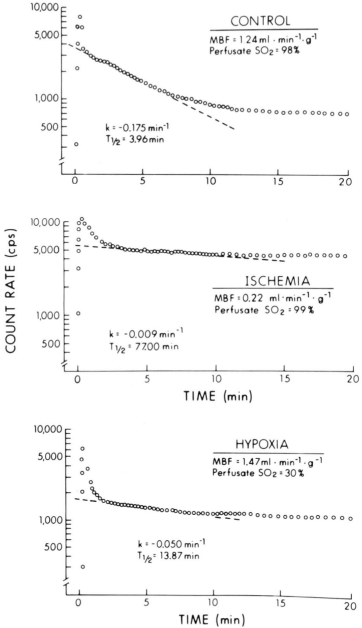

←

thrombolysis decreased to a varying extent compared to defect size observed during coronary occlusion, depending on the duration of ischemia (Figure 1) [19]. When coronary thrombolysis was induced 1–2 or 2–4 hours after coronary occlusion, defect size decreased by 51 ± 6 (SEM)% and $21 \pm 2\%$, respectively. In contrast, when reperfusion was delayed beyond 4 hours, no recovery of regional $(1-^{11}C)$-palmitate uptake was observed despite restoration of myocardial perfusion [19]. The time course of progression of irreversible depression of $(1-^{11}C)$-palmitate uptake in reperfused myocardium closely resembled that of the 'wave front' phenomenon of necrosis observed morphologically in canine models of myocardial infarction [20]. Even though serial studies with $(1-^{11}C)$-palmitate may permit the documentation of progression of irreversible injury as a function of the duration of coronary occlusion, the relationship between tissue viability and metabolism $(1-^{11}C)$-palmitate is still incompletely defined. Recent observations from our laboratory suggest that myocardial fatty acid uptake and oxidation may recover after reperfusion, at least transiently, in myocardium that undergoes irreversible injury either during ischemia or early after reperfusion [21].

Clearance of myocardial activity

Figure 2 depicts semilogarithmic plots of time activity curves recorded by a positron detector in open chest dogs after intracoronary injection of $(1-^{11}C)$-palmitate. In normal myocardium (top panel), the initial peak of vascular transit is followed by two slower clearance components reflecting egress of radioactivity from extracted $(1-^{11}C)$-palmitate. The slope of the first myocardial clearance component correlated with the rate of myocardial release of $^{11}CO_2$ [10]. This phase presumably reflects clearance of radioactivity from $(1-^{11}C)$-palmitate that rapidly is transferred into the mitochondria and oxidized [10–13, 22]. If not specified, in the following discussion the term 'clearance

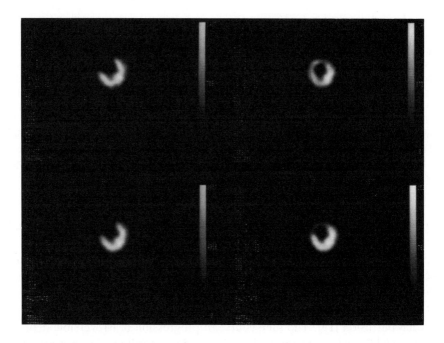

Figure 2. Semilogarithmic plots of regional time activity curves recorded in an open chest dog with perfusion of the left anterior descending coronary artery (LAD) by an extracorporeal bypass sytem. (1-^{11}C)-palmitate was injected intracoronarily and myocardial radioactivity monitored with a β^+-detector. Under control conditions (top) there exist three distinct components of (1-^{11}C)-clearance: (1) vascular transit, (2) early rapid clearance of radioactivity from extracted (1-^{11}C)-palmitate evident between 3 and 7 minutes, (3) late slow phase evident later than 10 minutes after tracer injection. During low flow ischemia (middle panel) the rate of the early myocardial clearance component is markedly decreased. A similar pattern of clearance is observed during perfusion with hypoxic blood at normal flow (bottom). MBF, myocardial blood flow; SO_2, hemoglobin saturation of blood entering the LAD; k, rate constant of early monoexponential ^{11}C-clearance; $T_{1/2}$, half-time of early monoexponential ^{11}C-clearance. (Adapted from Lerch RA, Bergmann SR, Ambos HD, Welch MJ, Ter-Pogossian MM, Sobel BE. Effect of flow-independent reduction of metabolism on regional myocardial clearance of ^{11}C-palmitate. Circulation 1982; 65: 731–8. Used by permission of the American Heart Association, Inc.)

rate' refers to the slope of this early component (without subtraction of the subsequent slow component). The second slow component of ^{11}C-clearance, which predominates later than 10 minutes after tracer injection, reflects turnover of the (1-^{11}C)-palmitate initially incorporated into triacylglycerols and phospholipids [10–13]. This interpretation has been corroborated by radiobiochemical analysis of serial myocardial biopsies [22].

Schelbert et al. [14, 23] have used compartmental analysis of the clearance curves to estimate the partition of extracted fatty acids between rapid oxidation and initial incorporation into lipid esters. In fasted dogs, 39 ± 17 (SD)% of extracted (1-^{11}C)-palmitate entered the fast turnover pool [23]. The size of this component decreased to $11 \pm 13\%$ after intravenous infusion of glucose and insulin, suggesting a reduction of oxidation of extracted (1-^{11}C)-palmitate and increased incorporation into lipid esters [23]. Thus, sequential imaging after injection of (1-^{11}C)-palmitate, allows noninvasive documentation of alterations of the intracellular fate of the labeled fatty acid in response to modification of the circulating substrate pattern.

The middle panel of Figure 2 depicts a time activity curve recorded after reduction of myocardial perfusion to 18% of control. Although a substantial fraction of (1-^{11}C)-palmitate is still retained in the myocardium after vascular transit, the early clearance component is virtually abolished [12]. Since a similar clearance pattern was observed when flow was maintained but oxygen supply reduced by hypoxia (bottom panel of Figure 2), slow clearance of radioactivity does not simply reflect to slow washout of labeled molecules during flow reduction but rather reflects altered metabolism [12]. Thus, impairment of fatty acid oxidation during reduction of oxygen supply is associated with a reduction of the rate of ^{11}C-clearance, irrespective of the level of myocardial perfusion. This observation is consistent with the known shift from oxidation to incorporation into triacylglycerol of fatty acids during ischemia and hypoxia [9, 24]. However, the rate of ^{11}C-clearance is not quantitatively related to the rate of residual fatty acid oxidation. Analysis of the coronary effluent revealed that, in contrast to the observation under control conditions, during ischemia and hypoxia back diffusion of non metabolized (1-^{11}C)-palmitate accounts for up to 50% of the release of myocardial radioactivity [10].

Schwaiger et al. [25, 26] have observed in dogs that, during postischemic reperfusion, the myocardial clearance rate of (1-^{11}C)-palmitate radioactivity remained depressed for hours [25] or days [26] depending on the duration of the preceding coronary occlusion. This observation seems at first to be at variance with a number of recent studies in isolated rat hearts [21, 27] and pig hearts in vivo [28] employing continuous labeling with ^{14}C-palmitate and direct measurement of [14]CO_2 release. These latter observations suggest rapid recovery of fatty acid oxidation within 15 minutes after reperfusion [21, 27, 28]. A possible explanation for the apparent discrepancy is provided by the observation of increased labeling of the triacylglycerol fraction after reperfusion in two of the studies employing continuous labeling [21, 27]. It is therefore conceivable that the slower myocardial clearance rate after bolus injection of (1-^{11}C)-palmitate may reflect passage of a larger fraction of the tracer into a slow-turnover lipid compartment, such as the triacylglycerols, rather than persistent reduction of fatty acid oxidation.

Clinical observations with (1-^{11}C)-palmitate

In normal subjects, PET images of the heart, recorded 5 to 10 minutes after (1-^{11}C)-palmitate injection, display a homogenous distribution of radioactivity throughout the left ventricular myocardium [29, 30]. The clearance of myocardial activity is biexponential which is consistent with previous observations in animals [31, 32]. The rate of early ^{11}C-clearance in normal myocardium depends on the availability of circulating substrates and the level of cardiac work.

Schelbert et al. [32] reported an increase of the clearance half-time by 46% after ingestion of glucose. On the other hand, the clearance half-time decreased by 40% during atrial pacing [31]. However, Geltman et al. [33] recently reported that the clearance half-time was even prolonged when cardiac work was increased by bicycle exercise. The most likely explanation for this observation is that fatty acid oxidation is inhibited by increased circulating levels of lactate, despite exercise-induced stimulation of overall oxidative metabolism [34].

Coronary artery disease

In patients with recent or remote myocardial infarction, the infarcted region is detected and localized with high accuracy based on reduced uptake of (1-^{11}C)-palmitate [29, 35, 36]. Among 24 patients with non-transmural infarction, Geltman et al. [36] observed an uptake defect in 23 patients (96%) with PET and (1-^{11}C)-palmitate, but only in 11 of a subgroup of 18 patients (61%) using scintigraphy with thallium-201. The size of the uptake defect in patients with transmural or nontransmural infarction correlated closely with infarct size estimated from MB-CK-determination in serial blood samples [29].

Sobel et al. [37] studied 19 patients immediately before and 48 to 72 hours after administration of a thrombolytic agent. Among the 11 patients with successful thrombolysis, the size of the (1-^{11}C)-palmitate uptake defect decreased by an average of 29%. The defect size did not change in patients without reperfusion. Thus, PET with (1-^{11}C)-palmitate may allow documentation of myocardial salvage in patients. However, the practical application of this approach in the clinical setting is difficult without delaying the onset of thrombolytic therapy.

Grover-McKay et al. [31] have studied 10 patients with exertional angina by sequential (1-^{11}C)-palmitate imaging at rest and during atrial pacing. At rest, clearance of (1-^{11}C)-palmitate radioactivity was homogeneous throughout the myocardium. Although the clearance half-time decreased in every region during pacing, the clearance rate remained significantly slower in regions supplied by an artery with a stenosis greater than 70% in diameter. However, the difference in the clearance half-time between critically supplied and control myocardium was rather small, 13.4 ± 2.5 (SD) minutes versus 15.6 ± 4.0 minutes.

Cardiomyopathy

Patients with dilated cardiomyopathy exhibit marked spatial heterogeneity of initial (1-^{11}C)-palmitate accumulation [30]. The 'patchy' pattern of (1-^{11}C)-palmitate uptake in these patients is distinguishable from that observed in patients with extensive coronary artery disease and depressed left ventricular function, who exhibit discrete zones of reduced uptake [38]. In the fasted state, the clearance rate did not differ significantly from that observed in normal individuals [32]. However, in almost half of the patients with dilated cardiomyopathy, the response to glucose ingestion was abnormal, with no change, or even an increase, in the rate of ^{11}C-clearance [32]. In patients with hypertrophic cardiomyopathy, initial accumulation of (1-^{11}C)-palmitate was reduced by 29% in the septal region when compared to the lateral wall, without modification of the clearance rate [39]. The pathophysiological significance of these observations in patients with dilated or hypertrophic cardiomyopathy are as yet unknown.

Limitations of metabolic imaging with (1-^{11}C)-palmitate

Despite the significant contribution of PET with (1-^{11}C)-palmitate to an improved understanding of regional fatty acid metabolism in both experimental animals and patients, a number of limitations of the approach to have also become apparent. While PET has the potential for quantification, information on fatty acid metabolism has remained qualitative. Estimation of the rate of fatty acid oxidation from clearance of ^{11}C-activity is complicated by at least three factors. First, back diffusion of nonmetabolized palmitate, which occurs at a similar rate to the release of [11]CO_2, compromises the relationship between early ^{11}C-clearance and oxidative metabolic rate [10]. Second, estimation of the overall rate of fatty acid oxidation based on analysis of the early rapid clearance component does not take into account the contribution of endogenous lipid esters, such as triacylglycerols, to fatty acid oxidation. This factor may, as emphasized above, explain the apparently contrasting results obtained with noninvasive and invasive estimates of fatty acid oxidation during reperfusion. Third, the variation of the size of the pool in which a labeled compound

Table 1. Synopsis of the effect of several conditions on myocardial kinetics of (1-^{11}C)-palmitate.

Condition	Regional uptake	Early clearance component		References
		Relative size	Clearance rate[a]	
Glucose	=	↓	↓	[16, 23, 32]
Lactate	=	↓	↓	[16]
Pacing	↑	↑	↑	[13, 31]
Ischemia	= or ↓	↓	↓	[11, 14, 31]
Hypoxia	= or ↓	↓	↓	[10, 12]
Reperfusion	= or ↓	↓	↓	[25, 26]
Cardiomyopathy	heterogenous	abnormal response to glucose		[30, 32]

[a] Clearance rate without subtraction of late phase.

resides may affect the turnover rate at unaltered metabolic flux. Sophisticated compartmental tracer kinetic models for the estimation of flux in selected metabolic segments [40] have not found significant application to date.

Structurally modified ^{11}C-labeled fatty acids

With the aim of facilitating quantification of the initial segments of fatty acid metabolism, a methyl group has been introduced in the β-position of (1-^{11}C)-heptadecanoic acid to prevent β-oxidation [41]. (1-^{11}C)-β-methyl-heptadecanoic acid exhibited, as anticipated, a prolonged myocardial clearance half-time [42]. However, cellular uptake and intracellular activation appears to differ from a naturally occurring fatty acid, as indicated by a lower extraction fraction and enhanced backdiffusion of nonmetabolized tracer when compared with (1-^{11}C)-palmitate [42].

In order to obviate the need for on-site tracer synthesis, fatty acids have also been labeled in the terminal position with fluorine-18. As yet, these tracers have not found clinical application [43].

Conclusion

Positron emission tomography with (1-^{11}C)-palmitate permits the noninvasive detection of regional differences in myocardial fatty acid metabolism (Table 1). Although this tracer is instrumental in clinical research, the diagnostic application has remained limited, in part because of the dependence of its metabolism on circulating substrate levels, and also because of the complex intracellular kinetics which makes interpretation of the tomographic observations rather difficult.

Acknowledgement

Supported by the Swiss National Science Foundation grant 32.26373.89.

References

1. Bergmann SR, Fox KA, Geltman EM, Sobel BE. Positron emission tomography of the heart. Prog Cardiovasc Dis 1985; 28: 165–94.
2. Bergmann SR. Clinical applications of assessments of myocardial substrate utilization with positron emission tomography. Mol Cell Biochem 1989; 88: 201–9.
3. Schwaiger M, Wolpers HG. Advances in the assessment of myocardial-metabolism by positron emission tomography. Coronary Artery Dis 1990; 1: 547–55.
4. Weiss ES, Hoffmann EJ, Phelps ME et al. External detection and visualization of myocardial ischemia with ^{11}C-substrates in vitro and in vivo. Circ Res 1976; 39: 24–32.
5. Welch MJ, Dence CS, Marshall DR, Kilbourn MR. Remote system for production of carbon-11 labeled palmitic acid. J Label Compounds Radiopharm 1983; 20: 1087–95.
6. Vasdev SC, Kako KJ. Incorporation of fatty acids into rat heart lipids. In vivo and in vitro studies. J Mol Cell Cardiol 1977; 9: 617–31.
7. Carlsten A, Hallgren B, Jagenburg R, Svanborg A, Werko L. Myocardial arteriovenous differences of individual free fatty acids in healthy human individuals. Metabolism 1963; 12: 1063–71.
8. Neely JR, Rovetto MJ, Oram JF. Myocardial utilization of carbohydrate and lipids. Prog Cardiovasc Dis 1972; 15: 289–329.
9. Liedtke AJ. Alterations of carbohydrate and lipid metabolism in the acutely ischemic heart. Prog Cardiovasc Dis 1981; 23: 321–36.
10. Fox KA, Abendschein DR, Ambos HD, Sobel BE, Bergmann SR. Efflux of metabolized and nonmetabolized fatty acid from canine myocardium. Implications for quantifying myocardial metabolism tomographically. Circ Res 1985; 57: 232–43.
11. Lerch RA, Ambos HD, Bergmann SR, Welch MJ, Ter-Pogossian MM, Sobel BE. Localization of viable, ischemic myocardium by positron-emission tomography with ^{11}C-palmitate. Circulation 1981; 64: 689–99.
12. Lerch RA, Bergmann SR, Ambos HD, Welch MJ, Ter-Pogossian MM, Sobel BE. Effect of flow-independent reduction of metabolism on regional myocardial clearance of ^{11}C-palmitate. Circulation 1982; 65: 731–8.
13. Schön HR, Schelbert HR, Robinson G et al. C-11 labeled palmitic acid for the noninvasive evaluation of regional myocardial fatty acid metabolism with positron-computed tomography. I. Kinetics of C-11 palmitic acid in normal myocardium. Am Heart J 1981; 103: 532–47.
14. Schelbert HR, Henze E, Keen R et al. C-11 palmitate for the noninvasive evaluation of regional myocardial fatty acid metabolism with positron-computed tomography. IV. In vivo evaluation of acute demand-induced ischemia in dogs. Am Heart J 1983; 106: 736–50.
15. Schwaiger M, Fishbein MC, Block M et al. Metabolic and ultrastructural abnormalities

during ischemia in canine myocardium: noninvasive assessment by positron emission tomography. J Mol Cell Cardiol 1987; 19: 259–69.

16. Wyns W, Schwaiger M, Huang SC et al. Effects of inhibition of fatty acid oxidation on myocardial kinetics of ^{11}C-labeled palmitate. Circ Res 1989; 65: 1787–97.

17. Trach V, Buschmans-Denkel E, Schaper W. Relation between lipolysis and glycolysis during ischemia in the isolated rat heart. Basic Res Cardiol 1986; 81: 454–64.

18. Weiss ES, Ahmed SA, Welch MJ, Williamson JR, Ter-Pogossian MM, Sobel BE. Quantification of infarction in cross sections of canine myocardium in vivo with positron emission transaxial tomography and ^{11}C-palmitate. Circulation 1977; 55: 66–73.

19. Bergmann SR, Lerch RA, Fox KA et al. Temporal dependence of beneficial effects of coronary thrombolysis characterized by positron tomography. Am J Med 1982; 73: 573–81.

20. Jennings RB, Reimer KA. Factors involved in salvaging ischemic myocardium: effect of reperfusion of arterial blood. Circulation 1983; 68 (2 Suppl): I25–36.

21. Görge G, Chatelain P, Schaper J, Lerch R. Effect of increasing degrees of ischemic injury on myocardial oxidative metabolism early after reperfusion in isolated rat hearts. Circ Res 1991; 68: 1681–92.

22. Rosamond TL, Abendschein DR, Sobel BE, Bergmann SR, Fox KA. Metabolic fate of radiolabeled palmitate in ischemic canine myocardium: implications for positron emission tomography. J Nucl Med 1987; 28: 1322–9.

23. Schelbert HR, Henze E, Schon HR, Keen R, Hansen H, Selin C et al. C-11 palmitate for the noninvasive evaluation of regional myocardial fatty acid metabolism with positron computed tomography. III. In vivo demonstration of the effects of substrate availability on myocardial metabolism. Am Heart J 1983; 105: 492–504.

24. Whitmer JT, Idell-Wenger JA, Rovetto MJ, Neely JR. Control of fatty acid metabolism in ischemic and hypoxic hearts. J Biol Chem 1978; 253: 4305–9.

25. Schwaiger M, Schelbert HR, Keen R et al. Retention and clearance of C-11 palmitic acid in ischemic and reperfused canine myocardium. J Am Coll Cardiol 1985; 6: 311–20.

26. Schwaiger M, Schelbert HR, Ellison D et al. Sustained regional abnormalities in cardiac metabolism after transient ischemia in the chronic dog model. J Am Coll Cardiol 1985; 6: 336–47.

27. Lopaschuk GD, Spafford MA, Davies NJ, Wall SR. Glucose and palmitate oxidation in isolated working rat hearts reperfused after a period of transient global ischemia. Circ Res 1990; 66: 546–53.

28. Liedtke AJ, DeMaison L, Eggleston AM, Cohen LM, Nellis SH. Changes in substrate metabolism and effects of excess fatty acids in reperfused myocardium. Circ Res 1988; 62: 535–42.

29. Ter-Pogossian MM, Klein MS, Markham J, Roberts R, Sobel BE. Regional assessment of myocardial metabolic integrity in vivo by positron-emission tomography with ^{11}C-labeled palmitate. Circulation 1980; 61: 242–55.

30. Geltman EM, Smith JL, Beecher D, Ludbrook PA, Ter-Pogossian MM, Sobel BE. Altered regional myocardial metabolism in congestive cardiomyopathy detected by positron tomography. Am J Med 1983; 74: 773–85.

31. Grover-McKay M, Schelbert HR, Schwaiger M et al. Identification of impaired metabolic reserve by atrial pacing in patients with significant coronary artery stenosis. Circulation 1986; 74: 281–92.

32. Schelbert HR, Henze E, Sochor H et al. Effects of substrate availability on myocardial C-11 palmitate kinetics by positron emission tomography in normal subjects and patients with ventricular dysfunction. Am Heart J 1986; 111: 1055–64.

33. Geltman EM, Kaiserauer S, Walsh MN, Ehsani AA. Effects of maximal and submaximal exercise on myocardial ^{11}C-palmitate clearance assessed with positron emission tomography [abstract]. J Am Coll Cardiol 1988; 11 (2 Suppl A): 211A.

34. Keul J, Doll E, Steim H, Homburger H, Kern H, Reindell H. Über den Stoffwechsel des menschlichen Herzens. I. Die Substratversorgung des gesunden menschlichen Herzens in Ruhe, während und nach körperlicher Arbeit. Pflügers Arch Ges Physiol 1965; 282: 1–27.

35. Sobel BE, Weiss ES, Welch MJ, Siegel BA, Ter-Pogossian MM. Detection of remote myocardial infarction in patients with positron emission transaxial tomography and intravenous ^{11}C-palmitate. Circulation 1977; 55: 853–7.

36. Geltman EM, Biello D, Welch MJ, Ter-Pogossian MM, Roberts R, Sobel BE. Characterization of nontransmural myocardial infarction by positron-emission tomography. Circulation 1982; 65: 747–55.

37. Sobel BE, Geltman EM, Tiefenbrunn AJ et al. Improvement of regional myocardial metabolism after coronary thrombolysis induced with tissue-type plasminogen activator or streptokinase. Circulation 1984; 69: 983–90.

38. Eisenberg JD, Sobel BE, Geltman EM. Differentiation of ischemic from nonischemic cardiomyopathy with positron emission tomography. Am J Cardiol 1987; 59: 1410–4.

39. Grover-McKay M, Schwaiger M, Krivokapich J, Perloff JK, Phelps ME, Schelbert HR. Regional myocardial blood flow and metabolism at rest in mildly symptomatic patients with hypertrophic cardiomyopathy. J Am Coll Cardiol 1989; 13: 317–24.

40. Schelbert HR, Phelps ME. Positron computed tomography for the in vivo assessment of regional myocardial function. J Mol Cell Cardiol 1984; 16: 683–93.

41. Livni E, Elmaleh DR, Levy S, Brownell GL, Strauss WH. Beta-methyl [1-^{11}C]heptadecanoic acid: a new myocardial metabolic tracer for positron emission tomography. J Nucl Med 1982; 23: 169–75.

42. Abendschein DR, Fox KA, Ambos HD, Sobel BE, Bergmann SR. Metabolism of beta-methyl[1-11C]heptadecanoic acid in canine myocardium. Int J Rad Appl Instrum [B] 1987; 14: 579–85.

43. Knust EJ, Kupfernagel C, Stöcklin G. Long-chain F-18 fatty acids for the study of regional metabolism in heart and liver; odd-even effects of metabolism in mice. J Nucl Med 1979; 20: 1170–5.

19. Myocardial metabolic imaging with fluorine-18 deoxyglucose

NEAL G. UREN and PAOLO G. CAMICI

Introduction

With the definition of coronary artery anatomy by angiography has come the need to characterize the pathophysiological consequences of coronary artery disease. In order to quantify the functional significance of an epicardial coronary stenosis, measurement of coronary blood flow and blood flow reserve has developed using invasive techniques such as Doppler catheterization [1] and coronary sinus thermodilution [2, 3]. Coronary sinus catheterization may also be used to measure the transmyocardial extraction of metabolic substrates by simultaneous catheterization of an artery and coronary sinus or great cardiac vein [4]. However, these invasive methods are limited by their inability to measure coronary blood flow or metabolism in different myocardial regions at the same time or in regions supplied by arteries other than the left anterior descending artery in the case of coronary sinus catheterization. This is an even greater limitation if one takes into account the intrinsic regionality of ischemic heart disease.

On the other hand, conventional single photon nuclear techniques can give information about the regional distribution of myocardial perfusion, but they do not allow absolute quantification of flow per unit mass of myocardium. Regional myocardial blood flow may now be measured noninvasively in absolute terms using positron emission tomography (PET) [5] often with the advantage of studying territory subtended by normal and diseased coronary arteries simultaneously. Regional myocardial metabolism may also be accurately defined using positron-emitting tracers with the improved spatial resolution achieved with PET [6].

Ernst E. van der Wall et al. (eds), What's new in cardiac imaging?, 263–276.
© *1992 Kluwer Academic Publishers. Printed in the Netherlands.*

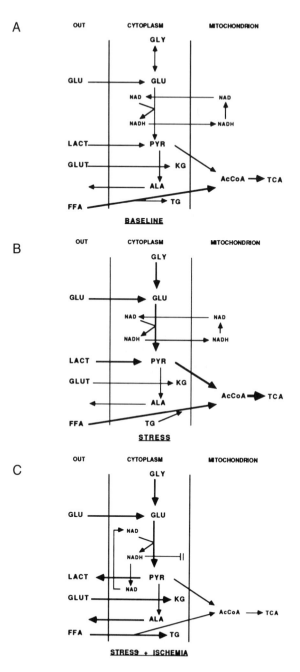

At a cellular level in the normoxic state, oxidative phosphorylation of metabolic substrates occurs in the mitochondria to generate high-energy phosphates, namely adenosine triphosphate (ATP), to fuel cellular function and myocardial contractility. Under fasting conditions, the heart preferentially uses free fatty acids (FFA) as its source of energy, using up to 10% of the whole body turnover despite receiving only 5% of cardiac output [7]. Oxidation of lipid-derived substrates accounts for up to 80% of myocardial oxygen consumption, with the majority of the remaining energy requirement provided by carbohydrates (glucose, pyruvate and lactate). However, with the increase in glucose loading in the fed state, glucose and insulin levels increase with subsequent reduction in fatty acid uptake through insulin inhibition of adipose tissue lipolysis [7]. With greater production of energy from glucose for each unit of oxygen consumed, there is improved efficiency of oxygen (O_2) usage after feeding (5.01 kcal/l of O_2 versus 4.66 kcal/l of O_2 from fatty acids) [7].

Normal cardiac metabolism of carbohydrates

At rest, normal subjects and patients with coronary artery disease have a similar metabolism to all major substrates (FFA, glucose, ketone bodies, pyruvate, lactate, and glutamate) extracted to generate acetyl Coenzyme A (acetyl CoA) to fuel the tricarboxylic acid cycle (Figure 1a).

←——

Figure 1. (a) Schematic representation of major metabolic pathways in resting human myocardium under fasting conditions. Most of the energy produced (> 80%) derives from oxidation of free fatty acids (FFA). Most of the pyruvate (PYR) formed from lactate (LACT) and glucose (GLU) through glycolysis is used aerobically and enters the trocarboxylic cycle (TCA) after conversion to acetyl coenzyme A (AcCoA). A small amount of ppyruvate is transaminated to alanine (ALA), which is then released at the expense of glutamate (GLUT) which is converted to alpha-ketoglutarate (KG). The reduced coenzyme nicotinamide adenine dinucleotide (NADH), which is formed during glycolysis in the cytosol, is normally reoxidized (NAD) in the mitochondrion by way of the malate-aspartate cycle. GLY, glycogen; TG, triglyceride.

(b) Metabolic changes during increased cardiac workload in normal myocardium. There is rapid activation of GLY breakdown and increased utilization of exogenous GLU and LACT. Carbohydrate (GLU, LACT, PYR, and ALA) oxidation is significantly increased and accounts for more than 60% of energy production, acting as a booster and contributing to the extra energy required during maximum stress.

(c) During stress-induced myocardial ischemia, there is a reduced oxidation of FFA with an increased storage of TG. GLU utilization is increased (both from exogenous GLU and from GLY), but the extra PYR formed cannot be oxidized. There is an increased production of ALA with a greater myocardial GLUT consumption. In addition, due to the accumulation of NADH, there is activation of the enzyme lactate dehydrogenase, with conversion of PYR to LACT that is then released; at the same time 1 mole of NADH is reoxidized to NAD.

Glucose is transported into the cell by a specific carrier system which is not energy-dependent. Myocardial glucose uptake is determined by cardiac workload, insulin concentration, glucose concentration, the degree of adrenergic activation, and tissue oxygen tension [7]. After trans-sarcolemmal transport, glucose is rapidly phosphorylated into glucose-6-phosphate by the enzyme hexokinase, even in conditions of high glucose transport such as tissue hypoxia. Normally, the rate of trans-sarcolemmal transport and hexokinase activity are the limiting steps for myocardial glucose utilization. Glucose-6-phosphate may then be converted to glycogen by glycogen synthetase or to pyruvate through the glycolysis by the Embden-Meyerhof pathway. Glucose-6-phosphate may also be metabolized via the pentose-phosphate pathway but this pathway, although very important for cellular survival, is of lesser quantitative importance.

Glycolysis is controlled by feedback from the distal products of aerobic and anaerobic glucose metabolism and by fatty acid metabolism at discrete sites [8], which depends on whether the subject is in the fed state, because of the increased levels of circulating glucose and insulin with increased glucose oxidation, or fasting state where oxidation of lipid-derived substrates provides most of the energy for ATP production [9]. Hexokinase activation shifts control of glucose metabolism to the enzyme phosphofructokinase, which is a major rate-limiting step.

Phosphofructokinase activity is amplified by reduced concentrations of ATP and creatine phosphate and increased concentrations of ADP, adenosine monophosphate (AMP) and inorganic phosphate (Pi). Citrate is also a powerful inhibitor of this enzyme. In the fasting state, fatty acid and ketone body oxidation lead to acetyl CoA production with the excess accumulation of citrate through the tricarboxylic acid cycle countering the usual positive feedback of high levels of fructose-6-phosphate (a subsequent product of glucose-6-phosphate) on phosphofructokinase, thus inhibiting glycolysis.

Pyruvate occupies a central role in the ultimate disposal of glucose: it may be reduced to lactate (completing anaerobic glycolysis); transaminated to alanine at the expense of glutamate which serves as amine group donor; or oxidized to acetyl CoA inside the mitochondrion by pyruvate dehydrogenase, which is the predominant route under aerobic conditions. A decreased ratio of [ATP]/[ADP], the fasting state, adrenaline, and increased cardiac workload all facilitate conversion of the enzyme from the inactive to the active form. Under aerobic conditions, there is also a net balance in favor of lactate extraction from the circulation into myocardium with conversion to pyruvate, underlining the versatility of the heart to use a variety of different substrates for energy production depending on their plasma concentration. In general, in both normal subjects and patients with coronary artery disease at rest under

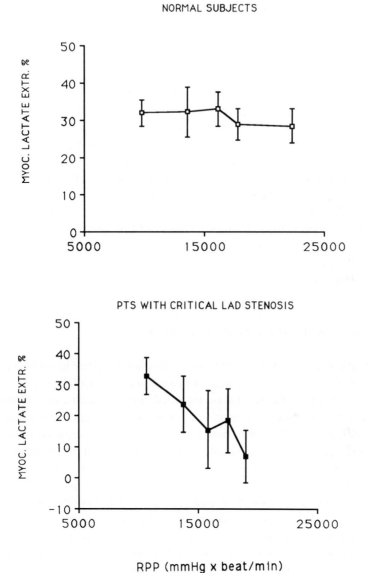

Figure 2. The values (mean ± SEM) of the rate-pressure product (RPP), obtained with incremental atrial pacing, are plotted against myocardial lactate extraction. No significant changes in lactate extraction are noted with increasing RPP in normal subjects. The same relationship was studied in a group of patients with coronary artery disease and isolated severe left anterior descending (LAD) coronary artery (P. Camici, unpublished data). Note the significant progressive decrease of lactate extraction with increasing RPP in patients with LAD disease.

fasting conditions, carbohydrate (mainly glucose) uptake exceeds oxidation (Figure 2), indicating nonoxidative disposal of these substrates.

The tricarboxylic (citric) acid cycle is tightly controlled in the mitochondria by extramitochondrial [ATP]/[ADP], intramitochondrial [NAD]/[NADH] (NAD, nicotinamide adenine dinucleotide) and oxygen tension. This prevents unnecessary utilization of substrate when ATP levels are adequate for cellular respiration. However, under conditions of stress such as exercise or atrial pacing, the heart needs to increase oxygen consumption and generate an increased amount of high energy phosphates. This is achieved by increasing utilization of exogenous substrates such as glucose and FFA whose delivery is facilitated by the increase in coronary blood flow. At moderate workload, FFA remain the preferential substrate providing acetyl-CoA for oxidative phosphorylation. With increasing cardiac workload, glucose uptake and utilization increases with no further change in FFA uptake (Figure 1b), with additional substrate for glycolysis derived from glycogen breakdown [10]. This may be because of the greater energy yield (amount of ADP phosphorylated per oxygen consumed) with glucose compared to FFA.

Metabolic consequences of myocardial ischemia

An epicardial coronary artery stenosis reduces the increase in coronary blood flow available during stress when an increase in myocardial oxygen demand occurs. Most of our knowledge on myocardial metabolism comes from work on isolated perfused animal hearts in normoxic and anoxic conditions. However, ischemia is the commonest situation leading to reduced myocardial oxygen delivery in man, and many different factors determine the duration, severity, and extent of ischemia [11]. During myocardial ischemia, major changes occur in intracellular substrate metabolism: there is an increased glycogen breakdown and exogenous glucose uptake which fuel glycolysis (Figure 1c) [7, 12]. Accumulation of reduced coenzymes ($NADH_2$) stimulate the conversion of pyruvate to lactate by lactate dehydrogenase (Figure 2). With mild ischemia, the transport of glucose into the cell is accelerated, as is glycolysis [7]. However, the distal products of glycolysis, lactate and reduced coenzymes, will finally inhibit the enzyme glyceraldehyde 3-phosphate dehydrogenase lower down the Embden-Meyerhof pathway [13]. Although there is an increase in glucose uptake, carbohydrate oxidation is negligible (Figure 3). With the return of myocardial oxygen delivery, lactate is oxidized back to pyruvate with restoration of glycogen to pre-ischemic values. The time required to return to the pre-ischemic metabolic pattern is prolonged with persisting high glucose uptake, probably for glycogen re-synthesis, more so in

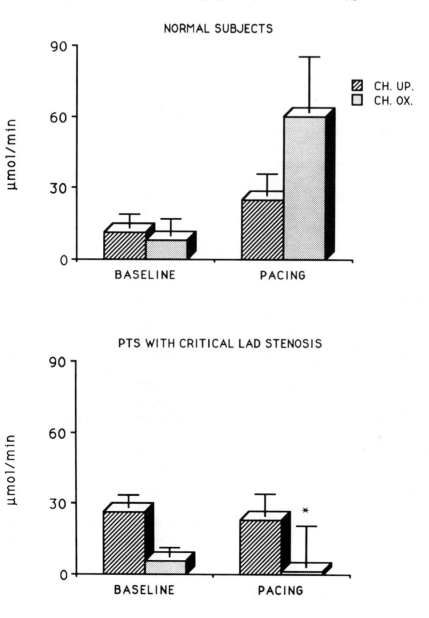

Figure 3. Myocardial uptake and oxidation of carbohydrates in normal subjects and patients with a critical lesion of the left anterior descending (LAD) coronary artery at baseline and during maximal atrial pacing (P. Camici et al., unpublished data). Carbohydrate uptake is the sum of glucose and lactate, pyruvate and alanine (expressed as glucose equivalents). Uptake and oxidation of carbohydrates are comparable in the two groups at baseline. During pacing, which induced angina and ST segment depression in patients with an LAD stenosis, despite comparable uptakes, carbohydrate oxidation is significantly increased in normal individuals and negligible in patients.

post-ischemic then normal myocardium [10]. This persistence of high glucose uptake in post-ischemic myocardium is the underlying principle which allows the identification of transiently ischemic myocardium using fluorine-18-fluoro 2-deoxyglucose (FDG) with PET.

During severe ischemia, the rate of exogenous glucose delivery is also reduced. Under these circumstances, the ischemic myocardium will rely almost exclusively on intracellular glycogen stores. However, the insufficient 'washout' of accumulated hydrogen ions and the ensuing intracellular acidosis will inhibit phosphofructokinase, and thus, glycolysis much earlier than with mild ischemia [14]. Thus, the uptake and intracellular utilization of glucose is modulated by the presence and severity of ischemia.

Positron emission tomography for the study of myocardial metabolism

Positron emission tomography (PET) has developed as one of the best noninvasive methods of quantifying absolute regional myocardial blood flow and metabolism [5, 6, 15]. Using a cyclotron (a particle accelerator), radioisotopes may be produced which emit positrons (positively charged electrons), each positron annihilating with an electron to produce two 511 keV gamma rays emitted in diametrically opposite directions. This may be detected over several transaxial slices by circular detector arrays [5]. Compared to conventional radio-imaging techniques, improved resolution of images is obtained from PET and, using specific tracer models, it is possible to derive quantitative data on myocardial blood flow and substrate utilization. The short half-lives of positron emitting tracers, for example, oxygen-15 (2 minutes), carbon-11 (20 minutes), allow serial studies to be performed to assess the response to an intervention, such as vasodilator stress or exercise, with a small dose of radioactivity for the patient. Several positron-emitting radioisotopes have been incorporated into physiological substrates (without altering their chemical structure) and may be used as metabolic tracers, such as FDG [16–18].

Clinical applications of deoxyglucose imaging

As described previously, under ischemic conditions, there is an increased utilization of glucose by the myocardium both from glycogen breakdown and from exogenous glucose. The glucose analogue 2-deoxyglucose, in which a hydroxyl group is substituted by a hydrogen atom on the second carbon atom, shares with glucose the same trans-sarcolemmal carrier and is a good substrate for hexokinase with production of deoxyglucose-6-phosphate. This will not be further metabolized and accumulates in the cell according to exogenous glucose utilization [16]. Global and regional changes in glucose utilization under controlled conditions may be studied using 2-deoxyglucose, labeled with the positron emitter fluorine-18 (FDG) [15–17]. Thus, FDG may be used to demonstrate regions of myocardial ischemia in different ischemic syndromes.

1. Chronic stable angina

At rest in the fasting state, myocardial FDG uptake is comparably low in normal controls and in patients with angiographically proven coronary artery disease and stable exertional angina. After supine exercise (sufficient to induce chest pain and significant ST segment depression), a marked increase in FDG uptake my be seen in both normals and patients [19].

In patients, FDG uptake in nonischemic regions (regions with a normal increment of coronary flow on exercise) was similar to that in control subjects. However, FDG uptake was significantly higher in regions with impaired flow during exercise. This disparity in FDG uptake was detected well into the post-exercise phase (Figure 4), after defects of the flow marker rubidium-82 (^{82}Rb) and the electrocardiogram had returned to baseline. This increased uptake is thought to be due to prolonged recovery of metabolic function with a continued preference for glucose in 'post-ischemic' myocardium, and may reflect increased glycogen synthesis to replenish glycogen stores that were depleted during ischemia and increased cardiac work [19]. However, the precise time course of this phenomenon and its possible relation to the severity of the ischemic episode is still to be elucidated.

Recovery of full contractile function after revascularization may also be delayed until tissue glucose metabolism returns to normal. In a preliminary study of 11 patients, Nienaber et al. demonstrated that segmental wall motion abnormalities did not improve 48 hours after coronary angioplasty despite improvement in perfusion [20]. However, wall motion scores had improved at two montws follow-up associated with improvement in blood flow-FDG mismatch, implying that normalization of the altered metabolic state is a prerequisite for contractile recovery. This may be evidence for slow normalization of a chronic metabolic adaptation to a persistent reduction in blood flow [21].

2. Unstable angina

PET scanning with FDG has also been done in patients with severe coronary artery disease and unstable angina characterized by frequent spontaneous episodes of ST segment depression at rest. Unlike patients with stable angina pectoris with an FDG uptake at rest similar to control subjects, patients with

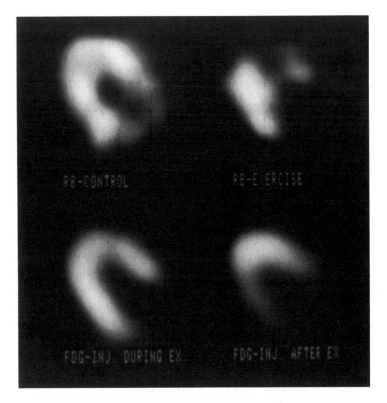

Figure 4. Positron computed tomographic images of rubidium-82 (^{82}Rb) and FDG uptake in the left ventricle (LV) of a patient with left anterior descending disease. Each image is a transaxial slice of the heart (1.6 cm thick). In each image, the LV free wall is in the 6 to 10 o'clock position, the anterior wall and septum are in the 10 to 3 o'clock position, and the remaining open area is in the plane of the mitral valve. The ^{82}Rb scan at rest (*top left*) shows a homogeneous cation uptake in all myocardial walls. The ^{82}Rb scan recorded during exercise (*top right*) shows a severely reduced cation uptake on the anterior LV wall. FDG was injected during exercise. An FDG scan recorded during exercise shows homogeneous glucose uptake consistent with increased glucose utilization (*bottom left*). Another FDG scan, recorded 60 minutes after tracer injection, shows a greater FDG uptake in the previously ischemic area (*bottom right*). FDG uptake in the anterior wall is 1.55 times higher than that in the nonischemic muscle.

unstable angina may have regional and even global increases in FDG uptake already at rest in the absence of perfusion abnormalities or transient myocardial ischemia [22]. As a control, glucose utilization was similar in chest-wall skeletal muscle in all groups studied. This increase in FDG uptake, of up to four times, occurred despite similar disease severity at angiography. No relationship was seen between FDG uptake and recent episodes of chest pain or ST segment depression. This has led to the concept of a metabolic adaptation to chronic ischemia (with preferential glucose utilization) which is sustained even in the absence of demonstrable myocardial ischemia [22].

It is of interest that an increase in glucose utilization may occur in areas not subtended by a stenotic artery. This may imply that the metabolic derangement in areas supplied by diseased vessels imposes a metabolic stress on a normal area such that there is also a move towards an increased glucose flux, possibly because of a necessary increase in cardiac work. Alternatively, this may be evidence for altered metabolism in territories subtended by angiographically normal arteries.

3. Myocardial infarction and tissue viability

With the advent of thrombolysis and reperfusion, myocardial salvage after acute myocardial infarction has increased, but often with a significant residual coronary artery stenosis and a variable degree of myocardial injury or 'myocardial stunning' – reversible left ventricular hypokinesis in the presence of normal coronary blood flow [23]. Characterization of residual metabolic function after acute ischemic injury in myocardial regions with reduced or normal perfusion is of additional value in predicting the recovery of mechanical function. Impairment of FFA metabolism with reduced oxidative metabolism leads to increased glycolytic flux and glucose uptake which manifest as enhanced FDG uptake with PET. This may also allow prediction of improvement of infarcted segments or those with wall motion abnormalities even in the absence of demonstrable infarction, measured as a recovery in contractile function after revascularization [24].

The concept of viability is based on the demonstration of a maintained glucose metabolism in areas of reduced perfusion ('mismatch'). On the other hand, a concordant reduction of myocardial blood flow and glucose uptake ('match') would indicate the presence of scar without any viable tissue and predict no recovery of function. Marshall et al. demonstrated that within the first weeks after myocardial infarction, preserved glucose metabolism (relative to flow measured with nitrogen-13 ammonia), i.e. mismatch, identified viable tissue [25].

In another study, Schwaiger et al. demonstrated that within three days of myocardial infarction, in hypoperfused regions with preserved glucose metabolism, it is not possible to differentiate these regions from those without residual metabolic viability according to myocardial perfusion alone, segmental wall motion abnormalities, or left ventricular ejection fraction [26]. However, on subsequent follow-up at 6 weeks, 8 of 16 mismatched segments improved their segmental wall motion (6 of 16 unchanged) compared to no change in the matched group. Thus, maintenance of metabolic activity in infarcted territory predicts a variable outcome consistent with the wide variation in residual perfusion, collateralization and borderline ischemia in within 72 hours of infarction.

Consistent with the added prognostic value of an open artery after thrombolysis, PET scanning with FDG has demonstrated increased uptake in 76% of regions subtended by such an artery, compared to 29% of regions with an occluded artery, despite significant collateral flow in the majority of these [27]. Conversely, reduced or absent FDG uptake in an infarct territory is predictive for no improvement in ventricular function [27, 28].

The use of blood flow to FDG uptake mismatch as an index of viability has been used to predict success of revascularization. In a study of 17 post-infarction patients, preservation of glucose uptake predicted recovery of 85% of hypokinetic segments after coronary artery bypass grafting. Decreased glucose uptake implied irreversibility of hypokinesis in 92% of cases [24]. This was confirmed by Tamaki et al. in another study of 22 patients before and 5–7 weeks after surgery with a positive predictive accuracy of 78% of blood flow-FDG mismatch [29]. They reported a lower negative predictive accuracy of 78% than the 92% quoted by Tillisch et al. [24]. This probably reflects studying patients in the fasted state with a much lower uptake by normal myocardium increasing the sensitivity of FDG uptake, but in areas with not sufficient viability to improve with revascularization.

These studies demonstrate the heterogeneity of myocardial infarction and reaffirm the importance of early recanalization of the infarct-related artery to reduce the extent of myocardial necrosis and maintain tissue viability. The additional value of PET with FDG is that it demonstrates jeopardized but viable myocardium where conventional techniques such as electrocardiography (pathological Q waves), gated radionuclide ventriculography, echocardiography (segmental ventricular asynergy) and thallium-210 redistribution scintigraphy (fixed perfusion defects) may indicate irreversibile myocardial injury [30].

Conclusions

Positron emission tomography with FDG may be used to complement the noninvasive measurement of myocardial blood flow in patients with acute and chronic myocardial ischemia and infarction. This has improved detection of significant coronary artery disease and increased understanding of the pathophysiological and metabolic consequences of myocardial ischemia. By defining tissue viability as the mismatch of persistent or increased glucose uptake with reduced blood flow, residual metabolic function may be detected in myocardial regions with the potential for recovery of contractile function in time, or after a revascularization procedure. This accurate detection of jeopardized but viable tissue may allow us to improve the selection of patients for bypass surgery or coronary angioplasty. With revascularization directed by the presence or absence of tissue viability, it may be possible to reduce morbidity and even mortality from coronary artery disease in the long term.

References

1. Wilson RF, Laughlin DE, Ackell PH et al. Transluminal, subselective measurement of coronary artery blood flow velocity and vasodilator reserve in man. Circulation 1985; 72: 82–92.
2. Ganz W, Tamura K, Marcus HS, Donoso R, Yoshida S, Swan HJ. Measurement of coronary sinus blood flow by continuous thermodilution in man. Circulation 1971; 44: 181–95.
3. Pepiine CJ, Mehta J, Webster WW Jr, Nichols WW. In vivo validation of a thermodilution method to determine regional left ventricular blood flow in patients with coronary artery disease. Circulation 1978; 58: 795–802.
4. Bing RJ. The metabolism of the heart. Harvey Lect 1954; 50: 27–70.
5. Phelps ME. Emission computed tomography. Semin Nucl Med 1977; 7: 337–65.
6. Phelps ME, Hoffman EJ, Huang SC, Kuhl DE. ECAT: a new computerized tomographic imaging system for positron-emitting radiopharmaceuticals. J Nucl Med 1978; 19: 635–47.
7. Camici P, Ferrannini E, Opie LH. Myocardial metabolism in ischemic heart disease: basic principles and application to imaging by positron emission tomography. Prog Cardiovasc Dis 1989; 32: 217–38.
8. Newsholme EA, Crabtree B. Theoretical principles in the approaches to control of metabolic pathways and their application to glycolysis in muscle [editorial]. J Mol Cell Cardiol 1979; 11: 839–56.
9. Randle PJ, Garland PB, Hales CN, Newsholme EA. The glucose fatty-acid cycle. Its role in insulin sensitivity and the metabolic disturbances of diabetes mellitus. Lancet 1963; 1: 785–9.
10. Camici P, Marraccini P, Marzilli M et al. Coronary hemodynamics and myocardial metabolism during and after pacing stress in normal humans. Am J Physiol 1989; 257: E309–17.
11. Maseri A. The changing face of angina pectoris: practical implications. Lancet 1983; 1: 746–9.
12. Opie LH, Owen P, Riemersma RA. Relative rates of oxidation of glucose and free fatty acids by ischaemic and non-ischaemic myocardium after coronary artery ligation in the dog. Eur J Clin Invest 1973; 3: 419–35.
13. Rovetto MJ, Lamberton WF, Neely JR. Mechanisms of glycolytic inhibition in ischemic rat hearts. Circ Res 1975; 37: 742–51.
14. Neely JR, Liedtke AJ, Whitmer JT, Rovetto MJ. Relationship between coronary flow and adenosine triphosphate production from glycolysis and oxidative metabolism. In: Roy EP, Harris P, editors. The cardiac sarcoplasm. München: Urban & Schwarzenberg, 1976: 301–21.
15. Bergmann SR, Fox KA, Geltman EG, Sobel BE. Positron emission tomography of the heart. Prog Cardiovasc Dis 1985; 28: 165–94.
16. Phelps ME, Hoffman EJ, Selin C et al. Investigation of [F18]2-fluoro-2-deoxyglucose for the measurement of myocardial glucose metabolism. J Nucl Med 1978; 19: 1311–9.
17. Gallagher BM, Ansari A, Atkins H et al. Radiopharmaceuticals XXVII. 18F-labelled 2--deoxy-2-fluoro-d-glucose 25 a radiopharmaceutical for measuring regional myocardial glu-

cose metabolism in vivo: tissue distribution and imaging studies in animals. J Nucl Med 1977; 18: 990–6.

18. Ratib O, Phelps ME, Huang SC, Henze SC, Selin CE, Schelbert HR. Positron tomography with deoxyglucose for estimating local myocardial glucose metabolism. J Nucl Med 1982; 23: 577–86.

19. Camici P, Araujo LI, Spinks T et al. Increased uptake of ^{18}F-fluorodeoxyglucose in postischemic myocardium of patients with exercise-induced angina. Circulation 1986; 74: 81–8.

20. Nienaber CA, Brunken RC, Sherman CT et al. Recovery of myocardial metabolism precedes functional improvement following relief of chronic myocardial ischemia by PTCA [abstract]. J Nucl Med 1989; 30 Suppl: 838.

21. Fedele FA, Gerwirtz H, Capone RJ, Sharaf B, Most AS. Metabolic response to prolonged reduction of myocardial blood flow distal to a severe coronary artery stenosis. Circulation 1988; 78: 729–35.

22. Araujo LI, Camici P, Spinks TJ, Jones T, Maseri A. Abnormalities in myocardial metabolism in patients with unstable angina as assessed by positron emission tomography. Cardiovasc Drugs Ther 1988; 2: 41–6.

23. Braunwald E, Kloner RA. The stunned myocardium: prolonged, post-ischemic ventricular dysfunction. Circulation 1982; 66: 1146–9.

24. Tillisch J, Brunken R, Marshall R. Reversibility of cardiac wall-motion abnormalities predicted by positron tomography. N Engl J Med 1986; 314: 884–8.

25. Marshall RC, Tillisch JH, Phelps ME et al. Identification and differentiation of resting myocardial ischemia in man with positron computed tomography, ^{18}F-labeled fluorodeoxyglucose and N-13 ammonia. Circulation 1983; 67: 766–78.

26. Schwaiger M, Brunken R, Grover-McKay M et al. Regional myocardial metabolism in patients with acute myocardial infarction assessed by positron emission tomography. J Am Coll Cardiol 1986; 8: 800–8.

27. Schwaiger M, Brunken RC, Kripokavich J et al. Beneficial effect of residual anterograde flow on tissue viability as assessed by positron emission tomography in patients with myocardial infarction. Eur Heart J 1987; 8: 981–8.

28. Pierard LA, de Landsheere CM, Berthe C, Rigo P, Kulbertus HE. Identification of viable myocardium by echocardiography during dobutamine infusion in patients with myocardial infarction after thrombolytic therapy: comparison with positron emission tomography. J Am Coll Cardiol 1990; 15: 1021–31.

29. Tamaki N, Yonekura Y, Yamashita K et al. Positron emission tomography using fluorine-18 deoxyglucose in evaluation of coronary artery bypass grafting. Am J Cardiol 1989; 64: 860–5.

30. Schwaiger M, Hicks R. The clinical role of metabolic imaging of the heart by positron emission tomography. J Nucl Med 1991; 32: 565–78.

31. Camici P, Marraccini P, Lorenzoni R et al. Metabolic markers of stress-induced ischaemia. Circulation 1991; 83 (suppl III): III-8–III-13.

20. Myocardial metabolic imaging with carbon-11-acetate

MARY NORINE WALSH

Introduction

The noninvasive quantification of regional myocardial oxygen consumption has long been an objective of cardiovascular research. It's potential utility lies primarily in the assessment of patients with ischemic heart disease where the delineation of viable myocardium is essential in determining which patients may benefit from percutaneous transluminal coronary angioplasty or coronary artery bypass grafting. In addition, the quantification of myocardial oxidative metabolism is important in defining the pathophysiology of many other cardiovascular diseases.

Despite the quantitative power of positron emission tomography (PET) and its sensitivity for detection of labeled physiologic substrates, quantification of carbohydrate or fatty acid metabolism alone (i.e. with ^{18}F-deoxyglucose or ^{11}C-palmitate) does not provide a direct measure of regional myocardial oxygen consumption [1, 2]. An admixture of diverse substrates obscures changes in myocardial oxygen consumption estimated on the basis of metabolism of individual substrates such as glucose or fatty acid [2]. The myocardial handling of either labeled palmitate or glucose (or the glucose analog, fluorodeoxyglucose) is critically dependent upon the level of arterial substrate content as well as on the hormonal milieu [2–5]. In addition, back diffusion of nonmetabolized ^{11}C-palmitate occurs in myocardial ischemia and contributes up to 50% of the total clearance of radioactivity from the myocardium, overestimating overall rates of oxidation [6].

Carbon-11-labeled acetate provides a noninvasive, indirect measure of myocardial oxygen consumption. In contradistinction to the case with glucose or

277

Ernst E. van der Wall et al. (eds), What's new in cardiac imaging?, 277–286.
© *1992 Kluwer Academic Publishers. Printed in the Netherlands.*

fatty acid, metabolism of acetate is confined virtually exclusively to mitochondrial oxidation. This chapter will review both the animal and clinical investigations that have been done to date with ^{11}C-acetate and PET as well as summarize its clinical utility.

Kinetics

Although the concentration of acetate in human plasma is low, acetate is oxidized readily by the heart [7–8]. All major myocardial oxidative fuels including free fatty acids, glucose, lactate, pyruvate, ketone bodies and some amino acids are oxidized via conversion to acetyl coenzyme A (CoA) and passage through the tricarboxylic acid (TCA) cycle [9]. Because TCA cycle turnover is tightly coupled to oxidative phosphorylation, measurement of TCA cycle flux provides an index of oxidative metabolism. In the myocardium, acetate is oxidized via the TCA cycle and is not metabolized by any other major pathways [7, 8]. The oxidation of acetate, therefore, provides an indirect measure of tricarboxylic cycle flux and serves as an index of oxidative metabolism.

Between 1980 and 1982, preliminary studies describing the kinetics of ^{11}C-acetate in a canine model, normal human subjects, and in patients with coronary artery disease were described [10–13]. No attempt was made to quantitatively correlate acetate kinetics to TCA cycle flux in these initial studies, but they did demonstrate that the clearance of extracted tracer from the heart after exercise was accelerated in normal myocardium and decreased in ischemic myocardium. These studies also demonstrated that the clearance of radioactivity from normal human myocardium of ^{11}C-acetate was monoexponential. In 1987, Brown et al. [14] reported studies with ^{14}C-acetate in an isolated perfused heart preparation demonstrating that the rate of flux of [14]CO_2 correlated very closely with myocardial oxygen consumption. This correlation was demonstrated in control hearts as well as ischemic and reperfused hearts. The clearance of ^{11}C-acetate was measured externally with a gamma probe in both normal and ischemic myocardium and this, too, correlated closely with overall myocardial oxygen consumption. Myocardial extraction of ^{14}C-acetate was high in all hearts and was not diminished by increasing the concentration of acetate to that found in plasma in vivo. These investigators also found that back diffusion of ^{14}C-acetate was minimal even in ischemic hearts. Similar studies by Buxton et al. [15] demonstrated that the presence of alternate substrates such as palmitate, lactate, and hydroxybutyrate had no significant effect on acetate clearance.

Studies in intact dogs from these same groups [16–18] demonstrated rapid

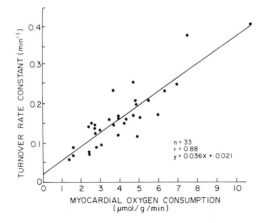

Figure 1. Correlation between the myocardial turnover rate constant measured noninvasively with PET after intravenous administration of ^{11}C-acetate and MVO_2 measured by direct arterial coronary venous sampling in intact dogs studied at rest, after myocardial work had been altered with sympathetic stimulation or blockade, or after the pattern of myocardial substrate use had been changed by altering arterial substrate content after infusion of either glucose or lipid. These data indicate that the turnover rate constant correlated closely with myocardial oxygen consumption. (Reproduced, with permission, from Walsh et al [22].)

clearance of ^{11}C-acetate from arterial blood and high extraction of ^{11}C-acetate by the myocardium. Good contrast was also seen between the myocardium and the surrounding lung parenchyma. Dogs were studied under baseline conditions, at high and low workloads [16–18], with ischemia, and after reperfusion [18]. In all studies the rate of clearance of ^{11}C radioactivity from the heart correlated closely with myocardial oxygen consumption (Figure 1) as well as with the rate pressure product. The clearance of ^{11}C radioactivity from the heart was biexponential and there was no significant difference found between the early rapid phase of ^{11}C clearance from the myocardium measured noninvasively with PET and the myocardial efflux of ^{11}CO$_2$ measured directly from the coronary sinus. The rate constant for the early rapid phase of ^{11}C clearance was found to correlate linearly with myocardial oxygen consumption. No correlation was found between myocardial oxygen consumption and the second rate constant. In contrast to ^{11}C-palmitate kinetics, estimates of myocardial oxygen consumption using ^{11}C-acetate were unchanged despite changes in the pattern of myocardial substrate utilization [17, 19]. Thus, all initial animal studies suggested that ^{11}C-acetate would be an ideal tracer in human studies for the noninvasive assessment of myocardial oxygen consumption assessed with PET.

Clinical studies

Normal controls

The uptake of ^{11}C-acetate in the hearts of normal human subjects has been found to be homogeneous throughout the left ventricular myocardium with little variation in regional clearance [20–23]. Because the rate pressure product has been shown to correlate closely with global myocardial oxygen consumption in animals [16, 19] and in humans [24–26], the rate pressure product has been used in human studies to evaluate the ability of ^{11}C-acetate to delineate changes in myocardial oxygen consumption. Although in animals, clearance of acetate was shown to be biexponential, at the lower myocardial workloads seen in resting human subjects, fitting of the second exponential is difficult due to the longer duration of the first clearance phase and is generally not clinically useful. As a result, most groups have used monoexponential fitting of the initial linear portion of the time-activity curve in human studies to correlate ^{11}C-acetate clearance and myocardial oxygen consumption. Even in subjects studied under high workload states after dobutamine infusion [20], or supine bicycle exercise [21], when acetate clearance becomes biexponential, fitting of the initial exponential has been found to be more useful for clinical applications.

Measurement of this rate constant for the first exponential of ^{11}C clearance following intravenous ^{11}C-acetate administration has accurately correlated with indirect measurements of regional myocardial oxygen consumption in normal volunteers over a wide range of hemodynamic and metabolic conditions [20–23]. As in previously performed animal experiments, glucose loading in normal volunteers proved to have no effect on overall acetate clearance [21, 23], corroborating the relative insensitivity of acetate clearance to changes in myocardial substrate supply and use. Henes et al. [20] calculated that estimates of myocardial oxygen consumption (MVO_2) in normal human subjects at rest averaged $0.92 \pm 0.38\,\mu$mol/g/min and increased to an average of $4.90 \pm 0.19\,\mu$mol/g/min after infusion of dobutamine. Although these estimated values are somewhat lower than those that have been measured invasively in human subjects [24–26] the ability of the rate constant k_1 to fairly accurately estimate changes in MVO_2 has clearly demonstrated the power of ^{11}C-acetate used with PET to noninvasively measure myocardial oxygen consumption in humans.

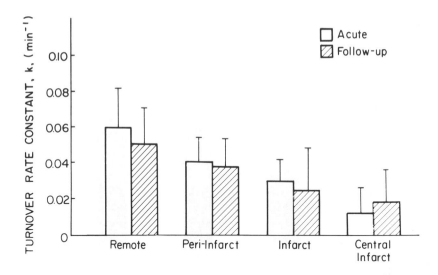

Figure 2. Histogram displaying the myocardial turnover rate constant, *k* from patients studied acutely and again at least 7 days after myocardial infarction. These data demonstrate that there was no change in estimated myocardial oxygen consumption over time. (Reproduced, with permission, from Walsh et al. [22].)

Patient studies

Walsh et al. [22] demonstrated that, in contrast to the homogeneous clearance observed in the hearts of normal control subjects, clearance of radioactivity from the myocardium is heterogeneous in patients with myocardial infarction. Uptake of tracer in the zone of infarction was decreased and the turnover rate constant within the infarct zone was markedly diminished, indicative of a profound decrease in regional MVO_2 (Plate 20.1). Regions immediately adjacent to the infarct zone also demonstrated diminished MVO_2 in comparison to those regions more remote from the infarct. In these patients who underwent no intervention during or after myocardial infarction (i.e., thrombolysis, percutaneous transluminal coronary angioplasty), the uptake of ^{11}C-acetate remained markedly diminished in the infarct zone, and the turnover rate constant (Figure 2), clearance half-time, and estimated myocardial oxygen consumption did not change over time. Thus, after myocardial infarction, regions that exhibit marked impairment of oxidative metabolism remain depressed over a prolonged interval. In other preliminary studies done soon after myocardial infarction [27, 28], myocardial regions that exhibited enhanced acetate clearance in spite of diminished myocardial blood flow gave evidence

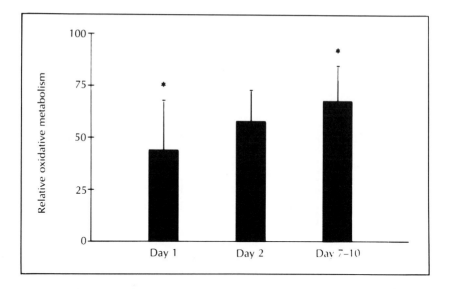

Figure 3. Mean rate of relative oxidative metabolism in jeopardized zones in patients with myocardial infarction treated with a thrombolytic agent. The rate of oxidative metabolism is expressed by the fraction of that in remote, normal zones and is expressed as a percentage of the remote myocardium. Progressive improvement of relative oxidative metabolism occurred between day 1 and delayed study on day 7–10. (Reproduced, with permission, from Henes et al. [31].)

of long-term improvement defined either as a recovery in contractile function [27], or an increase in ^{18}F-deoxyglucose uptake [28].

Gropler et al. [29] reported that in patients who underwent revascularization after myocardial infarction, the maintenance of oxidative metabolism as measured by ^{11}C-acetate predicted an improvement in regional wall motion after revascularization. In this study the uptake of ^{18}F-deoxyglucose proved to be more variable than that of ^{11}C-acetate in the prediction of functional recovery. This superiority over ^{18}F-deoxyglucose as a predictor of myocardial viability has also been shown in patients with coronary artery disease prior to coronary artery bypass surgery [30]. Acetate criteria of viability correctly predicted improvement in 68% of dysfunctional myocardial segments where lack of improvement was predicted in 80% of those who did not improve. Henes et al. [31] measured myocardial oxidative metabolism with ^{11}C-acetate sequentially in patients with acute myocardial infarction who received a thrombolytic agent. Clearance of ^{11}C from reperfused zones was initially depressed to 45% of normal. Clearance increased to 59% within 2 days and subsequently to 68% of normal within 9 days after thrombolysis (Figure 3). Regional wall motion was assessed in each patient and improvement in regional myocardial oxidative metabolism predicted improvement in regional left ventricular function. In general, patients who had the greatest improvement of oxidative metabolism exhibited the greatest improvement in wall motion. Conversely, those with the least improvement in metabolism exhibited the least improvement in wall motion.

Because significant clearance of ^{11}C activity does not occur until approximately 4 minutes after uptake of the tracer into the myocardium [19], recent reports have detailed the use of ^{11}C-acetate to estimate regional myocardial blood flow [32, 33]. As is the case with other metabolic tracers, initial myocardial uptake of ^{11}C-acetate is at least partially dependent on blood flow, and as a result, the initial portion of the time activity curve may be useful for evaluating regional flow. Gropler et al. [32] studied patients with coronary artery disease with both ^{11}C-acetate and the perfusion tracer ^{15}O-water in sequential fashion and found that the early myocardial uptake of ^{11}C-acetate correlated closely with perfusion. This correlation was found to be insensitive to changes in oxidative metabolism. In a similar study, Chan et al. [33] reported a close correlation between the early myocardial tissue activity of ^{11}C-acetate and the equilibrium tissue activity of ^{13}N-ammonia in patients with stable coronary artery disease at rest. Both of these reports suggest the feasibility of assessing myocardial perfusion and oxidative metabolism in a single study with ^{11}C-acetate. Recent reports from other investigators have detailed the use of ^{11}C-acetate and PET to assess myocardial oxidative metabolism in patients with chest pain and normal coronary arteries [34], in the right ventricle [35], in the pressure and volume loaded heart [36], in patients with idiopathic dilated cardiomyopathy [37] and in patients with myocardial infarction to assess the effect of vessel patency [38].

Conclusion

PET with ^{11}C-acetate has been shown to provide an accurate, noninvasive estimation of myocardial oxygen consumption in human subjects. Although studies have, thus far, been limited in numbers a fairly broad patient population has been studied by several different groups with reproducible results. Of particular interest are results that indicate that maintenance of oxidative metabolism in the setting of acute or chronic myocardial ischemia predicts functional recovery. It is this ability to serve as a marker of tissue viability that may soon bring PET with ^{11}C-acetate into the clinical arena.

Acknowledgements

The author is indebted to Steven R. Bergmann, MD, PhD, for advice and encouragement and to Cheryl Somers for preparation of the typescript.

References

1. Bergmann SR, Fox KA, Geltman EM, Sobel BE. Positron emission tomography of the heart. Prog Cardiovasc Dis 1985; 28: 165–94.
2. Myears DW, Sobel BE, Bergmann SR. Substrate use in ischemic and reperfused canine myocardium: quantitative considerations. Am J Physiol 1987; 253: H107–14.
3. Schelbert HR, Henze E, Schon HR et al. C-11 palmitate for the noninvasive evaluation of regional myocardial fatty acid metabolism with positron computed tomography. III. In vivo demonstration of the effects of substrate availability on myocardial metabolism. Am Heart J 1983; 105: 492–504.
4. Schelbert HR, Henze E, Sochor H et al. Effects of substrate availability on myocardial C-11 palmitate kinetics by positron emission tomography in normal subjects and patients with ventricular dysfunction. Am Heart J 1986; 111: 1055–64.
5. Phelps ME, Hoffman EJ, Selin C et al. Investigation of [^{18}F]2-fluoro-2-deoxyglucose for the measure of myocardial glucose metabolism. J Nucl Med 1978; 19: 1311–9.
6. Fox KA, Abendschein DR, Ambos HD, Sobel BE, Bergmann SR. Efflux of metabolized and nonmetabolized fatty acid from canine myocardium. Implications for quantifying myocardial metabolism tomographically. Circ Res 1985; 57: 232–43.
7. Williamson JR. Effects of insulin and starvation on the metabolism of acetate and pyruvate in the perfused rat heart. Biochem J 1964; 93: 97–105.
8. Randle PJ, England PJ, Denton RM. Control of the tricarboxylate cycle and its interactions with glycolysis during acetate utilization in rat heart. Biochem J 1970; 117: 677–95.
9. Taegtmeyer H. Myocardial metabolism. In: Phelps M, Mazziotta J, Schelbert H, editors. Positron emission tomography and autoradiography: principles and applications for the brain and heart. New York: Raven Press, 1986: 149–95.
10. Pike VW, Eakins MN, Allan RM, Selwyn AP. Preparation of [1-^{11}C] acetate – an agent for the study of myocardial metabolism by positron emission tomography. Int J Appl Radiat Isot 1982; 33: 505–12.
11. Allan RM, Selwyn AP, Pike VW, Eakins MN, Maseri A. In vivo experimental and clinical studies of normal and ischemic myocardium using ^{11}C-acetate [abstract]. Circulation 1980; 62 (4 Suppl III): III 74.
12. Allan RM, Pike VW, Maseri A, Selwyn AP. Myocardial metabolism of ^{11}C-acetate: experimental and patient studies [abstract]. Circulation 1981; 64 (4 Suppl IV): IV 75.
13. Selwyn AP, Allan RM, Pike V, Fox K, Maseri A. Positive labeling of ischemic myocardium: a new approach in patients with coronary disease [abstract]. Am J Cardiol 1981; 47: 481.
14. Brown M, Marshall DR, Sobel BE, Bergmann SR. Delineation of myocardial oxygen utilization with carbon-11-labeled acetate. Circulation 1987; 76: 687–96.
15. Buxton DB, Schwaiger M, Nguyen A, Phelps ME, Schelbert HR. Radiolabeled acetate as a tracer of myocardial tricarboxylic acid cycle flux. Circ Res 1988; 63: 628–34.
16. Brown MA, Myears DW, Bergmann SR. Noninvasive assessment of canine myocardial

oxidative metabolism with carbon-11 acetate and positron emission tomography. J Am Coll Cardiol 1988; 12: 1054–63.

17. Buxton DB, Nienaber CA, Luxen A et al. Noninvasive quantitation of regional myocardial oxygen consumption in vivo with [1-¹¹C]acetate and dynamic positron emission tomography. Circulation 1989; 79: 134–42.

18. Armbrecht JJ, Buxton DB, Schelbert HR. Validation of [1-¹¹C]acetate as a tracer for noninvasive assessment of oxidative metabolism with positron emission tomography in normal, ischemic, postischemic, and hyperemic canine myocardium. Circulation 1990; 81: 1594–1605.

19. Brown MA, Myears DW, Bergmann SR. Validity of estimates of myocardial oxidative metabolism with carbon-11 acetate and positron emission tomography despite altered patterns of substrate utilization. J Nucl Med 1989; 30: 187–93.

20. Henes CG, Bergmann SR, Walsh MN, Sobel BE, Geltman EM. Assessment of myocardial oxidative metabolic reserve with positron emission tomography and carbon-11 acetate. J Nucl Med 1989; 30: 1489–99.

21. Armbrecht JJ, Buxton DB, Brunken RC, Phelps ME, Schelbert HR. Regional myocardial oxygen consumption determined noninvasively in humans with [1-¹¹C]acetate and dynamic positron tomography. Circulation 1989; 80: 863–72.

22. Walsh MN, Geltman EM, Brown MA et al. Noninvasive estimation of regional myocardial oxygen consumption by positron emission tomography with carbon-11 acetate in patients with myocardial infarction. J Nucl Med 1989; 30: 1798–1808.

23. Kotzerke J, Hicks RJ, Wolfe E et al. Three-dimensional assessment of myocardial oxidative metabolism: a new approach for regional determination of PET-derived carbon-11-acetate kinetics. J Nucl Med 1990; 31: 1876–93.

24. Kitamura K, Jorgensen CR, Gobel FL, Taylor HL, Wang Y. Hemodynamic correlates of myocardial oxygen consumption during upright exercise. J Appl Physiol 1972; 32: 516–22.

25. Nelson RR, Gobel FL, Jorgensen CR, Wang K, Wang Y, Taylor HL. Hemodynamic predictors of myocardial oxygen consumption during static and dynamic exercise. Circulation 1974; 50: 1179–89.

26. Gobel FL, Nordstrom LA, Nelson RP, Jorgensen CR, Wang Y. The rate-pressure product as an index of myocardial oxygen consumption during exercise in patients with angina pectoris. Circulation 1978; 57: 549–56.

27. Hicks RJ, Dick RJ, Molina E, Wolpers HG, Al-Aouar ZR, Schwaiger M. Assessment of myocardial viability early following infarction using PET-derived C-11 acetate kinetics [abstract]. Circulation 1990; 82 (4 Suppl III): III 479.

28. Czernin J, Chan S, Brunken R, Porenta G, Phelps M, Schelbert H. Accuracy of early PET blood flow and metabolic measurements for predicting late improvement in the clinical infarct zone [abstract]. J Am Coll Cardiol 1991; 17 (2 Suppl A): 347A.

29. Gropler RJ, Siegel BA, Sampathkumaran K, Perez JE, Geltman EM. Maintenance of oxidative metabolism determines recovery of contractile and metabolic function after myocardial infarction [abstract]. Circulation 1990; 82 (4 Suppl III): III 479.

30. Gropler RJ, Siegel BA, Sampathkumaran K, Perez JE, Bergmann SR, Geltman EM. Comparison of positron emission tomography using C-11 acetate with F-18 fluorodeoxyglucose in predicting myocardial viability [abstract]. J Am Coll Cardiol 1991; 17 (2 Suppl A): 121A.

31. Henes CG, Bergmann SR, Perez JE, Sobel BE, Geltman EM. The time course of restoration of nutritive perfusion, myocardial oxygen consumption, and regional function after coronary thrombolysis. Coronary Artery Dis 1990; 1: 687–96.

32. Gropler RG, Siegel BA, Geltman EM. Myocardial uptake of carbon-11-acetate as an indirect estimate of regional myocardial blood flow. J Nucl Med 1991; 32: 245–51.

33. Chan SY, Brunken RC, Phelps ME, Schelbert HR. Use of the metabolic tracer carbon-11-acetate for evaluation of regional myocardial perfusion. J Nucl Med 1991; 32: 665–72.

34. Senneff MJ, Bergmann SR, Henes CG, Sobel BE, Geltman EG. Impaired myocardial oxidative metabolism assessed with positron emission tomography (PET) in patients with chest pain and normal coronary arteries [abstract]. J Nucl Med 1990; 31 Suppl: 713.

35. Hicks RJ, Kalff V, Savas V, Hutchins G, Kirsch M, Schwaiger M. C-11 acetate kinetics as a marker of right ventricular work [abstract]. J Am Coll Cardiol 1990; 15 (2 Suppl A): 81A.

36. Hicks RJ, Savas V, Currie PJ, Kalff V, Kuhl DE, Swaigher M. PET-derived C-11 acetate kinetics as a marker of metabolic performance in the pressure and volume loaded heart [abstract]. J Nucl Med 1990; 31 Suppl: 773.

37. Chan SY, Warner-Stevenson L, Brunken RC, Krivokapich J, Phelps ME, Schelbert HR. Myocardial oxygen consumption in patients with idiopathic dilated cardiomyopathy [abstract]. J Nucl Med 1990; 31 Suppl: 773.

38. Czernin J, Porenta G, Brunken RC, Wong BL, Tillisch J, Phelps ME et al. Infarct vessel patency benefits both oxidative and glycolytic metabolism in acute myocardial infarction [abstract]. Circulation 1990; 82 (4 Suppl III): III 85.

SECTION THREE

Infarct-avid imaging

21. Infarct-avid imaging:
usefulness, problems and limitations

ERNEST K.J. PAUWELS

Physicians working in coronary care units may face problems in diagnosing infarction in patients with electrocardiographic conduction disturbances or when electrocardiographic data are in conflict with enzyme data. Under such circumstances, noninvasive diagnostic imaging may be of help.

In the early seventies, technetium-99m (Tc-99m)-pyrophosphate, Tc-99m-tetracycline, Tc-99m-glucoheptonate and (sodium-fluorine-18) NaF-18 were all shown to localize in areas of acute myocardial infarction. The infarct/background ratio and the hepatic uptake varied for various agents. Tc-99m-pyrophosphate (Tc-99m-PYP) appeared to be the clinical agent of choice for infarct-avid imaging due to its better clearance characteristics, higher target to background ratios, availability and low cost. A historical review of these studies has been published by Wynne et al. [1]. Of these compounds, only Tc-99m-PYP has been studied extensively.

Tc-99m-pyrophosphate

Apparently, patients without acute infarction or with unstable arteriosclerotic heart disease show no or nonfocal ill-defined accumulation of Tc-99m-PYP, whereas cases with acute transmural infarction displayed a well-defined area of tracer uptake [2]. The sensitivity reported for this examination is higher than 85% [3–4]. The interesting behavior of this radiopharmaceutical can be clinically used for the assessment of reperfusion: if reperfusion occurs as a result of, e.g., successful thrombolytic therapy, localization of Tc-99m-PYP takes place within 1–2 hours of the infarct development [5]. In case of perma-

Ernst E. van der Wall et al. (eds), What's new in cardiac imaging?, 289–294.

nent coronary artery occlusion, uptake of Tc-99m-PYP can be noticed within 12 hours of the event and tracer accumulation increases in the 24–72 hours following infarction. Histological studies have shown excellent correlation between the area of Tc-99m-PYP concentration and irreversible tissue injury [6].

Most literature on Tc-99m-PYP 'hot-spot' imaging dates from the seventies and early eighties. During that period, experimental studies have thrown some light on the biochemical mechanism responsible for the accumulation of Tc-99m-PYP in an acutely infarcted myocardium. It is tempting to ascribe Tc-99m-PYP localization to binding in a calcium phosphate crystalline structure. Indeed, after the function of the mitochondriae in the infarcted zone is reduced or even ceases, mitochondrial calcification is observed [7]. There is a firm experimental basis to explain Tc-99m-PYP uptake in acutely infarcted myocardium by selective accumulation in damaged or necrotic tissue. Also Dewanjee and Kahn [8] have demonstrated that Tc-99m-PYP uptake is associated with the status of the mitochondriae, but in subcellular localization studies they showed that Tc-99m-PYP is primarily bound to soluble proteins. Thus the uptake of Tc-99m-PYP may be due to complexing with calcium deposits as well as organic (denaturated) macromolecules. A survey of pathophysiological mechanisms, responsible for Tc-99m-PYP uptake in areas of myocardial infarction has been given by Buja et al. [9].

Whatever the mechanism of Tc-99m-PYP localization, the use of Tc-99m-PYP has shown to be a valuable technique in localizing and assessing the extent of myocardial tissue injury. On the other hand, the uptake kinetics of Tc-99m-PYP involve the major drawback of this compound in its ability to help the clinician to definitely diagnose myocardial infarction within a time spend of a few hours. In addition to this unfortunate characteristic of Tc-99m-PYP, clinicians may be held back from the use of this agent in view of the reported equivocal scintigrams, both in the group of transmural infarction and in cases with no evidence of acute myocardial infarction [10]. Such disturbing results may be due to the fact that local concentration of Tc-99m-PYP is proportional to the product of the degree of necrosis and local blood flow. Whereas uptake is directly related to the degree of tissue damage, it is inversely related to the extent of the reduction in blood flow [9]. Furthermore, Tc-99m-PYP, being primarily developed as a bone-scanning agent, localizes in the ribs and the sternum, thereby obscuring smaller infarcts.

With Tc-99m-PYP 'false positive' results have been reported [11]. Noncardiac causes of positive Tc-99m-PYP scintigrams occur infrequently but may be due to inadequate data processing, rib fractures, skin lesions, and breast disorders. Positive results under noninfarct heart conditions occur more frequently and have been reported in patients with heart diseases in which myocardial necrosis is likely to be present [2, 12]. These entities include unstable angina, aneurysm of the left ventricle and cardiomyopathy. Poliner et al. [12] have emphasized that in some instances scintigraphic imaging provides evidence of chronic and severe ischemia causing infarction of small islands of cells. This cardiac necrosis is probably not detectable by other imaging techniques. Nondiagnostic images and problems in interpreting Tc-99m-PYP images arise in patients with excessive residual radioactivity in and around the heart. This occurs in elderly patients and in cases of congestive heart failure and renal failure. These scintigrams are characterized by the visualization of blood pool compartments as heart chambers and great vessels.

Antimyosin

In view of the mentioned limitations, researchers have focused their efforts on the development of a new class of agents based upon the hall-mark of myocardial infarction, viz. myocyte necrosis. Whereas the intact myocyte is surrounded by an impermeable cell membrane, the damaged myocyte allows exposure of intracellular myosin. The unique antigenicity of this protein has made it possible to develop monoclonal antibodies against this intracellular material [13].

Over the past decade Haber [14] and Khaw et al. [15] have set the stage for the clinical use of indium-111 (In-111) labeled to antimyosin as a marker of acute myocardial infarction (see Chapter 22). Experimental and clinical studies have shown that tracer accumulation is greatest in regions with the lowest myocardial blood flow. This is in contrast with Tc-99m-PYP behavior, which has its greatest uptake in areas at 20 to 40% of maximum myocardial blood flow [9]. The doughnut pattern, reported for Tc-99m-PYP accumulation at the periphery of an infarct, is not seen with the use of radiolabeled antimyosin. With this agent positive images can be seen at 12 hours after injection but usually high-quality images are obtained only at 24 to 48 hours post-injection. This means that patients, needing antimyosin imaging for infarct-evaluation should be injected as soon as clinically possible. The half-life of In-111 ($T^{1}/_{2} =$ 2.8 days) is long enough to obtain diagnostic images at 48 hours post-injection. In-111 antimyosin can detect myocardial damage a week after infarction [16]. In the days following infarction, cardiac myosin disappears gradually [17] which makes uptake of the radiopharmaceutical less intense. Usually, no uptake of radiolabeled antibody is observed in old infarcts, but incidentally positive images have been obtained at various stages up till 9 months after the acute event [18].

In a selected group of patients with proven acute myocardial infarction, a sensitivity of 96% (52 out of 54 patients) was found [15]. A similar sensitivity has been reported by Liu et al. [19] who used a quantitative approach for the detection of pathological accumulation of radiolabeled antimyosin. In this study, sufficient evidence came out to prove the capacity of antimyosin to delineate zones of acute myocardial necrosis in a clinical setting. Furthermore, there is experimental evidence that a more diffuse antimyosin accumulation corresponds with a patchy or subendocardial infarction, whereas intense, well-delineated and homogeneous accumulation corresponds with homogeneous transmural infarction. A review on the clinical utility of In-111 antimyosin has been presented by Morguet et al. [20].

Future aspects

The interpretation of antimyosin images may be hampered by the fact that liver uptake is prominent with this agent. This may limit the detection possibilities of inferior infarcts. Also for other infarct-locations, data processing is often necessary to reduce nontarget activity and to enhance contrast. Viewing of three-dimensional structures as obtained by single photon emission tomography may help the interpreter, but the decision whether pathologic tracer uptake occurs can sometimes not be taken without extensive data processing and, as indicated earlier, this procedure is a potential source for false negative or false positive results. Therefore, future radiopharmaceutical design should be directed towards agents with little or virtually no liver uptake. To play a more prominent role in clinical decision-making, infarct avid agents should be able to delineate the infarcted areas a few hours after injection so that prospects for salvaging myocardium are still present. This kinetic behavior would also allow the use of Tc-99m with its short half-life of 6 hours and better imaging characteristics than In-111.

In high-risk patients, repeated injections could throw light on the presence or absence of new infarctions or reinfarction. Therefore, one would wish to use tracers that do not concentrate in old infarctions. An important consideration in evaluating positive Tc-99m-PYP images is the fact that in about 10–45% of cases, an abnormal scintigram is present for at least 6 months after the clinical event [21–22]. Scintigraphy with antibodies do cause concern on immunologic response when a tracer is administered more than once. Human or humanized antibodies should diminish this concern, but agents without the chance of immunologic reactions should be preferred (see Chapter 23 for myocardial infarct imaging with cardiac troponin-I antibodies). The development of synthetic peptides or simple chemical entities for positive infarct imaging should have priority. In this respect, it is to be expected that a number of Tc-99m labeled compounds show affinity for necrotic myocardial tissue. Tc-99m glucaric acid, the first compound of this class, not showing liver or osseous activity, has been reported recently and holds promise for future myocardial imaging [23].

References

1. Wynne J, Holman BL, Lesch M. Myocardial scintigraphy by infarct-avid radiotracers. Prog Cardiovasc Dis 1978; 20: 243–66.
2. Perez LA, Hayt DB, Freeman LM. Localization of myocardial disorders other than infarction with ^{99m}Tc-labeled phosphate agents. J Nucl Med 1976; 17: 241–6.
3. Joseph SP, Pereira-Prestes AV, Ell PJ, Donaldson R, Sommerville W, Emanuel RW. Value of positive myocardial infarction imaging in coronary care units. Br Med J 1979; 1: 372–4.
4. Tetalman MR, Foley LC, Spencer CP, Bishop SP. A critical review of the efficacy of ^{99m}Tc pyrophosphate in detecting myocardial infarction in 103 patients. Radiology 1977; 124: 431–2.
5. Parkey RW, Kulkarni PV, Lewis SE et al. Effect of coronary blood flow and site of injection of Tc-99m PPi detection of early canine myocardial infarcts. J Nucl Med 1981; 22: 133–7.
6. Izquierdo C, Devous MD Sr, Nicod P et al. A comparison of infarct identification with technetium-99m pyrophosphate and staining with triphenyl tetrazolium chloride. J Nucl Med 1983; 24: 492–7.
7. Buja LM, Parkey RW, Stokely EM, Bonte FJ, Willerson JT. Pathophysiology of technetium-99m stannous pyrophosphate and thallium-201 scintigraphy of acute anterior myocardial infarcts in dogs. J Clin Invest 1976; 57: 1508–22.
8. Dewanjee MK, Kahn PC. Mechanism of localization of ^{99m}Tc-labeled pyrophosphate and tetracycline in infarcted myocardium. J Nucl Med 1976; 17: 639–46.
9. Buja LM, Tofe AJ, Kulkarni PV et al. Sites and mechanisms of localization of technetium-99m phosphorous radiopharmaceuticals in acute myocardial infarcts and other tissues. J Clin Invest 1977; 60: 724–40.
10. Berman DS, Amsterdam EA, Hines HH et al. New approach to interpretation of technetium-99m pyrophosphate scintigraphy in detection of acute myocardial infarction. Am J Cardiol 1977; 39: 341–6.
11. Cowley MJ, Mantle JA, Rogers WJ, Russell RO Jr, Rackley CE, Logic JR. Technetium-99m stannous pyrophophate myocardial scintigraphy. Reliability and limitations in assessment of acute myocardial infarction. Circulation 1977; 56: 192–8.
12. Poliner LR, Buja LM, Parkey RW, Bonte FJ, Willerson JT. Clinicopathologic findings in 52 patients studied by technetium-99m stannous pyrophosphate myocardial scintigraphy. Circulation 1979; 59: 257–67.
13. Khaw BA, Fallon JT, Strauss HW, Haber E. Myocardial infarct imaging of antibodies to canine cardiac myosin with indium-111-diethylenetriamine pentaacetic acid. Science 1980; 209: 295–7.
14. Haber E. Immunological probes in cardiovascular disease. Br Heart J 1982; 47: 1–10.
15. Khaw BA, Yasuda T, Gold HK et al. Acute myocardial infarct imaging with indium-111-labeled monoclonal antimyosin Fab. J Nucl Med 1987; 28: 1671–8.
16. Nakata T, Sakakibara T, Noto T et al. Myocardial distribution of indium-111-antimyosin Fab in acute inferior and right ventricular infarction: comparison with technetium-99m-pyrophosphate imaging and histologic examination. J Nucl Med 1991; 32: 865–7.

17. Fishbein MC, MacLean D, Maroko PR. The histopathologic evolution of myocardial infarction. Chest 1978; 73: 843–9.
18. Tamaki N, Yamada T, Matsumori A et al. Indium-111-antimyosin antibody imaging for detecting different stages of myocardial infarction; comparison with technetium-99m-pyrophosphate imaging. J Nucl Med 1990; 31: 136–42.
19. Liu XJ, Jain D, Senior R, Broadhurst P, Lahiri A. ^{111}In-antimyosin antibody imaging for detection of myocardial infarction: a quantitative approach. Nucl Med Commun 1990; 11: 667–75.
20. Morguet AJ, Munz DL, Kreuzer H, Emrich D. Immunoscintigraphy with ^{111}In antimyosin Fab. Nucl Med Commun 1990; 11: 727–35.
21. Olson HG, Lyons KP, Aronow WS, Kuperus J, Orlando J, Hughes D. Prognostic value of a persistently positive technetium-99m stannous pyrophosphate myocardial scintigram after myocardial infarction. Am J Cardiol 1979; 43: 889–98.
22. Croft CH, Rude RE, Lewis SE et al. Comparison of left ventricular function and infarct size in patients with and without persistently positive technetium-99m pyrophosphate myocardial scintigrams after myocardial infarction: analysis of 357 patients. Am J Cardiol 1984; 53: 421–8.
23. Orlandi C, Crane PD, Edwards S et al. Early scintigraphic detection of experimental myocardial infarction in dogs with technetium-99m-glucaric acid. J Nucl Med 1991; 32: 263–8.

22. Myocyte necrosis-avid imaging with radiolabeled antimyosin antibody: experimental and clinical acute myocardial infarction, myocarditis and heart transplant rejection

BAN AN KHAW, JAGAT NARULA and PHILIP NICOL

Introduction

The underlying amalgam in coronary disease, myocarditis and cardiac transplant rejection is myocyte necrosis. Since cell necrosis is the hall mark of cell death, this principle has been used to develop a noninvasive immunoscintigraphic diagnostic approach. The entry of antibodies in diagnostic cardiology was launched by the development of antimyosin antibody for localization and targeting of acute experimental myocardial infarction [1]. Normal myocardium with intact sarcolemma will not permit extracellular macromolecules to enter the cells. This barrier no longer exists in myocytes with cell membrane disruption and will permit free access to the once privileged sites. If the extracellular macromolecules were to be antimyosin antibody molecules, then the regions of myocyte necrosis can be determined by the assessment of the regions of antimyosin accumulation. This principle was demonstrated in neonatal murine myocyte culture studies where normal myocytes did not accumulate antimyosin linked beads whereas antimyosin beads were bound to myofilaments exposed to the extracellular environment through regions of sarcolemmal disruption (Figure 1) [2].

Acute experimental myocardial infarction

The first antimyosin antibody used to demonstrate the feasibility of in vivo visualization by gamma imaging of acute experimental myocardial infarction was a F(ab')$_2$ of polyclonal rabbit anti-canine cardiac myosin antibody labeled

Ernst E. van der Wall et al. (eds), What's new in cardiac imaging?, 295–315.
© *1992 Kluwer Academic Publishers. Printed in the Netherlands.*

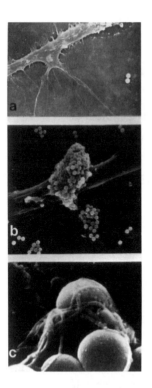

Figure 1. Scanning electron micrograph of an intact myocyte in culture showing lack of antimyosin-bead binding (a). Antimyosin-bead attachment to extruded intracellular contents in the area of a tear in the membrane of a necrotic myocyte (b). Higher magnification (100,000 ×) showing binding of antimyosin-beads to the exposed myofibrils of a necrotic myocyte (c). (From [2] with permission of the American Association for the Advancement of Science.)

with radioiodine [3]. Localization of I-125 labeled antimyosin F(ab′)$_2$ in the necrotic myocardium was highly specific relative to the accumulation of simultaneously administered I-131 labeled control F(ab′)$_2$ [3]. The mean ratio of specific antimyosin uptake in the infarct center was 32:1, whereas control fragments had a mean uptake ratio of only 6.5:1 in the same tissue samples.

Specificity alone, however, may not be a sufficient condition for successful imaging of acute myocardial infarction. As illustrated in Figure 2, the images of canine experimental myocardial infarction obtained after injection with a low affinity antimyosin Fab designated 3H3 (Ka = 5 × 10^6 L/M) (left panels) did not show unequivocal infarct localization whereas the images of another dog obtained after injection with identically radiolabeled antimyosin Fab

$\longrightarrow$

Figure 2. Serial left lateral gamma scintigrams of two dogs with acute experimental myocardial infarction. The dogs were injected with In-111-antimyosin R11D10 Fab with a K$_a$ of 5 × 10^8 L/M (right) and In-111-antimyosin 3H3 Fab with K$_a$ of 5 × 10^6 L/M (left). The one hour image with R11D10 already showed delineation of the infarct (top right), which was more clearly seen at 5 hours after intravenous administration of the radiolabeled antibody. The animal injected with 3H3 Fab showed only minimal delineation of the infarct. This comparison shows the necessity of high affinity for successful visualization by gamma scintigraphy.

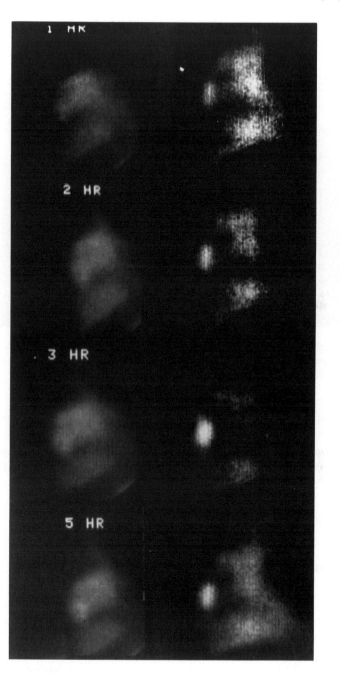

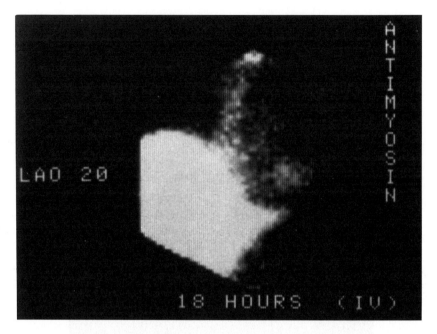

Figure 3. Left anterior oblique (20°) image of a patient with a small apical acute myocardial infarction obtained at 18 hours after intravenous administration of Tc-99m-labeled monoclonal antimyosin Fab. Note the liver and sternal activities as well as the infarct activity.

designated R11D10 (Ka = 5×10^8 L/M) showed unequivocal infarct delineation (right panels) [4].

Thus localization and visualization of experimental myocardial infarction were demonstrated to be highly specific. Furthermore, antimyosin delineated infarction corresponded to thallium-201 [5] and radiolabeled microsphere [6] perfusion defects, and was in agreement with histochemically and histologically delineated regions of myocyte necrosis [7].

Identification of acute myocardial infarction

To enable the transition from experimental to clinical applications of antimyosin for non-invasive imaging of acute myocardial infarction, a method of radiolabeling antimyosin Fab with technetium-99m (Tc-99m) was developed [8]. Tc-99m is a generator eluted radioisotope which has an ideal peak energy of emission of 140 keV for single photon emission gamma scintigraphy with an all purpose collimator and a physical half-life of 6 hours. It is eluted as a stable Tc-99m-pertechnitate, which must be reduced to a lower valency state before

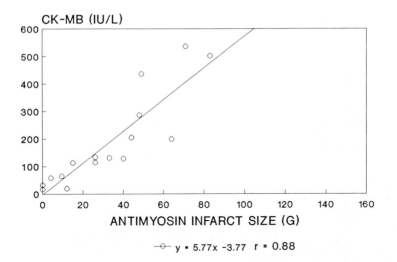

Figure 4. Relationship between peak CK-MB values in IU/l to SPECT antimyosin infarct size in grams in 12 patients with acute myocardial infarction who had successful thrombolytic therapy [8].

it can be chelated. A method of dithionite reduction of pertechnitate was developed to label DTPA linked antimyosin Fab. Tc-99m-labeled antimyosin Fab proved to be 87% sensitive for the diagnosis of acute myocardial infarction by planar gamma scintigraphy (Figure 3) which increased to 90% when single photon emission computed tomography (SPECT) was added to the imaging protocol [8]. SPECT imaging enabled quantitative determination of the infarct size which was observed to be directly correlated to the peak CK-MB values (Figure 4) and the length of the hypokinetic segments (Figure 5). Due to high hepatic activity with Tc-99m labeled antimyosin Fab, detection of small inferior myocardial infarcts was difficult. All false negative images in this study of 30 patients were of small inferior myocardial infarcts.

In order to improve the sensitivity and simplify the radiolabeling protocol, In-111 labeling method using citrate at pH 5–6 as a weak transchelator was developed [9]. This switch in the radioisotope from Tc-99m to indium-111 (In-111) enabled the sensitivity of antimyosin scintigraphy for the diagnosis of acute myocardial infarction to increase to 96% in our study of 54 patients [9]. It was observed that the intensity of tracer localization was related to the extent and density of myocyte necrosis and was independent of the perfusion status of the offending coronary vessel. Figure 6 demonstrates anterior and left anterior oblique gamma images of two patients, one with persistent left anterior descending coronary artery occlusion and the other after successful thrombolysis. Both images showed comparable tracer intensity in the infarct territories. Johnson et al., however, observed that the faint antimyosin uptake was

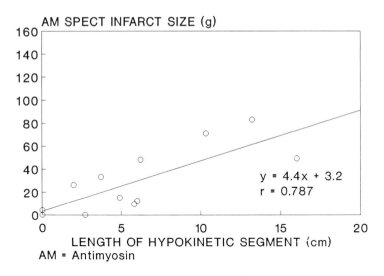

Figure 5. Relationship between SPECT antimyosin infarct size in grams to length of the hypokinetic segment in cm determined 10–14 days after the acute event, by cineangiography. (From [8] with permission of the American Heart Association, Circulation.)

related to the absence of collateral blood flow in a persistently occluded coronary territory [10].

In reperfused infarcts, Taki and co-workers reported that the intensity of antimyosin localization quantitated as count density ratios (CDI = count density in infarct/count density in the left lung) can predict small or incomplete infarcts within 1–2 days of thrombolytic therapy [11]. CDI > 2.2 in 15 patients was associated with a mean akinetic segment length of 9.7 ± 4.7 cm as determined from cine left ventriculogram 10 days after the acute coronary event which was greater than 3.7 ± 3.6 cm in another 15 patients with CDI < 2.2 (p < 0.005).

Specificity of antimyosin for delineation of acute myocardial infarction was further demonstrated in three case reports where antemortem In-111-antimyosin delineated infarcts showed a high correlation with postmortem histochemical and histologic infarcts [12–14].

Diagnostic accuracy of antimyosin imaging for acute myocardial infarction

High sensitivity of antimyosin scintigraphy for localization of myocyte necrosis associated with myocardial infarction was confirmed by various subsequent studies [15–18]. Braat et al. [15] demonstrated antimyosin uptake in all anterior and all but one inferior myocardial infarcts. Cox et al. [16] identified

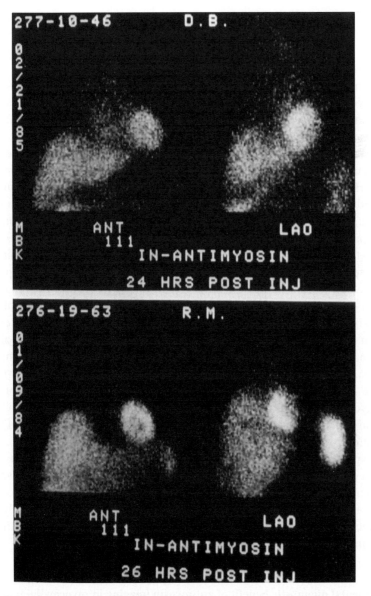

Figure 6. Anterior and left anterior oblique In-111-antimyosin Fab gamma scintigraphic images of two patients, one with persistent LAD occlusion (top panels, peak CK = 1820 IU/l, CK-MB = 11%) and one with successful reperfusion 5.8 hours after the acute onset of chest pain (bottom panels, peak CK = 1443, CK-MB = 15%). The intensity of radiotracer localization in both patients was very similar irrespective of the status of the left anterior descending coronary arteries.

myocardial infarction in 19 of the 21 patients with electrocardiographic myocardial infarcts. Antunes et al. [17] observed antimyosin uptake in all 27 patients with transmural myocardial infarction and the estimated infarct sizes correlated with the left ventricular wall motion score. Volpini et al. [18] performed indium-111 antimyosin scintigraphy in 57 patients with chest pain. Antimyosin scintigraphy was positive in 49/50 patients with Q wave myocardial infarction, and 6/7 patients with unstable angina pectoris did not demonstrate antimyosin uptake. Ten healthy volunteers also had negative scans. While the feasibility of the technique was clearly established, multicenter trials were launched for the evaluation of the diagnostic accuracy of antimyosin scintigraphy. Fifty patients with acute Q-wave myocardial infarction were entered into a phase I/II trial involving three centers [10]. In-111-antimyosin Fab fragments were injected intravenously 27 ± 16 hours after the onset of chest pain and planar and tomographic images were obtained 27 ± 9 hours there after. Forty-six patients showed myocardial uptake of antimyosin antibody (sensitivity: 92%). Focal myocardial uptake of antimyosin corresponded to the electrocardiographic infarct localization. No patient had adverse reaction to antimyosin administration. In addition, 125 serum samples, collected up to six weeks after the antimyosin injection, tested negative for presence of human anti-mouse antibody titers [10]. To determine the specificity of antimyosin scintigraphy for the diagnosis of acute myocardial infarction, phase III trial was undertaken at 26 centers which produced a study of 492 patients [19]. Of the 202 patients with Q wave infarct, 190 patients had regional uptake of antimyosin Fab (sensitivity 94%). Forty-eight of 57 patients with non-Q wave myocardial infarction also had positive antimyosin scans (sensitivity 84%). In 41 patients with chest pain but no infarct the specificity was 93%. Focal antimyosin uptake was observed in 21 of the 44 patients (48%) with unstable angina pectoris, which was identical to myocardial infarction in the suspected coronary territory providing an overall incremental diagnostic benefit of 74%. Thus, all clinical studies established that antimyosin imaging is a highly accurate technique for the detection of myocardial necrosis associated with acute myocardial infarction.

Incremental diagnostic benefit of antimyosin imaging in myocardial infarction

In most patients with chest pain, the clinical history, electrocardiographic and enzymatic changes are sufficient to prove or rule out acute myocardial infarction. However, antimyosin imaging may find a clinical value in the diagnosis of acute myocardial infarction when the patient is admitted several days after the onset of chest pain, or in the presence of conduction disorders such as left bundle branch block or pre-excitation syndromes or subsequent to coronary bypass surgery [20–22] when electrocardiographic changes are nondiagnostic. Incremental diagnostic utility of antimyosin imaging was demonstrated in a recent study of 75 patients with suspected acute myocardial infarction which included 7 patients with no diagnostic electrocardiographic changes [20]. Antimyosin immunoscintigraphy disclosed localized myocyte necrosis in all seven cases which was corroborated by abnormal wall motion or abnormal thallium images at the sites of antimyosin uptake. Moreover, the extent and intensity of antimyosin uptake have been proposed as prognostic indicators, which were predominantly based on quantitation of the necrotic myocardial tissue or transmurality of the infarction. Antimyosin uptake in at least 50% of the myocardium significantly predicted the incidence of sudden cardiac death after acute myocardial infarction [23]. Similarly, the count density index of the antimyosin uptake has been demonstrated to predict the severity of the wall motion abnormality [11] and the probability of improvement in wall motion abnormality [24].

Duration of antimyosin positivity subsequent to acute myocardial infarction

Indium-111 antimyosin Fab can be used to image acute myocardial infarction up to 2–3 weeks after the acute event. In the study by Johnson et al. [10], 14 of the 50 patients had evidence of prior myocardial infarction, In-111 antimyosin did not localize in areas of previous myocardial necrosis which occurred more than 2 weeks before the current episode. Similarly Volpini et al. [18] reported that in nine patients with > 3 months old myocardial infarction, no antimyosin uptake was observed in the remote infarcts. Antunes et al. [17] also reported that in nine patients with clinical or electrocardiographic evidence of old infarction did not demonstrate antimyosin uptake. However, recent reports have indicated that antimyosin may localize at sites of necrosis long after the acute event [25]. This observation may reduce the specificity of this modality for imaging acute onset of myocyte necrosis. Due to the specific mechanism of localization of antimyosin, brief but not prolonged positivity would be understandable. Similar uptake of pyrophosphate weeks to months after the acute event has been demonstrated. The cause for this positivity has been attributed to myocytolysis within the regions of fibrosis, and clinically with episodes of recurrent angina, congestive heart failure or sudden cardiac death [26–28]. However, the exact mechanism is not clear.

Studies of the evolution of myocardial infarcts have not produced histologic evidence of necrotic myocytes in any infarcts that were 36–90 days old [29, 30]. However, necrosis was observed in 35% of infarcts that were 22–35 days old

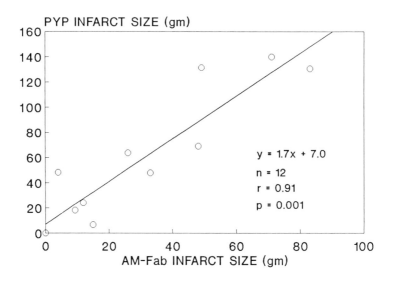

Figure 7. Relationship between infarct sizes in grams determined by pyrophosphate SPECT and antimyosin SPECT in 12 patients with acute myocardial infarction. Both reagents were labeled with Tc-99m, however, antimyosin images were obtained at about 24 hours and pyrophosphate images were obtained on day 3 of the acute event. A good correlation was observed between the two methods of infarct size determination. (From [8] with permission of the American Heart Association, Circulation.)

[29]. Large infarcts and subendocardial infarcts healed less rapidly. The rate of healing also depended on the competency of the remaining circulation [30]. In rare instances, islands of necrotic myocytes may remain longer (mummified myocytes) in the midst of thick, strong fibrous scar tissues. Whether anti-myosin can diffuse through fibrous scar tissue, or for that matter, whether mummified myocyte is still antimyosin-avid is unknown. Although the introduction of thrombolytic therapy may facilitate healing of necrotic tissues due to the restoration of blood flow, it may also permit survival of pockets of myocardial tissue that may be amenable to intermittent ischemic insults, resulting in prolonged antimyosin positivity. It is logical to expect that the intense localization of antimyosin would occur in fresh infarcts and that the intensity would decrease with diminution of antigenic determinants as the infarcts undergo the processes of healing.

Tc-99m-pyrophosphate and In-111 antimyosin

Tc-99m-pyrophosphate and In-111-antimyosin are two of the most successful infarct-avid imaging agents. The pharmacokinetics and the mechanism of tracer localization of the two agents are different. Pyrophosphate has a short plasma half life of less than one hour whereas antimyosin has a half life of 4 hours (slow component being $\simeq 12$ hours). The mechanism of antimyosin localization has already been discussed, whereas pyrophosphate uptake is believed to be associated with the calcium concentration in the compromised myocardium [31]. Due to these differences, it is inevitable that the two tracers show differences in in-vivo distribution when compared in the same patients or animals.

In our initial clinical study, infarct sizes were determined with Tc-99m-labeled antimyosin Fab on day 1 and with Tc-99m pyrophosphate on day 3 in 12 patients. Although, Tc-99m pyrophosphate SPECT infarct size was observed to bear a linear correlation to the antimyosin SPECT infarct size, pyrophosphate infarct size was larger than the antimyosin infarct size [11] (Figure 7). This was in agreement with our experimental data where localization of the two tracers was correlated to histochemically delineated infarcts. Mean pyrophosphate infarct size was approximately 1.5 times larger than either histochemical or antimyosin-delineated infarct sizes (Table 1). Other investiga-

Table 1. Comparison of infarct sizes by TTC, antimyosin and pyrophosphate (after intravenous administration).[a]

Dog no. (weight kg)	Infarct size (sq cm)				
	TTC	Antimyosin	Counts[b]	Pyrophosphate	Counts[b]
1 (30)	17.4	34.5	71,488	45.3	96,540
2 (32)	28.6	30.7	77,556	40.8	82,271
3 (22)	12.0	8.0	53,269	9.7	81,121
4 (23)	0.0	0.1	19,227	1.6	18,121
5 (22)	6.3	6.1	45,858	16.0	54,326
6 (21)	19.0	9.9	58,222	20.4	102,274
7 (22)	13.8	15.2	29,114	17.2	28,493
8 (18)	10.3	11.6	18,274	14.2	24,968
9 (20)	14.8	11.9	38,755	16.4	41,119
Mean ±	13.9 ±	14.2 ±	45,751 ±	20.2 ±	58,804 ±
s.d	8.0	11.3[c]	20,194	14.1[d,e]	30,576

[a] Linear correlation between: (a) TTC infarct size (x axis) and antimyosin infarct size (y axis) $y = 1.09x - 0.61$, $n = 9$, $r = 0.78$; (b) TTC infarct size (x axis) and pyrophosphate infarct size (y axis) $y = 1.38x + 1.43$, $n = 9$, $r = 0.79$; (c) Antimyosin infarct size (x axis) and pyrophosphate infarct size (y axis) $y = 1.208x + 3.01$, $n = 9$, $r = 0.97$.
[b] Total counts in the image/5 min.
[c] No significant difference between TTC and antimyosin infarct sizes.
[d] $p = 0.05$ Relative to mean TTC infarct size.
[e] $p = 0.05$ Relative to mean antimyosin infarct size.

tors have also reported pyrophosphate infarct size to be larger than antimyosin infarct size in the same patients [25]. Localization of pyrophosphate in reversibly injured myocardium has been previously reported [32–34], and Jansen et al. [35] confirmed that pyrophosphate bound to reperfused myocardium which was not irreversibly compromised. Recently, Takeda and co-workers [36] reported that the areas of experimental myocardial infarcts delineated by In-111-antimyosin and Tc-99m-pyrophosphate were identical by ex vivo tissue counting and that the overestimation of the pyrophosphate infarct size was probably due to very high uptake of pyrophosphate in necrotic tissue. This conclusion may be due to experimental oversight. Takeda et al. [36] used a gamma scintillation counter setting of 400 to 500 keV to count In-111 tissue activity and a setting of 60–156 keV for Tc-99m activity. Since In-111 has two photopeaks of emission at 173.5 and 247 keV, and no high energy emission in the range of 400–500 keV window, it is possible that counts were from the cross-talk of Nb-95 and Sc-46 which were used in the microsphere forms in their study.

Volpini and co-workers [18] in a study of 15 patients (10 Q wave and 5 non-Q wave infarcts) reported that antimyosin was positive in all 15 but pyrophosphate was positive in only 12 patients. In this study antimyosin was administered within 4–72 hours of the onset of chest pain and pyrophosphate 24 hours after antimyosin imaging. The reason for the lower sensitivity of pyrophosphate in this group of patients is not known.

Antimyosin scintigraphy for the detection of diffuse myocyte necrosis

Discrete and intense localization of antimyosin have been the rule in imaging of acute myocardial infarction. Tracer accumulation also corresponded to the myocardial region of the occluded coronary artery. Since diffuse myocyte necrosis is a common manifestation in idiopathic or secondary myocarditis as well as cardiac allograft rejection [37, 38], it was reasoned that the application of antimyosin immunoscintigraphy should provide a noninvasive diagnostic modality for these cardiac disorders.

Identification of myocyte necrosis associated with myocarditis

The feasibility of imaging diffuse myocardial necrosis was demonstrated in experimental murine myocarditis models [9–41]. These studies reported selective localization of monoclonal antimyosin antibody in the damaged myocytes which significantly correlated with the extent of histopathological myocardial damage [39, 40] as well as to the left ventricular dysfunction [41].

Yasuda et al. [42] investigated 28 patients of acute onset dilated cardiomyopathy suspected to be due to myocarditis. Presenting symptoms included heart failure in 21 patients, complex ventricular tachyarrhythmias in four and chest pain in three patients. All patients were documented to have normal coronary arteriograms. Twenty-five patients had left ventricular ejection fraction of less than 45%. All patients underwent In-111-antimyosin imaging and right ventricular endomyocardial biopsy. An antimyosin study was interpreted as positive when focal or diffuse uptake of the tracer was present in the planar image and in at least two of the three tomographic reconstructions. The study was judged negative when no tracer uptake was demonstrated in the planar or tomographic images. Seventeen patients had positive and 11 had negative antimyosin scans. None of the patients with negative scans had histological evidence of myocarditis. Nine patients with positive scans also had positive biopsy for myocarditis. Eight of the patients with abnormal scans did not have histological evidence of myocarditis. This study demonstrated the feasibility and potential utility of antimyosin antibody imaging as a non-invasive screening test for the diagnosis of myocarditis. Figure 8 shows 48 hours (post intravenous antimyosin injection) anterior and 60° LAO planar images (a) and SPECT transverse and coronal reconstructed images (b) of a patient with biopsy confirmed myocarditis. Antimyosin scan was originally performed on this patient at the time of admission three months previously. Antimyosin scan was positive but the original biopsy was nondiagnostic [43]. Similar results were reported in a subsequent study [44]. These studies have been corroborated by a larger study of Dec et al. [45], which provided more precise estimates of the diagnostic accuracy of this technique. In 82 patients with suspected myocarditis, the sensitivity of antimyosin imaging was 83%, specificity 53% and predictive value of the normal scan 92% relative to histopathological biopsy data. Although the positive predictive value of abnormal antimyosin scan of 33% was not impressive, an abnormal scan was proposed as a useful screening tool, since right ventricular endomyocardial biopsy in the patients who did not undergo antimyosin imaging averaged only 13% [45].

A negative scan reliably predicts a negative biopsy. A positive scan may be associated either with a positive or a negative biopsy. It has been demonstrated that the semi-quantitative antimyosin uptake as determined by the heart to lung ratios in scan-positive, biopsy-positive as well as scan-positive, biopsy-negative cases is similar, suggesting an identical underlying pathology [46]. The question to be resolved is whether these discordant results represent false positives or whether the scan is more accurate than the biopsy. Myocarditis

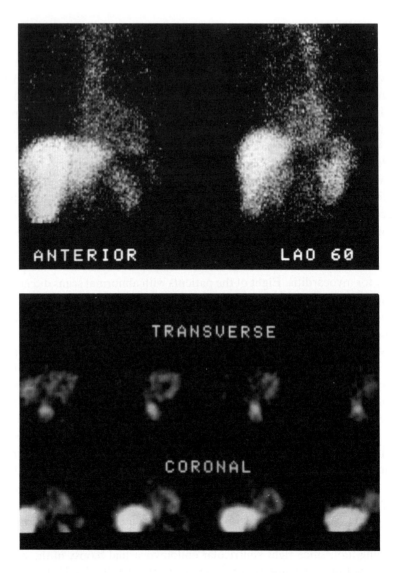

Figure 8. Planar anterior and 60° LAO (a), and SPECT transverse and coronal (b) antimyosin images of a patient with biopsy proven myocarditis. The images were obtained 48 h after intravenous administration of In-111-antimyosin Fab. (From [43] with permission of the Society of Nuclear Medicine, J Nucl Med.)

frequently presents as a focal or multifocal process, and the true frequency with which myocarditis occurs but is not detected by endomyocardial biopsy is not known [47–49]. In a postmortem simulated biopsy study, with five biopsy specimens from each of the 50 hearts with myocarditis, diagnosis of myocarditis could be made only in nine hearts [47]. In a similar study with 14 hearts, myocarditis was diagnosed in 79% of cases with more than 17 biopsy samples per heart [50]. The incidence of myocarditis in clinical dilated cardiomyopathy, as diagnosed by endomyocardial biopsy, has varied from as low as 2% to as high as 80% [47]. Underestimation of the incidence of myocarditis by endomyocardial biopsy thus appears to be a distinct possibility. Since the histopathological evidence of myocarditis by endomyocardial biopsy is currently accepted as the gold standard for evaluation of the diagnostic accuracy of other investigative techniques for the detection of myocarditis, it presents a methodological problem. The new test with a better sensitivity than the endomyocardial biopsy will be judged inevitably to have poor specificity for the diagnosis of myocarditis.

Spontaneous improvement in cardiac functions is a recognized feature of active myocarditis [51, 52] and one of the ways to validate a new diagnostic method would be to demonstrate that patients diagnosed to have myocarditis by the new test, on follow-up, may have different clinical outcome from those diagnosed not to have myocarditis. Dec et al. [45] demonstrated a higher likelihood of improvement in left ventricular function in patients with abnormal antimyosin scans. An increase in left ventricular ejection fraction of 10% or more occurred in 54% of patients with positive antimyosin scan within 6 months of treatment, as compared to 18% of those patients with negative antimyosin scans. In addition to the follow-up evaluation of the left ventricular functions, a subgroup of patients underwent repeat antimyosin scintigraphy after six months of treatment. Seventy-five percent of the patients with subsequent follow-up negative antimyosin scans had significant improvement in the ejection fraction [45]. Therefore, it appears that the discordant antimyosin uptake (at least in a subgroup of patients with improved ejection fraction) may in fact have identified myocarditis which the right ventricular biopsy failed to detect.

Surveillance role of antimyosin scintigraphy in cardiac transplant rejection

Since the histological evidence of myocyte necrosis is an obligatory component for the diagnosis of acute cardiac transplant rejection [38], the avidity of antimyosin antibody for acutely necrotic myocardium offers an additional application. The efficacy of antimyosin imaging for the detection of cardiac transplant rejection has been well demonstrated in experimental studies [53, 54]. In a pilot study for the detection human cardiac transplant rejection, 20 antimyosin images were obtained, seven days to nine years after transplantation (Figure 9) [55]. Eight patients had positive antimyosin images confirmed

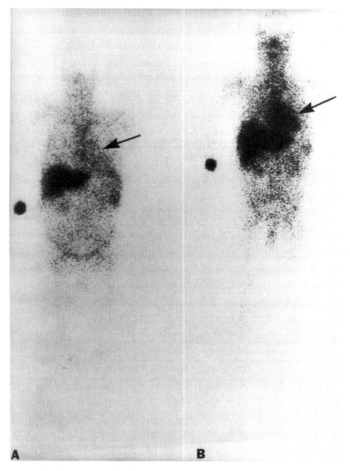

Figure 9. Anterior whole body In-111-antimyosin Fab gamma scintigraphic images of two heart transplant patients obtained 48 hours after antibody administration. The patient on the left had no clinical criteria for acute rejection and the myocardial activity (arrow) was minimal. The patient on the right with biopsy evidence of acute rejection showed intense myocardial uptake of In-111-antimyosin Fab (arrow). (From [54] with permission of the American Heart Association, Circulation.)

by biopsy to be undergoing acute rejection, and eight patients had negative images with no biopsy evidence of rejection. Discordance was observed in four studies, two with positive images and negative biopsy and two vice-versa. The sensitivity and specificity of the technique were 80% each [55]. De Nardo et al. [56] performed 30 antimyosin scintigraphic studies in 10 transplant recipients and compared the image results to endomyocardial biopsies. Antimyosin scintigraphy was negative in 19 instances; none of the images was false negative. Eleven positive images correlated with mild rejection ($n = 2$), moderate rejection ($n = 2$), myocyte necrosis due to ischemic damage ($n = 6$) and cytotoxic myocyte damage ($n = 1$) on the basis of endomyocardial biopsy data. Fifty-three antimyosin imaging studies in 21 patients from 7 to 40 months after transplantation were performed by Ballester et al. [57]. Heart to lung ratios of antimyosin uptake, signifying the intensity of myocyte necrosis, were significantly higher in patients demonstrating histologic evidence of rejection. Antimyosin uptake ratios were comparatively higher at one to three months after transplantation than after one year. A decrease in antimyosin uptake on follow-up studies in five patients correlated with uneventful clinical course while two transplant recipients with persistent antimyosin myocardial activity developed congestive failure. The feasibility of using multiple antimyosin scans in an attempt to reduce the frequency of biopsies for identification of rejection episodes was also demonstrated [58]. Since the recognition of myocyte necrosis and not mononuclear cell infiltrations forms the cut-off point for therapeutic intervention in allograft rejection, antimyosin imaging holds promise.

Antimyosin scintigraphy for identification of cardiac involvement in systemic disorders or secondary myocardial involvement

Cardiac involvement happens to be a significant component of various systemic disorders. Clinical diagnosis of carditis in this situation may be difficult when cardiac involvement is subclinical or is the only manifestation of the disorder. Demonstration of myocardial involvement may not only aid in establishing the diagnosis but may also offer serial evaluation of the efficacy of therapeutic intervention. The usefulness of antimyosin scintigraphy has also been reported in patients with rheumatic fever [59], Lyme's disease [60, 61], polymyositis [62], and Whipple's disease [63]. Secondary myocardial involvement has also been demonstrated by antimyosin scintigraphy in pheochromocytoma [64] and subsequent to adriamycin toxicity [65, 66].

Conclusions

Antimyosin immunoscintigraphy appears to be highly sensitive and specific for the diagnosis of acute myocardial infarction. It is safe and does not appear to be immunogenic. Although its primary utility may not be in the diagnosis of run of the mill acute myocardial infarction, its extreme sensitivity should make antimyosin invaluable in the diagnosis of equivocal infarcts. Furthermore, its utility in the assessment of the efficacy of thrombolytic intervention in preservation of viable myocardium must be considered. The ultimate worth of antimyosin immunoscintigraphy may be in the diagnosis of cardiac disorders of diffuse myocyte necrosis. To date, unequivocal diagnosis of myocarditis and heart transplant rejection utilizes the endomyocardial biopsy gold standard. Due to the insensitivity and invasiveness of the biopsy procedure, antimyosin imaging has gained increased utility and preference in the diagnosis of these two cardiac disorders. Studies can be performed without danger of immunological reactions to multiple antimyosin administrations. Therefore, efficacy of therapeutic interventions can be followed without clinical complications. Diagnosis of other clinical situations such as in dilated-phase hypertrophic cardiomyopathy, adriamycin cardiotoxicity and rheumatic carditis should all benefit from the availability of antimyosin immunoscintigraphy.

References

1. Khaw BA, Beller GA, Haber E, Smith TW. Localization of cardiac myosin-specific antibody in myocardial infarction. J Clin Invest 1976; 58: 439–46.
2. Khaw BA, Scott J, Fallon JT, Cahill SL, Haber E, Homcy C. Myocardial injury: quantitation by cell sorting initiated with antimyosin fluorescent spheres. Science 1982; 217: 1050–3.
3. Khaw BA, Gold HK, Leinbach RC et al. Early imaging of experimental myocardial infarction by intracoronary administration of ^{131}I-labeled anticardiac myosin (Fab′)$_2$ fragments. Circulation 1978; 58: 1137–42.
4. Khaw BA, Strauss HW. Haber E. Production and characterization of monoclonal antimyosin antibody: immunoscintigraphic visualization of necrotic myocardium. In: Chatal JF, editor. Monoclonal antibodies in immunoscintigraphy. Boca Raton: CRC Press, 1989: 339–56.
5. Khaw BA, Mattis JA, Melincoff G, Strauss HW, Gold HK, Haber E. Monoclonal antibody to cardiac myosin: imaging of experimental myocardial infarction. Hybridoma 1984; 3: 11–23.
6. Khaw BA, Beller GA, Haber E. Experimental myocardial infarct imaging following intravenous administration of Iodine-131 labeled antibody (Fab′)$_2$ fragments specific for cardiac myosin. Circulation 1978; 57: 743–50.
7. Khaw BA, Fallon JT, Beller GA, Haber E. Specificity of localization of myosin-specific antibody fragments in experimental myocardial infarction. Histologic, histochemical, autoradiographic and scintigraphic studies. Circulation 1979; 60: 1527–31.
8. Khaw BA, Gold HK, Yasuda T et al. Scintigraphic quantification of myocardial necrosis in patients after intravenous injection of myosin-specific antibody. Circulation 1986; 74: 501–8.
9. Khaw BA, Yasuda T, Gold HK et al. Acute myocardial infarct imaging with indium-111-labeled monoclonal antimyosin Fab. J Nucl Med 1987; 28: 1671–8.
10. Johnson LL, Seldin DW, Becker LC et al. Antimyosin imaging in acute transmural myocardial infarctions: results of a multicenter clinical trial. J Am Coll Cardiol 1989; 13: 27–35.
11. Taki J, Yasuda T, Gold HK et al. Prediction of extent of akinesis at 10 days from acute antimyosin scintigraphy [abstract]. J Nucl Med 1988; 29 Suppl: 851–2.
12. Jain D, Lahiri A, Crawley JC, Raftery EB. Indium-111 antimyosin imaging in a patient with

acute myocardial infarction: postmortem correlation between histopathologic and autoradiographic extent of myocardial necrosis. Am J Card Imaging 1988; 2: 158–61.

13. Jain D, Crawley JC, Lahiri A, Raftery EB. Indium-111-antimyosin images compared with triphenyl tetrazolium chloride staining in a patient six days after myocardial infarction. J Nucl Med 1990; 31: 231–3.

14. Hendel RC, McSherry BA, Leppo JA. Myocardial uptake of indium-111-labeled antimyosin in acute subendocardial infarction: clinical, histochemical, and autoradiographic correlation of myocardial necrosis. J Nucl Med 1990; 31: 1851–3.

15. Braat SH, de Zwaan C, Teule J, Heidendal G, Wellen HJ. Value of indium-111 monoclonal antimyosin antibody for imaging in acute myocardial infarction. Am J Cardiol 1987; 60: 725–6.

16. Cox PH, Schonfeld D, Remme WF, Pillay M, Brons R. A comparative study of myocardial infarct detection using Tc-99m pyrophosphate and In-111 antimyosin (R11D10 Fab). Int J Card Imaging 1987; 2: 197–8.

17. Antunes ML, Seldin DW, Wall RM, Johnson LL. Measurement of acute Q-wave myocardial infarct size with single photon emission computed tomography imaging in indium-111 antimyosin. Am J Cardiol 1989; 63: 777–83.

18. Volpini M, Guibbini R, Gei P et al. Diagnosis of acute myocardial infarction by indium-111 antimyosin antibody and correlation with traditional techniques for the evaluation of extent and localization. Am J Cardiol 1989; 63: 7–13.

19. Berger H, Lahiri A, Leppo J et al. Antimyosin imaging in patients with ischemic chest pain: initial results of phase III multicenter trial [abstract]. J Nucl Med 1988; 29 Suppl: 805–6.

20. Matsumori A, Yamada T, Tamaki N et al. Persistent uptake of indium-111 antimyosin monoclonal antibody in patients with myocardial infarction. Am Heart J 1990; 120: 1026–34.

21. Jain D, Lahiri A, Raftery EB. Immunoscintigraphy for detecting acute myocardial infarction without electrocardiographic changes [published erratum appears in BMJ 1990; 300: 306]. BMJ 1990; 300: 151–3.

22. van Vlies B, van Royen EA, Visser CA et al. Frequency of myocardial indium-111 antimyosin uptake after uncomplicated coronary artery bypass surgery. Am J Cardiol 1990; 66: 1191–5.

23. Berger HJ. Prognostic significance of the extent of antimyosin uptake in unstable ischemic heart disease: early risk stratification [abstract]. Circulation 1988; 78 (4 Suppl II): II 131.

24. van Vlies B, Baas J, Visser CA et al. Predictive value of indium-111 antimyosin uptake for improvement of left ventricular wall motion after thrombolysis in acute myocardial infarction. Am J Cardiol 1989; 64: 167–71.

25. Tamaki N, Yamada T, Matsumori A et al. Indium-111-antimyosin antibody imaging for detecting different stages of myocardial infarction: comparison with technetium-99m-pyrophosphate imaging. J Nucl Med 1990; 31: 136–42.

26. Buja LM, Poliner LR, Parkey RW et al. Clinicopathological study of the persistently positive technetium-99m stannous pyrophosphate myocardial scintigram and myocytolytic degeneration after myocardial infarction. Circulation 1977; 56: 1016–23.

27. Olson HG, Lyons KP, Aronow WS, Kupers J, Orlando J, Hughes D. Prognostic value of persistently positive technetium-99m stannous pyrophosphate myocardial scintigram after myocardial infarction. Am J Cardiol 1979; 43: 889–98.

28. Nicod P, Lewis SE, Corbett JC et al. Increased incidence and clinical correlation of persistently abnormal technetium pyrophosphate myocardial scintigrams following acute myocardial infarction in patients with diabetes mellitus. Am Heart J 1982; 103: 822–9.

29. Fishbein MC, MacLean D, Maroko PR. The histopathological evolution of myocardial infarction. Chest 1978; 73: 843–9.

30. Mallory GK, White PD, Salcedo-Salgar J. The speed of healing of myocardial infarction: a study of the pathological anatomy in 72 cases. Am Heart J 1939; 18: 647–71.
31. Buja LM, Tofe AJ, Kulkarni PV et al. Sites and mechanisms of localization of technetium-99m phosphorus radiopharmaceuticals in acute myocardial infarcts and other tissues. J Clin Invest 1977; 60: 724–40.
32. Bianco JA, Kemper AJ, Taylor A, Lazewatsky J, Tow DE, Khuri SF. Technetium-99m (Sn^{2+})pyrophosphate in ischemic and infarcted dog myocardium in early stages of acute coronary occlusion: histochemical and tissue-counting comparisons. J Nucl Med 1983; 24: 485–91.
33. Schelbert HR, Ingwall JS, Sybers HD, Ashburn WL. Uptake of infarct-imaging agents in reversibly and irreversibly injured myocardium in cultured fetal mouse heart. Circ Res 1976; 39: 860–8.
34. Zaret BL, DiCola VC, Donabedian RK et al. Dual radionuclide study of myocardial infarction. Relationships between myocardial uptake of potassium-43, technetium-99m stannous pyrophosphate, regional myocardial blood flow and creatine phosphokinase depletion. Circulation 1976; 53: 422–8.
35. Jansen DE, Corbett JR, Buja LM et al. Quantification of myocyte injury produced by temporary coronary artery occlusion and reflow with technetium-99m-pyrophosphate. Circulation 1987; 75: 611–7.
36. Takeda K, LaFrance ND, Weisman HF, Wagner HN Jr, Becker LC. Comparison of indium-111 antimyosin antibody and technetium-99m pyrophosphate localization in reperfused and nonreperfused myocardial infarction. J Am Coll Cardiol 1991; 17: 519–26.
37. Aretz HT, Billingham ME, Edwards WD et al. Myocarditis. A histopathologic definition and classification. Am J Cardiovasc Pathol 1987; 1: 3–14.
38. Billingham ME. Diagnosis of cardiac rejection by endomyocardial biopsy. Heart Transplant 1981; 1: 25–30.
39. Matsumori A, Ohkusa T, Matoba Y et al. Myocardial uptake of antimyosin monoclonal antibody in a murine model of viral myocarditis. Circulation 1989; 79: 400–5.
40. Rezkalla S, Kloner RA, Khaw BA et al. Detection of experimental myocarditis by monoclonal antimyosin antibody, Fab fragment. Am Heart J 1989; 117: 391–5.
41. Kishimoto C, Hung GL, Ishibashi M et al. Natural evolution of cardiac function, cardiac pathology, and antimyosin scan in a murine myocarditis model. J Am Coll Cardiol 1991; 17: 821–7.
42. Yasuda T, Palacios IF, Dec GW et al. Indium 111-monoclonal antimyosin antibody imaging in the diagnosis of acute myocarditis. Circulation 1987; 76: 306–11.
43. Narula J, Southern JF, Abraham SA, Pieri P, Khaw BA. Myocarditis simulating myocardial infarction. Clinicopathological conferences. J Nucl Med 1991; 32: 312–8.
44. Carrio I, Berna L, Ballester M et al. Indium-111 antimyosin scintigraphy to assess myocardial damage in patients with suspected myocarditis and cardiac rejection. J Nucl Med 1988; 29: 1893–1900.
45. Dec GW, Palacios IF, Yasuda T et al. Antimyosin antibody cardiac imaging: its role in the diagnosis of myocarditis. J Am Coll Cardiol 1990; 16: 97–104.
46. Narula J, Yasuda T, Southern JF et al. Antimyosin scintigraphy in myocarditis: evaluation of diagnostic methodology [abstract]. J Am Coll Cardiol 1991; 17 (2 Suppl A): 342A.
47. Lie JT. Myocarditis and endomyocardial biopsy in unexplained heart failure: a diagnosis in search of disease. Ann Intern Med 1988; 109: 525–8.
48. Baandrup U, Florio RA, Olsen EG. Do endomyocardial biopsies represent the morphology of the rest of the myocardium? A quantitative light microscopic study of single v. multiple biopsies with the King's bioptome. Eur Heart J 1982; 3: 171–8.

49. Ferrans VJ, Roberts WC. Myocardial biopsy: a useful diagnostic procedure or only a research tool [editorial]? Am J Cardiol 1978; 41: 965–7.
50. Chow LH, Radio SJ, Sears TD, McManus BM. Insensitivity of right ventricular endomyocardial biopsy in the diagnosis of myocarditis. J Am Coll Cardiol 1989; 14: 915–20.
51. Dec GW Jr, Palacios IF, Fallon JT et al. Active myocarditis in spectrum of acute dilated cardiomyopathies. Clinical features, histologic correlates, and clinical outcome. N Engl J Med 1985; 312: 885–90.
52. Johnson RA, Palacios IF. Dilated cardiomyopathies of the adult (first of two parts). N Engl J Med 1982; 307: 1051–8; Dilated cardiomyopathies of the adult (second of two parts). N Engl J Med 1982; 307: 1119–26.
53. Nishimura T, Sada M, Sasaki H et al. Assessment of severity of cardiac rejection in heterotopic heart transplantation using indium-111 labeled antimyosin and magnetic resonance imaging. Cardiovasc Res 1988; 22: 108–12.
54. Isobe M, Haber E, Khaw BA. Early detection of rejection and assessment of cyclosporine therapy by indium-111 antimyosin imaging in mouse heart allografts. Circulation. In press.
55. Frist W, Yasuda T, Segall G et al. Noninvasive detection of human cardiac transplant rejection with indium-111 antimyosin (Fab) imaging. Circulation 1987; 67 (5 Suppl): V 81–5.
56. De Nardo D, Scibilia G, Macchiarelli AG et al. The role of indium-111 antimyosin (Fab) imaging as a noninvasive surveillance method of human heart transplant rejection. J Heart Transplant 1989; 8: 407–12.
57. Ballester-Rodes M, Carrio-Gasset I, Abadal-Berini L, Obrador-Mayol D, Berna-Roqueta L, Caralps-Riera JM. Patterns of evolution of myocyte damage after human heart transplantation detected by indium-111 monoclonal antimyosin. Am J Cardiol 1988; 62: 623–7.
58. Ballester RM, Obrador D, Carrio I et al. Indium-111-monoclonal antimyosin antibody studies after the first year of heart transplantation. Identification of risk groups for developing rejection during long-term follow-up and clinical implications. Circulation 1990; 82: 2100–8.
59. Malhotra A, Narula J, Yasuda T et al. Indium-111 monoclonal antimyosin antibody imaging for diagnosis of rheumatic myocardis [abstract]. J Nucl Med 1990; 31 Suppl: 841.
60. Kimball SA, Janson PA, LaRaia PJ. Complete heart block as the sole manifestation of Lyme disease. Arch Intern Med 1989; 149: 1897–8.
61. Casans I, Villar A, Almenar V, Blanes A. Lyme myocarditis diagnosed by indium-111-antimyosin antibody scintigraphy. Eur J Nucl Med 1989; 15: 330–1.
62. De Geeter F, Deleu D, Debeukelaere S, De Coninck A, Somers G, Bossuyt A. Detection of muscle necrosis in dermatomyositis by ^{111}In labelled antimyosin Fab fragments. Nucl Med Commun 1989; 10: 603–7.
63. Southern JF, Moscicki RA, Magro C, Dickersin GR, Fallon JT, Bloch KJ. Lymphedema, lymphocytic myocarditis, and sarcoidlike granulomatosis. Manifestations of Whipple's disease. JAMA 1989; 261: 1467–70.
64. Case records of the Massachusetts General Hospital. Weekly clinicopathologic exercises. Case 15–1988. A 26-year-old women with cardiomyopathy, multiple shakes, and an adversal mass. N Engl J Med 1988; 318: 970–81.
65. Estorch M, Carrio I, Berna L et al. Indium-111-antimyosin scintigraphy after doxorubicin therapy in patients with advanced breast cancer. J Nucl Med 1990; 31: 1965–9.
66. Yamada T, Matsumori A, Tamaki N et al. Detection of adriamycin cardiotoxicity with indium-111 labeled antimyosin monoclonal antibody imaging. Jpn Circ J 1991; 55: 377–83.

23. Myocardial infarct imaging with cardiac troponin-I antibodies

PETER CUMMINS

Introduction

The proteins of the myofibril exist in many different forms which vary in their tissue distributions. Particular attention has focused on those forms which are located preferentially or even specifically in the heart as possible markers of myocardial tissue injury.

Troponin-I (Tn-I) is part of the calcium regulatory complex of the myofibril and exists as cardiac, fast or slow skeletal muscle isoforms (Figure 1) [1, 2]. The cardiac form with a molecular mass of 23,000 daltons is specifically located in the human adult heart [3, 4] and distributed uniformly throughout the atria and ventricles. It has the properties of an ideal intracellular cardiac specific marker. As Tn-I is located externally on the myofibril it is easily accessible inside necrotic cells to antibody targeting.

Methodology

Both polyclonal and monoclonal antibodies can be produced to cardiac Tn-I which are highly cardiac specific and which do not react with the other skeletal Tn-I isoforms. The protein is highly antigenic. When first prepared, some cross-reactivity of polyclonal antisera with skeletal muscle Tn-I isoforms is occasionally observed. This arises from the homology of 60% in primary amino acid sequence between cardiac and skeletal Tn-I isoforms [2]. However, this cross reactivity is usually no more than 10% of the reactivity with

317

Ernst E. van der Wall et al. (eds), What's new in cardiac imaging?, 317–326.
© *1992 Kluwer Academic Publishers. Printed in the Netherlands.*

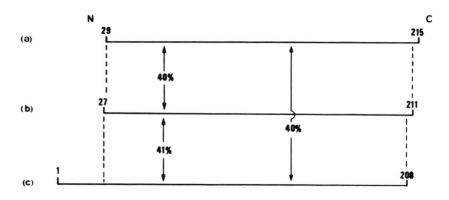

Figure 1. Representation of isoforms of troponin-I. (a) slow skeletal: (b) fast skeletal, (c) cardiac. Percentage figures indicate degree of sequence heterogeneity between isoforms. Numbers indicate residue positions. From [16].

cardiac Tn-I and is easily removed by immunoaffinity absorption chromatography on a mixed fast and slow skeletal Tn-I isoform immunoaffinity column.

Studies using radiolabeled Tn-I antibodies have been conducted in which both whole immunoglobulin and Fab fragments have been employed. It has been argued that the reduced molecular size of the latter (50.000 compared with 150.000 for whole IgG) is more suited for in vivo administration [5]. Smaller molecules are thought to be both more likely to gain intracellular access to damaged cells via compromised membranes and also to be cleared faster from the circulation leading to reduced background uptake. When Fab antibodies are produced from sheep anti-cardiac Tn-I sera about 10% of the overall immunological activity is retained. Both Fab and whole IgG from polyclonal antibodies have been radiolabeled with iodine-131 and indium-111 using the chloramine-T and DTPA methods respectively [6, 7] and examined for their ability to localize in necrotic myocardial tissue using an experimental canine model of myocardial infarction [8, 9].

Dogs (20–30 kg) were anaesthetized with pentobarbital sodium and a left lateral thoracotomy made. The left anterior descending coronary artery was ligated below the first major branch. Radiolabeled antibody was administered via an indwelling catheter in the left jugular vein. A mean of 1.88 mCi of iodine-131 or 0.57 mCi of indium-111 labeled Fab (200–300 g) was injected into the animals approximately 5 hours after ligation of the coronary artery. In those animals injected with iodine-131 labeled antibodies, these were also co-injected with iodine-125 labeled nonimmune Fab at the same time after ligation to examine nonspecific antibody uptake. Technetium 99m (Tc-99m) labeled human albumin was also injected 24 hours after Fab administration to visualize the whole blood pool. Animals were imaged in the left lateral view for 10 minutes using an Anger type gamma camera with a medium energy collimator for Tc-99m followed immediately by imaging for iodine-131. Imaging was performed between 24 and 40 hours after injection of Fab.

Regional blood flow within the myocardium was determined by injection of 0.5 mCi of cerium-141 labeled microspheres slowly into the left atrium of the anaesthetized animal 10 minutes before termination. In order to identify precisely where the uptake of radiolabeled antibody occurred, studies were also conducted on individual heart slices and biopsies from selected slices within the infarcted region. After animals were terminated, hearts were removed and washed with ice-cold physiologically buffered saline and partially frozen before being imaged for 10 minutes for either iodine-131 or indium-111. The area of necrotic tissue was visualized using nitroblue tetrazolium staining. Hearts were cut into 3–5 mm sections, incubated for 20 minutes in 0.5 mg/ml nitroblue tetrazolium, 0.1 M Sorensen's phosphate buffer pH 7.4 [10] after which healthy myocardium stained dark blue and necrotic myocardium remained unstained. The extent of necrosis was then determined graphically.

Heart slices were imaged for iodine-131 for 60 minutes and indium-111 for 10 minutes. Infarcted tissue was outlined directly on the computer display by comparison with histochemical and imaged views. Isotope counts and doses within necrotic zones were determined with reference to activity standards. Counts were corrected for background contribution and normalized to determine infarct to normal heart uptake ratios. Uptake ratios in heart biopsies from individual slices were differentially counted for iodine-131, iodine-125, indium-111 and cerium-141 with correction for possible overlap using correction factors obtained with isotope standards.

In-vivo imaging

In-vivo images for both iodine-131 and indium-111 (after whole body blood pool subtraction) demonstrated positive uptake in the left lateral view immediately overlying the ventricular chambers with no significant difference between administered Fab or whole IgG (Figure 2). The images obtained at 40 hours showed a similar distribution although in the case of iodine there was significant nonspecific uptake by the kidneys and spleen prior to clearance. The specificity of the antibodies for the cardiac isoform of Tn-I was clearly demonstrated when the incision from the thoracotomy was examined. Although this caused significant skeletal muscle trauma immediately overlying the heart no evidence of antibody uptake was visible in any images.

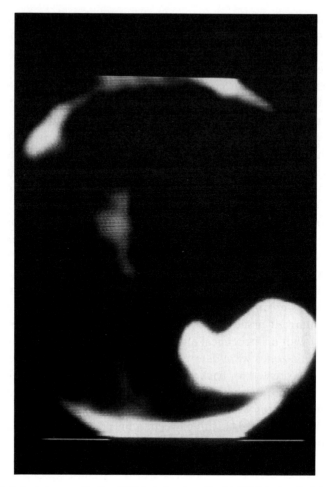

Figure 2. Whole body image of iodine-131 labeled anti-cardiac Tn-I Fab in dog. Left lateral whole body view. Head uppermost. The area of increased radioactivity in the centre corresponds to the apical region of heart.

Isolated heart imaging

When hearts were excised and re-imaged there was clear evidence of cardiac uptake localized to the apical region usually overlying the left ventricle (Figure 3). These areas coincided with the externally visible ischemic areas in isolated hearts. Subsequent identification of necrotic areas in histochemically stained heart slices confirmed that infarcted areas were confined to the apical regions of the left ventricle. This was further confirmed on subsequent imaging of the individual slices which clearly demonstrated that antibody uptake was

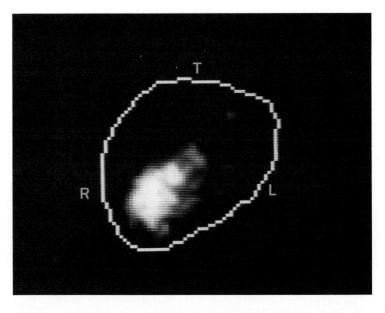

Figure 3. Isolated heart scintigram for iodine-131 labeled anti cardiac Tn-I Fab. Uptake is localized in the apical region of the ventricles. R: right; L: left; T: top.

localized to the areas of infarction outlined by nitroblue tetrazolium (Figure 4).

Specificity of antibody uptake and relation to blood flow

Confirmation that antibody in infarcted areas binds directly to Tn-I was confirmed by dual administration of iodine-131 labeled immune cardiac specific Tn-I Fab and iodine-125 labeled nonimmune Fab. Maximum immune Fab uptake alone, normalized for biopsy weight, was confined to biopsies within or immediately on the border of histochemically defined infarcted areas. Normalized counts for iodine-131 immune Fab in biopsies within the infarct zone were up to 24 times greater than the mean of those within the normal posterior left ventricle. Specific antibody uptake in biopsies due to antigen binding was determined by subtracting the relative uptake of nonimmune Fab (iodine-125 uptake in each biopsy/mean iodine-125 uptake in normal posterior left ventricle) from the relative uptake of immune Fab (iodine-131 uptake in each biopsy/mean iodine-131 uptake in normal posterior left ventricle). The antigen specific uptake of I-131 immune Fab was found to be up to 14 times greater than iodine-125 nonimmune Fab in biopsies near the centre of the infarct.

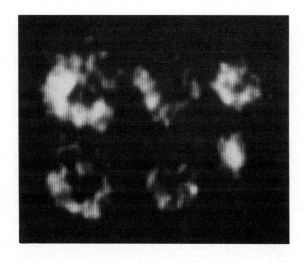

a

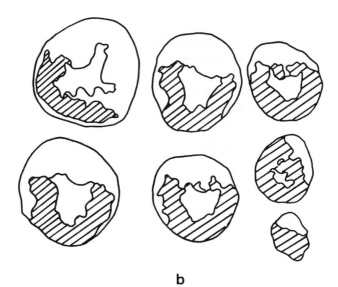

b

Figure 4. Iodine-131 Fab uptake in histochemically stained heart slices. (a) Iodine-131 labeled anti-cardiac Tn-I Fab scintigram of seven heart slices. (b) Corresponding heart slices to (a) in which areas identified as necrotic by nitroblue tetrazolium staining are hatched.

Specific antibody uptake also correlated well with areas of reduced blood flow as determined by cerium-141 microsphere uptake. Excised whole hearts imaged for both iodine-131 and cerium-141 showed apical localization only of the anti-cardiac Tn-I Fab. The cerium-141 microsphere distribution extended to all areas of the heart with the exception of the areas of increased iodine-131 activity. Blood flow in individual biopsies as determined by cerium-141 microsphere distribution was also compared in all biopsies. Flow was at the lowest levels in the majority of biopsies within the histochemical infarct. Over 95% of biopsies outside this area demonstrated the highest blood flow. Biopsies containing the highest relative uptake of specific Fab exhibited the most severe blood flow reductions. The highest ratio of antibody uptake between infarcted and normal myocardium (mean value of 9.9) was present in biopsies which exhibited the most severe blood flow reduction of between 0 and 10% of normal.

Dose and uptake ratios for iodine-131 and indium-111 labeled antibodies

Visualisation of targeted cells in vivo depends on the amount of antibody reaching the target (i.e. % of injected dose/g of infarcted tissue) and on the infarct: background antibody uptake ratio. Scintigrams of heart slices were used to calculate the amount of iodine-131 and indium-111 cardiac Tn-I Fab present in infarcted areas. When corrected for infarct size which ranged between 5.2 and 22.1% of the whole heart (mean = 14.7%), a mean of $0.003 \pm 0.002\%$ of the injected dose for iodine-131 Fab was present per gram of infarcted tissue. Uptake ratios of iodine-131 Fab activities in the whole infarct compared with activities in a similar mass of normal myocardium were determined directly from scintigrams. These ranged between 1.39 and 3.94 with a mean uptake ratio of 2.48 for infarcted:normal myocardium. When indium-111 labeled Fab was injected, % injected dose/g of infarct increased sevenfold to $0.021 \pm 0.016\%$ and uptake ratio increased to 4.67 ± 1.79.

The extent of cardiac Tn-I Fab uptake in damaged skeletal muscle was estimated from biopsies taken from injured skeletal muscles at the site of the thoracotomy. The ratio of uptake of immune iodine-131 Fab in this region when compared to normal skeletal or cardiac muscle was not significantly different to the uptake ratios of nonimmune iodine-125 Fab in the same tissues.

Some antibodies in polyclonal antibody mixtures may be unable to bind to Tn-I epitopes due to myofibrillar protein interactions. A panel of cardiac Tn-I monoclonal antibodies was analyzed for epitope availability using both isolated myocytes and myofibrils. Only 50% of antibodies gained access to Tn-I epitopes. Injection of an indium-111 labeled Fab monoclonal antibody to cardiac Tn-I which was shown to gain access to Tn-I epitopes inside damaged myocytes gave similar results. The % injected dose/g infarcted tissue was 0.019 and uptake ratio was 2.53. These values increased to 0.037% and 5.46, respectively when labeled Fab was co-injected with a 10-fold bolus of unlabeled monoclonal IgG.

Discussion

Other myofibrillar proteins such as actin, myosin and troponin-T also exist as cardiac isotypes although their strict cardiac localization is less well established. Cardiac actin is present in skeletal muscle [11] and the large number of troponin-T isotypes resulting from differential gene splicing [12] have not allowed precise tissue distributions to be established to date in the heart. Myosin light and heavy chain subunits display varying levels of cross reactivity with corresponding skeletal subunit isotypes [13–15].

The success of in-vivo imaging of targetted tissues using radiolabeled antibodies ultimately depends on both the tissue content of antibody (i.e. absolute dose of injected radiolabeled antibody attaching to the target site) and the uptake ratio (ratio of labeled antibody uptake in abnormal compared with normal tissue). Cellular Tn-I is known to be lost to the circulation for up to 7–10 days after myocardial infarction both in this model [8] and clinically [16] which would reduce the available levels progressively. Moreover, by comparison with myosin, which has been used as a successful in-vivo imaging target and which comprises 40–50 mg/g of cardiac muscle, Tn-I represents only 2–3 mg/g.

However, injected radiolabeled antibodies to Tn-I do localize in necrotic myocardium and this localization is mainly due to direct antigen binding. The uptakes are comparable to those obtained clinically with injected radiolabeled antibodies to tumour markers in which maximum tumour contents of around 0.005% of injected dose/g are achieved [5, 17]. Biodistribution studies of Tc-99m labeled antimyosin Fab 24 hours after intravenous injection in canine experimental infarction have demonstrated tissue contents of 0.017% injected dose/g infarcted myocardium which is increased three-fold after reperfusion [18]. Direct injection of antimyosin Fab into the coronary arteries increased the % injected dose four-fold. This could reflect the greater tissue content of myosin compared with Tn-I and/or the affinity of antibody employed.

The uptake ratios of antibody between infarcted and normal myocardium ranged from 1.39 to 3.94 when the whole infarcted area was considered which also compares with tumour antibody uptake ratios of usually less than 5 [5, 17].

Uptake of Tn-I in infarcted tissue is inversely related to blood flow and presumably in some direct way to the extent of damage. This confirms previous findings with myosin antibodies [14, 19, 20] and contrasts with that seen for cardiac avid imaging agents such as Tc-99m pyrophosphate. In the latter case uptake is maximal where flow is moderately reduced but minimal at infarct centres with neglible flow [20]. This could be due to the time for accumulation of calcium deposits which are the supposed targets for Tc-99m pyrophosphate. In the case of Tn-I and presumably with myosin antibodies, there is sufficient blood flow due to development of collateral circulation that numbers of target sites are not a limiting factor and uptake reflects numbers and development of necrotic cells. In contrast, blood flow in tumours is usually thought to be increased so the similarity in uptake ratios between tumour and myofibrillar markers is probably due more to numbers of target sites available.

References

1. Syska H, Perry SV, Trayer IP. A new method of preparation of troponin-I (inhibitory protein) using affinity chromatography. Evidence for three different forms in striated muscle. FEBS Lett 1974; 40: 253–7.
2. Wilkinson JM, Grand RJA. Comparison of amino acid sequence of troponin-I from different striated muscles. Nature 1978; 271: 31–5.
3. Cummins P, Perry SV. Troponin-I from human skeletal and cardiac muscles. Biochem J 1978; 171: 251–9.
4. Humphreys JE, Cummins P. Atrial and ventricular tropomyosin and troponin-I in the developing and adult bovine and human heart. J Moll Cell Cardiol 1984; 16: 643–57.
5. Thomas GD, Chappell MJ, Dykes PW et al. Effect of dose, molecular size, affinity, and protein binding on tumour uptake of antibody or ligand: a biomathematical model. Cancer Res 1989; 49: 3290–6.
6. Greenwood FC, Hunter WM, Glover JS. The preparation of I131 labelled human growth hormone of high specific radioactivity. Biochem J 1963; 89: 114–23.
7. Hnatowich DJ, Layne WW, Childs RL. The preparation and labelling of DTPA-coupled albumin. Int J Appl Radiat Isot 1982; 33: 327–32.
8. Cummins B, Cummins P. Cardiac specific troponin-I release in canine experimental myocardial infarction: development of a sensitive enzyme-linked immunoassay. J Mol Cell Cardiol 1987; 19: 999–1010.
9. Cummins B, Russell GJ, Chandler ST, Pears DJ, Cummins P. Uptake of radioiodinated cardiac specific troponin-I antibodies in myocardial infarction. Cardiovasc Res 1990; 24: 317–27.
10. Ramkissoon RA. Macroscopic identification of early myocardial infarction by dehydrogenase alterations. J Clin Pathol 1966; 19: 479–81.
11. Swynghedauw B. Developmental and functional adaptation contractile proteins in cardiac and skeletal muscles. Physiol Rev 1986; 66: 710–71.
12. Breitbart RE, Andreadis A, Nadal-Ginard B. Alternative splicing: a ubiquitous mechanism

for the generation of multiple protein isoforms from single genes. Annu Rev Biochem 1987; 56: 467–95.

13. Katus HA, Yasuda T, Gold HK et al. Diagnosis of acute myocardial infarction by detection of circulating cardiac myosin light chains. Am J Cardiol 1984; 54: 964–70.

14. Khaw BA, Beller G, Haber E, Smith TW. Localization of cardiac myosin specific antibody in myocardial infarction. J Clin Invest 1976; 58: 439–46.

15. Haber E, Katus HA, Hurrell JG et al. Detection and quantitation of myocardial cell death: application of monoclonal antibodies specific for cardiac myosin. J Mol Cell Cardiol 1982; 14 Suppl 3: 139–46.

16. Cummins B, Auckland ML, Cummins P. Cardiac-specific troponin-I radioimmunoassay in the diagnosis of acute myocardial infarction. Am Heart J 1987; 113: 1333–44.

17. Dykes PW, Bradwell AR, Chapman CE, Vaughan ATM. Radioimmunotherapy of cancer: clinical studies and limiting factors. Cancer Treat Rev 1987; 14: 87–106.

18. Khaw BA, Mattis JA, Melincoff G, Strauss HW, Gold HK, Haber E. Monoclonal antibody to cardiac myosin: Imaging of experimental myocardial infarction. Hybridoma 1984; 3: 11–23.

19. Khaw BA, Beller GA, Haber E. Experimental myocardial infarct imaging following intravenous administration of iodine-131 labelled antibody (Fab')$_2$ fragments specific for cardiac myosin. Circulation 1978; 57: 743–50.

20. Beller GA, Khaw BA, Haber E, Smith TW. Localisation of radiolabelled cardiac myosin specific antibody in myocardial infarcts: comparison with technetium-99m stannous pyrophosphate. Circulation 1977; 55: 74–8.

Function

24. Radionuclide imaging in the evaluation of cardiac function: new developments?

ERNST E. VAN DER WALL and BERTHE L.F. VAN ECK-SMIT

Summary

Evaluation of cardiac function by radionuclide techniques seems to have reached a phase of consolidation in nuclear cardiology. Nevertheless, there have been new developments and applications for radionuclide imaging of cardiac function. These developments regard the manufacturing of new tracers, the different ways of acquisition and analysis, new imaging devices, and the potential to simultaneously combine perfusion and function studies. These new attainments are an important step forward in the domain of radionuclide assessment of cardiac function.

Introduction

The evaluation of cardiac function by nuclear cardiology techniques seems to have reached a phase of consolidation. At present, radionuclide angiography has proved to be an accurate, noninvasive method to assess left ventricular function at rest and during exercise. Both left ventricular ejection fraction and wall motion abnormalities can be readily assessed in patients with suspected or known coronary artery disease, valvular heart disease, cardiomyopathies, and congenital heart disease. Furthermore, it allows the evaluation of drug therapy and interventional procedures. The major value of radionuclide angiography is currently its ability to stratify patients into high and low risk patients. Left ventricular ejection fraction at rest and its response during exercise have shown to be utmost important predictors of morbidity and mortality following

329

Ernst E. van der Wall et al. (eds), What's new in cardiac imaging?, 329–339.
© *1992 Kluwer Academic Publishers. Printed in the Netherlands.*

myocardial infarction. Despite the apparent consolidation phase of radionu-clide angiography, several new developments and applications have appeared at the horizon for the evaluation of cardiac function. These developments are: first, the manufacturing of new tracers; second, the mode of acquisition; third, the mode of analysis; fourth, new imaging devices; and lastly, the appropriate combination of function with perfusion studies.

Evolution of tracer development

(A) Single photon emission agents

Radionuclide angiography started in 1958 [1] with radioiodinated iodine-131 labeled human serum albumin for the detection of pericardial effusion. In the early seventies, first pass and equilibrium gated blood pool imaging were developed to measure regional and global ventricular function. At that time, radionuclide angiography was described as a 'noninvasive scintiphotographic method for measuring left ventricular function in man' [2, 3]. This procedure required radiopharmaceuticals that could provide a high photon flux with an acceptable radiation to permit recording of several million events in an accept-able interval of time. First studies were performed with technetium-99m labeled human serum albumin as the imaging compound.

Technetium-99m labeled human serum albumin
Technetium-99m-labeled human serum albumin, an agent originally intro-duced as a blood pool tracer for placental imaging in 1964, was initially selected for cardiac blood pool imaging [4].

Although technetium-99m labeled albumin was widely used, it was far from an ideal compound due to its complex preparation, poor quality control, and little stability in vivo. There are several specific disadvantages to the use of technetium-99m albumin. First, due to poor analytical techniques in the separation of the end product, technetium-99m albumin contained several unwarranted impurities. Second, the compound leaks out of the vascular compartment to equilibrate with the total-body albumin space. Third, the high concentration of labeled albumine in the liver may interfere with visualization of the inferior wall of the cardiac blood pool. Lastly, the lungs have a larger albumin space than red cell volume which contribute to the lower target/ background activity seen with albumin imaging.

Technetium-99m labeled red cells
The introduction of technetium-99m labeled red cells by an in vitro method in

1973 [5] and an in vivo method in 1977 [6] circumvented most of the problems encountered with labeled albumin. The labeling procedure is based on the observation that the reduced technetium ion cannot move in or out of the red cell, while pertechnetate can diffuse freely in and out of the red cell. Technetium-99m labeled to red blood cells is prepared by reducing the pertechnetate ion inside the cell with a reducing agent such as stannous ion, already present in the cell.

Technetium-99m labeled red cells maintain a higher concentration in the vascular space. The liver has a relatively small red cell volume and does not usually interfere with visualization of the inferior wall, while the spleen has a high hematocrit and is frequently the site of the highest red cell concentration. Currently, technetium-99m in vivo labeled red blood cells are standardly used in nuclear medicine practice for assessment of cardiac function.

Technetium-99m diethylenetriamine-pentaacetic acid conjugated with human serum albumin

Nishimura et al. [7] reported in 1991 on the use of technetium-99m chelated diethylenetriamine-pentaacetic acid (DTPA) conjugated to human serum albumin cardiac imaging. They compared the performance of technetium-99m DTPA human serum albumin with in vivo labeled red blood cells in 31 patients with various heart diseases and found that both labels offer similar results for the determination of ventricular function. It was demonstrated that the left ventricular ejection fraction obtained with this compound was comparable to that of contrast angiography. Spleen uptake with technetium-99m DTPA-human serum albumin is lower than that of technetium-99m labeled red blood cells, but in contrast to labeled blood cells, the activity of technetium-99m DTPA-human serum albumin does not remain constant long enough in circulation. The compound escapes from the vascular space into the extracellular fluid system, contributing to the slightly higher uptake noticed in the liver. However, technetium-99m DTPA human serum albumin seems to be considerably better than the previously used technetium-99m stannous-human serum albumin preparations.

Technetium-99m sestaMIBI

In the mid-eighties, technetium-99m labeled isonitriles were developed for cardiac imaging purposes and one of these compounds, technetium-99m sestaMIBI, became available for clinical use. Although technetium-99m sestaMIBI is predominantly used for myocardial perfusion imaging (see Chapters 6 and 7), several studies have shown its value in assessing ventricular function [8, 9]. Derived from first pass studies, close linear correlations have been observed between ejection fraction determined by standard technetium-99m and technetium-99m sestaMIBI ejection fraction [8]. It was also demonstrated that first pass technetium-99m studies can be used to assess regional left ventricular wall motion. Using treadmill exercise, it was shown that first pass technetium-99m sestaMIBI procedures were feasible and that there was no difference between one-day and two-day rest-exercise protocols for the assessment of left and right ventricular ejection fraction [9]. Of course, most information will be obtained by combination of perfusion and function studies when using technetium-99m sestaMIBI (see Chapter 26).

Krypton-81m
Apart from technetium-99m labeled radiopharmaceuticals, other single photon emitting radionuclides have been developed for imaging of cardiac function. Krypton 81m, an inert gas radionuclide with an ultra-short half-life of 13 seconds, has been shown to be ideally suited to right heart imaging. Krypton-81m is eluted from its parent rubidium-81 (half-life 4.7 hours) and it decays to stable krypton-81 by emitting 190 keV gamma photons that allow excellent imaging with standard gamma equipment. With continuous intravenous infusion of krypton-81m, the technique is better described as an equilibrium technique comparable to technetium-99m blood pool ventriculography to image the left ventricle. Following infusion, there is substantial accumulation of krypton-81m activity within the lungs, which necessitates background subtraction. A static technetium-99m perfusion lung image is used to subtract lung activity, resulting in excellent definition of right heart structures. With the application of this technique of image analysis, good correlations are found between right ventricular ejection fractions derived from krypton-81m imaging and right ventricular contrast angiography. Furthermore, krypton-81m equilibrium ventriculography allows the evaluation of right ventricular systolic and diastolic indices, and the estimation of right ventricular volumes [10]. Krypton-81m equilibrium ventriculography therefore offers the potential for repeatable noninvasive assessment of important parameters of right ventricular function (Chapter 25). The value of krypton-81m in delineating myocardial perfusion is addressed in Chapter 5.

Aurium-195m, iridium-191m, tantalum-178
Also other tracers for the evaluation of cardiac function have been developed, such as aurium-195m, iridium-191m, and tantalum-178. Since these tracers are currently not available for clinical use, they will be not further addressed in this chapter.

(B) Positron emitting agents

Cardiac function imaging can now also be performed using positron emission tomography (PET). While PET blood pool imaging is not a common procedure, the enhanced resolution of PET and its ability to provide tomographic delineation of the cardiac structure has the potential to improve the quality of diagnostic information that can be gleaned from the PET study. Several positron emitting agents have been developed to characterize cardiac function.

Carbon-11 labeled carbon monoxide

In the past, the major red cell label was carbon-11 labeled carbon monoxide. Following inhalation, this agent binds to hemoglobin, forming carboxyhemoglobin. While this is an excellent red cell label, it suffers from gradual dissociation from the red cell and requires the use of an on-site cyclotron to manufacture the radionuclide. Therefore, clinical acceptance of carbon-11 carbon dioxide is low and applications are limited.

Copper-62

In a study by Mathias et al. [11] in 1991, the use of the positron-emitting radionuclide copper-62 (copper-62 benzyl-TETA-human serum albumin) for blood pool imaging with PET was reported. Copper-62 is a positron-emitting nuclide with a half-life of 9.7 minutes, which is obtained from a zinc-62 generator (half-life of zinc is 9.2 hours). Copper is found in both serum albumin and ceruloplasmin in plasma. The copper must be complexed with a protein through a ligand to form a stable bond complex that remains intravascularly. The new biologic tracer copper-62 benzyl-tetraazacyclotetra decane-N,N',N'',N'''-tetraacetic acid (TETA) human serum albumin seems to be stable in vitro in serum, possibly due to both square planar structure and macrocylic effects. The copper-62 benzyl-TETA-human serum albumin complex stays in the blood pool in an appreciable quantity even after 1 hour which is sufficient to record high quality blood pool images. The tomographic nature of PET imaging overcomes the potential problems from radiotracer uptake in the lungs, liver, and spleen, which would contribute to the background activity if the data were recorded with planar techniques. As a blood pool tracer, copper-62 benzyl-TETA-human serum albumin performs better when compared to other copper-62 radiopharmaceuticals tested. The use of copper-62 benzyl-TETA-human serum albumin as a subtraction agent in conjunction with copper-62 pyruvaldehyde bis(N^4-methylthiosemicarbazone) (^{62}Cu-PTSM) [12] in perfusion studies of brain and myocardium offers another interesting development that needs further investigation (Chapter 13). An advantage of the use of copper-62 is that no cyclotron is needed for doing PET studies. The combination of available radiopharmaceutical and PET imaging devices will make the copper-62 benzyl-TETA human serum albumin blood pool imaging and the copper-62-PTSM perfusion measurements competitive with single photon techniques in the near future.

Acquisition mode

Gated tomographic radionuclide angiography

A new area is the potential to perform gated blood pool imaging using photon emission computed tomography (SPECT). It allows the automated identification of the left ventricular surface in gated tomographic radionuclide ventriculograms, whereby the data can be displayed in three dimensions. Global volumes computed from these surfaces corresponded well with known volumes [13]. Ohtake et al. [14] showed that the regurgitation fraction in patients with mitral and aortic insufficiency could be accurately measured by gated radionuclide angiography SPECT imaging. Although the resolution of gated SPECT is not as high as magnetic resonance imaging, it is relatively inexpensive and provides an accurate picture of ventricular function.

New detection devices

VEST

The recent development of miniature detection devices that can be used for assessing ventricular function on a ambulatory basis seems promising. A device called the cardiac 'VEST' has been developed and is reported to allow ambulatory assessment of left ventricular ejection fraction and ventricular volumes over a period up to 8 hours following the injection of technetium-99m labeled red blood cells. Preliminary clinical results indicate that this method can be used to track changes in ejection fraction that occur during daily activities and during exercise. Kayden et al. showed that, both in patients following thrombolytic therapy [15] and in patients during balloon angioplasty [16], continuous monitoring using the 'VEST' was sensitive for the detection of silent ischemia and provided important prognostic information beyond that obtained by electrocardiographic changes. Despite these encouraging findings, considerable more work is needed to determine the general clinical use of the 'VEST'.

New ways of analysis

Quantitative approaches

At present, increased quantitation provided by the application of computers has been universally recognized as an important advance in nuclear cardiology. The first radionuclide angiography studies consisted of only enddiastolic and endsystolic images but permitted evaluation of left ventricular ejection fraction and regional wall motion using manually drawn outlines of the left ventricle and area-length methods. Subsequent application of computer technology has led to the development of multi-image gated studies, easy storage and retrieval of digitized images, semi- or fully-automated methods for detecting left ventricular edges, and count-based methods for measuring left ventricular ejection fraction and other functional parameters, such as left ventricular ejection and filling rates. Although for most clinical applications qualitative assessment of global and regional wall motion appears to be quite adequate, in some clinical situations more precise quantitative estimates of regional ventricular function are required. A number of approaches have been described including stroke count, ejection fraction, and paradox images [17]. These functional images utilize the enddiastolic and endsystolic frames from a multiframe gated study and display volume changes on a pixel-by-pixel basis. Regional ejection fractions can be determined by dividing the left ventricle in the left anterior oblique view into multiple sectors using radial coordinates drawn from the center of the ventricle. Another approach characterizes regional wall motion by the extent of movement of the endocardial boundary along multiple radial profiles, similar to the quantitative analysis of contrast ventriculograms. Both the regional ejection fraction and radial chord shortening approaches have been validated against contrast ventriculograms in animal models and patients, with generally good results considering the differences in methodology.

Fourier analysis

Fourier analysis of the radionuclide ventriculogram for assessment of regional left ventricular function was first proposed in 1979 [18]. Temporal Fourier analysis involves mathematically fitting sine and cosine waves to the time-activity data for each pixel over the cardiac cycle. Since most of the changes in activity within the heart occur at the fundamental heart frequency, the amplitude of the fundamental frequency is proportional to stroke volume and the phase is related to the time in the cardiac cycle when emptying begins. Phase and amplitude images are formed by mapping the calculated values to the corresponding pixel locations in the image matrix. Impaired regional function is characterized by reduced amplitude and delayed phase over a significant number of contiguous pixels.

Results in a given patient must be compared to previously determined normal limits, since regional function is normally inhomogeneous, with reduced emptying along the septum and in the area of the outflow tract. Brateman et al. [19] in 1991 compared the ability of the conventional cinematic display and Fourier image analysis of radionuclide ventriculograms to detect regional wall motion abnormalities as identified by biplane contrast ventriculograms in patients with suspected coronary artery disease. They found that the Fourier images had higher sensitivity and accuracy for identifying abnormal wall motion and they suggested that Fourier analysis could replace the cine display for routine clinical purposes. However, the radionuclide views were not totally similar to the contrast angiographic views. If these views do not match precisely, different areas of myocardium are represented on the edges of the left ventricular blood pool. Validation studies in animal models employing truly matched views have demonstrated that abnormal wall motion produced by regional myocardial ischemia can generally be assessed equally well by cine display of contrast and radionuclide ventriculograms [20, 21]. When the ischemic region is small (< 4 g), however, the contrast ventriculogram is more sensitive, probably because of the better spatial resolution available with the radiographic technique.

There are many other reasons why it is essential to view the cine display of a radionuclide ventriculogram. The cine display provides information about the quality of the study: the adequacy of blood pool labeling, the positioning of the patient, and the degree of separation of the cardiac chambers. Without an assessment of the quality of the original data, one cannot be confident about the validity of the processed data, including Fourier analysis or regional ejection fraction calculations. Such analyses may provide misleading information about regional function where the right and left ventricles overlap, or where the left atrium is not clearly separated from the left ventricle. The cine display also allows assessment of the position of the heart in the thorax, the size of the cardiac chambers, and the presence of left ventricular hypertrophy, right ventricular or dysfunction. The information contained in the cine display is critical for a full evaluation of cardiac function and cannot be replaced by a few functional Fourier images. Therefore, Fourier analysis cannot replace the cine display, but it can enhance the reading of radionuclide ventriculograms by calling attention to subtle areas of abnormal wall motion that might have been missed by visual analysis alone. Abnormal myocardial segments located inside the left ventricular blood pool image and not represented on the edge of silhouette in a particular view should be detected more readily by Fourier analysis. Quantitation should not be a replacement for visual analysis, but instead should represent an important adjunct.

Combination of function and perfusion

Simultaneous assessment of perfusion and function studies have been proven advantageous in studying patients with cardiac disease (Chapter 26). An explicit advantage of the combination of perfusion and function is that it increases the observer's confidence in interpreting the results especially in the presence of subtle changes. A minimal perfusion abnormality in the presence of a normal wall motion and a normal ejection fraction during exercise is unlikely to be important. The presence of a normal perfusion, normal wall motion and normal exercise ejection fraction will decrease the need for separate resting studies and will therefore diminish cost, inconvenience and radiation burden to the patient. Most experience has been obtained with technetium-99m sestaMIBI using the gating SPECT procedure. The combination of the gated function information with the perfusion information reflects both exercise and rest information [22]. This approach is of considerable interest since changes from resting to peak exercise ejection fraction have been shown to be most powerful prognostic indicators. Gating the technetium-99m sestaMIBI images (this holds similarly for gated rubidium-82 and copper-62 images) provides simultaneous information on function and perfusion. This combined information is an important new step in the evaluation of cardiac function by radionuclide techniques.

Conclusion

Evaluation of cardiac function by radionuclide techniques seems to have reached a phase of consolidation in nuclear cardiology. In many institutions determination of radionuclide ejection fraction and wall motion has become a routine procedure both in research investigations that involve cardiac function studies and in studies that are pertinent to patient management. Nevertheless, there have been new developments and applications for radionuclide imaging of cardiac function. These developments regard the manufacturing of new tracers, the different ways of acquisition and analysis, new imaging devices, and the potential to simultaneously combine perfusion and function studies. These new attainments are an important step forward in the domain of radionuclide assessment of cardiac function.

References

1. Rejali AM, MacIntyre WJ, Friedell HL. Radioisotope method of visualization of blood pools [abstract]. Am J Roentgenol Radium Ther Nucl Med 1958; 79: 129.
2. Zaret BL, Strauss HW, Hurley PJ, Natarajan TK, Pitt B. A noninvasive scintiphotographic method for detecting regional ventricular dysfunction in man. N Engl J Med 1971; 284: 1165–70.
3. Strauss HW, Zaret BL, Hurley PJ, Natarajan TK, Pitt B. A scintophotographic method for measuring left ventricular ejection fraction in man without cardiac catheterization. Am J Cardiol 1971; 28: 575–80.
4. McAfee JG, Stern HS, Fueger GF et al. Tc-99m-labeled human serum albumin for scintillation scanning of the placenta [abstract]. J Nucl Med 1964; 5: 936.
5. Atkins HL, Eckelman WC, Klopper JF, Rickards P. Vascular imaging with 99mTc red blood cells. Radiology 1973; 106: 357–60.
6. Pavel DG, Zimmer M, Patterson VN. In vivo labeling of red blood cells with 99mTc: a new approach to blood-pool visualization. J Nucl Med 1977; 18: 305–8.
7. Nishimura T, Hamada S, Hayshida K, Uekara T, Katabuchi T, Hayashi M. Cardiac blood-pool scintigraphy using technetium-99m in DTPA-HSA: comparison with in vivo technetium-99m-RBC labeling. J Nucl Med 1989; 30: 1713–7.
8. Baillet GY, Mena IG, Kuperus JH, Robertson JM, Freech WJ. Simultaneous technetium-99m-MIBI angiography and myocardial perfusion imaging. J Nucl Med 1989; 30: 38–44.
9. Borges-Neto S, Coleman RE, Jones RH. Comparison of one and two day rest and treadmill cardiolite tests [abstract]. J Nucl Med 1989; 30: 790.
10. Oliver RM, Gray JM, Challenor VF, Fleming JS, Waller DG. Krypton-81m equilibrium radionuclide ventriculography for the assessment of right heart function. Eur J Nucl Med 1990; 16: 89–95.
11. Mathias CJ, Welch MJ, Green MA et al. In vivo comparison of copper blood-pool agents: potential radiopharmaceuticals for use with copper-62. J Nucl Med 1991; 32: 475–80.
12. Mathias CJ, Welch MJ, Raichle ME et al. Evaluation of a potential generator-produced PET tracer for cerebral perfusion imaging: single-pass cerebral extraction measurements and imaging with radiolabeled Cu-PTSM. J Nucl Med 1990; 31: 351–9.
13. Faber TL, Stokely EM, Templeton GH, Akers MS, Parkey RW, Corbett JR. Quantification of three-dimensional left ventricular segmental wall motion and volumes from gated tomographic radionuclide ventriculograms. J Nucl Med 1989; 30: 638–49.
14. Ohtake T, Nishikawa J, Machida K et al. Evaluation of regurgitant fraction in the left ventricle by gated cardiac blood-pool scanning using SPECT. J Nucl Med 1987; 28: 19–24.
15. Kayden DS, Wackers FJTh, Zaret BL. Silent left ventricular dysfunction during routine activity after thrombolytic therapy for acute myocardial infarction. J Am Coll Cardiol 1990; 15: 1500–7.
16. Kayden DS, Remetz MS, Cabin HS et al. Validation of continuous radionuclide left ventricular functioning monitoring in detecting silent myocardial ischemia during balloon angioplasty of the left anterior descending coronary artery. Am J Cardiol 1991; 67: 1339–43.
17. Corbett JR, Jansen DE, Willerson JT. Radionuclide ventriculography. II. Anatomic and physiologic aspects. Am J Physiol Imaging 1987; 2: 85–104.
18. Adam WE, Tarkowska A, Bitter F, Stauch M, Geffers H. Equilibrium (gated) radionuclide ventriculography. Cardiovasc Radiol 1979; 2: 161–73.
19. Brateman L, Buckley K, Keim SG, Wargovich TJ, Williams CM. Left ventricular regional

wall motion assessment by radionuclide ventriculography: a comparison of cine display with Fourier analysis. J Nucl Med 1991; 32: 777–82.

20. Kronenberg MW, Born ML, Smith CW et al. Comparison of radionuclide and contrast ventriculography for detection and quantitation of regions of myocardial ischemia in dogs. J Clin Invest 1981; 67: 1370–82.

21. Doss JK, Hillis LD, Curry G et al. A new model for the assessment of regional ventricular wall motion. Radiology 1982; 143: 763–70.

22. Villanueva-Meyer J, Mena I, Narahara KA. Simultaneous assessment of left ventricular wall motion and myocardial perfusion with technetium-99m-methoxy isobutyl isonitrile at stress and rest in patients with angina: comparison with thallium-201 SPECT. J Nucl Med 1990; 31: 457–63.

25. Krypton-81m equilibrium radionuclide ventriculography for the assessment of right ventricular function

RICHARD M. OLIVER

Introduction

The study of right ventricular function is hampered by the complex and variable anatomical configuration of the right ventricle. Radionuclide imaging techniques permit the study of right ventricular function without assumptions concerning the exact right ventricular configuration, and do not involve measurement of right ventricular dimensions. The assessment of right ventricular function is, however, dependent upon the technique used, and the ability to reliably identify and separate right heart structures is crucial to the accurate calculation of right ventricular ejection fraction (RVEF).

Krypton-81m, an inert gas radionuclide with ultra-short half-life, is ideally suited to right heart imaging. This chapter describes how krypton-81m equilibrium ventriculography has been applied to the detailed evaluation of right ventricular function.

Technical aspects of krypton-81m production

The short half-life of krypton-81m means it must be continuously eluted from a rubidium-81 radionuclide generator. The rubidium-81 parent is prepared by alpha bombardment of bromine-79 in a cyclotron. Rubidium-81 decays (half-life 4.7 hours) by electron capture and positron emission to the krypton-81m daughter. Rubidium-81 is adsorbed in a macroporous cation exchange column from which krypton-81m can be eluted using 5% dextrose for intravenous infusion. Krypton-81m decays by isomeric transition to stable krypton-81m

341

Ernst E. van der Wall et al. (eds), What's new in cardiac imaging?, 341–351.
© *1992 Kluwer Academic Publishers. Printed in the Netherlands.*

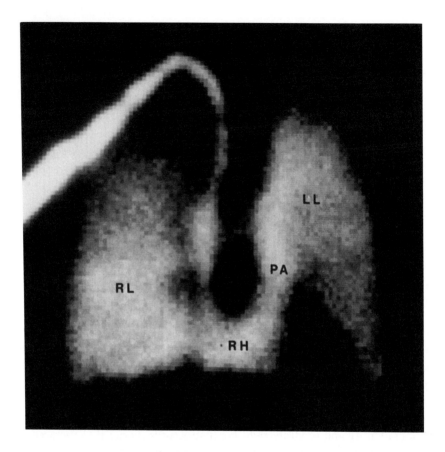

Figure 1. Distribution of krypton-81m when given by peripheral intravenous infusion via a right forearm vein. (LL = left lung; PA = pulmonary artery; RH = right heart; RL = right lung).

(half-life 13 seconds), emitting 65% unconverted 190 keV gamma photons that allow excellent imaging with standard gamma camera equipment available in most nuclear medicine departments.

Distribution of krypton-81m following infusion

Krypton-81m in solution is infused intravenously and after passage through the right heart, enters the pulmonary circulation where, because of its insolubility, if diffuses across the alveolar membrane and is exhaled. The first-pass elimination in the lungs combined with its ultra-short half-life, ensures that negligible radionuclide activity reaches the left heart. This enables the right heart to be imaged in isolation and allows imaging projection to be optimized without interference from left heart structures. The distribution of krypton-81m when given by intravenous infusion via a right forearm vein is illustrated in Figure 1.

The half-life of krypton-81m and its elimination during first-pass through the pulmonary circulation ensures that the radiation burden to the patient during imaging is low (Appendix).

**Krypton-81m ventriculographic imaging of the right heart–
image acquisition and analysis**

Krypton-81m ventriculography has often been regarded as a first-pass technique for imaging the right heart and some investigators have used short duration bolus infusions [1, 2]. During continuous infusion of krypton-81m, the technique is better described as an equilibrium technique comparable to technetium-99m blood-pool ventriculography used to image the left ventricle. All radionuclide techniques are dependent upon uniform mixing of infused activity within the heart. This assumption may not be entirely justified following a short duration radionuclide bolus for first-pass studies. The mixing of krypton-81m within the right heart following continuous peripheral intravenous infusion has been shown to be uniform and almost instantaneous [3].

Most investigators have used similar techniques for image acquisition. Krypton-81m is continuously eluted in 5% dextrose from an 800–1200 MBq rubidium-81 generator. The eluate is passed through a short length of fine bore tubing before infusion into a medial right antecubital fossa vein. An infusion rate of 10 ml/min and a small dead-space within the infusion system minimises krypton-81m decay during passage to the heart. Images are usually acquired as ECG-gated frames and imaging performed over 8–15 minutes depending upon the activity of the generator.

Following intravenous infusion of krypton-81m, there is substantial accumulation of radionuclide activity within the lungs (Figure 1). Although the right anterior oblique imaging projection should produce optimal separation of right heart structures, some investigators have used the anterior projection to reduce the overlay of right heart on lung [1, 4]. In addition, the anterior imaging projection allows the gamma camera to be positioned closer to the chest wall to improve radionuclide count acquisition. A preliminary description of the comparison of the right anterior oblique and anterior imaging projections suggested that calculated RVEF was similar [5]. However, the author has shown that the contribution of radionuclide counts arising from lung is similar in the two projections and that the anterior imaging projection may lead to problems with image analysis as result of superimposition of right

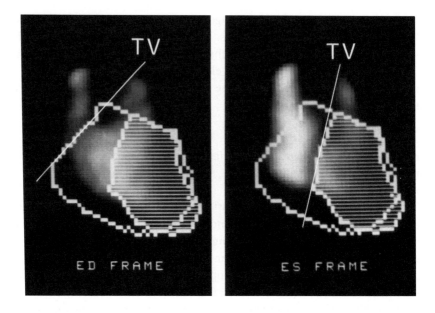

Figure 2. End-diastolic (ED) and end-systolic (ES) frames from a krypton-81m equilibrium ventriculographic study in the right anterior oblique projection following 'anatomical' lung subtraction with both ED and ES regions of interest superimposed to demonstrate the substantial movement of the tricuspid valve (TV) plane during cardiac systole.

atrium and right ventricle [6]. It is now generally agreed that a 20–30° right anterior oblique imaging projection results in optimal spatial separation of right heart structures during image acquisition.

Many different techniques for the analysis of krypton-81m ventriculographic images have been described and a detailed discussion of their advantages and limitations is beyond the scope of this chapter. However, a few important aspects of image analysis will be discussed.

Early methodology involved the definition of a single fixed region of interest defined over the right ventricle. A single region of interest technique has been shown to produce significantly lower values for RVEF than when separate end-diastolic and end-systolic regions of interest are used [7]. This is due to the substantial movement of the tricuspid valve plane during the cardiac cycle [5, 8, 9]. It is now accepted that separate end-diastolic and end-systolic regions of interest must be defined over the right ventricle to take account of tricuspid valve plane movement during cardiac systole (Figure 2).

The substantial accumulation of radionuclide activity within lung means that it is generally agreed that background correction is essential during image analysis [3, 7]. Conventional background correction analytical techniques employ an empirically defined region of interest around the septum and free wall of the right ventricle to approximate the contribution of radionuclide activity arising from lung to the right ventricular regions of interest. This contribution may be quite substantial and may be as high as 25% [6]. In an attempt to more accurately correct for the scatter of lung activity to right ventricular regions of interest, 'anatomical' lung subtraction using technetium-99m lung perfusion scintigraphy has been described [3, 6, 9]. A static technetium-99m perfusion lung image is used to subtract lung activity from each ECG-gated frame during analysis. This technique of image analysis results in excellent definition of right heart structures and enhances the accurate identification of tricuspid and pulmonary valve planes (Plate 25.1). Using the technetium-99m lung image, at least 30% of counts are subtracted from the right ventricular regions of interest during image processing. This accounts for the observation that RVEF derived using 'anatomical' lung subtraction is greater than that derived using a background region of interest technique [6]. 'Anatomical' lung subtraction is difficult to apply to studies during dynamic exercise since movement artifact precludes accurate lung subtraction. Studies during exercise are usually analyzed using a conventional background correction technique.

Most investigators have shown a good correlation between RVEF derived using krypton-81m equilibrium ventriculography and that derived using a first-pass radionuclide technique [7, 9, 10]. However, the formal validation of krypton-81m ventriculographic imaging has been hampered by the lack of an accepted 'gold standard' with which to evaluate right ventricular function. An acceptable correlation has been demonstrated between RVEF derived using krypton-81m ventriculography and that derived using right ventricular contrast cineangiography [8].

Indices of systolic ejection and diastolic filling for the right ventricle

The measurement of ejection fraction is a useful index of global ventricular function but additional information about ventricular function may be obtained by deriving indices of systolic ejection and diastolic filling.

Preliminary observations by Sugrue et al. [10] using krypton-81m equilibrium ventriculography suggested that indices of systolic ejection for the right ventricle could be defined. A fixed region of interest and conventional background correction analytical technique was employed. The author has used krypton-81m equilibrium ventriculography images acquired at a high frame rate (32 frames/cardiac cycle) and analysis following 'anatomical' lung subtraction to generate a high resolution time-activity curve for the right ventricle

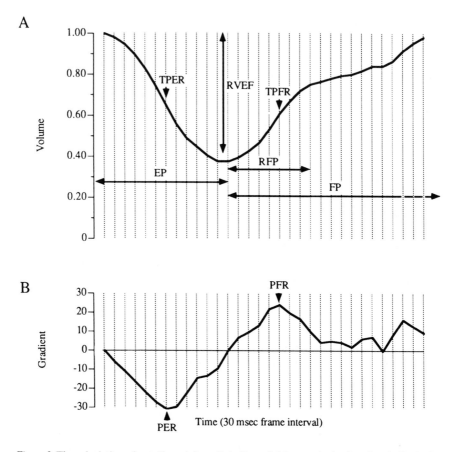

Figure 3. The calculation of systolic and diastolic indices of right ventricular function derived using krypton-81m equilibrium ventriculography. (A) Smoothed time-activity curve (volume curve) for the right ventricle and (B) gradient curve derived from the smoothed time-activity curve. (EP = ejection period; FP = filling period; PER = peak ejection rate; PFR = peak filling rate; RFP = rapid filling period; RVEF = right ventricular ejection fraction; TPER = time to peak ejection rate; TPFR = time to peak filling rate).

(unpublished methodology). The tricuspid valve plane displacement during cardiac systole requires the definition of a separate right ventricular region of interest on each frame during the cardiac cycle. The identification of the tricuspid valve plane on each frame is improved by lung subtraction and facilitates the creation of accurate right ventricular regions of interest crucial to the generation of a 'physiological' time-activity curve from which indices of sytolic ejection and diastolic filling can be derived (Figure 3).

At present, the application of the technique is limited to resting studies since the activity of the rubidium generator available currently dictates a minimum imaging time of 10 minutes to acquire adequate counts per frame for reliable definition of separate right ventricular regions of interest. Sustained exercise over this duration of imaging, even at a submaximal level, inevitably introduces some movement artifact resulting in technical problems with image analysis.

Using krypton-81m equilibrium ventriculography, values for resting right ventricular systolic and diastolic indices (Table 1) are comparable to those previously defined for the left ventricle in normal subjects (author's unpublished data).

Estimation of right ventricular volumes

Radionuclide techniques are potentially useful for the measurement of cardiac volumes since, at steady-state, externally detected radionuclide counts are directly proportional to volume. Technetium-99m blood-pool ventriculography has been applied to the estimation of volumes for the left ventricle but, because of difficulty in obtaining spatial separation of right heart structures using this technique, right ventricular volumes cannot readily be derived.

A technique for measuring right ventricular volumes using krypton-81m equilibrium ventriculography has been described [11]. The preliminary validation of the technique showed a good correlation between right ventricular stroke volume estimated by krypton-81m equilibrium ventriculography and that derived using the thermodilution technique during right heart catheterization. The technique was capable of demonstrating the anticipated changes

Table 1. Systolic ejection and diastolic filling indices for the right ventricle derived using krypton-81m gated equilibrium ventriculography in 23 normal subjects (age 20–63 years).

		Mean ± SD	Range
Systolic ejection indices:			
RVEF[a]		0.57 ± 0.05	0.48–0.64
PER	(EDV/sec)	2.9 ± 0.4	2.1–3.9
TPER	(msec)	200 ± 40	120–300
EP	(msec)	363 ± 33	300–450
Diastolic filling indices:			
FP	(msec)	541 ± 131	347–815
RFP	(msec)	235 ± 37	150–300
PFR	(EDV/sec)	2.5 ± 0.6	1.7–3.5
TPFR	(msec)	163 ± 38	80–240

[a] For explanation of abbreviations, see Figure 3.

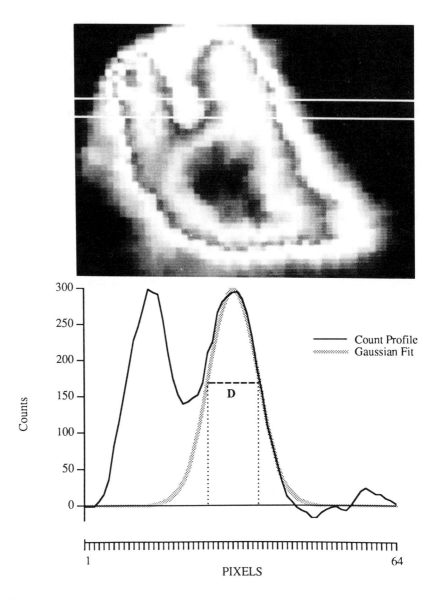

Figure 4. The estimation of right ventricular volumes from krypton-81m equilibrium ventriculo-graphic imaging using an in-vivo count to volume calibration technique calculated using an internal reference region of interest in the right ventricular outflow tract at the level of the pulmonary valve plane on the end-diastolic frame. The Gaussian fit to the count profile across the right ventricular outflow tract is shown and the diameter of the reference region of interest (D) is computed at 61% of the maximum Gaussian fit.

in right ventricular volumes during maneuvres which alter right ventricular loading.

The calculation of right ventricular volumes from krypton-81m equilibrium ventriculographic images following 'anatomical' lung subtraction involves the application of an in-vivo count to volume calibration factor calculated using an internal reference region of interest in the right ventricular outflow tract [11, 12]. The internal region of interest delineated at the level of the pulmonary valve approximates to a right-angle cylinder in three dimensions, the diameter of which is computed at 61% of the maximum Gaussian fit to the count profile across the right ventricular outflow tract (Figure 4). The volume represented by this internal region of interest is derived from the expression: $\pi \times (D/2)^2 \times H$, where D is the diameter of the internal region of interest and H is the height of the internal region of interest. Counts derived from the internal region of interest are calculated from the area under the Gaussian curve. Counts within the right ventricular region of interest at end-diastole and end-systole are used to derive right ventricular end-diastolic volume and stroke volume.

Difficulties with imaging the right ventricle mean there is no universally accepted technique for right ventricular volume estimation and few references to normal values. However, right ventricular volumes estimated using krypton-81m equilibrium ventriculography are comparable to those derived from contrast cineangiography and magnetic resonance imaging [12].

Conclusions

Right heart krypton-81m equilibrium ventriculography is ideally suited to the non-invasive evaluation of right ventricular function and overcomes many of the technical limitations of other radionuclide imaging techniques. In addition to the measurement of RVEF, a more detailed evaluation of ventricular function may be obtained by using the technique to derive specific indices of systolic ejection and diastolic filling for the right ventricle. The imaging technique is also uniquely suited to the noninvasive determination of right ventricular volumes.

Krypton-81m equilibrium ventriculography offers the potential for repeatable noninvasive evaluation of right ventricular function. Detailed information may be derived concerning the response of the right ventricle to changes in loading conditions, particularly following therapeutic intervention.

Appendix: radiation dosimetry for krypton-81m ventriculography

Problems with quantification of absorbed radiation dose to the patient following intravenous infusion of krypton-81m mean that few authors have quoted formal radiation dosimetry [2, 10]. The author has made dosimetry measurements based on a krypton-81m infusion generator of nominal activity 1000 MBq eluted at 10 ml/minute. Attenuation corrected gamma camera count rates from three source organs (vein contents between injection site and central veins, the heart and the lungs) were used. The application of MIRD principles showed the effective dose equivalent for a 10 minute intravenous infusion of krypton-81m to be 0.365 mSv. The effective dose equivalent due to the principal radionuclide impurity, rubidium-81, is small and can be discounted (0.004 mSv) (unpublished data).

References

1. Knapp WH, Helus F, Lambrecht RM, Elfner R, Gasper H, Vollhaber HH. Kr-81m for determination of right ventricular ejection fraction (RVEF). Eur J Nucl Med 1980; 5: 487–92.
2. Wong DF, Natarajan TK, Summer W et al. Right ventricular ejection fraction measured by first-pass intravenous krypton-81m: reproducibility and comparison with technetium-99m. Am J Cardiol 1985; 56: 776–80.
3. Ham HR, Franken PR, Georges B, Delcourt E, Guillaume M, Piepsz A. Evaluation of the accuracy of steady-state krypton-81m method for calculating right ventricular ejection fraction. J Nucl Med 1986; 27: 593–601.
4. Horn M, Witztum K, Neveu C, Perkins G, Walsh B. Krypton-81m imaging of the right ventricle. J Nucl Med 1985; 26: 33–6.
5. Ham HR, Piepsz A, Vandevivere J, Guillaume M, Goethals P, Lenaers A. The evaluation of right ventricular performance using krypton-81m. Clin Nucl Med 1983; 8: 257–60.
6. Oliver RM, Gray JM, Challenor VF, Fleming JS, Waller DG. Krypton-81m equilibrium radionuclide ventriculography for the assessment of right heart function. Eur J Nucl Med 1990; 16: 89–95.
7. Caplin JL, Flatman WD, Dymond DS. Gated right ventricular studies using krypton-81m: comparison with first-pass studies using gold-195m. J Nucl Med 1986; 27: 602–8.
8. Nienaber CA, Spielmann RP, Wasmus G, Mathey DG, Montz R, Bleifeld WH. Clinical use of ultrashort-lived radionuclide krypton-81m for noninvasive analysis of right ventricular performance in normal subjects and patients with right ventricular dysfunction. J Am Coll Cardiol 1985; 5: 687–98.
9. Franken PR, Delcourt E, Ham HR. Right ventricular ejection fraction: comparison of technetium-99m first pass technique and ECG-gated steady state krypton-81m angiocardiography. Eur J Nucl Med 1986; 12: 365–8.
10. Sugrue DD, Kamal S, Deanfield JE et al. Assessment of right ventricular function and anatomy using peripheral vein infusion of krypton-81m. Br J Radiol 1983; 56: 657–63.
11. Franken PR, Mols P, Delcourt E, Dobbeleir A, Georges B, Ham HR. Measurement of right

ventricular volumes from ECG-gated steady-state krypton-81m angiocardiography. Nucl Med Commun 1987; 8: 365–73.
12. Oliver RM, Peacock AJ, Challenor VF, Fleming JS, Waller DG. The effect of acute hypoxia on right ventricular function in healthy adults. Int J Cardiol 1991; 31: 235–41.

26. Simultaneous assessment of myocardial function and perfusion

ABDULMASSIH S. ISKANDRIAN

Introduction

The radionuclide techniques that may be used to assess function are listed in Table 1 [1–3]. Assessment of both myocardial function and perfusion in the past was done using two different radionuclides (for example, thallium-201 and technetium-99m pertechnetate) and two separate exercise studies [1, 4–13]. For a short period of time, thallium-201 and aurium-195m were simultaneously used for perfusion/function assessment but aurium-195m is no longer available for clinical use [4, 14]. Thallium-201 is injected 20 seconds before peak exercise and then, at peak exercise, radionuclide ventriculography is obtained with aurium-195m. The short half-life of aurium-195m (30.5 seconds) makes simultaneous dual isotope imaging possible and substantially reduces the radiation exposure from the isotope angiography. Narahara and associates [4] studied 24 subjects with coronary artery disease and 20 healthy volunteers, using such a dual technique. They were able to obtain high-quality first-pass angiograms in all patients. The exercise thallium images provided a sensitivity of 83% and a specificity of 95% suggesting that its diagnostic accuracy was not altered by simultaneous dual isotope imaging. The dual isotope technique permits simultaneous analysis of regional and global ventricular function in relation with regional thallium redistribution. Other short-lived isotopes, though available, have not received widespread interest or require specially designed gamma cameras such as tantalum-178. The methods available to assess both perfusion and function are summarized in table 2.

Lessons from the past: The primary reason for doing both perfusion and function studies was to compare the sensitivity and specificity of both tech-

Ernst E. van der Wall et al. (eds), What's new in cardiac imaging?, 353–365.
© *1992 Kluwer Academic Publishers. Printed in the Netherlands.*

niques in diagnosing coronary artery disease and, thus, to determine which of the two tests is preferred. Many of these studies were done on highly selected groups of patients and, in general, it was found that both of these tests (perfusion and function) provided a comparable degree of accuracy in the diagnosis of coronary artery disease. Caldwell and co-workers [6] studied 11 healthy persons and 41 patients with coronary artery disease and found that the sensitivity of radionuclide ventriculography was higher and the specificity lower than those of exercise thallium imaging. Both tests combined identified all patients with coronary artery disease.

In other studies by Eklayam [1] and Jungo [8] and their associates, the sensitivity and specificity of exercise thallium imaging and radionuclide angiography were found to be identical. Either test was more sensitive than exercise ECG. In 39 patients with coronary artery disease, Johnstone and colleagues [7] found that the sensitivity of exercise thallium imaging was 62%, while that of radionuclide ventriculography was 85%. Both test results were normal in only three patients with one-vessel disease.

Similarly, Uhl and colleagues [11] studied 32 asymptomatic Air Force personnel in whom subsequent catheterization showed coronary artery disease in 13; they found that both exercise thallium and radionuclide ventriculography

Table 1. Assessment of left ventricular function by radionuclide angiography.

I.   Techniques
  1.   First-pass: gated and ungated
  2.   Gated equilibrium
  3.   Non imaging devices: nuclear probe; ambulatory nuclear monitor (vest); miniature nuclear probe system (Cardioscint)

II.   Types of studies
  1.   Rest
  2.   Exercise: Bike or treatmill; supine or upright
  3.   Pharmacologic stressors
  4.   Pacing

III. Radionuclides used
  1.   Tc-99m pertechnetate
  2.   Short lived agents: Ir-191m; krypton-81; aurium-195m; tantalum-178

IV. Types of measurements
  1.   Ejection fraction
  2.   Wall motion
  3.   Volumes: EDV, ESV, SV, CO
  4.   Filling and emptying rates and times: SER, PFR, time to PFR

EDV: end-diastolic volume; ESV: end-systolic volume; SV: stroke volume; CO: cardiac output; SER: systolic ejection rate; PFR: peak filling rate.

were abnormal in all patients with coronary artery disease but in none of the patients without coronary artery disease. Kirshenbaum and associates [9] evaluated the presence and nature of perfusion defects on thallium scintigraphy in relation to the changes in exercise ejection fraction. They found that patients with reversible thallium defects had a decrease in ejection fraction during exercise, whereas those with fixed defects had no change in ejection fraction. In patients with both fixed and reversible defects, the rsponse of ejection fraction was variable. Our results correlating the presence or absence of reversible defects and the change in ejection fraction during exercise in patients with normal or abnormal left ventricular function at rest also suggest that patients with reversible perfusion defects have abnormal ejection fraction response to exercise [1]. Osbakken and colleagues [5] performed exercise thallium imaging and gated equilibrium blood pool scintigraphy in 120 patients with chest pain syndrome. Based on coronary arteriography, 86 had coronary disease and 34 did not. The results indicate that the sensitivity and specificity of both techniques were comparable. Since both exercise scintigraphy and radionuclide ventriculography are extremely sensitive, the combination of both tests is expected to identify all patients with coronary artery disease.

The selected nature of patients is reflected by specificity results in excess of 90% with radionuclide angiography. It was also appreciated that a host of other cardiac and noncardiac diseases can impair left ventricular performance during exercise though such patients may have a normal perfusion pattern.

Table 2. Types of imaging techniques to assess myocardial perfusion and function

---

1.* Non-simultaneous
    a. Thallium-201: perfusion
    b. Tc-99m pertechnetate: first pass or MUGA

2.* Simultaneous
    a. SestaMIBI: perfusion and first pass RNA
    b. SestaMIBI: gated perfusion
    c. Teboroxime: perfusion and first pass RNA

3.* Simultaneous nuclear + 2DE
    a. Thallium-201 + 2DE
    b. SestaMIBI + 2DE
    c. Teboroxime + 2DE

4. Simultaneous: investigational
    a. Thallium + contrast left ventriculography
    b. SestaMIBI + contrast left ventriculography

---

*Rest, exercise, dipyridamole, adenosine. 2DE: two dimensional echocardiography. RNA: radionuclide angiography.

These disorders are characterized by impairment of myocardial contractility or inappropriate changes in preload or afterload which are the two other determinants of myocardial performance [1]. It is also clear that post-referral bias is an importaant factor that affects specificity, but obviously this bias is applicable for both perfusion and function studies. In fact, it is the recognition that exercise ejection fraction may be abnormal in a number of noncoronary artery disease patients that resulted in a noticeable decline in the interest and use of radionuclide angiography. The previous methods were also plagued by two problems. First, these tests required two separate exercise studies, and second, the mode of exercise was often different. For example, the perfusion studies were done on the treadmill while the function studies were done on the bicycle in either supine, semi-erect, or erect position.

Important observations from these studies are:

1. Most patients with coronary artery disease with reversible thallium abnormalities have a decrease in left ventricular ejection fraction with exercise. This was true in patients with normal as well as those with abnormal resting left ventricular ejection fraction.

2. There is a fair correlation between the extent of reversible perfusion abnormality and the degree of change in ejection fraction response to exercise.

3. There is a segmental agreement between the presence of regional perfusion abnormality and corresponding regional wall motion abnormality.

4. Radionuclide techniques provide information on exercise right ventricular performance which could not so easily be evaluated by perfusion imaging.

5. Radionuclide studies made it possible to evaluate serial changes in regional and global left ventricular performance during exercise and the recovery period. Such serial changes are not possible with perfusion studies.

6. Localization of coronary artery disease is better accomplished with perfusion than function studies because multiple views are examined while only one projection is available with the function studies except, of course, in studies that utilize biplane radionuclide angiography or two separate function studies in different projections but these studies are tedious and have not received wide acceptance. Generally, there is a fair correlation between the extent of coronary artery disease and the absolute left ventricular exercise ejection fraction; the more extensive the disease the lower the ejection fraction.

7. Assessment of the ejection fraction is less operator-dependent and is quantitative and reproducible while perfusion imaging is highly dependent on the expertise of the observer although, more recently, with the use of tomographic (SPECT) imaging computer-derived quantitative assessment is also available.

8. The level of exercise affects both test results and, therefore, should be considered when interpreting these results [1, 15].
9. Perfusion abnormalities are rather specific markers for coronary artery disease while the change in ejection fraction from rest to exercise as discussed earlier is affected by myocardial contractility, preload and afterload. For example, roughly 50% of patients with essential hypertension have abnormal ejection fraction response to exercise even though the coronary angiograms in these patients are normal and the perfusion pattern is normal.
10. In rare situations such as patients with isolated left main disease, it is conceivable that the perfusion pattern may be normal while the function study is abnormal. This, in fact, is distinctly unusual because most patients with left main disease have associated coronary artery disease and diffuse ischemia as a cause for false negative thallium scans is very rare.

When the results of radionuclide angiographic studies were examined for risk assessment, a clear picture emerged about the power and usefulness of these data. From our experience and those by others, notably by the Duke investigators, the following conclusions can be drawn:

1. Exercise radionuclide variables are more important than the rest variables [1, 16–19].
2. By multivariate analysis, the exercise left ventricular ejection fraction appears to be the strongest predictor of future events defined as cardiac death, nonfatal acute myocardial infarction, or all cause mortality.
3. The radionuclide data provide information that are just as important, if not more important, than those obtained by coronary angiography. Further, the combined catheterization and radionuclide data are even stronger predictors of future events than either alone. It is clear, for example, from these data that patients with an exercise ejection fraction of 50% or greater have a low event rate at follow-up for as long as seven years. On the other hand, in patients with exercise ejection fraction below 50%, the risk increases proportionately to the absolute level of exercise ejection fraction. Patients with exercise ejection fraction of less than 30% are at higher risk than those with ejection fraction of 30–50%. These studies were obtained using bicycle exercise with either a multicrystal camera using the first pass technique or with a single crystal camera using the gated equilibrium technique. Our experience and that of Duke has been with the first pass technique with the multicrystal camera. The newer version of the multicrystal camera appears to be less sturdy during exercise studies but an algorithm has been developed for motion artifact correction.

Having emphasized the prognostic value of radionuclide angiography, we and others have also shown the usefulness of thallium data in risk assessment.

Depending on patient selection and definition of endpoints, various thallium descriptors are prognostically important (Table 3) [20–25]. The extent thallium abnormality is the most important predictor of cardiac events; this parameter is comparable to the exercise ejection fraction which is a measure of the resting ejection fraction and the change in ejection fraction from rest to exercise. It is possible that the change in ejection fraction and the presence of reversible thallium defects are important markers of subsequent nonfatal acute myocardial infarction as they denote the presence of jeopardized myocardium. However, the exercise ejection fraction or size of perfusion defect is a marker of future cardiac mortality. These issues have been recently discussed elsewhere [25].

Current options: The availability of the newer technetium labeled myocardial imaging agents (sestaMIBI and teboroxime) allows for simultaneous assessment of perfusion and function using the same agents in a single exercise study. Either agent can be injected as a bolus and a first pass radionuclide angiogram is obtained and then the perfusion imaging is done using either planar or SPECT imaging. These studies can be done at rest, upright bicycle exercise, upright treadmill exercise, or during pharmacologic testing such as dipyridamole or adenosine infusions. Both the multicrystal camera and the newer digital single crystal cameras with high counting efficiency have been used (Plates 26.1 and 26.2) [26–37]. The specific features of these two agents are discussed elsewhere by Drs Rigo, De Swart and Hendel.

Using sestaMIBI it has been found that:
1. Left ventricular ejection fraction at rest and exercise is reproducible using either the one-day or two-day protocol.
2. There is a good correlation between the left ventricular ejection fraction and the right ventricular ejection fraction compared to similar measurement obtained with technetium-99m pertechnetate; even with single crystal camera, a correlation of 0.93 for left ventricular ejection fraction and 0.92 for right ventricular ejection fraction has been found in patients with coronary artery disease [33].
3. There is a linear and inverse correlation between ejection fraction at rest

Table 3. Table 3. The thallium predictors of cardiac events.

1. Presence of redistribution (reversible defects)
2. The extent of reversible abnormality
3. The extent of the total perfusion deficit (reversible and fixed defect)
4. Increased lung thallium uptake
5. Number of vascular territories with abnormal thallium uptake
6. Left ventricular dilatation during exercise

and exercise with the extent of the perfusion abnormality [32]. The perfusion abnormality is determined from SPECT images using the polar maps. There also appears to be a correlation between the perfusion abnormality and the regional wall motion abnormality obtained and between the (first pass) radionuclide wall motion and contrast angiographic wall motion. Nevertheless, at any given level of ejection fraction, a considerable variability in the size of the perfusion abnormality is apparent. The reason or reasons for such a variability is not clear but several issues need to be considered.

(a) SPECT imaging may result in inaccuracy in measuring the size of th perfusion abnormality. The use of 180° tomography with no attenuation correction may introduce a margin of error in such measurement [38]. In general, however, this measurement appears reproducible and agrees with independent methods to measure infarct size and muscle mass in man and animal.

(b) The ejection fraction measurement is inaccurate especially during exercise because of motion artifact. This also is unlikely as these measurements have been well validated and were reproducible.

(c) The differences in the time at which these images are obtained may be important. For example, the ejection fraction is obtained at peak exercise while the SPECT images are obtained one to two hours later. Although sestaMIBI shows negligible redistribution others have found that some redistribution may occur and may account for a decrease in the perfusion size in some of these studies [30, 36].

(d) The degree of wall motion may differ from perfusion. For example, hyperkinesis may compensate for regions with hypokinesis. Yet the normal and hyperkinetic areas have similar perfusion pattern. A difference in the degree of hypo perfusion and hypo function in abnormal areas may also exists.

An advantage of the combination of the perfusion/function studies that may not be apparent is that it increases the observer's confidence in interpreting the results, especially in the presence of subtle changes. For example, a subtle perfusion abnormality in the presence of a normal wall motion and a normal ejection fraction during exercise is unlikely to be important. It may also be that the presence of the normal perfusion, normal wall motion and normal exercise ejection fraction will decrease the need for separate rest studies and, therefore, decrease the cost, inconvenience, and radiation burden to the patient, and improve the throughput of the laboratory.

Gated perfusion sestaMIBI studies

Gating of the images can be done with planar and SPECT imaging; it provides regional information on wall motion and thickening. The electrocardiogram is used as the physiological marker for gating. In the previous experience, gated studies were done to improve the image quality by decreasing the blurring due to cardiac action. In fact the gated diastolic thallium images were of better quality than conventional images, however, the diagnostic accuracy did not change and, therefore, this technique did not receive wide acceptance. Gating the sestaMIBI images is done for a different purpose. It is assumed that the perfusion image reflects the events at peak exercise, however, since imaging is done 30 to 60 minutes later, the gated information reflects resting rather than exercise information as ischemia has subsided. The combination of the gated information with the perfusion information, in essence, reflects exercise plus rest information. The presence of a perfusion abnormality during exercise in a region that shows normal wall thickening and normal wall motion is likely to indicate that the perfusion abnormality is reversible and the muscle in that region is viable. On the other hand, a perfusion abnormality associated with akinesia and no thickening is likely to indicate a fixed abnormality and non-viable myocardium. There are computer programs that depict the regional thickening and wall motion in a manner similar to circumferential profile analysis used to depict extent and severity of the perfusion abnormality. Normal profiles have been developed against which the patient profiles can be compared. One concern using this type of analysis is that areas with severe perfusion defects may have low count statistics and, therefore, precise assessment of thickening and wall motion may not be accurate. Therefore, it is still unclear whether these studies will replace or supplement the information obtained from separate rest studies. Nevertheless, the concept that gating the images can provide simultaneously function information to that obtained from the perfusion information is indeed intriguing. Some observers have even measured the ejection fraction of the left ventricle from these gated images and have found that it correlates fairly well with those obtained with echocardiography. Nevertheless, I believe the method of first pass radionuclide angiography is the preferred method for more precise assessment of left ventricular ejection fraction.

Teboroxime perfusion function studies

These studies may be done on bicycle or treadmill. A multicrystal camera was used for both the perfusion and function imaging (using different collimators).

It is feasible to do these studies in a manner similar to sestaMIBI studies where the perfusion images are obtained with SPECT (using either a single headed or triple headed gamma camera) and the function studies are obtained with either a single crystal or a multicrystal camera [37]. However, the experience with this agent has not been as extensive as that with sestaMIBI in this regard.

Simultaneous perfusion and two-dimensional echocardiographic assessment

Several groups have reported that echocardiographic assessment of left ventricular function including ejection fraction, volume and wall motion is feasible during exercise and pharmacologic testing such as adenosine and dipyridamole infusion [38, 39]. It is, therefore, possible to combine the perfusion studies with either thallium, sestaMIBI, or teboroxime with a nonnuclear technique using two-dimension echocardiography to assess the ventricular function. It is also possible to combine Doppler studies to assess left ventricular diastolic function. With this approach, we have found that during adenosine thallium imaging, most areas of perfusion abnormalities are associated with hyperkinesis rather hypokinesis and, in fact, regional wall motion abnormalities were very unusual during adenosine infusion. Other groups have reported different results showing higher incidence of wall motion abnormalities with either adenosine, dipyridamole, or during exercise [40]. In general, pharmacologic testing provides better two-dimensional echocardiographic images than exercise because there is less patient motion. The reason for these disparities between our results and many other groups, especially those reported by echocardiographers is not clear but may be related to personal biases, preconceived notions, lack of quantitative assessment of wall motion, expertise, and patient selection.

To better understand these controversies, we have recently obtained contrast left ventriculograms in the catheterization laboratory in conjunction with simultaneous adenosine thallium scans and have found results similar to our echocardiographic studies. Adenosine produces hyperkinesis with hyperdynamic left ventricular function even though these regions have extensive perfusion abnormalities. Wall motion abnormality is rare, and when present is localized and far smaller than corresponding perfusion abnormality. This technique is another example of simultaneous perfusion and function assessment albeit being for investigational purposes. Therefore, in my experience, I think perfusion abnormalities are far more frequent during pharmacologic testing than corresponding wall motion abnormalities no matter how these wall motion abnormalities are examined, i.e. radionuclide angiography, two-dimensional echocardiography, or contrast left ventriculography.

Conclusion

Which patients need both simultaneous perfusion and function studies? Patients with suspected coronary artery disease who have other associated diseases that may affect left ventricular performance such as hypertension and valvular heart disease; patients with stable coronary artery disease for risk stratification; patients with borderline isolated left main disease; patients with previously equivocal perfusion studies; resting studies after acute myocardial infarction to assess infarct size and biventricular function [41]; patients after coronary artery bypass grafting to assess perioperative infarction and biventricular function and possibly also to assess physiological principles such as coronary artery steal during coronary vasodilatation. The development of definite wall motion abnormality although unusual is probably a good marker of coronary artery steal.

Acknowledgement

The author would like to thank Susan Kelchner for her expert secretarial assistance in the preparation of this manuscript.

References

1. Iskandrian AS. Thallium-201 myocardial imaging and radionuclide ventriculography. In: Iskandrian AS, editor. Nuclear cardiac imaging: principles and applications. Philadelphia: F.A. Davis, 1986: 81–122.
2. Broadhurst P, Cashman P, Crawley J, Raftery E, Lahiri A. Clinical validation of a miniature nuclear probe system for continuous on-line monitoring of cardiac function and ST-segment. J Nucl Med 1991; 32: 37–43.
3. Ishibashi M, Tamaki N, Yasuda T, Taki J, Strauss HW. Assessment of ventricular function with an ambulatory left ventricular function monitor. Circulation 1991; 83 (4 Suppl): II 166–72.
4. Narahara KA, Mena I, Maublant JC, Brizendine M, Criley JM. Simultaneous maximal exercise radionuclide angiography and thallium stress perfusion imaging. Am J Cardiol 1984; 53: 812–7.
5. Osbakken MD, Okada RD, Boucher CA, Strauss HW, Pohost GM. Comparison of exercise perfusion and ventricular function imaging: an analysis of factors affecting the diagnostic accuracy of each technique. J Am Coll Cardiol 1984; 3: 272–83.
6. Caldwell JH, Hamilton GW, Sorensen SG, Ritchie JL, Williams DL, Kennedy JW. The detection of coronary artery disease with radionuclide techniques: a comparison of rest-exercise thallium imaging and ejection fraction response. Circulation 1980; 61: 610–9.
7. Johnstone DE, Sands MJ, Berger HJ et al. Comparison of exercise radionuclide angiocar-

diography and thallium-201 myocardial perfusion imaging in coronary artery disease. Am J Cardiol 1980; 45: 1113–9.

8. Jengo JA, Freeman R, Brizendine M, Mena I. Detection of coronary artery disease: comparison of exercise stress radionuclide angiocardiography and thallium stress perfusion scanning. Am J Cardiol 1980; 45: 535–41.

9. Kirshenbaum HD, Okada RD, Boucher CA, Kushner FG, Strauss HW, Pohost GM. Relationship of thallium-201 myocardial perfusion pattern to regional and global left ventricular function with exercise. Am Heart J 1981; 101: 734–9.

10. Elkayam U, Weinstein M, Berman D et al. Stress thallium-201 myocardial scintigraphy and exercise technetium ventriculography in the detection and location of chronic coronary artery disease: comparison of sensitivity and specificity of these noninvasive tests alone and in combination. Am Heart J 1981; 101: 657–66.

11. Uhl GS, Kay TN, Hickman JR Jr. Comparison of exercise radionuclide angiography and thallium perfusion imaging in detecting coronary disease in asymptomatic men. J Card Rehabil 1982; 2: 118–24.

12. Massie BM, Botvinick EH, Brundage BH, Greenberg B, Shames D, Gelberg H. Relationship of regional myocardial perfusion to segmental wall motion. A physiologic basis for understanding the presence and reversibility of asynergy. Circulation 1978; 58: 1154–63.

13. Narahara KA, Mena I, Maublant JC, Brizendine M, Criley JM. Simultaneous maximal exercise radionuclide angiography and thallium stress perfusion maging. Am J Cardiol 1984; 53: 812–7.

14. Mena I, Narahara KA, de Jong R, Maublant J. Gold-195m, an ultra-short-lived generator-produced radionuclide: clinical application in sequential first pass ventriculography. J Nucl Med 1983; 24: 139–44.

15. Iskandrian AS, Heo J, Kong B, Lyons E. Effect of exercise level on the ability of thallium-201 tomographic imaging in detecting coronary artery disease: analysis of 461 patients. J Am Coll Cardiol 1989; 14: 1477–86.

16. Johnson SH, Bigelow C, Lee KL, Pryor DB, Jones RH. Prediction of death and myocardial infarction by radionuclide angiography in patients with suspected coronary artery disease. Am J Cardiol 1991; 67: 919–26.

17. Bonow RO, Kent KM, Rosing DR et al. Exercise-induced ischemia in mildly symptomatic patients with coronary-artery disease and preserved left ventricular function. Identification of subgroups at risk of death during medical therapy. N Engl J Med 1984; 311: 1339–45.

18. Iskandrian AS, Hakki AH, Schwartz JS, Kay H, Mattleman S, Kane S. Prognostic implications of rest and exercise radionuclide ventriculography in patients with suspected or proven coronary heart disease. Int J Cardiol 1984; 6: 707–18.

19. Iskandrian AS, Hakki AH, Goel I et al. The use of rest and exercise radionuclide ventriculography in risk stratification in patients with suspected coronary artery disease. Am Heart J 1985; 110: 864–72.

20. Iskandrian AS, Heo J, DeCoskey D, Askenase A, Segal BL. Use of exercise thallium-201 imaging for risk stratification of elderly patients with coronary artery disease. Am J Cardiol 1982; 61: 269–72.

21. Iskandrian AS, Hakki AH, Kane-Marsch S. Prognostic implications of exercise thallium-201 scintigraphy in patients with suspected or known coronary artery disease. Am Heart J 1985; 110: 135–43.

22. Iskandrian AS, Hakki AH. Thallium-201 myocardial scintigraphy. Am Heart J 1985; 109: 113–29.

23. Boucher CA, Zir LM, Beller GA et al. Increased lung uptake of thallium-201 during exercise

myocardial imaging: clinical, hemodynamic and angiographic implications in patients with coronary artery disease. Am J Cardiol 1980; 46: 189–96.

24. Brown KA. Prognostic value of thallium-201 myocardial perfusion imaging. A diagnostic tool comes of age. Circulation 1991; 83: 363–81.

25. Iskandrian AS. Appraisal of clinical models based on results of stress nuclear imaging in risk stratification [editorial]. Am Heart J 1990; 120: 1487–90.

26. Meerdink DJ, Leppo JA. Myocardial transport of hexakis(2-methoxyisobutylisonitrile) and thallium before and after coronary reperfusion. Circ Res 1990; 66: 1738–46.

27. Beanlands RS, Dawood F, Wen WH et al. Are the kinetics of technetium-99m methoxy-isobutyl isonitrile affected by cell metabolism and viability? Circulation 1990; 82: 1802–14.

28. Villanueva-Meyer J, Mena I, Narahara KA. Simultaneous assessment of left ventricular wall motion and myocardial perfusion with technetium-99m-methoxy isobutyl isonitrile at stress and rest in patients with angina: comparison with thallium-201 SPECT. J Nucl Med 1990; 31: 457–63.

29. Okada RD, Glover D, Gaffney T, Williams S. Myocardial kinetics of technetium-99m--hexakis-2-methoxy-2-methylpropyl-isonitrile. Circulation 1988; 77: 491–8.

30. Taillefer R, Primeau M, Costi P, Lambert R, Léveillé J, Latour Y. 99-m-Tc-Sestamibi myocardial perfusion imaging in detection of coronary artery disease: comparison between initial (1 hours) and delayed (3 hours) post-exercise images. J Nucl Med 1991; 32: 1961–5.

31. Narahara KA, Villanueva-Meyer J, Thompson CJ, Brizendine M, Mena I. Comparison of thallium-201 and technetium-99m hexakis 2-methyisobutyl isonitrile single-photon emission computed tomography for estimating the extent of myocardial ischemia and infarction in coronary artery disease. Am J Cardiol 1990; 66: 1438–44.

32. Jones RH, Borges-Neto S, Potts JM. Simultaneous measurement of myocardial perfusion and ventricular function during exercise from a single injection of technetium-99m Sestamibi in coronary artery disease. Am J Cardiol 1990; 66: 68E–71E.

33. Baillet GY, Mena IG, Kuperus JH, Robertson JM, French WJ. Simultaneous technetium-99m MIBI angiography and myocardial perfusion imaging. J Nucl Med 1989; 30: 38–44.

34. Marcassa C, Marzullo P, Parodi O, Sambuceti G, L'Abbate A. A new method for noninvasive quantitation of segmental myocardial wall thickening using technetium-99m 2--methoxy-isobutyl-99m 2-isonitrile scintigraphy – results in normal subject. J Nucl Med 1990; 31: 173–7.

35. Borges-Neto S, Coleman RE, Jones RH. Perfusion and function at rest and treadmill exercise using technetium-99m-sestamibi: comparison of one- and two-day protocols in normal volunteers. J Nucl Med 1990; 31: 1128–32.

36. Iskandrian AS, Heo J, Kong B, Lyons E, Marsch S. Use of technetium-99m isonitrile (RP-30A) in assessing left ventricular perfusion and function at rest and during exercise in coronary artery disease, and comparison with coronary arteriography and exercise thallium-201 SPECT imaging. Am J Cardiol 1989; 64: 270–5.

37. Iskandrian AS, Heo J, Nguyen T, Mercuro J. Myocardial imaging with Tc-99m teboroxime: technique and initial results. Am Heart J 1991; 121: 889–94.

38. Iskandrian AS, Heo J, Askenase A, Segal BL, Helfant RH. Thallium imaging with single photon emission computed tomography. Am Heart J 1987; 114: 852–65.

39. Nguyen T, Heo J, Ogilby JD, Iskandrian AS. Single photon emission computed tomography with thallium-201 during adenosine-induced coronary hyperemia: correlation with coronary arteriography, exercise thallium imaging, and two-dimension echocardiography. J Am Coll Cardiol 1990; 16: 1375–83.

40. Iskandrian AS, Heo J, Askenase A, Segal BL, Auerbach N. Dipyridamole cardiac imaging. Am Heart J 1988; 115: 432–43.

41. Hakki AH, Nestico PF, Heo J, Unwala AA, Iskandrian AS. Relative prognostic value of rest thallium-201 imaging, radionuclide ventriculography and 24 hour ambulatory electrocardiographic monitoring after acute myocardial infarction. J Am Coll Cardiol 1987; 10: 25–32.

SECTION FIVE

Sympathetic nerve system

27. Radiolabeled metaiodobenzylguanidine (I-123 MIBG): value in clinical cardiology?

CORINNE KLÖPPING and ERNST E. VAN DER WALL

Summary

The relative distribution of radiolabeled metaiodobenzylguanidine (MIBG) in the heart is similar to that of endogenous norepinephrine and therefore represents the distribution of sympathetic nerve endings with a preserved uptake process. Various diseases of the heart can cause (regional) sympathetic denervation and may alter the levels of MIBG in the myocardium. Scintigraphic patterns of MIBG obtained from hearts of patients provide a very useful tool for studying noninvasively alterations in sympathetic cardiac innervation. The use of MIBG offers several potential advantages for applications in clinical cardiology: first, it may yield prognostic information in patients with congestive heart failure; second, it may be valuable in patients with hypertrophic cardiomyopathy; third, it will guide electrophysiologic studies and anti-arrhythmic therapy in patients with myocardial infarction, and lastly, the use of MIBG may give information about reinnervation in cardiac transplant patients. In this chapter, the most salient findings with MIBG are summarized and the clinical utility of the use of MIBG in cardiological practice will be discussed. Detailed information about this issue is given in the chapters written by Dae (Chapter 28) and Bourguignon et al. (Chapter 29).

Introduction

Imaging with radioiodinated metaiodobenzylguanidine (MIBG labeled with iodine-123), an analogue of the adrenergic blocking agent guanethidine, was

369

originally described by Wieland et al. in 1980 [1]. Research over the last decade has been helpful in clarifying mechanisms of uptake, storage, and release of MIBG and has led to its development as a useful clinical tool to visualize various neuro-endocrine tumors. In additon, organs with rich adrenergic innervation, such as the heart, have been noted to have substantial MIBG uptake offering great potential for scintigraphic imaging. Therefore, it allows the study of the cardiac adrenergic nervous system, which is felt to play an important role in several cardiac diseases. MIBG is taken up by sympathetic nerve endings in the heart. Depressed neuronal uptake function, e.g. in mechanical overload heart failure or reduced sympathetic innervation following infarction, produces smaller uptake intraneuronally and relatively larger accumulation in the extraneuronal compartment which is subjected to faster washout. The degree of sympathetic denervation and catecholamine depletion can be visualized noninvasively with MIBG in a variety of disease states. It is the most suitable and widely tested imaging agent for the evaluation of sympathetic axonal catecholamine transport. As would be expected from the metabolism of norepinephrine, localization of MIBG, particularly in the heart, is affected by the presence of sympathomimetic agents, especially catecholamines and sympatholytic compounds such as anti-adrenergic drugs. Nakajo et al. [2] demonstrated an inverse relationship between cardiac accumulation of radioiodinated MIBG and circulating catecholamines in patients with pheochromocytoma.

Experimental and clinical investigations

Studies in healthy volunteers

Kline et al. [3], in 1981, were the first to demonstrate, in five normal volunteers, myocardial uptake of MIBG after intravenous administration. The distribution of MIBG most closely represented the distribution of sympathetic nerve endings with a preserved uptake process. In most cases, the image patterns in normal hearts showed reduced uptake in the apex of the heart, possibly because of relative denervation of a limited area of the apex. Studies that have evaluated the myocardial distribution of norepinephrine have shown similar patterns with a reduction in norepinephrine content at the apex. To optimize MIBG imaging of the myocardium, single photon emission computed tomography (SPECT) is the preferred investigative method.

Studies in patients with various cardiac diseases

For the evaluation of cardiac adrenergic integrity and function, MIBG has been mainly employed in four subgroups of cardiac diseases: patients with (1) idiopathic dilated cardiomyopathy, (2) hypertrophic cardiomyopathy, (3) ischemic heart disease, and (4) cardiac transplantation.

(1) Idiopathic dilated cardiomyopathy
In patients with chronic congestive heart failure associated with increased sympathetic tone, neuronal uptake function in the heart is depressed, resulting in decreased cardiac MIBG uptake. Three recent reports have evaluated MIBG uptake and kinetics in patients with dilated cardiomyopathy [4, 7, 8].

Schofer et al. [4], in 1988, made the first description of a relatively large number of patients ($n = 28$) with idiopathic dilated cardiomyopathy and with various degrees of left ventricular dysfunction in whom MIBG scintigraphic data were examined in relation to clinical and hemodynamic variables, as well as to plasma and myocardial catecholamine concentrations. It was shown that the scintigraphically determined MIBG activity in the septal region significantly correlated with MIBG activity from the endomyocardial biopsy samples out of the same region. The calculated myocardial versus mediastinal MIBG activity ratio was significantly related to myocardial norepinephrine concentration and to left ventricular ejection fraction, although did not correlate with the New York Heart Association functional class or with plasma catecholamine concentration. Whether these findings are also applicable to patients with heart failure due to valvular or coronary artery disease, could not be answered with certainty. However, biopsy studies showed the same myocardial norepinephrine depletion as in patients with idiopathic dilated cardiomyopathy [5]. Therefore, one might also expect a correlation between myocardial MIBG activity and left ventricular ejection fraction in these patients. Cohn et al. [6], in patients with chronic congestive heart failure, were able to correlate plasma catecholamine levels with the risk of death. Yet, the severity of myocardial adrenergic dysfunction – as demonstrated by a low MIBG uptake – has not been directly linked to the risk of morbidity or mortality in patients with cardiomyopathy. Whether the scintigrahic data can serve as a prognostic indicator in patients with cardiomyopathy remains to be investigated.

Henderson et al. [7], in 1988, showed that patients with idiopathic dilated cardiomyopathy ($n = 16$) compared with controls ($n = 14$) had greater intra-image heterogeneity of the myocardial MIBG activity. Focal attribution of adrenergic neurons, interstitial scar, and fibrosis could be responsible for this inhomogeneity in the cardiomyopathy images. The initial images demonstrated no significant differences in MIBG concentration between patients and controls, but the myocardial retention of MIBG was significantly reduced in the patients with cardiomyopathy. The patients with cardiomyopathy had a $28 \pm 12\%$ washout rate compared with $6 \pm 8\%$ in the controls ($p < 0.001$).

Similar to Henderson et al. [7], Glowniak et al. [8], in 1989, demonstrated rapid washout of MIBG from the heart in patients with idiopathic congestive cardiomyopathy ($n = 6$) compared with controls ($n = 8$), suggesting increased cardiac sympathetic nerve activity in patients with cardiomyopathy.

From these studies, it can be concluded (1) that MIBG scintigraphy is a useful noninvasive method to assess the severity of myocardial adrenergic disintegrity in patients with dilated cardiomyopathy, and (2) that the myocardial distribution and kinetics of MIBG in images obtained from patients with dilated cardiomyopathy differ significantly from those of controls.

(2) Hypertrophic cardiomyopathy
Taki et al. [9] and Nakajima et al. [10], in 1988, performed studies with MIBG scintigraphy in patients with hypertrophic cardiomyopathy. None of the patients showed signs of heart failure. Myocardial washout of MIBG proved significantly faster in the severely hypertropic heart (septum thickness $> 20\,mm$), and there was a significant positive correlation ($r = 0.52, p < 0.01$) between the washout rate of MIBG from the heart and the thickness of the septal wall, while the initial myocardial uptake was similar. From these points of view, the faster washout of MIBG in the severely hypertrophic heart suggests that a larger proportion of the MIBG appears to be accumulated in the extravesicular space compared to the less affected heart. Hence, cardiac adrenergic neuronal innervation or activity is depressed in severe hypertrophic cardiomyopathy. It was concluded that quantitative MIBG scintigraphy may be a useful parameter for evaluating the severity of altered cardiac innervation and activity in hypertrophic cardiomyopathy.

(3) Ischemic heart disease
Experimental findings. Minardo et al. [11], in 1988, demonstrated, in their scintigraphic and electrophysiological study in dog hearts, that the correlation between the scintigraphic findings and the known electrophysiological characteristics of denervated myocardium was excellent. Sympathetic reinnervation after phenol- and infarction-induced denervation occurred at 8–17 weeks. The MIBG images after transmural infarction revealed areas of myocardium apical to the infarct that did not take up MIBG but had normal perfusion, as demonstrated by uptake of thallium-201 (i.e. MIBG/thallium mismatch pattern). These areas exhibited efferent denervation as well as supersensitivity to norepinephrine at subsequent electrophysiologic testing. Based on these findings, it can be concluded that denervation in dogs is followed by denervation

supersensitivity, which elicits inhomogeneous autonomic and electrophysi-ologic changes and makes the heart more vulnerable to electrical induction of ventricular arrhythmias.

Dae et al. [12], in 1989, compared in dog hearts the myocardial distribution of sympathetic nerve endings using MIBG with the distribution of thalli-um-201 following regional denervation. Regional denervation was performed by left or right stellate ganglion removal or by application of phenol to the epicardial surface. They showed reduced MIBG uptake in both stellectomized and phenolpainted hearts, whereas thallium-201 distribution remained homo-geneous and normal. Norepinephrine content was greater in regions showing normal MIBG compared with regions showing reduced MIBG, confirming the presence of regional denervation. The observations of a mismatch between MIBG and thallium-201 uptake in the myocardium were recently underscored by Dae et al. [13] in dog experiments, whereby regional sympathetic denerva-tion was observed in both infarcted and noninfarcted myocardium. In partic-ular, transmural myocardial infarction showed reduced MIBG but normal thallium-201 uptake in distal myocardial regions. The mismatch of MIBG and thallium-201 cardiac images suggests interruption of the efferent sympathetic nerves to noninfarcted viable areas of the heart.

These animal studies indicate that denervated but viable myocardium can be demonstrated using scintigraphic techniques following myocardial infarction. By simultaneously comparing distribution of sympathetic nerves (MIBG) with regional perfusion (thallium-201) new insights into neuronal mechanisms are provided, whereby an imbalance in sympathetic activity may relate to clinical disorders.

Clinical findings. Few clinical studies in patients with acute myocardial in-farction have been reported. Fagret et al. [14], in 1989, studied 30 patients following myocardial infarction and compared myocardial uptake of MIBG with the distribution of blood flow assessed by thallium-201. It was found that when a defect was detected on the thallium-201 scintigram, its localization was mostly identical to the defect on the MIBG scintigram. In three cases, how-ever, a defect was found on the MIBG scintigram corresponding to the electrocardiographic localization of the infarct, whereas the thallium-201 scin-tigram was normal. In five patients with transmural inferior wall infarction, a complete absence of MIBG uptake in the heart was observed whilst the thallium-201 scintigrams showed only defects in the inferior cardiac region. These MIBG/thallium mismatches are probably explained by the temporary depletion of tissue norepinephrine in noninfarcted areas, or by the drugs taken by these patients. At the moment the scintigraphic study was performed, patients were taking adrenergic receptors antagonists, calcium antagonists, or amiodarone, i.e. drugs which are known to act on neuronal norepinephrine transport. The authors concluded that most of the myocardial infarction patients showed matched defects of MIBG and thallium-201 uptake in the infarct region, but that any interpretation of the MIBG scintigram should take into account the treatment administered.

Stanton et al. [15], in 1989, showed that regional sympathetic denervation may occur in noninfarcted myocardium apical and lateral to the infarct site. They studied 19 patients of whom 12 patients with spontaneous ventricular arrhythmias after myocardial infarction and seven patients without known arrhythmias following myocardial infarction. Ten (83%) of the 12 post-infarction patients with arrhythmias had areas of MIBG/thallium mismatch, but also two (29%) of the seven patients without arrhythmias demonstrated a region of mismatch. In the case of a mismatch, MIBG uptake was invariably absent and thallium uptake was normal; the reverse uptake pattern was never observed. Eleven of the 12 patients with arrhythmias had ventricular tachycardia induced at electrophysiologic study and metoprolol never prevented induction. They concluded that although the presence of sympathetic denervation may be related to the onset of spontaneous ventricular tachyarrhythmias in some patients, it does not appear to be related to sustained ventricular tachycardia induced at electrophysiologic study.

To summarize, in humans the importance of regional sympathetic denervation in viable and perfused myocardium after myocardial infarction, as demonstrated by MIBG/thallium mismatch, is not yet known and its relation to the genesis of ventricular tachyarrhythmias remains uncertain. The partial denervation may produce imbalanced sympathetic innervation which during enhanced sympathetic tone can predispose the heart to arrhythmias. The ability to detect the distribution of innervation scintigraphically and to correlate these imaging findings with electrophysiologic assessment of vulnerability to arrhythmias, may provide important new understanding of the interaction of the sympathetic nerves and cardiac pathophysiology. A noninvasive method may be found to detect patients at risk for sudden death after myocardial infarction and this will possibly lead to a basis for more rational approaches to therapy.

(4) Cardiac transplants
Several investigators studied patients with cardiac transplants, in whom apparently all cardiac nerves have been destroyed [8, 16]. Glowniak et al. [8], in 1989, showed that within 4 months after surgery, no myocardial MIBG activity was visible in any of the four patients they examined. Iturralde et al. [16], in 1988, described one patient after orthotopic heart transplantation who showed increased MIBG uptake in the myocardium during an episode of rejection

which disappeared after adequate therapy. A clear explanation for this finding will need further study.

Conclusion

Imbalances in sympathetic function are thought to play an important role in the etiology and outcome of several clinical cardiac disorders and may be pivotal in the cause of sudden death. However, the pathophysiologic mechanisms relating abnormalities in sympathetic activity to these various clinical disorders are poorly understood and, relatively unexplored, and therefore in need of further investigation. The new ability to noninvasively visualize with MIBG the distribution of sympathetic nerves in the heart, may provide important new insights into mechanisms relating the sympathetic nervous system to cardiac disease pathogenesis. It may well give us the ability to stratify patients with heart failure for future serious complications and it will enhance our knowledge of the origin of ventricular arrhythmias following myocardial infarction. The images can be performed with 40 MBq I-123 MIBG, which will give an effective dose equivalence of 0.7 mSv (Category II of the World Health Organization). The costs of a MIBG-scintigraphic imaging study will be approximately $ 400, which is relatively expensive compared to other noninvasive modalities. However, the information gained in a wide variety of cardiac diseases may prove cost-effective and of important value in clinical practice.

References

1. Wieland DM, Wu JL, Brown LE, Mangnet TJ, Swanson DP, Beierwaltes WH. Radiolabeled adrenergic neuron-blocking agents: adrenomedullary imaging with [131-I] iodobenzylguanidine. J Nucl Med 1980; 21: 349–53.
2. Nakajo M, Shapiro B, Glowniak JV, Sisson JC, Beierwaltes WH. Inverse relation between cardiac accumulation of meta-[131]iodobenzylguanidine (I-131 MIBG) and circulating catecholamines in suspected pheochromocytoma. J Nucl Med 1983; 24: 1127–34.
3. Kline RC, Swanson DP, Wieland DM et al. Myocardial imaging in man with I-123 meta-iodobenzylguanidine. J Nucl Med 1981; 22: 129–32.
4. Schofer J, Spielmann R, Schuchert A, Weber K, Schlüter M. Iodine-123 meta-iodobenzylguanidine scintigraphy: a noninvasive method to demonstrate myocardial adrenergic nervous system disintegrity in patients with idiopathic dilated cardiomyopathy. J Am Coll Cardiol 1988; 12: 1252–8.
5. Dequattro V, Nagatsu T, Mendez A, Verska J. Determinants of cardiac noradrenaline depletion in human congestive heart failure. Cardiovasc Res 1973; 7: 344–50.

6. Cohn JN, Levine TB, Olivari MT et al. Plasma norepinephrine as a guide to prognosis in patients with chronic congestive heart failure. N Engl J Med 1984; 311: 819–23.

7. Henderson EB, Kahn JK, Corbett JR et al. Abnormal I-123 metaiodobenzylguanidine myocardial washout and distribution may reflect myocardial adrenergic derangement in patients with congestive cardiomyopathy. Circulation 1988; 78: 1192–9.

8. Glowniak JV, Turner FE, Gray LL, Palac RT, Lagunas-Solar MC, Woodward WR. Iodine-123 metaiodobenzylguanidine imaging of the heart in idiopathic congestive cardiomyopathy and cardiac transplants. J Nucl Med 1989; 30: 1182–91.

9. Taki J, Nakajima K, Bunko H, Simizu M, Muramori A, Hisada K. Whole-body distribution of iodine 123 metaiodobenzylguanidine in hypertrophic cardiomyopathy: significance of its washout from the heart. Eur J Nucl Med 1990; 17: 264–8.

10. Nakajima K, Bunko H, Taki J et al. Evaluation of hypertrophic cardiomyopathy with I-123 metaiodobenzylguanidine. Jpn J Nucl Med 1990; 27: 33–8.

11. Minardo JD, Tuli MM, Mock BH et al. Scintigraphic and electrophysiological evidence of canine myocardial sympathetic denervation and reinnervation produced by myocardial infarction or phenol application. Circulation 1988; 78: 1008–19.

12. Dae MW, O'Connell JW, Botvinick EH et al. Scintigraphic assessment of regional cardiac adrenergic innervation. Circulation 1989; 79: 634–44.

13. Dae MW, Herre JM, O'Connell JW, Botvinick EH, Newman D, Munoz L. Scintigraphic assessment of sympathetic innervation after transmural versus nontransmural myocardial infarction. J Am Coll Cardiol 1991; 17: 1416–23.

14. Fagret D, Wolf JE, Comet M. Myocardial uptake of meta-[123I]-iodobenzylguanidine ([123I]-MIBG) in patients with myocardial infarct. Eur J Nucl Med 1989; 15: 624–8.

15. Stanton MS, Tuli MM, Radtke NL et al. Regional sympathetic denervation after myocardial infarction in humans detected noninvasively using I-123-metaiodobenzylguanidine. J Am Coll Cardiol 1989; 14: 1519–26.

16. Iturralde M, Novitzky D, Cooper DKC et al. The role of nuclear cardiology procedures in the evaluation of cardiac function following heart transplantation. Semin Nucl Med 1988; 18: 221–40.

28. Scintigraphic assessment of cardiac innervation using iodine-123 metaiodobenzylguanidine

MICHAEL W. DAE

Introduction

Autonomic imbalance, through differential effects of catecholamines, has long been hypothesized as a major mechanism leading to a number of clinical disorders, particularly those involving the heart [1]. The largest source of catecholamines is found in the sympathetic nerves of the heart, which are distributed on a regional basis [2]. Only in the past few years has it been possible to evaluate abnormalities in heart innervation in the intact animal. Recent developments in cardiac imaging have led to the ability to map the distribution of the sympathetic nerves in vivo. As a result, the pathophysiologic mechanisms relating alterations in sympathetic nerve activity to disease processes are now being explored.

Radionuclide assessment of sympathetic innervation

Myocardial sympathetic nerves have been shown to take up exogenously administered catecholamines. Early studies in rat hearts showed rapid accumulation of tritiated norepinephrine [3]. The labeled compound was subsequently shown to enter the sympathetic nerve endings by a high affinity uptake process (uptake 1), however, a low affinity, high capacity nonneuronal uptake process was also found (uptake 2) [4]. Subsequent studies showed that the neuronally bound catecholamine was retained in storage vescicles for long periods of time, whereas the nonneuronally bound compound was rapidly metabolized and subsequently washed out of the heart at a fairly rapid rate [5].

Ernst E. van der Wall et al. (eds), What's new in cardiac imaging?, 377–385.
© *1992 Kluwer Academic Publishers. Printed in the Netherlands.*

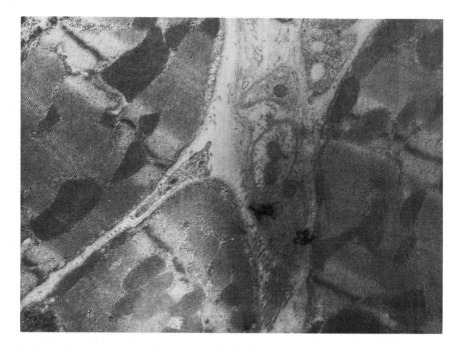

Figure 1. Shown is an electron microscopic autoradiograph of a rat heart. The two silver grains are localized over a sympathetic nerve terminal and are formed by I-125 MIBG.

Numerous other substances with chemical structures similar to norepine-phrine were also shown to enter sympathetic nerves (false adrenergic transmit-ters) [6].

Several years ago, metaiodobenzylguanidine (MIBG), an analogue of the false adrenergic transmitter, guanethidine, was developed [7]. Radioiodinated MIBG was shown to localize to the heart and other organs in several animal species and in man [8].

Radiolabeled metaiodobenzylguanidine – validation of neuronal uptake

MIBG is thought to share similar uptake and storage mechanisms as norepine-phrine [9, 10], but is not metabolized by monoamine oxidase or catechol-*o*-methyl transferase (Figure 1). Numerous studies have evaluated the character-istics of MIBG uptake and distribution in experimental models designed to alter global and regional function of myocardial sympathetic nerves.

Global myocardial neuronal uptake

Sisson et al. [11] assessed the myocardial uptake of 125I-MIBG in rats treated with either 6-hydroxydopamine, which causes a chemical degeneration of sympathetic nerves, and desmethylimipramine, an uptake-1 inhibitor. Significant reductions in MIBG uptake occurred with both treatments. The responses of MIBG to pertubations of sympathetic nerves were qualitatively similar to the responses of 3H-norepinephrine.

We studied the effects of 6 hydroxydopamine treatment on MIBG uptake in dog hearts [12]. Dogs were studied at baseline and one week after the intravenous injection of 50 mg/kg of 6-OH dopamine. Images were acquired at 5 minutes and 3 hours after injection of I-123 MIBG. At baseline, there was homogeneous myocardial uptake of MIBG on initial images, with homogeneous retention of MIBG at 3 hours. These results suggest that the initial accumulation of MIBG in the denervated hearts represented nonneuronal localization, and support the conclusion that MIBG localization on the delayed images in the normally innervated hearts represents accumulation in sympathetic nerve endings.

In another study, Sisson et al. [13] evaluated acute changes in adrenergic nerve activity of the heart by measuring the rates of loss of triated norepinephrine and MIBG in rat and dog hearts. Rates of loss of norepinephrine were considered to be proportional to norepinephrine secretion and to adrenergic function. They used yohimbine, an alpha-2 adrenergic receptor antagonist, to increase the function of the sympathetic nerves; and, clonidine, an alpha-2 agonist, to decrease the activity of the sympathetic nerves. In rat hearts, yohimbine induced similar increases in rates of loss of 3H-NE and I-125 MIBG; while, clonidine induced similar decreases in rates of loss of 3H-NE and I-125 MIBG. Imaging studies in dog hearts with I-123 MIBG showed similar responses to yohimbine and clonidine. These results suggest that it may be possible to noninvasively assess acute changes in sympathetic tone.

Regional neuronal uptake

We evaluated the ability of MIBG to detect regional denervation in dog hearts [14]. We compared the distribution of I-123 MIBG to thallium-201 in dogs that underwent prior left or right stellectomy, or applications of phenol to the epicardial surface. These regionally denervated hearts showed reduced uptake of MIBG relative to thallium in the posterior left ventricle in left stellectomized hearts (Figure 2 and Plate 28.1), and the anterior left ventricle in right stellectomized hearts (Plate 28.1). Phenol-treated hearts showed reduced MIBG uptake within and beyond the region of phenol application. Control

MIBG

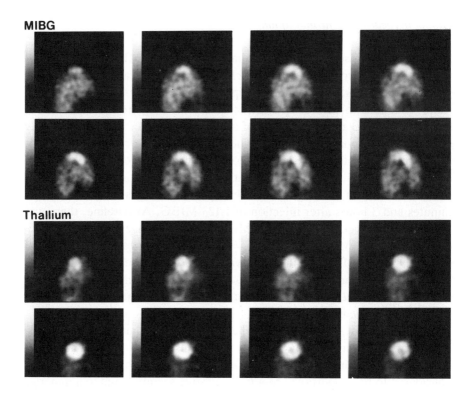

Thallium

Figure 2. Shown here are dual isotope emission computed tomograms from a dog with left stellectomy. MIBG images (upper rows) show a region of decreased uptake at the posterior left ventricle, whereas the corresponding thallium images show normal perfusion to this area, indicating regional denervation of the posterior left ventricle. (Reproduced from Circulation with permission.)

hearts showed similar and homogeneous distributions of MIBG and thallium (Plate 28.2). There was a significant difference in tissue norepinephrine content between areas showing reduced MIBG uptake versus areas showing normal MIBG uptake, confirming regional denervation (Figure 3). Others have also shown reduced MIBG uptake in regionally denervated dog hearts [15].

In another series of experiments, we evaluated the contractile responses of hearts showing regional denervation by MIBG imaging [16]. Regional denervation was produced by epicardial phenol treatment. Regions showing normal MIBG uptake showed enhanced contractile responses during stellate stimulation, after infusion of tyramine, and after isoproterenol infusion. Regions showing reduced MIBG uptake showed no augmentation in contractile response during stellate stimulation or infusion of tyramine, confirming dener-

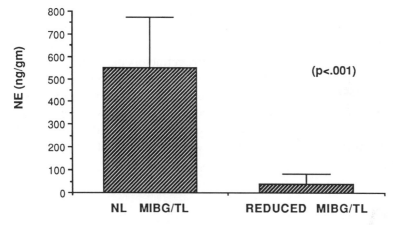

Figure 3. Bar graph of tissue norepinephrine (NE) contents in regionally denervated (reduced MIBG/TL) and innervated (normal MIBG/TL) areas of myocardium. (Reproduced from circulation with permission.)

vation. There was, however, increased contractile response to isoproterenol infusion, indicating intact post synaptic responses to beta-receptor stimulation.

Regional neuronal uptake after experimental myocardial infarction

Recent studies have shown that transmural myocardial infarction can lead to a partially denervated ventricle [17], which may predispose the heart to arrhythmias [18]. We assessed MIBG uptake in dogs with transmural and non-transmural myocardial infarction [19]. Transmural myocardial infarction was produced by the injection of vinyl latex into the left anterior descending coronary artery, and nontransmural myocardial infarction was produced by ligation of the left anterior descending coronary artery. Hearts with transmural infarction showed zones of absent MIBG and thallium, indicating scar. Adjacent and distal regions showed reduced MIBG but normal thallium uptake, indicating viable but denervated myocardium (Plate 28.3). Nontransmural myocardial infarction also showed regional denervation. There were zones of wall thinning with decreased thallium uptake and a greater reduction of MIBG localized to the region of the infarct. These findings demonstrate that, in experimental myocardial infarction, the relative uptake of MIBG shows a spectrum: no uptake in the center of an infarct with no flow and relative decreased MIBG uptake in the border zone of an infarct. This border zone may be transmural or nontransmural.

Minardo et al. [20] also found evidence of regional denervation after myocardial infarction. They correlated MIBG scintigraphy with electrophysiologic responses to sympathetic stimulation. Areas of viable myocardium with diminished MIBG uptake showed reduced shortening of effective refractory period compared to normal basal myocardium, during sympathetic stimulation. However, enhanced shortening of effective refractory period was found in the regions showing reduced MIBG uptake during norepinephrine infusion, indicating supersensitivity of the denervated regions. MIBG images returned to normal a mean of 14 weeks after infarction, consistent with reinnervation. Other studies have shown increased susceptibility to induced ventricular fibrillation or ventricular tachycardia in dogs with myocardial infarction and denervation [18, 21].

Clinical applications

Patients studied with MIBG early after cardiac transplantation show an absence of MIBG uptake as expected [22]. The unexpected finding, however, was that there was an absence of MIBG uptake on the early images (5 to 15 minutes) after injection of MIBG. These findings suggest that nonneuronal uptake is not significant in human hearts, unlike other species. Interestingly, some patients studied a year or more after cardiac transplantation, show evidence of partial reinnervation (unpublished observations), of which the functional significance is unknown.

Partial denervation has been shown to occur in humans after myocardial infarction. We studied the distribution of MIBG and thallium in patients studied 2 weeks to 7 years after myocardial infarction [23]. Infarct patients showed reduced MIBG relative to thallium in a zone of myocardium generally apical and lateral to scar, indicating the presence of viable but denervated myocardium (Plate 28.4). Stanton et al. [24] have also reported denervated myocardium in patients after myocardial infarction. They found a relationship between the presence of sympathetic denervation and the occurrence of spontaneous ventricular tachyarrhythmias, but not to sustained ventricular tachycardia induced at electrophysiologic testing.

Several studies have examined the kinetics of MIBG washout in various patient populations. Patients with generalized automonic neuropathy [25], generalized adrenergic dysfunction [26], dilated cardiomyopathy [27], and severe hypertrophic cardiomyopathy [28] have all shown enhanced washout of MIBG from the heart. Whether this enhanced washout is due to denervation or to enhanced sympathetic activity is not entirely clear at present. Schofer et al. [29] found a significant correlation between reduced MIBG uptake and reduced myocardial norepinephrine content and ejection fraction in patients with idiopathic dilated cardiomyopathy. Richalet et al. [30] found reduced cardiac MIBG uptake after exposure to high altitude hypoxia, suggesting the presence of an hypoxia induced reduction of adrenergic neurotransmitter reserve in the heart.

Gohl et al. [31] recently reported reduced MIBG uptake in the inferior wall and posterior septal regions of the left ventricle in patients with idiopathic long QT syndrome. They found that quantitative MIBG tomographic imaging had greater diagnostic validity than QT interval measurements in identifying patients at high risk of sudden cardiac death in this clinical condition.

Conclusions

There is an increasing body of literature confirming the feasibility of imaging the sympathetic innervation of the intact heart. These early studies suggest that the numerous hypotheses relating enhanced autonomic tone and autonomic imbalance to increased risk of arrhythmias and sudden death can be successfully tested. Future studies to compare functional abnormalities of the sympathetic nerves to myocardial perfusion, metabolism, and adrenergic receptor density, may provide a more comprehensive understanding of the action of the autonomic nervous system in disease states. The ability to detect the distribution of innervation scintigraphically and to correlate these imaging findings with electrophysiologic assessment of vulnerability may provide important new understanding of the interaction of the sympathetic nerves and cardiac pathophysiology. In addition, a noninvasive means may be found to detect patients at risk for sudden death, and possibly provide a basis for more rational approaches to therapy.

References

1. Manger WM. Adrenergic involvement in cardiac pathophysiology. Adv Cardiol 1982; 30: 74–107.
2. Randall WC. Nervous control of cardiovascular function. New York: Oxford University Press, 1984.
3. Whitby LG, Axelrod J, Weil-Malherbe H. The fate of 3H-norepinephrine in animals. J Pharmacol Exp Ther 1961; 132: 193–201.
4. Iversen LL. Role of transmitter uptake mechanisms in synaptic neurotransmission. Br J Pharmacol 1971; 41: 571–91.
5. Lightman SL, Iversen LL. The role of uptake in the extraneuronal metabolism of catecholamines in the isolated rat heart. Br J Pharmacol 1969; 37: 638–49.
6. Kopin I. False adrenergic transmitters. Annu Rev Pharmacol 1968; 8: 377–94.
7. Wieland DM, Wu JL, Brown LE, Mangner TJ, Swanson DP, Beierwalters WH. Radiola-

beled adrenergic neuron-blocking agents: adrenomedullary imaging with (131-I) Iodoben-zylguanidine. J Nucl Med 1980; 21: 349–53.

8. Kline RC, Swanson DP, Wieland DM et al. Myocardial imaging in man with I-123 meta-iodobenzylguanidine. J Nucl Med 1981; 22: 129–32.

9. Manger WM, Hoffman BB. Heart imaging in the diagnosis of pheochromocytoma and assessment of catecholamine uptake [editorial]. J Nucl Med 1983; 24: 1194–6.

10. Wieland DM, Brown LE, Rogers WL et al. Myocardial imaging with a radioiodinated norepinephrine storage analog. J Nucl Med 1981; 22: 22–31.

11. Sisson JC, Wieland DM, Sherman P, Mangner TJ, Tobes MC, Jacques S. Metaiodoben-zylguanidine as an index of the adrenergic nervous system integrity and function. J Nucl Med 1987; 28: 1620–4.

12. Dae MW, O'Connell W, Chin MC, Herre JM, Huberty JP, Botvinick EH. Scintigraphic assessment of global adrenergic nerve density with MIBG washout maps [abstract]. J Am Coll Cardiol 1988; 11 (2 Suppl A): 214A.

13. Sisson JC, Bolgas G, Johnson J. Measuring acute changes in adrenergic nerve activity of the heart in the living animal. Am Heart J 1991; 121: 1119–23.

14. Dae MW, O'Connell JW, Botvinick EH et al. Scintigraphic assessment of regional cardiac adrenergic innervation. Circulation 1989; 79: 634–44.

15. Sisson JC, Lynch JJ, Johnson J et al. Scintigraphic detection of regional disruption of adrenergic neurons in the heart. Am Heart J 1988; 116: 67–76.

16. Mori H, Pisarri TE, Aldea GS et al. Usefulness and limitations of regional cardiac sympa-thectomy by phenol. Am J Physiol 1989; 257: H1523–33.

17. Barber MJ, Mueller TM, Henry DP, Felten SY, Zipes DP. Transmural myocardial infarction in the dog produces sympathectomy in noninfarcted myocardium. Circulation 1983; 67: 787–96.

18. Herre J, Wetstein L, Lin YL, Mills AS, Dae M, Thames MD. Effect of transmural versus nontransmural myocardial infarction on inducibility of ventricular arrhythmias during sympa-thetic stimulation. J Am Coll Cardiol 1988; 11: 414–21.

19. Dae M, Herre J, O'Connell J, Botvinick E, Newman D, Munoz L. Scintigraphic assessment of sympathetic innervation after transmural versus nontransmural myocardial infarction. J Am Coll Cardiol 1991; 17: 1416–23.

20. Minardo JD, Tuli MM, Mock BH et al. Scintigraphic and electrophysiologic evidence of canine myocardial sympathetic denervation and reinnervation produced by myocardial in-farction or phenol application. Circulation 1988; 78: 1008–19.

21. Inoue H, Zipes D. Results of sympathetic denervation in the canine heart: supersensitivity that may be arrhythmogenic. Circulation 1987; 75: 877–87.

22. Dae MW, DeMarco T, Botvinick EH, Hattner RH, Ratzlaff NW, Huberty JH. Absence of extraneuronal uptake of MIBG following cardiac transplantation [abstract]. J Nucl Med 1990; 31: 792.

23. Dae M, Herre J, Botvinick E et al. Scintigraphic assessment of adrenergic innervation after myocardial infarction [abstract]. Circulation 1986; (4 Suppl II): II 297.

24. Stanton MS, Tuli MM, Radtke NL et al. Regional sympathetic denervation after myocardial infarction in humans detected noninvasively using I-123-metaiodobenzylguanidine. J Am Coll Cardiol 1989; 14: 1519–26.

25. Sisson JC, Shapiro B, Meyers L et al. Metaiodobenzylguanidine to map scintigraphically the adrenergic nervous system in man. J Nucl Med 1987; 28: 1625–36.

26. Nakajo M, Shimabukuro K, Miyaji N et al. Rapid clearance of iodine-131 MIBG from the heart and liver of patients with adrenergic dysfunction and pheochromocytoma. J Nucl Med 1985; 26: 357–65.

27. Henderson EB, Kahn JK, Corbett JR et al. Abnormal I-123 metaiodobenzylguanidine myocardial washout and distribution may reflect myocardial adrenergic derangement in patients with congestive cardiomyopathy. Circulation 1988; 78: 1192–9.

28. Taki J, Nakajima K, Bunko H, Simizu M, Muramori A, Hisada K. Whole-body distribution of iodine 123 metaiodobenzylguanidine in hypertrophic cardiomyopathy: significance of its washout from the heart. Eur J Nucl Med 1990; 17: 264–8.

29. Schofer J, Spielmann R, Schuchert A, Weber K, Schluter M. Iodine-123 meta-iodobenzylguanidine scintigraphy: a noninvasive method to demonstrate myocardial adrenergic nervous system disintegrity in patients with idiopathic dilated cardiomyopathy. J Am Coll Cardiol 1988; 12: 1252–8.

30. Richalet J, Merlet P, Bourguignon J et al. MIBG scintigraphic assessment of cardiac adrenergic activity in response to altitude hypoxia. J Nucl Med 1990; 31: 34–7.

31. Gohl K, Feistel H, Weikl A, Bachman K, Wolf F. Congenital myocardial sympathetic dysinnervation – a structural defect of idiopathic long QT syndrome. PACE 1991; 14: 1544–53.

29. Clinical experience with iodine-123 metaiodobenzylguanidine

PASCAL MERLET, HÉRIC VALETTE,
MICHEL H. BOURGUIGNON, ALAIN CASTAIGNE
and ANDRÉ SYROTA

Introduction

Considerable data ara available on abnormalities of the function of sympathetic system in heart disease. These alterations are of interest for pathophysiological understanding, therapy evaluation and patient management. I-123 labeled to metaiodobenzylguanidine (MIBG) scintigraphy provides the opportunity to explore noninvasively the adrenergic neuronal function in vivo.

I-123 MIBG imaging has been used in humans primarily to localize pheochromocytoma [1]. The first report of the use of I-123 MIBG in cardiology is due to Kline et al. [2] who imaged the myocardium of normal volunteers.

The potential of I-123 MIBG scintigraphy in the exploration of patients with heart disease is examined in this chapter.

Congestive heart failure

The prognosis of patients with congestive heart failure is poor despite the introduction of new and active pharmacologic agents and cardiac transplantation may represent the only therapeutic option for the most severe patients. Unfortunately, a striking discrepancy exists between the number of candidates for heart transplantation and the availability of donors. The discrimination between high and low risk patients with regard to mortality is needed to rationalize the indication of cardiac transplantation and its timing. Of the available prognostic indices, a diminished left ventricular ejection fraction has been showed to be one of the most potent predictors of mortality [3, 4].

Ernst E. van der Wall et al. (eds), What's new in cardiac imaging?, 387–397.
© *1992 Kluwer Academic Publishers. Printed in the Netherlands.*

However, all these indices are not discriminatory enough and the decision of heart transplantation remains difficult in individuals. We feel that cardiac MIBG imaging can help the physicians for heart transplantation decision-making.

Decreased MIBG uptake in the failing heart

In canine mechanical overload heart failure at the decompensated state, left ventricular accumulation and retention of the tracer were reduced, suggesting that MIBG imaging represents a new tool to assess adrenergic presynaptic activity in the failing heart [5]. Similar results were found in patients with idiopathic cardiomyopathy who showed a noticeable global decrease in cardiac uptake associated with an increase in MIBG washout and a greater heterogeneity of the cardiac MIBG distribution in comparison with controls [6].

The ability of scintigraphy to measure MIBG uptake has been tested in patients with idiopathic cardiomyopathy.

I-123 MIBG activity scintigraphically determined correlated with MIBG activity measured from endomyocardial biopsy samples [7]. Interestingly, this diminished MIBG uptake has been repeatedly related to indices of left ventricular dysfunction. The cardiac MIBG uptake has been found to be correlated with left ventricular ejection fraction in ischemic or idiopathic dilated cardiomyopathy [7, 8]. In patients with idiopathic cardiomyopathy, MIBG cardiac uptake also correlated with right and left catheterization data such as cardiac index, left ventricular ejection fraction, and with left ventricular end-diastolic pressure. A similar relationship between markers of left ventricular dysfunction and other adrenergic disorders has been previously reported in heart failure [9–11]. Moreover, elevated circulating norepinephrine concentration has been shown in a large population of patients with heart failure to be a potent prognostic marker [10]. Therefore, the relationship repeatedly found between decreased MIBG uptake and altered indices of left ventricular function suggests that MIBG imaging may be a prognostic marker.

Results of a prospective study from our group concerning 90 patients with congestive heart failure related to a dilated cardiomyopathy either idiopathic or ischemic have already supported this consideration [12]. In these patients, the following parameters were initially assessed: cardiac MIBG uptake, radionuclide left ventricular ejection fraction, X-ray cardio-thoracic ratio and echocardiographic M-mode data. Cardiac MIBG uptake was assessed as the heart to mediastinum activity ratio measured on the chest anterior view image obtained 4 hours after intravenous injection (Plate 29.1). Patients were mostly treated with diuretics, anti-converting-enzyme-inhibitors or nitrates and followed-up during 1 to 27 months: 10 patients were transplanted, 22 died and 58 were still alive at the end of the study. After discarding the transplanted patients from the analysis, the multivariate stepwise regression discriminant analysis showed that cardiac MIBG uptake was more potent to predict survival than other indices and, when using a cutoff value of 120% for heart to mediastinum ratio, MIBG imaging had a high predictive value for survival. Moreover, also multivariate life-table analysis showed that the best predictor for life duration was cardiac MIBG uptake. Thus, MIBG imaging can be helpful in patients with heart failure to both make heart transplantation decision and to evaluate its timing. Further information is needed to evaluate the prognostic value of MIBG imaging in comparison with that of right heart catheterization data and circulating norepinephrine concentrations.

Patho-physiological importance of the myocardial neuronal norepinephrine uptake

The neuronal norepinephrine uptake function is the principal means for terminating the action of the neurotransmitter. Therefore, an impairment of this process may induce an increase in the stimulation of the myocytes by the norepinephrine either released from the adrenergic nerve terminal or delivered by the coronary blood circulation. If prolonged, this may induce myocardial overexposure to norepinephrine and subsequent deleterious effects such as myocyte calcium overload, arrhythmias, desensitization of β-adrenergic receptor pathway which are thought to participate in the evolution of cardiomyopathies.

Mechanisms of neuronal norepinephrine and MIBG uptake in the heart

MIBG shares the same uptake and storage mechanisms as norepinephrine and is unmetabolizable by catechol-*o*-methyl transferase or monoamine-oxidase [13].

Two types of uptake systems for norepinephrine and MIBG have been identified in adrenergic tissues: the uptake-1 system (neuronal uptake) that dominates at low concentrations of the substrates, is sodium and ATP-dependent, and is inhibited by tricyclic antidepressants; the uptake-2 system (extraneuronal uptake), a diffusion system that dominates at high concentrations of norepinephrine or MIBG and is slightly inhibited by tricyclic agents [14–16]. Besides, neurons of the heart may also sequester MIBG by the diffusion pathway.

Indeed, quantitative differences between tritiated norepinephrine and MIBG have been identified and may be attributable to partial neuronal uptake of MIBG by the diffusion pathway [15]. However, MIBG administered at the low doses used for clinical applications may enter mainly through the uptake-1 pathway to be stored in the presynaptic vesicles [17].

The exact proportion of the neuronal uptake in the amount of MIBG fixed by the myocardium in a given physiologic or pathologic condition is probably the most important question to be addressed to evaluate the potential of MIBG imaging for the investigation of patients suffering from heart disease. MIBG uptake measured at least 4 hours after injection, appears to be the best index of neuronal accumulation of the tracer because, in a reserpine blocking study of the rat heart, the intravesicular accumulation to total tissue concentration was found to represent 50% of the MIBG uptake from 4 to 24 hours after injection [18]. Similar results were reported in the canine heart [13]. The neuronal uptake seems to therefore represent only half of the total MIBG uptake in these models, the remaining quantity of MIBG being fixed by the uptake-2 pathway.

In humans, the uptake-2 pathway is probably much lower than in these laboratory species: a ten-fold difference of cardiac MIBG uptake was found between heart transplanted patients and normal subjects, suggesting that MIBG uptake through uptake-2 pathway is low in the human heart [19].

Cause of decreased MIBG uptake in the failing heart

This decrease is mainly related to an impairment of the neuronal norepinephrine uptake or storage function or to neuronal disintegrity. In canine experiments designed to disrupt the adrenergic neurons in the heart (phenolization of left ventricular epicardium, denervation either by stellectomy or autotransplantation), a diminished MIBG uptake was found and the regional distribution of the tracer was comparable to that of endogenous norepinephrine contents [5, 20, 21]. Similarly, in heart transplanted patients, a dramatic decrease in MIBG uptake has been observed [19]. Interestingly, in patients with idiopathic dilated cardiomyopathy, the cardiac MIBG uptake significantly correlated with myocardial endogenous norepinephrine concentration. These findings are in agreement with previous studies which demonstrated that in the failing heart, different alterations of the function of cardiac adrenergic innervation occurred, including decrease in catecholamine content, impairment of norepinephrine uptake function and lesions of nerve terminals [22–26].

On the other hand, a decrease in MIBG uptake may be caused by other factors. Indeed, elevation of norepinephrine concentration at the synaptic level may compete the MIBG uptake. This elevation may be a result of an increase in either circulating norepinephrine level or neuronal norepinephrine release. In congestive heart failure, the circulating norepinephrine concentration is elevated in proportion to the severity of the disease and may therefore be a factor involved in the decrease in MIBG uptake observed in congestive heart failure. Support for this hypothesis has been provided by the observation that in patients with pheochromocytoma, the cardiac accumulation at 24 and 48 hours after injection was inversely related to plasma concentrations of catecholamines [18]. However, increased circulating concentration of norepinephrine is not the only factor involved in the decrease of cardiac MIBG uptake. In patients with moderate heart failure, we found that a significant decrease in cardiac MIBG uptake could coexist with normal circulating concentrations of norepinephrine [27]. Finally, an increase in the presynaptic release of norepinephrine has been reported in some studies, and could theoretically participate in the diminished MIBG uptake. It is not easy to assess in vivo the presynaptic release of norepinephrine and conflicting data are reported in the literature: an increased norepinephrine release was found in some studies in heart failure patients [28, 29] while opposite findings were shown by other authors [22, 23].

Quantification of myocardial uptake

Quantification of myocardial MIBG activity on scintigraphic images has technical limitations. Tomographic imaging provides an opportunity to study the myocardial distribution of MIBG uptake [6]. However, in our experience, the marked decrease in MIBG uptake in severe patients induces difficulties for image reconstruction, therefore hindering the use of tomographic imaging in routine examination. This discrepancy with Henderson's report may be due to the low doses of MIBG used in our laboratory (10 mCi versus 4, respectively).

We use planar imaging to compare cardiac MIBG uptake of different patients. However, planar imaging has limitations of its own. The ideal cardiac region of interest should include myocardial activity and exclude adjacent lung and liver activities. Ventricular enlargement may induce an underestimation of the myocardial activity. Pulmonary crosstalk in the cardiac region of interest may induce an overestimation of the myocardial activity. The activity measured over a cardiac region of interest is therefore a crude estimate of the actual activity. For these reasons and to minimize the effects of individual attenuation, cardiac activity has to be normalized to enable comparisons between different subjects. No anatomic structure showing MIBG uptake can be individualized in the upper mediastinum on scintigraphic images, suggesting that this is a nontarget area for MIBG. The upper mediastinum can therefore be used for normalization and cardiac MIBG uptake can be evaluated as a heart to mediastinum activity ratio. Several investigators have used the heart to mediastinum activity ratio as an index of MIBG uptake [7, 30]. Such an index may allow to evaluate a large number of patients with a simple and reproducible test.

Ischemic heart disease

Background

Experimental studies have demonstrated the extensive myocardial catecholamine depletion and the adrenergic denervation in the infarcted area [31–35]. The relationship between alteration of the autonomic nervous system and the mortality in coronary heart disease has been extensively studied [36].

The ability of MIBG scintigraphy to noninvasively map the distribution of sympathetic nerve endings with the simultaneous comparison to regional perfusion has been experimentally validated in dogs [21].

The uptake of both tracers, MIBG and thallium-201, is ATP-dependent [16, 37], but the needed amount of ATP should be different for the myocyte Na-K ATPase and for the neuronal norepinephrine reuptake. Experimental studies [31, 32, 35] demonstrated that myocardial neuronal injury was a two-step process induced by energy deficiency. As a first step, norepinephrine is lost from the storage vesicles, leading to an increase in the axoplasmic concentrations; the second step is the rate-limited transport of intracellular norepinephrine through the cellular membrane by the uptake-1 carrier. After a prolonged period of ischemia, the latter has reversed its normal net transport direction. This phenomenon is likely to occur in patients with chronic coronary artery disease.

MIBG, an analog of guanethidine, shares similar uptake and storage mechanism as norepinephrine. The decrease of MIBG uptake in the ischemic myocardium is likely to be related to the nerve energy deficiency and to the consequent alteration in the uptake-1 function. Acute ischemia as seen in the myocardial areas vascularized by a stenotic vessel, leads to a cathecholamine depletion as a first step, during which the net transport direction of the uptake-1 system is reversed. With the prolongation of ischemia over at least months, the uptake-1 system could be chronically impaired. This phenomenon leads to a low MIBG uptake by the cardiac nerve endings. Sympathetic nerve endings appeared to be more sensitive to ischemia than the myocytes. Denervated myocardium with absent MIBG uptake was shown to be suprasensitive to adrenergic stimulation [38].

In patients, radiolabeled I-123 MIBG has been successfully used for the nuclear imaging of the normal myocardium and of the denervated area after myocardial infarction [2, 39]. Acute effects of ischemia has been studied in animal models with the same imaging technique [38], but the ischemic situation, as seen in patients with chronic coronary artery disease, has not been extensively studied [8, 40, 419.

Prognosis after myocardial infarction is related to the degree of left ventricular dysfunction and the presence of ventricular arrhythmias. Abnormalities in cardiac adrenergic function occur with heart failure and have been implicated as a possible contributing mechanism to arrhythmogenesis [42, 43].

Studies in patients recovering from acute myocardial infarction suggested that the neuronal damage was more extensive than the perfusion defect and was correlated with left ventricular regional wall motion abnormalities or with the occurrence of ventricular arrhythmias.

Information about these chronic ischemic areas could offer new insights on the physiopathology of numerous cardiac disorders. This approach may be a different appreciation of endangered but viable myocardium than the estimation of jeopardized myocardial area by thallium-201 flow imaging.

Clinical studies

In a normal heart, the left ventricle shows a similar and parallel distribution of MIBG and thallium activity, either on planar or on tomographic images [2].

In infarcted patients with a single vessel disease, the same pattern is observed. In these patients, the MIBG uptake by myocardium, after the initial acute global depression, can partially recover after a period of about two months. The extent of the MIBG defect size has been found to be larger than the thallium defect size [8, 39, 40] 2 weeks after infarction. The conclusion of these studies suggested that the myocardial nerve endings were more sensitive than the myocytes to the effect of acute ischemia induced by coronary occlusion.

We have studied 53 pattients, 1 to 3 months after a myocardial infarction. A dual isotope tomographic imaging protocol was used. To obtain extensive data in one day, patients were imaged with thallium alone after intravenous injection of dipyridamole and I-123 MIBG was injected one hour later after completion of the tomographic thallium imaging (Plate 29.2). A significant difference between the uptake of the tracers in the necrotic, ischemic and normal areas was found. The defect sizes were significantly different for post-dipyridamole thallium, for the delayed thallium and for the MIBG images. In few patients, MIBG uptake was higher than delayed thallium uptake in the border zone of the necrotic area and in ischemic area. This higher uptake was not correlated with the presence of a redistribution of thallium-201. The difference in the defect size was smaller than in other studies, suggesting a partial reinnervation as observed in dogs [33]. A mismatch uptake of thallium and MIBG was also found in patients with a remote myocardial infarction and ventricular tachycardia [41]. MIBG myocardial uptake was also found to correlate with left ventricular dysfunction from dilated cardiomyopathies [6, 7] or from infarction [8]. This may be explained in part by the size of the myocardial infarction, since the perfusion defect (thallium) also correlated with the left ventricular dysfunction.

On a clinical point of view, a study using thallium-MIBG imaging can be a powerful tool in making the decision for a mechanical revascularization. Furthermore, the MIBG cardiac imaging, used alone, had also a potent prognostic value [12] in ischemic heart disease.

Primary hypertrophic cardiomyopathy

Primary hypertrophic cardiomyopathy represents a totally different clinical entity from dilated cardiomyopathy, including mainly asymmetric hypertrophy associated with hyperdynamic contractility and diastolic filling abnormalities [44, 45]. Different clinical features may have a prognostic value such as the importance of clinical symptoms, a family history of sudden death, and the importance of hypertrophy and its mechanical consequences, the presence of arrhythmias. However, the prognosis of this disease remains to be defined, especially in individuals.

The pathophysiological importance and the nature of the adrenergic disorders in primary hypertrophic cardiomyopathy is controversial. In animal models, abnormalities of the cardiac adrenergic function includes mostly changes in catecholamine synthesis or turnover, alterations of norepinephrine release or uptake, decreased myocardial catecholamine content and impairment of β-receptor pathways [25, 26, 46]. In humans, conflicting data are available concerning most of these abnormalities. However, a decreased norepinephrine uptake function has been found when using pharmacologic in-vivo techniques [47].

Data from MIBG scintigraphy studies are congruent with this finding, since a significant decrease in the tracer fixation has been evidenced. Tomographic quantitative analysis of MIBG uptake combined with thallium-201 tomographic imaging has suggested that this decrease predominates in the most hypertrophic myocardial area [48]. These findings have provided support for the 'catecholamine hypothesis' of primary hypertrophic cardiomyopathy. Moreover, a link between the severity of the disease and the decrease in MIBG uptake has been suggested [49]. Thus, MIBG scintigraphy could provide helpful information on a clinical and pathophysiological viewpoint. Further study is necessary to determine the prognostic value of MIBG imaging in patients with primary hypertrophic cardiomyopathy.

Conclusion

I-123 MIBG is an example of the potential of radiochemistry applied to nuclear medicine. The noninvasive assessment of the uptake-1 neuronal pathway is a useful tool for physiological and physiopathological studies. In patients with congestive heart failure, MIBG scintigraphy is a simple, reliable means for the prognostic evaluation. Further studies are needed to determine the clinical relevance of MIBG scintigraphy in the other cardiac diseases.

References

1. Sisson JC, Frager MS, Valk TW et al. Scintigraphic localization of pheochromocytoma. N Engl J Med 1981; 305: 12–7.
2. Kline RC, Swanson DP, Wieland DM et al. Myocardial imaging in man with I-123 meta-iodobenzylguanidine. J Nucl Med 1981; 22: 129–32.
3. Likoff MJ, Chandler SL, Kay HR. Clinical determinants of mortality in chronic congestive heart failure secondary to idiopathic cardiomyopathy or to ischemic cardiomyopathy. Am J Cardiol 1987; 59: 634–8.
4. Keogh AM, Freund J, Baron DW, Hickie JB. Timing of cardiac transplantation in idiopathic cardiomyopathy. Am J Cardiol 1988; 61: 418–22.
5. Rabinovitch MA, Rose CP, Rouleau JL et al. Metaiodobenzylguanidine (131I) scintigraphy detects impaired myocardial sympathetic neuronal transport function of canine mechanical-overload heart failure. Circ Res 1987; 61: 797–804.
6. Henderson EB, Kahn JK, Corbett JR et al. Abnormal I-123 myocardial washout and distribution may reflect myocardial adrenergic derangement in patients with congestive cardiomyopathy. Circulation 1988; 78: 1192–9.
7. Schofer J, Spielmann R, Schubert A, Weber K, Schlüter M. Iodine-123 metaiodoben-zylguanidine scintigraphy: a non invasive method to demonstrate myocardial adrenergic system disintegrity in patients with idiopathic dilated cardiomyopathy. J Am Coll Cardiol 1988; 12: 1252–8.
8. McGhie AI, Corbett JR, Akers MS et al. Regional cardiac adrenergic function using I-123 metaiodobenzylguanidine tomographic imaging after acute myocardial infarction. Am J Cardiol 1991; 67: 236–42.
9. Rector TS, Olivari MT, Levine TB, Francis GS, Cohn JN. Predicting survival for an individual with congestive heart failure using the plasma norepinephrine concentration. Am Heart J 1987; 114: 148–52.
10. Cohn JN, Levine TB, Olivari MT et al. Plasma norepinephrine as a guide to prognosis in patients with chronic congestive heart failure. N Engl J Med 1984; 311: 819–23.
11. Fowler MB, Laser JA, Hopkins GL, Minobe W, Bristow MR. Assessment of the adrenergic

receptor pathway in the intact failing human heart: progressive receptor down-regulation and subsensitivity to agonist response. Circulation 1986; 74: 1290–302.

12. Merlet P, Valette H, Dubois-Rande JL et al. Prognostic value of cardiac metaiodoben-zylguanidine imaging in patients with heart failure. J Nucl Med. In press.
13. Wieland DM, Brown LE, Rogers WL et al. Myocardial imaging with a radioiodinated norepinephrine storage analog. J Nucl Med 1981; 22: 22–31.
14. Jaques S Jr, Tobes MC, Sisson JC. Comparison of the sodium dependency of uptake of metaiodobenzylguanidine and norepinephrine into cultured bovine adrenomedullary cells. Mol Pharmacol 1984; 26: 539–46.
15. Sisson JC, Wieland DM, Sherman P, Mangner TJ, Tobes MC, Jaques S Jr. Metaiodoben-zylguanidine as an index of the adrenergic nervous system integrity and function. J Nucl Med 1987; 28: 1620–4.
16. Tobes MC, Jaques S Jr, Wieland DM, Sisson JC. Effect of uptake one inhibitors on the uptake of norepinephrine and metaiodobenzylguanidine. J Nucl Med 1985; 26: 897–907.
17. Gasnier B, Roisin MP, Scherman D, Coornaert S, Desplanches G, Henry JP. Uptake of meta-iodobenzylguanidine by bovine chromaffin granule membranes. Mol Pharmacol 1986; 29: 275–80.
18. Nakajo M, Shimabukuro K, Yoshimura H et al. Iodine-131 metaiodobenzylguanidine intra- and extravesicular accumulation in the rat heart. J Nucl Med 1986; 27: 84–9.
19. Glowniak JV, Turner FE, Palac RT, Lagunas-Solar MC, Woodward WR. Iodine-123 meta-iodobenzylguanidine imaging of the heart in idiopathic congestive cardiomyopathy and cardiac transplants. J Nucl Med 1989; 30: 1182–91.
20. Sisson JC, Shapiro B, Meyers L et al. Metaiodobenzylguanidine to map scintigraphically the adrenergic nervous system in man. J Nucl Med 1987; 28: 1625–36.
21. Dae MW, O'Connell JW, Botvinick EH et al. Scintigraphic assessment of regional cardiac adrenergic innervation. Circulation 1989; 79: 634–44.
22. Rose C, Burgess JH, Cousineau D. Tracer norepinephrine kinetics in coronary circulation of patients with heart failure secondary to chronic pressure and volume overload. J Clin Invest 1985; 76: 1740–7.
23. Sandoval AB, Gilbert EM, Rose CP, Bristow MB. Cardiac norepinephrine uptake and release is decreased in dilated cardiomyopathy [abstract]. Circulation 1989; 80 (4 Suppl II): II 393.
25. Chidsey CA, Braunwald E, Morrow AG. Catecholamine excretion and cardiac stores of norepinephrine in congestive heart failure. Am J Med 1965; 39: 442–51.
26. Spann JF, Chidsey CA, Pool PE, Braunwald E. Mechanism of norepinephrine depletion in experimental heart failure produced by aortic constriction in the guinea pig. Circ Res 1965; 17: 312–21.
27. Merlet P, Dubois-Randé JL, Adnot S et al. Myocardial beta adrenergic desensitization and neuronal norepinephrine uptake function in idiopathic cardiomyopathy. J Cardiovasc Pharmacol 1992; 19: 10–16.
28. Swedberg K, Viquerat C, Rouleau JL et al. Comparison of myocardial catecholamine balance in chronic congestive heart failure and in angina pectoris without failure. Am J Cardiol 1984; 54: 783–6.
29. Hasking GJ, Esler MD, Jenning GL, Burton D, Johns JA, Korner PI. Norepinephrine spillover to plasma in patients with congestive heart failure: evidence of increased overall and cardiorenal sympathetic nervous activity. Circulation 1986; 73: 615–21.
30. Fagret D, Wolf JE, Comet M. Myocardial uptake of meta-(I123)-iodobenzylguanidine (MIBG) in patients with myocardial infarct. Eur J Nucl Med 1989; 15: 624–8.

31. Schömig A, Dart AM, Dietz R, Mayer E, Kübler W. Release of endogenous catecholamines in the ischemic myocardium of the rat. Part A: Locally mediated release. Circ Res 1984; 55: 689–701.

32. Dart A, Schömig A, Dietz R, Mayer E, Kübler W. Release of endogenous catecholamines in the ischemic myocardium of the rat. Part B: Effect of sympathetic nerve stimulation. Circ Res 1984; 55: 702–6.

33. Inoue H, Zipes DP. Time course of denervation of efferent sympathetic and vagal nerves after occlusion of the coronary artery in the canine heart. Circ Res 1988; 62: 1111–20.

34. Wollenberg A, Shahab L. Anoxia-induced release of noradrenaline from the isolated perfused heart. Nature 1965; 207: 88–91.

35. Schömig A, Fischer S, Kurz T, Richardt G, Schömig E. Nonexocytocic release of endogenous noradrenaline in the ischemic and anoxic rat heart: mechanism and metabolic requirements. Circ Res 1987; 60: 194–205.

36. McCance AJ. The autonomic nervous system and mortality in coronary heart disease. CV World Rep 1989; 2: 148–53.

37. Carlin RD, Jan K. Mechanism of thallium extraction in pump perfused canine hearts. J Nucl Med 1985; 26: 165–9.

38. Minardo JD, Tulli MM, Rock BH et al. Scintigraphic and electrophysiological evidence of canine myocardial sympathetic denervation and reinnervation produced by myocardial infarction or phenol application. Circulation 1988; 78: 1008–19.

39. Eisen HJ, Nader RG, Reilley J et al. Assessment of regional myocardial adrenergic activity following myocardial infarction using I-123 metaiodobenzylguanidine [abstract]. Circulation 1989; 80: (4 Suppl II): II 514.

40. Tulli MM, Stanton MS, Mock BH et al. Comparative SPECT I-123-metaiodobenzyl guanidine (MIBG) and thallium 201 (TL) cardiac imaging following myocardial infarction [abstract]. J Nucl Med 1989; 29: 840.

41. Stanton MS, Tulli MM, Radtke NL et al. Regional sympathetic denervation after myocardial infarction in human detected noninvasively using I-123-metaiodobenzylguanidine. J Am Coll Cardiol 1989; 14: 1519–26.

42. Han J, Garcia de Jalon P, Moe GK. Adrenergic effects on ventricular vulnerability. Circ Res 1964; 14: 516–24.

43. Inoue H, Zipes DP. Results of sympathetic denervation in the canine heart: supersensitivity that may be arrhythmogenic. Circulation 1987; 75: 877–87.

44. Wigle ED, Sasson Z, Henderson MA et al. Hypertrophic cardiomyopathy. The importance of the site and the extent of hypertrophy. A review. Prog Cardiovasc Dis 1985; 28: 1–83.

45. Maron BJ, Bonow RO, Cannon RO, Leon MB, Epstein SE. Hypertrophic cardiomyopathy. N Engl J Med 1987; 316: 780–9.

46. Ganguly PK, Lee SL, Beamisch RE, Dhalla NS. Altered sympathetic system and adrenoreceptors during the development of cardiac hypertrophy. Am Heart J 1989; 18: 520–5.

47. Brush JE Jr, Eisenhofer G, Garty M et al. Cardiac norepinephrine kinetics in hypertrophic cardiomyopathy. Circulation 1989; 79: 836–44.

48. Nakajima K, Bunko H, Taki J, Shimizu M, Muramori A, Hisada K. Quantitative analysis of 123I-metaiodobenzylguanidine (MIBG) uptake in hypertrophic cardiomyopathy. Am Heart J 1990; 119: 1329–37.

49. Bourguignon M, Valette H, Merlet P et al. I-123 metaiodobenzylguanidine (MIBG) cardiac imaging as an index of the severity of cardiomyopathies. In: Schmidt HAE, Buraggi GL, editors. Trends and possibilities in nuclear medicine. Stuttgart: Schattauer, 1989: 281–3.

30. Studies of cardiac receptors by positron emission tomography

AREN VAN WAARDE, PAUL K. BLANKSMA,
JOAN G. MEEDER, GERBEN M. VISSER
and WIEK H. VAN GILST

Cardiac receptor imaging: why?

New concepts regarding neurohumoral regulation of cardiac function by myocardial receptors in health and disease have become prominent during the last two decades. Radioligand binding studies have greatly advanced our knowledge of hormone and neurotransmitter binding sites. Changes in the number and/or affinity of cardiac receptors have been assessed by in vitro techniques and shown to be associated with congestive heart failure [1–3], myocardial ischemia and infarction [4–9], cardiomyopathy [10, 11], hypertension [12, 13], chronic drug administration [14–17] and ageing [18]. In vivo assays may improve our understanding of the time course of diseases and enable better prognosis.

Different approaches for the study of myocardial receptors

Cardiac receptors are normally studied in membranes isolated from biopsy material which is collected during surgery and heart catheterization, or acquired post mortem. If biopsies are not available, binding sites on the surface of blood cells are examined. These in vitro methods suffer from the following disadvantages: (1) isolated receptors have lost their relationships with other components of the tissue, so their properties may have been altered or they may correspond to a selective fraction of the total population; (2) the limited size of biopsies makes it possible to detect *global* changes in receptor number but *regional* changes remain elusive; (3) since tissue samples are only taken

Ernst E. van der Wall et al. (eds), What's new in cardiac imaging?, 399–411.

from certain classes of patients, they provide only limited information; (4) alterations in blood cells do not always reflect similar changes in the heart [19–21]; and (5) it is usually impossible to study the relation between receptor occupancy and function.

The development of positron emission tomography (PET) has made it possible to directly measure densities and affinities of receptors in human beings. Selective receptor agonists or antagonists are labeled with carbon-11 (^{11}C) or fluorine-18 (^{18}F) and their regional binding is studied by assessment of the kinetics of association, dissociation and displacement in vivo. PET thus offers the following unique oportunities: (1) receptors are studied in situ in the target organ; (2) relatively detailed information is acquired on their spatial distribution in the heart; (3) many classes of patients can be examined, even healthy volunteers; and (4) the low burden of radiation of short-lived isotopes means that multiple studies are allowed in a single patient. The progress of disease and the influence of therapy may therefore be evaluated which will certainly improve our understanding of the involvement of receptor populations in the pathophysiology and pathogenesis of heart diseases.

Information available from a PET study

A PET camera detects 511 keV gamma radiation which arises when a positron meets an electron and the total mass of the two particles is converted to energy. The fact that two quanta are simultaneously emitted in 180° opposed directions makes it possible to correct for absorption and scattering in the surrounding tissues. PET provides quantitative information on tracer uptake (i.e. binding expressed as pmoles/ml), in contrast to a technique like SPECT where attenuation is not accurately known.

Although the amount of radioactivity in a region of interest can be precisely determined, PET images do not show the molecular form and subcellular localization of the tracer. Drugs are usually rapidly metabolized in vivo. Some metabolites bind to the receptor of interest, whereas others have negligible affinity. Binding can be mainly *specific* (when it occurs as a unique receptor), or *nonspecific* (when it is not receptor-mediated). The ligand and its metabolites may remain outside, but they can also be transported into the cell where they can bind to internalized receptors or other intracellular proteins. Information on these subjects must be obtained before the PET images can be interpreted.

A radiolabeled molecule has to meet several criteria to be a useful PET ligand: (1) uptake by the tissue of interest must be largely due to specific binding (i.e. it must be saturable, stereo-specific, and displaceable); (2) bind-

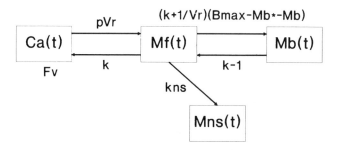

Figure 1. Tracer-kinetic model of the interaction of ¹¹C-MQNB with muscarinic receptors in dog heart. Ca(t) arterial ligand concentration, Mf(t) free ligand in interstitium, Mb(t) ligand bound to receptors, Mns(t) nonspecifically bound ligand, Fv fraction of tissue volume which consists of blood, Vr fraction of tissue volume in which the ligand can interact with receptors. The PET camera measures {Mf(t) + Mb(t) + Mns(t) + Fv.Ca(t)}. Ca(t) is determined by analysis of blood samples. (Reproduced from [22] with permission.)

ing must be to the desired receptor only (e.g. when β-receptors are to be quantified, the compound should not also bind to alpha-adrenergic or dopaminergic sites); (3) the tracer should be rapidly cleared from the circulation to obtain sufficient contrast between tissue and blood; (4) radiolabeled metabolites must be formed slowly (or be absent) and they should not be taken up by the organ under study; and (5) binding must occur with high affinity (K_d $< 10^{-8}$ M) to a signal-transducing site (i.e. displacement of bound radioactivity by a drug should produce a physiological effect).

After biodistribution studies and preliminary PET experiments on animals have shown that these basic conditions are sufficiently fulfilled, it remains necessary to develop a suitable protocol for tracer injection and a mathematical model of the ligand-receptor interaction in vivo. A large number of receptors with low affinity or a small number of high-affinity binding sites may result in a similar amount of bound radioactivity in the heart. Low uptake in a certain region may be due to a reduced number of receptors, but also to reduced blood flow. The injection protocol and the tracer-kinetic model must be carefully designed (using pilot studies on animals and computer simulations) so that such ambiguities of interpretation are avoided.

The models used in PET studies of receptors usually consist of 2–4 compartments (e.g. ligand in arterial blood, ligand in the interstitial fluid, ligand bound to receptors and nonspecifically bound ligand, see Figure 1). Exchange between the compartments is described by a set of differential equations. The PET camera measures the 'tissue response', i.e. the time course of radioactivity in a selected region of the heart, which comprises specifically and nonspecifically bound tracers, tracer in the insterstitium and in plasma, since a significant fraction of the observed volume consists of blood. The time course of the arterial ligand concentration (the 'input function' of the model) is determined by measuring the amount of radioactivity and the percentage of unmetabolized tracer in arterial plasma.

A typical PET experiment consists of 1–3 injections of the ligand at different specific activities, combined with analysis of blood samples and observation of the tissue response. The mathematical model is then solved by a computer using the measured input function. The model parameters (i.e. the values of k, k_{+1}, k_{-1}, k_{ns}) are adjusted via an iterative search procedure and a nonlinear regression program until the predicted response fits the data observed by the PET camera.

As one might expect, a relationship exists between the complexity of model and experimental protocol. A model with many parameters also requires multiple tracer injections [23, 24]. When the protocol does not produce enough perturbations of the system, most parameters are unidentifiable, or there are several solutions which all produce an acceptable fit of the PET data. Careful experimental design must result in a unique solution of the model and a sufficiently accurate estimation of the parameters of interest.

Cardiac receptors studied by PET

Beta-adrenergic receptors

Beta-receptors are involved in the positive regulation of coronary blood flow, cardiac rate, and contractile force via a stimulatory G-protein and adenylate cyclase. The natural ligands (catecholamines: noradrenaline and adrenaline) are neurotransmitters of the sympathetic nervous system and are also produced by the adrenal glands in 'stress, fight, and flight' situations. Myocardial β-adrenoreceptors can be classified in at least two subtypes: the $β_1$ which are mainly found on myocytes, and the $β_2$ which are predominantly localized in smooth muscle cells. $β_1$-adrenoreceptors are the major subclass in the human heart [25], although a relative high proportion of $β_2$-receptors (up to 50%) is also present [26]. Controversies exist regarding the relative amount of both subtypes, especially in disease. Congestive heart failure is accompanied by high circulating levels of endogenous noradrenaline [27] and this heightened activity of the adrenergic system seems to be associated with a loss (down-regulation) of postsynaptic β-receptors [28]. On the contrary, treatment with β-blocking agents causes up-regulation [16, 17]. Up- and down-regulation may be considered as adaptive mechanisms which enable the cell to amplify or attenuate its response upon prolonged exposure to an agonist or antagonist. PET studies may elucidate the physiological significance of these regulatory processes and they may answer the question whether only β_1, or β_1 and β_2-receptors are progressively down-regulated during heart failure. PET may also assist in drug design, since the time course of receptor occupancy by unlabeled compounds can be assessed in vivo [29].

As shown in Table I, several commercially available β-blockers have been labeled with ^{11}C but most of these do not meet the criteria for a good PET ligand. The most promising agent for β-receptor imaging seems to be CGP 12177, an experimental drug produced by Ciba-Geigy. This ligand only binds to receptors on the cell surface [30], it produces clear images of the heart [31], its accumulation is saturable and displacement by unlabeled pindolol is accompanied by a decrease of the heart rate [31]. Biodistribution studies in rats confirm that cardiac uptake is largely ($>85\%$) receptor-mediated and stable for extended periods of time (>20 min), whereas the clearance from plasma is extremely rapid [32–34]. Metabolites of CGP-12177 are not taken up by the heart [34, 35], which facilitates interpretation of the PET data. A simple graphical method for the measurement of myocardial β-receptor density in dogs has been published, using a racemic mixture of ^{11}C-CGP 12177 and a triple injection protocol [36]. Clinical studies therefore seem within reach, but considerable research efforts are still directed towards the synthesis of the pure S($-$)isomer of ^{11}C-CGP 12177 which may metabolize more slowly than the racemate and may enable tracer-kinetic modeling in vivo [37]. Biodistribution studies with a β_1-selective ligand, CGP 26505, in our laboratory indicate that it is more lipophilic than CGP 12177, resulting in higher nonspecific binding [34]. We are now evaluating both ligands for use in humans.

Table I. Positron-emitting beta-adrenoreceptor ligands.

Compound	Subtype	Perspectives for cardiac imaging	Refs.
Atenolol	β_1	Affinity for binding site too low	[38]
Carazolol	β	Meets some criteria for useful ligand	[39, 40]
Metoprolol	β_1	Affinity for binding site too low	[38]
Pindolol	β	Meets some criteria for useful ligand	[41, 42]
Practolol	β_1	Affinity for binding site too low	[43]
Propranolol	β	Heart invisible due to uptake in lungs	[38, 44]
CGP 12177	β	Meets most criteria for useful ligand	[33, 45]
CGP 26505	β_1	Meets some criteria for useful ligand	[34]

All compounds have been labeled with ^{11}C, but ^{18}F analogs of carazolol and pindolol have also been prepared.

Sympathetic innervation

The interaction between neurotransmitter and receptor leads to a cascade of molecular events via the second messenger system, resulting in the physiological response. However, there is also a complex sequence of events that takes place within the nerve terminal and in the synaptic space. It includes synthesis and release of the neurotransmitter, binding to receptors, hydrolysis of the neurotransmitter in the synaptic cleft, and neurotransmitter reuptake. These mechanisms might be better understood if one could measure sympathetic function in vivo. Clinical interest stems also from the fact that injury to adrenergic neuron terminals without injury to postsynaptic β-receptors predisposes to arrhythmias [46, 47].

The sympathetic innervation of the heart and the functioning of the neurotransmitter reuptake system may be visualized after injection of radiolabeled catecholamine analogs. Three of these compounds have been thoroughly characterized: 6-fluorometaraminol (FMR, [46–51]), *m*-hydroxyephedrine (HED, [52–56]) and 6-fluorodopamine (FD, [57–58[). All behave like 'false neurotransmitters', which are transported by the same carrier and stored in the same vesicles as authentic noradrenaline. Their accumulation in the heart is blocked by inhibitors of the noradrenaline carrier and vesicular catecholamine storage [48, 49, 52, 53, 57]. Regional uptake is reduced when adrenergic neurons are destroyed by toxic drugs [47–49, 53] or an ischemic insult [50], and is closely related to the local noradrenaline concentration in the myocardium [47, 48, 53]. Uptake is virtually absent in denervated transplanted hearts [55]and inhomogeneous in patients suffering from dilated cardiomyopathy [56]. The compunds can therefore be used to image sympathetic nerve endings in vivo.

Since the specific activity of ^{18}F-FMR is < 10 Ci/mmol, injection of a measurable amount of radioactivity produces pharmacological effects. FMR therefore cannot be used for clinical studies [47]. HED can be prepared with high specific activity [52], but its rapid metabolism complicates quantitative imaging [54]. FD is a unique drug because it is not only taken up by neurons and stored in synaptic vesicles, but also released from nerve endings when the sympathicus is activated [57]. FD can therefore be used to measure the turnover rate of endogenous noradrenaline and it may be administered to humans at specific activities > 2000 Ci/mmol [58].

Alpha-adrenergic receptors

Alpha-receptors are present on cardiac myocytes and vascular smooth muscle cells. Alpha-agonists cause smooth muscle contraction, leading to vasoconstriction, increased vascular resistance, and a rise of blood pressure. The receptors can be divided in an α_1 subtype which binds the antagonist prazosin, and an α_2 type which binds yohimbine. Myocardial alpha-adrenoreceptors are mainly of the α_1 type and their stimulation causes a (relatively small) increase of the contractile force of the heart due to increased calcium influx across the sarcolemma, in contrast to the large β-effect which is mediated by an increase of myocardial cAMP. The responses to α-agonists are markedly reduced in myocytes of the failing heart, but there is no evidence of α_1-receptor down-regulation [1]. Although α-adrenergic vasoconstriction seems to be involved in the initiation and aggravation of myocardial ischemia, the precise role of α-receptors in coronary vessels remains to be established. PET studies may significantly contribute to our knowledge in this field.

[11]C-Prazosin has been prepared but the ligand is unsuitable due to high nonspecific binding in vivo [59]. No other α-specific imaging agents are available at the time of writing.

Muscarinic cholinergic receptors

Parasympathetic nerves innervating the heart release acetylcholine, which exerts negative inotropic and chronotropic effects via muscarinic receptors. The sympathetic and parasympathetic control systems enable rapid and reversible alteration of cardiac performance to meet variations in demand. Muscarinic receptors can be classified into at least two subtypes: M_1 and M_2. M_1-receptors are primarily located in the CNS, whereas M_2-receptors are found in peripheral effector organs like the heart. The density and affinity of M_2 receptors have been reported to be altered during ischemia, changes of thyroid status, heart failure, diabetes, and ageing. PET now makes it possible to investigate such processes in vivo [60].

[11]C-methyl quinuclidinyl benzilate (MQNB) is the only ligand which has been thoroughly characterized. This compound binds in a saturable and stereospecific fashion to a physiologically active site in the human heart [60–63]. Syrota and co-workers have developed a quadruple injection protocol and a tracer-kinetic model which enable quantification of cardiac muscarinic receptors in dogs [22]. They expect that a simplified protocol using two injections will be sufficient to measure M_2 receptors in humans. A preliminary study has indicated that MQNB-PET can detect changes of receptor density caused by hyper- or hypothyroidism [64].

Benzodiazepine receptors

Benzodiazepine receptors can be classified in a central subtype which binds clonazepam and Ro-15-1788, and a peripheral type which binds PK 11195 and Ro 5-4864. The central type is limited to the CNS, whereas the peripheral type occurs in kidney, liver, skeletal, and smooth muscles, lung, heart, and glia. The function of cardiac benzodiazepine receptors is poorly understood, but they are known to be coupled to Ca^{2+}-channels and their antagonists counteract the effect of calcium channel blockers [65].

Three ligands are available for PET imaging of peripheral benzodiazepine sites: ^{11}C-PK 11195 [65–67], ^{18}F-PK 14105 [68], and ^{11}C-Ro 5-4864 [69]. Only the in vivo binding of PK 11195 has been thoroughly characterized. Binding of the compound in dog heart is saturable, displacable by the proper antagonists, and it takes place to receptors which are physiologically active [65]. The use of PET and PK 11195 may thus enable investigation of benzodiazepine receptor function in the human heart.

Histamine receptors

The positive effect of histamine on the rate and contractile force of the heart is mediated by H_2 receptors in both ventricles. Thus far, there have been few attempts to visualize these binding sites by PET. The H_2 antagonist ranitidine has been labeled with ^{11}C and is now under study [70].

Adenosine receptors

Adenosine has negative inotropic and chronotropic effects in the heart which are probably mediated by myocardial A1 receptors. ^{11}C-cyclopentyltheophylline and a fluorinated methylxanthine, ^{18}F-FMB-XCC, are currently tested as A1 ligands [71, 72].

Inhibitors of angiotensin-converting enzyme (ACE)

The renin-angiotensin system plays a major role in the pathogenesis of congestive heart failure, the local regulation of vascular tone and the development of arterial wall hypertrophy in normal and pathological conditions. The synthesis of ^{18}F-captopril has been reported and this compound may prove to be useful for imaging of the local ACE concentration which is hard to assess by any alternative method [73].

Conclusion

Quantitative imaging of cardiac receptors is a rapidly expanding field. Research on the β-adrenergic and cholinergic systems seems to have progressed to the point that clinical studies will soon be feasible. In other cases, the search for suitable ligands continues, and a workable injection protocol and tracer-kinetic model must still be developed to enable quantitation of receptor density and affinity. There is a large scope for fundamental research in this area but major developments can be expected during this decade.

Acknowledgement

Aren van Waarde was supported by a grant from the Inter-University Cardiological Institute of the Netherlands (ICIN).

References

1. Bristow MR, Minobe W, Rasmussen R, Hershberger RE, Hoffman BB. Alpha-1 adrenergic receptors in the nonfailing and failing human heart. J Pharmacol Exp Ther 1988; 247: 1039–45.
2. Bristow MR, Ginsburg R, Umans V et al. β_1 and β_2-adrenergic subpopulations in nonfailing and failing human ventricular myocardium: coupling of both receptor subtypes to muscle contraction and selective β_2 receptor downregulation in heart failure. Circ Res 1986; 59: 297–309.
3. Brodde OE, Zerkowski HR, Borst HG, Maier W, Michel MC. Drug- and disease-induced changes of human cardiac β_1 and β_2 adrenoreceptors. Eur Heart J 1989; 10 (Suppl B): 38–44.
4. Mukherjee A, Bush LR, McCoy KE et al. Relationship between beta-adrenergic receptor numbers and physiological responses during experimental canine myocardial ischemia. Circ Res 1982; 50: 735–41.
5. Maisel AS, Motulsky HJ, Insel PA. Externalization of beta-adrenergic receptors promoted by myocardial ischemia. Science 1985; 230: 183–6.
6. Strasser RH, Krimmer J, Marquetant R. Regulation of beta-adrenergic receptors: impaired desensitization in myocardial ischemia. J Cardiovasc Pharmacol 1988; 12: S15–S24.
7. Mukherjee A, Wong TM, Buja LM et al. Beta-adrenergic and muscarinic cholinergic receptors in canine myocardium. Effects of ischemia. J Clin Invest 1979; 64: 1423–8.
8. Ohyanagi M, Matsumori Y, Iwasaki T. Beta-adrenergic receptors in ischemic and non-ischemic canine myocardium: relation to ventricular fibrillation and effects of pretreatment with propranolol and hexamethonium. J Cardiovasc Pharmacol 1988; 11: 107–14.
9. Freissmuth M, Schutz W, Weindlmayer-Gottel N et al. Effects of ischemia on the canine myocardial beta-adrenoreceptor-linked adenylate cyclase system. J Cardiovasc Pharmacol 1987; 10: 568–74.
10. Amorim DS, Heer K, Jenner D et al. Is there autonomic impairment in congestive (dilated) cardiomyopathy? Lancet 1981; 1: 525–7.
11. Amorim DS, Olsen EGJ. Assessment of heart neurons in dilated (congestive) cardiomyopathy. Br Heart J 1982; 47: 11–8.
12. Yamada S, Ishima T, Tomita T, Hayashi T, Okada T, Hayashi E. Alterations in cardiac

alpha- and beta-adrenoreceptors during the development of spontaneous hypertension. J Pharmacol Exp Ther 1984; 228: 454–9.

13. Hurwitz ML, Rosendorff C. Cardiovascular adrenoreceptor number and function in experimental hypertension in the baboon. J Cardiovasc Pharmacol 1985; 7 (Suppl 6): S172–7.

14. Kenakin TP, Beek D. In vitro studies on the cardiac activity of prenalterol with reference to its use in congestive heart failure. J Pharmacol Exp Ther 1982; 220: 77–85.

15. Gengo P, Skattebol A, Moran JF, Gallant S, Hawthorn M, Triggle DJ. Regulation by chronic drug administration of neuronal and cardiac calcium channel, beta-adrenoreceptor and muscarinic receptor levels. Biochem Pharmacol 1988; 37: 627–33.

16. Golf S, Hansson V. Effects of beta blocking agents on the density of beta-adrenoreceptors and adenylate cyclase response in human myocardium: intrinsic sympathomimetic activity favours receptor regulation. Cardiovasc Res 1986; 20: 637–44.

17. van den Meiracker AH, in 't Veld AJ, Boomsma F, Fischberg DJ, Molinoff PB, Schalekamp MADH. Hemodynamic and beta-adrenergic receptor adaptations during long-term beta-adrenoreceptor blockade. Circulation 1989; 80: 903–14.

18. Narayanan N, Derby J. Effects of age on muscarinic cholinergic receptors in rat myocardium. Can J Physiol Pharmacol 1983; 61: 822–9.

19. Michel MC, Beckeringh JJ, Ikezono K, Kretsch R, Brodde OE. Lymphocyte beta-2 adrenoreceptors mirror precisely beta-2-adrenoreceptor, but poorly beta-1 adrenoreceptor changes in the human heart. J Hypertens 1986; 4 (Suppl 6): S215–S218.

20. Maisel AS, Ziegler MG, Carter S, Insel PA, Motulsky HJ. In vivo regulation of beta-adrenergic receptors on mononuclear leukocytes and heart. Assessment of receptor compartmentation after agonist infusion and acute aortic constriction in guinea pigs. J Clin Invest 1988; 82: 2038–44.

21. Maisel AS, Phillips C, Michel MC, Ziegler MG, Carter SC. Regulation of cardiac beta-adrenergic receptors by captopril. Implications for congestive heart failure. Circulation 1989; 80: 669–75.

22. Delforge J, Janier M, Syrota A et al. Noninvasive quantification of muscarinic receptors in vivo with positron emission tomography in the dog heart. Circulation 1990; 2: 1494–504.

23. Delforge J, Syrota A, Mazoyer BM. Experimental design optimisation: theory and application to estimation of receptor model parameters using dynamic positron emission tomography. Phys Med Biol 1989; 34: 419–35.

24. Delforge J, Syrota A, Mazoyer BM. Identifiability analysis and parameter identification of an in vivo ligand-receptor model from PET data. IEEE Trans Biomed Engin 1990; 37: 653–61.

25. Heitz A, Schwartz J, Velly J. β-adrenoreceptors of the human myocardium: determination of β_1 and β_2 subtypes by radioligand binding. Br J Pharmacol 1983; 80: 711–7.

26. Robberecht P, Delhaye M, Taton G et al. The human heart β-adrenergic receptors I. Heterogeneity of the binding sites. Presence of 50% β_1- and 50% β_2-adrenergic receptors. Mol Pharmacol 1983; 24: 169–73.

27. Cohn JN, Levine TB, Olivari MT et al. Plasma norepinephrine as a guide to prognosis in patients with chronic congestive heart failure. N Engl J Med 1984; 311: 819–23.

28. Bristow MR, Ginsburg R, Minobe W et al. Decreased catecholamine sensitivity and β-adrenergic receptor density in failing human hearts. N Engl J Med 1982; 307: 205–11.

29. Wagner HN. Positron emission tomography in assessment of regional stereospecificity of drugs. Biochem Pharmacol 1988; 37: 51–9.

30. Staehelin M, Hertel C. [^{3}H] CGP-12177, a β-adrenergic ligand suitable for measuring cell surface receptors. J Receptor Res 1983; 3: 35–43.

31. Seto M, Syrota A, Crouzel C et al. Beta-adrenergic receptors in the dog heart characterized by ^{11}C-CGP 12177 and PET [abstract]. J Nucl Med 1986; 27: 949.

32. Law MP, Burgin J. Evaluation of CGP-12177 for characterization of β-adrenergic receptors by PET: in vivo studies in rat [abstract]. J Nucl Med 1989; 30: 766–7.

33. Law MP. Characterization of β-adrenoreceptors in vivo using [³H]CGP-12177. In: Szabadi E, Bradshaw CM, editors. Pharmacology of adrenoreceptors. Basel: Birkhauser Verlag, 1990: 7–8.

34. Van Waarde A, Meeder JG, Blanksma PK et al. Suitability of CGP 12177 and CGP 26505 for quantitative imaging of β-adrenoceptors. Nucl Med Biol (Submitted).

35. Delforge J, Nakajima K, Syrota A et al. PET investigation of β-adrenergic receptors using CGP 12177 [abstract]. J Nucl Med 1989; 30: 825.

36. Delforge J, Syrota A, Lançon JP et al. Cardiac β-adrenergic receptor density measured in vivo using PET, CGP 12177, and a new graphical method. J Nucl Med 1991; 32: 739–48.

37. Brady F, Luthra SK, Tochon-Danguy H et al. Towards a chiral precursor for the automated radiosynthesis of carbon-11 labelled S-CGP 12177 [abstract]. J Label Compounds Radiopharm 1991; 30: 251.

38. Antoni G, Ulin J, Långström B. Synthesis of the ¹¹C-labelled β-adrenergic receptor ligands atenolol, metoprolol and propranolol. Int J Appl Radiat Isotop 1989; 40: 561–4.

39. Berridge MS, Terris AH, Vesselle JM. [C-11]-carazolol: Synthesis and biodistribution of a ligand for imaging beta-adrenergic receptors [abstract]. J Nucl Med 1991; 32: 1097.

40. Kinsey BM, Tewson TJ. Fluorine-18 fluoroalkyl derivatives of carazolol: Potential ligands for the in vivo studies of the β-adrenergic receptor [abstract]. J Label Compounds Radiopharm 1991; 30: 385–6.

41. Prenant C, Sastre J, Crouzel C, Syrota A. Synthesis of ¹¹C-pindolol. J Label Compounds Radiopharm 1987; 24: 227–32.

42. Tewson TJ, Kinsey BM, Franceschini MP. Synthesis of fluorine-18 fluoroalkyl pindolol derivatives: ligands for the β-adrenergic receptor [abstract]. J Label Compounds Radiopharm 1991; 30: 385–6.

43. Berger G, Prenant C, Sastre J, Syrota A, Comar D. Synthesis of a β blocker for heart visualization: [¹¹C]Practolol. Int J Appl Radiat Isotop 1983; 34: 1556–7.

44. Berger G, Mazière M, Prenant C, Sastre J, Syrota A, Comar D. Synthesis of ¹¹C-propranolol. J Radioanal Chem 1982; 74: 301.

45. Boullais C, Crouzel C, Syrota A. Synthesis of 4-(3-t-butylamino--2-hydroxypropoxy)--benzimidazol-2-(¹¹C)-one (CPG 12177). J Label Compounds Radiopharm 1986; 23: 565–7.

46. Sisson JC, Wieland DM, Johnson JW et al. Scintigraphy of adrenergic receptors and neurons in myocardial infarcts [abstract]. J Nucl Med 1989; 30: 767.

47. Wieland DM, Rosenspire KC, Hutchins GD et al. Neuronal mapping of the heart with 6-[¹⁸F]fluorometaraminol. J Med Chem 1990; 33: 956–64.

48. Wieland DM, Rosenspire KC, Hutchins GD, Schwaiger M. Validation of 6-[¹⁸F] fluorometaraminol (FMR) for positron tomography [abstract]. Circulation 1988; 78 (Suppl 2): 598.

49. Mislankar SG, Gildersleeve DL, Wieland DM, Massin CC, Mulholland GK, Toorongian SA. 6-[¹⁸F] Fluorometaraminol: a radiotracer for in vivo mapping of adrenergic nerves of the heart. J Med Chem 1988; 31: 362–6.

50. Schwaiger M, Guibourg H, Rosenspire KC et al. Effect of regional myocardial ischemia on sympathetic nervous system as assessed by fluorine-18-metaraminol. J Nucl Med 1990; 31: 1352–7.

51. Rosenspire KC, Gildersleeve DL, Massin CC, Mislankar SG, Wieland DM. Metabolic fate of the heart agent [¹⁸F]6-fluorometaraminol. Nucl Med Biol 1989; 16: 735–9.

52. Rosenspire KC, Haka MS, Van Dort ME et al. Synthesis and preliminary evaluation of carbon-11-meta-hydroxyephedrine: A false transmitter agent for heart neuronal imaging. J Nucl Med 1990; 31: 1328–34.

53. Wieland DM, Hutchins GD, Rosenspire KC et al. [C-11]hydroxyephedrine (HED): A high specific activity alternative to 6-[F-18]fluorometaraminol (FMR) for heart neuronal imaging. J Nucl Med 1989; 30: 767–9.

54. Wieland DM, Rosenspire KC, Van Dort ME, Haka MS, Jung YW, Gildersleeve DL. Search for a non-metabolizable PET tracer for heart neuronal imaging [abstract]. J Label Compounds Radiopharm 1991; 30: 283.

55. Schwaiger M, Kalff V, Rosenspire KC et al. Noninvasive evaluation of sympathetic nervous system in human heart by positron emission tomography. Circulation 1990; 82: 457–64.

56. Schwaiger M, Hutchins G, Rosenspire KC, Haka M, Wieland DM. Quantitative evaluation of the sympathetic nervous system by PET in patients with cardiomyopathy [abstract]. J Nucl Med 1990; 31: 792.

57. Goldstein DS, Chang PC, Eisenhofer G et al. Positron emission tomographic imaging of cardiac sympathetic innervation and function. Circulation 1990; 81: 1606–21.

58. Ding YS, Fowler JS, Gatley SJ, Dewey SL, Wolf AP, Schlyer DJ. Synthesis of high specific activity 6-[^{18}F]fluorodopamine for positron emission tomography studies of sympathetic nervous tissue. J Med Chem 34: 861–3.

59. Ehrin E, Luthra SK, Crouzel C, Pike VW. Preparation of carbon-11 labelled prazosin, a potent and selective alpha$_1$-adrenoreceptor antagonist. J Label Compounds Radiopharm 1988; 25: 177–83.

60. Mazière M, Comar D, Godot JM, Collard P, Cepeda C, Naquet R. In vivo characterization of myocardium muscarinic receptors by positron emission tomography. Life Sci 1981; 29: 2391–7.

61. Syrota A, Dormont D, Berger A et al. C-11 ligand binding to adrenergic and muscarinic receptors of the human heart studied in vivo by PET [abstract]. J Nucl Med 1983; 24: P20.

62. Syrota A, Paillotin G, Davy JM, Aumont MC. Kinetics of in vivo binding of antagonist to muscarinic cholinergic receptor in the human heart studied by positron emission tomography. Life Sci 1984; 35: 937–45.

63. Syrota A, Comar D, Paillotin G et al. Muscarinic cholinergic receptor in the human heart evidenced under physiological conditions by positron emission tomography. Proc Natl Acad Sci USA 1985; 82: 584–8.

64. Syrota A, Le Guludec D, Prenant C et al. PET investigation of myocardial muscarinic cholinergic acetylcholine receptor in patients with hyper- and hypothyroidism [abstract]. J Nucl Med 1988; 29: 808.

65. Charbonneau P, Syrota A, Crouzel C, Valois JM, Prenant C, Crouzel M. Peripheral-type benzodiazepine receptors in the living heart characterized by positron emission tomography. Circulation 1986; 73: 476–83.

66. Camsonne R, Crouzel C, Comar D et al. Synthesis of N-(^{11}C)-methyl,N-(methyl-1--propyl),(chloro-2-phenyl)-1-isoquinoline carboxamide-3 (PK 11195). A new ligand for peripheral benzodiazepine receptors. J Label Compounds Radiopharm 1984; 21: 985–91.

67. Hashimoto K, Inoue O, Suzuki K, Yamasaki T, Kojima M. Synthesis and evaluation of ^{11}C-PK 11195 for in vivo study of peripheral-type benzodiazepine receptors using positron emission tomography. Ann Nucl Med 1989; 3: 63–71.

68. Pascali C, Luthra SK, Pike VW et al. The radiosynthesis of [^{18}F]PK 14105 as an alternative radioligand for peripheral-type benzodiazepine binding sites. Int J Rad Appl Instrum [A] 1990; 41: 477–82.

69. Watkins GL, Jewett DM, Mudholland GK, Kilbourn MR, Toorongian SA. A captive solvent method for rapid N-[^{11}C]methylation of secondary amides: application to the benzodiazepine, 4'-chlorodiazepam (Ro 5-4864). Int J Rad Appl Instrum [A] 1988; 39: 441–4.

70. Le Breton C, Crouzel C. Synthesis of [^{11}C]ranitidine: a potential PET imaging agent for H2 receptors in heart. J Label Compounds Radiopharm 1991; 30: 256–7.

71. Yorke JC, Prenant C, Crouzel C. Synthesis of carbon-11 labelled cyclopentyltheophylline: a radioligand for PET studies of adenosine receptors. J Label Compounds Radiopharm 1991; 30: 262–3.

72. Channing MA, Dunn BB, Boring DL, Jacobson KA. Development of a F-18 labeled antagonist for the AI adenosine receptor [abstract]. J Label Compounds Radiopharm 1991; 30: 244.

73. Hwang DR, Mathias CJ, Welch MJ, Lloyd J, Petrillo EW, Eckelman WC. Synthesis and biodistribution of [F-18]-labeled angiotensin converting enzyme inhibitor [F-18]fluorocaptopril [abstract]. J Nucl Med 1990; 31: 738.

31. Heart neuronal imaging with carbon-11- and fluorine-18-labeled tracers

DONALD M. WIELAND

Introduction

Radiotracers for positron emission tomographic (PET) studies of cardiac nerve integrity and function have been developed only within the past four years [1–8]. The first clinical PET studies were reported in 1990 [9, 10]. This chapter will discuss the design considerations that led to presently available neuronal tracers and will comment briefly on possible future directions in this area of research.

Autonomic nervous system of the heart

The autonomic or involuntary nervous system consists of two divisions, the sympathetic and parasympathetic. These two nerve divisions, compared in Table 1, are also referred to as the adrenergic and cholinergic divisions based on their respective transmitters norepinphrine (NE) and acetylcholine (ACh). The sympathetic nerves approach the heart along the anterior great vessels, course into the epicardium, and then penetrate gradually into the underlying endocardium as they descend towards the apex in much the same fashion as do the coronary vessels [11]. Based mainly on tissue NE measurements, the mammalian heart has been shown to have a dense network of adrenergic nerves with atria >> right ventricle > left ventricle [12–14]. Within the left ventricle itself, the base is 1.5–3 times more innervated than the apex. An average adrenergic neuron has approximately 100 mm of terminal axon with about 25,000 varicosities; each varicosity contains an estimated 250 pg of NE [15].

413

Ernst E. van der Wall et al. (eds), What's new in cardiac imaging?, 413–426.
© *1992 Kluwer Academic Publishers. Printed in the Netherlands.*

In contrast to their rich adrenergic innervation, the ventricles of the heart have sparse cholinergic innervation. Although adrenergic and cholinergic nerve fibers are sometimes closely apposed in the heart and may share a common Schwann sheath, surgical and regional chemical denervation studies [16] suggest that most of the efferent cholinergic nerves servicing the ventricles pass through the superficial layers of the atrioventricle groove and then dive deeper into the walls of the left ventricle [17, 18]. Sympathetic nerves of the ventricles tend to travel in the epicardium, but the parasympathetic nerves generally course deeper into the endocardium. Choline acetyltransferase (ChAT) concentrations indicate that cholinergic nerve density in the heart also decreases in the order atria $>>$ right ventricle $>$ left ventricle with the highest focal concentrations in the sinoatrial and atrioventricular nodes [19–22].

The authonomic nervous system is characterized by the reciprocity of its two divisions [23]. This chemical reciprocity subserves opposing physiological roles in heart regulation; the adrenergic nerves stimulate, the cholinergic nerves inhibit. Interaction occurs at both the neuronal and posynaptic membranes. The major post-junctional interaction has usually been thought to occur through adenylyl cyclase with sympathetic activity stimulating a rise in intracellular levels of cyclic AMP, and cholinergic activity stimulating a decrease [23]. In short, the agonist action of ACh on postsynaptic muscarinic receptors is thought to attenuate the rise in cyclic AMP that would otherwise be induced by the concurrent action of NE on the beta adrenergic receptors. Recent work using inside-out membrane patches of sinoatrial node cells suggests that, at least in the pacemaker cells, the adrenergic and cholinergic receptors are directly coupled to current channels by G protein [24]. By not utilizing second messengers such as cyclic AMP, these two postsynaptic receptor systems are able to modulate the nervous system within a single heartbeat.

Table 1. General characteristics of autonomic nerves of heart.

	Adrenergic	Cholinergic
Transmitter	NE	ACh
Density	high	low
Pattern	diffuse	focal
LV Locus	epicardium	endocardium
Marker	NE	ChAT
Uptake system	nonselective	selective
Action	stimulatory	inhibitory
Termination of action	reuptake by uptake-1	hydrolysis by ACh esterase

Mapping the adrenergic neurons of the heart

The availability of high specific activity [3H]-norepinephrine in the late 1950's opened the way for the first physiologically relevant studies of the in vivo fate of this catecholamine. Pioneering work by Axelrod demonstrated that intravenous [^{3}H]norepinephrine rapidly disappears from the circulation and is avidly sequestered by sympathetic nerves in the heart and other peripheral tissues [25]. Up to 60% of injected tracer localizes in peripheral tissues mainly as unchanged norepinephrine [26]. Thus, it became evident nearly 30 years ago that sympathetic nerves not only synthesize and release norepinephrine, but they also take up and store it as well. In healthy heart tissue the adrenergic neurons synthesize most of the norepinephrine needed for signal transmission [27]. It has been estimated that approximately 80% of endogenous norepinephrine in mammalian heart originates from synthesis within this organ [28].

The uptake of NE into the sympathetic nerve ending is by means of an ATP-requiring amine pump located in the plasma membrane. This amine pump, the uptake-1 carrier, transports NE into the cytosol of the nerve terminal where it rapidly enters the synaptic vesicles via an energy-requiring transporter located on the vesicle membrane. A comparison of the major features of the uptake-1 and vesicular transport systems is presented in Table 2. Stored within the confines of the vesicle, NE is protected from metabolic degradation by mitochondrial monoamine oxidase (MAO) and packaged for quantal release in response to nerve impulse. The rapid removal of cytosolic NE by the storage vesicles in effect lowers the concentration gradient of NE across the plasma membrane of the neuron thus amplifying the overall uptake process.

Advances in the 1970's in carbon-11 ($T_{1/2} = 20$ min) chemistry especially with [^{11}C]cyanide, were applied to the synthesis of racemic [^{11}C]norepinephrine [29]. The first in vivo image of mammalian heart based on adrenergic

Table 2. Comparison of adrenergic uptake systems.

		Uptake$_1$	Uptake$_2$	Vesicular
Locus		neuronal	extraneuronal	intraneuronal
L-NE	Km	0.27 μM	252 μM	5.3 μM
	V$_{max}$	1.18 nmol/min/g	100	870
Inhibitors		desipramine	phenoxybenzamine	reserpine
		cocaine	steroid hormones	tetrabenazine
Major function		terminate signal	metabolism	storage, synthesis
Energy required		yes	no	yes
Stereo-specificity		yes	no	yes

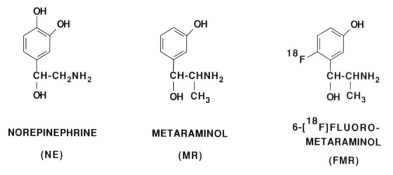

Figure 1. Chemical structures of adrenergic neuron markers.

nerve accumulation of a radiotracer was accomplished with this radiotracer in 1976 [30]. Labeled on the alpha carbon by synthetic incorporation of [^{11}C]cyanide, racemic [^{11}C]norepinephrine provided planar images of the dog heart using a standard gamma camera. PET imaging systems were in their infancy at the time so tomographic neuronal imaging of the heart would be delayed for another decade when commercial whole body PET imaging systems became available.

Initial efforts at the University of Michigan to develop adrenergic neuronal mapping agents focused on the false neurotransmitter metaraminol, a phenolamine and close structural analog of NE (Figure 1). Metaraminol is a high affinity substrate for the amine pump [31]; in addition, its quantitation in tissue or perfused organ preparations is not complicated by metabolism. The metabolic refractoriness of metaraminol relative to NE is due to the presence of the alpha methyl group which effectively blocks the action of monoamine oxidase (MAO), and to the absence of a catechol group which confers resistance to catechol-O-methyltransferase (COMT). Once in the cytoplasm, metaraminol is cosequestered with NE in the synaptic vesicles. Upon nerve impulse, both NE and metaraminol are released by exocytosis [32]. There has been controversy over the time course, extent, and mechanism by which metaraminol is sequestered in the intraneuronal storage vesicles. However, based on the work of Anton and Berk [33], as well our recent studies, it is clear that, in vivo at least, metaraminol in tracer amounts accumulates in the storage vesicle via the energy-requiring and reserpine-sensitive vesicular transport carrier, the same carrier that transports NE into the vesicles. Metarminol's appeal is also enhanced by its structural similarity to NE. Studies with [3H]-metarminol confirmed that this false transmitter is a highly selective in vivo marker for the adrenergic nerves of the heart [2]. Electrophilic ^{18}F-fluorination was one of the first techniques to be refined at the University of Michigan in the mid-1980's [34], so it was natural to evaluate this labeling approach to develop a positron-

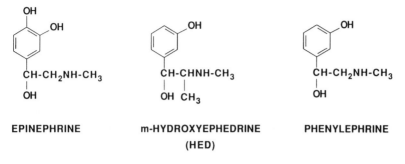

Figure 2. Chemical structures of three *N*-methyl sympathomimetic amines.

labeled derivative. Thus 6-[¹⁸F]fluorometaraminol (FMR) was earmarked for synthesis; the 6-position was chosen for the site of ¹⁸F incorporation based on studies with fluorodopa [35] and other catecholamines [36] which demonstrate that fluorine in this position minimally alters the biochemistry of the parent compound. A regiospecific synthesis of FMR was achieved by reaction of acetylhypo-[¹⁸F]fluorite with the respective 6-acetoxymercurio derivative [1]. The synthesis was unique in that no groups were used to protect either the phenolic or hydroxylic functionalities; no racemization occurred during the synthesis. Purification required only rapid elution of a small solid-phase column.

Studies were performed in animals to assess the tissue distribution of FMR and to validate its neuronal affinity [2]. Screening results in rats showed that [³H]MR and FMR had similar affinities for heart tissue and, more importantly, the two tracers had nearly identical heart neuronal selectivities as determined in the 6-hydroxydopamine sympathectomized rat model. PET/FMR analyses of closed-chest dogs bearing phenol-induced, regional neuronal defects in the left ventricle clearly delineated the region of neuronal impairment [2]. Blood perfusion in the heart was normal in these dogs as shown by [¹³N]NH₃ tomograms. The accumulation of FMR in these regionally denervated dog hearts correlated closely ($r = 0.88$) with endogenous norepinephrine concentrations.

Based on these very promising preclinical studies, evaluation of FMR was warranted. However, it was observed during the course of our studies with dogs that FMR sometimes produced a vasopressor response with the doses used for tomographic imaging. The mass of unlabeled FMR in projected clinical doses was subsequently determined to be too close to pharmacological levels to be safely used in human subjects. The specific activity of FMR made at our facility by the [¹⁸F]AcOF technique was 1–15 Ci/mmol. Fortunately, high specific activity [¹¹HC]CH₃I had just become available at the University of Michigan Medical Cyclotron Facility. Access to this versatile radiosynthetic agent made possible a change in our tracer design strategy. Three *N*-methyl sympathomimetic amines were designated for evaluation as possible successors to FMR: epinephrine, phenylephrine, and *meta*-hydroxyephedrine (Figure 2). All three of these amines could be theoretically labeled by methylation of their respective desmethyl precursors with [^{11}C]CH$_3$I. In order to quickly determine which of the three amines was the most promising, they were tritium labeled [37] and then screened in rats. Table 3 compares the heart affinities and neuronal selectivities of these three [^{3}H] labeled tracers. Epinephrine and *meta*-hydroxyephedrine (HED) were superior to phenylephrine in heart neuronal imaging potential. Epinephrine, although clearly an excellent marker for cardiac nerves, would present radiolabeling difficulties because of the high in vitro chemical reactivity of its catechol group and tracer kinetic modeling problems due to its rapid in vivo metabolism. [^{3}H]HED, also an

Table 3. Heart neuronal imaging potential of ^{3}H-labeled *N*-methyl sympathomimetic amines.

^{3}H-tracer	Tissue concentration (% dose/g ± S.D.)							LV drug blockade	
	RA	RV	LA	LV	Lung	Blood	LV/ blood	DMI	Reserpine
Meta-hydroxyephedrine	3.82 ± 0.55	4.06 ± 0.08	4.09 ± 0.62	3.65 ± 0.36	0.49 ± 0.11	0.07 ± 0.01	36.5	− 93%	− 70%
Epinephrine	2.60 ± 0.37	2.58 ± 0.50	2.88 ± 0.65	2.56 ± 0.46	0.34 ± 0.06	0.17 ± 0.03	15.1	− 93%	− 90%
Phenylephrine	1.89 ± 0.29	2.20 ± 0.51	1.87 ± 0.40	1.62 ± 0.32	1.02 ± 0.12	0.47 ± 0.03	3.5	− 71%	− 74%

Both *meta*-hydroxyephedrine and phenylephrine were tritium labeled in the 4-position of the aromatic ring; specific activities were 22 and 29 Ci/mmol, respectively [42]. [^{3}H]Epinephrine was obtained from Dupont/NEN with tritium label on the *N*-methyl group; specific activity was 67 Ci/mmol. RA = right atrium; RV = right ventricle; LA = left atrium; LV = left ventricle. N = 4–6 female Sprague-Dawley rats (150–200 mg) per data point. Tissue radioactivity concentrations are normalized to a 200 g rat. Animals under light ether anesthesia received femoral vein injections of 10–20 µCi of tracer and were sacrificed 30 minutes later. The uptake-1 blocker DMI (10 mg/kg, i.p.) was administered 30 minutes prior to tracer injection and the vesicular uptake blocker reserpine (1 mg/kg, i.p.) was given 3 hours before tracer injection. Control animals received vehicle prior to tracer injection. All animals were sacrificed 30 minutes after tracer injection. The values are given as % decrease in the left ventricle tritium concentration compared to control animals. The relatively low blockade of *meta*-hydroxyephedrine (− 70%) by reserpine pretreatment compared to epinephrine (− 90%) should not be interpreted as indicating that a smaller fraction of *meta*-hydroxyephedrine is stored in the vesicular compartment. Unlike epinephrine, false neurotransmitters bearing an alpha methyl group such as *meta*-hydroxyephedrine are resistant to degradation by cytoplasmic MAO and thus will clear less rapidly from reserpinized neurons.

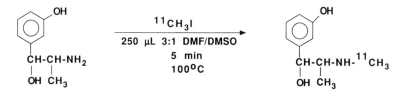

Figure 3. [¹¹C]HED synthesized by direct methylation of metaraminol.

excellent neuronal marker as shown in Table 3, shares the same in vivo characteristics as [³H]metaraminol and FMR. It is perhaps not surprising that HED and metaraminol display similar in vivo dispositions since norepinephrine and epinephrine, which share the same structural homology, also display similar in vivo distributions [38]. Thus, based on our screening studies with the three ³H-labeled *N*-methylamines, HED was chosen for ¹¹C labeling and evaluation as a high specific activity alternative to FMR.

As shown in Figure 3, [¹¹C]HED was synthesized in remarkably simple fashion by direct reaction of the free base form of metaraminol with [¹¹C]CH₃I in DMF/DMSO (3/1) and purified by radio-HPLC [3]. Radiochemical yields approached 40% in a total synthesis time of 40 minutes; specific activity ranged from 500 to 2000 Ci/mmol – over 50 times higher than was achieved with FMR. In all animal models tested, [¹¹C]HED behaved identically to FMR. Metabolic studies with [¹¹C]HED in guinea pigs showed that only unchanged tracer was present in heart tissue [3]. These findings agree with our earlier metabolic study with FMR [39]. However, [¹¹C]HED, like FMR, does show the presence of two metabolites in blood. Based on the studies of metaraminol by Fuller and coworkers [40], the two blood metabolites derived from HED are most likely alpha-methylepinephrine and the 3-*O*-methyl derivative of alpha-methylepinephrine. Reference standards need to be synthesized before definite identifications can be made. A rapid Sep-Pak determination of [¹¹C]HED blood levels has been developed which will permit correction of the arterial input function [3].

The Michaelis-Menten kinetics of vesicular HED uptake have been determined using bovine chromaffin granule membranes: a Ki of 134 μM was obtained for unlabeled HED inhibition of [³H]NE uptake compared to values of 23 and 27 μM for metaraminol and 6-fluorometaraminol, respectively [41]. The in vitro kinetics of neuronal (uptake-1) HED uptake using bovine adrenomedullary cells have not yet been evaluated. Despite the fairly high affinity of HED for the vesicular transporter, it has been found, as discussed below, that retention of [¹¹C]HED in the neuron does not require vesicular storage.

Mechanism of HED neuronal localization

The localization of HED in the heart requires neurons that have intact plasma membranes with functioning uptake-1 carriers requiring a constant supply of ATP. But are storage vesicles required for the neuronal localization of HED? The answer seems to be 'no', at least not on the ^{11}C/PET time scale maximum of 1–2 hours. We know this because HED showed only 10–50% decrease in heart localization in reserpine-pretreated rats compared to controls 5–30 min after tracer injection whereas DMl-pretreated rats showed a 90–95% decrease; [^{3}H]NE in this same experiment showed an 80–95% decrease in both reserpine- and DMl-pretreated rats [42]. Reserpine is a very selective blocker of vesicular uptake; DMl is a very selective uptake-1 blocker. To understand this result it must be remembered that vesicles not only store NE for subsequent quantal release, but they also protect NE from degradation by mitochondrial MAO. In fact, the neuronal localization of exogenous NE is not blocked when rats are pretreated with both reserpine and an MAO inhibitor [43]. HED is inherently resistant to the action of MAO by virtue of its alpha methyl group so when reserpine blocks entry into storage vesicles, HED finds relatively safe harbor in the cytosol. Passive diffusion or 'leakage' of HED into the synapses might occur but the efficient uptake-1 transporter would capture most of the HED before it escaped into interstitial space. Additional evidence for this concept comes from preliminary findings in our laboratory: (1) administration of DMl *after* radiotracer injection markedly shortens the heart $T_{1/2}$ of [^{11}C]HED but not [^{3}H]NE suggesting that nonvesicular release of HED occurs from the neuron; (2) a stereoisomer of HED, [^{11}C]*threo*-(1S,2S)HED, a drug known not to displace NE from the neuron and thus not likely stored in the vesicles, shows initial accumulation in the dog heart nearly equal to [^{11}C]HED; however, in contrast to HED, the *threo* form rapidly effluxes from the dog heart [44].

What relevance does the forgoing discussion have? It may have importance in mapping the reinnervation process in adult heart and the normal innervation process in neonatal heart, and, more importantly, in interpreting what the map means. Using mature dogs with surgically denervated hearts, Kaye and Tyce found during reinnervation that the development of the storage mechanism lags far behind development of the membrane amine pump [45]. Their conclusion was based on a comparison of endogenous NE and [^{3}H]NE heart levels following a 5 minute infusion of [^{3}H]NE into the inferior vena cava. The work of others has suggested that only a small number of adrenergic neuron fibers is needed in reinnervated heart tissue to generate large functional responses [46]. If, in fact, regenerated nerves can be functional prior to the development of storage vesicles, then [^{11}C]HED is likely to give a better functional map of the heart than radiolabeled NE or dopamine. However, this prediction is based on the pivotal presumption that mitochondrial MAO activity also returns before functional storage vesicles develop. If this presumption is incorrect [45], then [^{11}C]HED may have no obvious advantage over the labeled catecholamines other than its relative ease of synthesis.

Defining reinnervation in the human heart is still a controversial topic with important clinical implications [47]. Although most animal species show functional reinnervation 3–6 months after heart transplantation [48, 49], a very recent report concluded, based on myocardial catecholamines levels, that the transplanted human heart remains denervated for as long as five years after transplantation [50]. Our work with [^{11}C]HED [51], tyramine challenge studies [52], and reports that transplant patients can experience angina pectoris [53], suggest that some level of functional reinnervation is occurring. Further studies with [^{11}C]HED and with soon-to-be-developed PET radiotracers should serve an important role in defining the natural history of the reinnervation process in the human heart.

Radiotracer design – the cholinergic neuron

Development of cholinergic nerve markers constitute a far greater challenge for radiopharmaceutical chemists than do markers for the adrenergic neuron. When radiolabeled NE or a structurally related amine is injected intravenously, over half of the dose accumulates unchanged in tissues. In contrast, intravenous acetylcholine is completely hydrolyzed almost immediately by blood and tissue cholinesterases. Another complicating factor is the low density of cholinergic neurons in the heart. However, the bad news doesn't stop there. The design of a radiolabeled catecholamine, phenolic false transmitter, or structurally dissimilar false transmitter that will associate with the intraneuronal storage vesicles of the adrenergic nerve ending is fairly straightforward. Most of these candidate tracers enter the neuron via the amine pump and then quickly enter the NE storage vesicle through the vesicular transporter in exactly the same manner as does NE itself. Both transporters involved with the sequestration process of the adrenergic neuron are very forgiving. In contrast, the cholinergic nerve ending is a stern schoolmaster. Choline enters the cytosol of the nerve ending via the high affinity choline uptake (HACU) system, is rapidly acetylated by ChAT, and is then shuttled into storage vesicles. The HACU system is very restrictive [54]. Even close structural analogs of choline are poor substrates for the HACU system; esters of choline are even poorer substrates. Although ChAT has fairly broad specificity for choline-like analogs, the vesicular uptake system does not [55]. Thus, a choli-

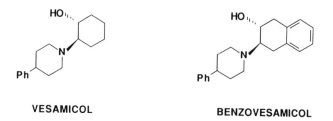

VESAMICOL   **BENZOVESAMICOL**

Figure 4. Chemical structures of vesamicol and benzovesamicol.

nergic false neurotransmitter can enter the acetylcholine storage vesicle only if it satisfies the structural requirements of three systems: (1) HACU; (2) ChAT; and (3) vesicular uptake. In other words, the tracer must jump through a very narrow hoop, undergo a costume change, and then jump through a flaming hoop. That's why review chapters on cholinergic false transmitters are very short [56].

Despite the sparse distribution and the stringent biochemical gauntlets of myocardial cholinergic nerves, preliminary findings with a new class of in-traneuronal receptor-binding agents suggest that there is hope for developing successful markers. Stanley Parsons and colleagues have characterized a unique binding site on the outer membrane surface of the ACh storage vesicle [57–59]. They have characterized this site with vesamicol (Figure 4), a compound first synthesized in the late 1960's as a possible analgesic [60]. Vesamicol binds to *Torpedo* electric organ synaptic vesicles with high affinity. The binding is noncompetitive, occurring at a locus allosteric to the ACh binding site. Benzo derivatives of vesamicol have been found to be even more potent than vesamicol [61, 62]. Both [^{11}C]- and [^{18}F]-labeled benzovesamicol analogs have been synthesized and their distribution in mammalian brain shown to correlate with cholinergic nerve density [63–65]. These tracers hold considerable promise as markers for the cholinergic neurons of the heart.

Future heart neuronal tracers

Two ^{18}F-labeled catecholamine tracers, 6-fluorodopamine and 6-fluoronorepi-nephrine, have been developed recently for heart neuronal mapping [4–8]. The use of these two PET tracers in humans has not been reported but they give excellent heart images in dog and baboon. More detailed studies should help determine whether specific biochemical processes occurring within the neurons of the heart can be attributed to specific features of the tracer kinetic patterns that were obtained with these two new tracers. As pointed out by

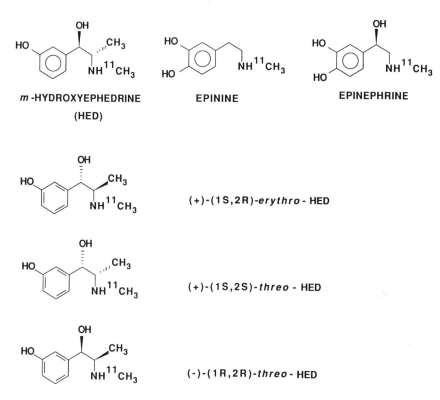

Figure 5. ^{11}C-labeled biogenic amines.

Ding and coworkers, it is important to develop a radiotracer that will be sensitive to a range of sympathetic neuronal activities [8]. This approach is being systematically evaluated in our laboratory. Both the enantiomeric and diastereomeric forms of [11C]HED, as well as the *N*-methyl catecholamines [11C]epinine and [11C]epinephrine (Figure 5), have been synthesized and are undergoing careful study for their comparative abilities to detect neuronal alterations of the heart [66, 67]. Hopefully HED, 6-[18F]fluorodopamine, [11C]epinine, or some future PET tracer will find important, routine applications in diagnosing and understanding cardiac disease.

References

1. Mislankar SG, Gildersleeve DL, Wieland DM, Massin CC, Mulholland GK, Toorongian SA. 6-[18F]Fluorometaraminol: a radiotracer for in vivo mapping of adrenergic nerves of the heart. J Med Chem 1988; 31: 362–6.

2. Wieland DM, Rosenspire KC, Hutchins GD et al. Neuronal mapping of the heart with 6[^{18}F]fluorometaraminol. J Med Chem 1990; 33: 956–64.

3. Rosenspire KC, Haka MS, Van Dort ME et al. Synthesis and preliminary evaluation of carbon-11-meta-hydroxyephedrine: a false transmitter agent for heart neuronal imaging. J Nucl Med 1990; 31: 1328–34.

4. Eisenhofer G, Hovevey-Sion D, Kopin IJ et al. Neuronal uptake and metabolism of 2- and 6-fluorodopamine: false neurotransmitters for positron emission tomographic imaging of sympathetically innervated tissues. J Pharmacol Exp Ther 1989; 248: 419–27.

5. Goldstein DS, Chang PC, Eisenhofer G et al. Positron emission tomographic imaging of cardiac sympathetic innervation and function. Circulation 1990; 81: 1606–21.

6. Chang PC, Szemeredi K, Grossman E, Kopin IJ, Goldstein DS. Fate of tritiated 6-fluorodopamine in rats: a false neurotransmitter for positron emission tomographic imaging of sympathetic innervation and function. J Pharmacol Exp Ther 1990; 255: 809–17.

7. Ding YS, Fowler JS, Gatley SJ, Dewey SL, Wolf AP. Synthesis of high specific activity (+) and (−) 6-[^{18}F]fluoronorepinephrine via the nucleophilic aromatic substitution reaction. J Med Chem 1991; 34: 767–71.

8. Ding YS, Fowler JS, Gatley SJ, Dewey SL, Wolf AP, Schlyer DJ. Synthesis of high specific activity 6-[^{18}F]fluorodopamine for PET studies of sympathetic nervous tissue. J Med Chem 1991; 34: 861–2.

9. Schwaiger M, Kalff V, Rosenspire K et al. Noninvasive evaluation of sympathetic nervous system in human heart by positron emission tomography. Circulation 1990; 82: 457–64.

10. Schwaiger M, Hutchins GD, Kalff V et al. Evidence for regional catecholamine uptake and storage sites in the transplanted human heart by positron emission tomography. J Clin Invest 1991; 87: 1681–90.

11. Randall WC, Ardell JL. Functional anatomy of the cardiac efferent innervation. In: Kulbertus HE, Franck G, editors. Neurocardiology. New York: Futura Publishing Co., 1988: 3–24.

12. Angelakos ET, King MP, Millard RW. Regional distribution of catecholamines in the hearts of various species. Ann N Y Acad Sci 1969; 156: 219–40.

13. Angelakos ET. Regional distribution of catecholamines in the dog heart. Circ Res 1965; 16: 39–44.

14. Pierpont GL, DeMaster EG, Reynolds S, Pederson J, Cohn JN. Ventricular myocardial catecholamines in primates. J Lab Clin Med 1985; 106: 205–10.

15. Bevan JA. Some bases of differences in vascular response to sympathetic activity. Circ Res 1979; 45: 161–71.

16. Ehinger B, Falck B, Sporrong B. Possible axo-axonal synapses between peripheral adrenergic and cholinergic nerve terminals. Z Zellforsch Mikrosk Anat 1970; 107: 508–21.

17. Takahashi N, Barber MJ, Zipes DF. Efferent vagal innervation of canine ventricle. Am J Physiol 1985; 248: H89–97.

18. Inque H, Mahomed Y, Kovacs RJ, Zipes DP. Surgery for Wolff-Parkinson-White syndrome interrupts efferent vagal innervation to the left ventricle and to the atrioventricular node in the canine heart. Cardiovasc Res 1988; 22: 163–70.

19. Schmid PG, Greif BJ, Lund DD, Roskoski R Jr. Regional choline acetyltransferase activity in the guinea pig heart. Circ Res 1978; 42: 657–60.

20. Stanley RL, Conatser J, Dettbarn WD. Acetylcholine, choline acetyltransferase and cholinesterases in the rat heart. Biochem Pharmacol 1978; 27: 2409–11.

21. Slavikova J, Tucek S. Choline acetyltransferase in the heart of adult rats. Pflugers Arch 1982; 392: 225–9.

22. Loffelholz K, Pappano AJ. The parasympathetic neuroeffector junction of the heart. Pharmacol Rev 1985; 67: 1–24.

23. Levy MN. Sympathetic-parasympathetic interactions in the heart. In: Kulbertus HE, Franck G, editors. Neurocardiology. New York: Futura Publishing Co., 1988: 85–98.

24. Yatani A, Okabe K, Codina J, Birnbaumer L, Brown AM. Heart rate regulation by G proteins acting on the cardiac pacemaker channel. Science 1990; 249: 1163–5.

25. Whitby LG, Axelrod J, Weh-Malherbe H. The fate of H^3-norepinephrine in animals. J Pharmacol Exp Ther 1961; 132: 193–201.

26. Iversen LL, Whitby LG. Retention of injected catecholamines by the mouse. Br J Pharmacol Chemother 1962; 19: 355–64.

27. Crout JR. The uptake and release of 3H-norepinephrine by the guinea-pig heart in vivo. Naunyn Schmiedeberg Arch Exp Pathol Pharmacol 1964; 248: 85–98.

28. Kopin IJ, Gordon EK. Origin of norepinephrine in the heart. Nature 1963; 199: 1289.

29. Fowler JS, MacGregor RR, Ansari AN. Radiopharmaceuticals XII. A new rapid synthesis of ^{11}C-norepinephrine hydrochloride. J Med Chem 1974; 17: 246–8.

30. Fowler JS, Wolf AP, Christman DR, MacGregor RR, Ansari A, Atkins H. Carrier-free ^{11}C-labeled catecholmaines. In: Subramanian G, Rhodes BA, Cooper JF, Sodd VJ, editors. Radiopharmaceuticals. New York: Society of Nuclear Medicine, 1975: 196–204.

31. Ross SB. Structural requirements for uptake into catecholamine neurons. In: Paton DM, editor. The mechanism of neuronal and extraneuronal transport of catecholamines. New York: Raven Press, 1969: 67–93.

32. Crout JR, Alpers HS, Tatum EL, Shore PA. Release of metaraminol (Aramine) from the heart by sympathetic nerve stimulation. Science 1964; 145: 828–9.

33. Anton AH, Berk AI. Distribution of metaraminol and its relation to norepinephrine. Eur J Pharmacol 1977; 44: 161–7.

34. Jewett DM, Potocki JF, Ehrenkaufer RE. A gas-solid-phase microchemical method for the synthesis of acetyl hypofluorite. J Fluorine Chem 1984; 24: 477–84.

35. Firnau G, Garnett ES, Chirakal R, Sood S, Nahmias C, Schrobilgen G. ^{18}F-Fluoro-L-dopa for the in vivo study of intracerebral dopamine. Int J Rad Appl Instrum [A] 1986; 37: 669–75.

36. Kirk KL, Cantacuzene D, Nimitkitpaisan Y. Synthesis and biological properties of 2-, 5- and 6-fluoronorepinephrines. J Med Chem 1979; 22: 1493–7.

37. Van Dort ME, Gildersleeve DL, Wieland DM. Synthesis of 3H-labeled sympathomimetic amines for neuronal mapping. J Label Compounds Radiopharm 1990; 28: 832–40.

38. Axelrod J, Weil-Malherbe H, Tomchick R. The physiological disposition of 3H-epinephrine and its metabolite metanephrine. J Pharmacol Exp Ther 1959; 127: 251–6.

39. Rosenspire KC, Gildersleeve DL, Massin CC, Mislanker S, Wieland DM. Metabolic fate of the heart agent 6-[18F]fluorometaraminol. Int J Rad Appl Instrum [B] 1989; 16: 735–9.

40. Fuller RW, Snoddy HD, Perry KW, Bernstein JR, Murphy PJ. Formation of α-methyl-norepinephrine as a metabolite of metaraminol in guinea pigs. Biochem Pharmacol 1981; 30: 2831–6.

41. Wieland DM, Sherman PS, Haka MS, Van Dort ME, Njus D, Kelley PM. Mechanistic studies of the heart agent [C-11]metahydorxyephedrine (HED) [abstract]. J Nucl Med 1990; 31: 707.

42. Wieland DM, Van Dort M, Hutchins G, Sherman P, Toorongian S: Unpublished findings (1990).

43. Malmfors T. Studies on adrenergic nerves. Acta Physiol Scand 1965; 64 Suppl 248: 1–93.

33. Hutchins G, Van Dort M, Toorongian S, Wieland DM. Unpublished findings (1990).

45. Kaye MP, Tyce GM. Norepinephrine uptake as an indicator of cardiac reinnervation in dogs. Am J Physiol 1978; 235: H289–94.

46. Peiss CN, Cooper T, Willman VL, Randall WC. Circulatory response to electrical and reflex activation of the nervous system after cardiac denervation. Circ Res 1966; 16: 153–66.

47. Bristow MR. The surgical denervated, transplanted human heart. Circulation 1990; 82: 658–60.
48. Willman VL, Cooper T, Hanlon CR. Return of neural responses after autotransplantation of the heart. Am J Physiol 1964; 207: 187–9.
49. Kontos HA, Thames MD, Lower RR. Responses to electrical and reflex autonomic stimulation in dogs with cardiac transplantation before and after innervation. J Thorac Cardiovasc Surg 1970; 59: 382–92.
50. Regitz V, Bossaller C, Strasser R, Schuler S, Hetzer R, Fleck E. Myocardial catecholamine content after heart transplantation. Circulation 1990; 82: 620–3.
51. Schwaiger M, Hutchins GD, Kalff V et al. Evidence for regional reinnervation of the transplanted human heart by positron emission tomography. J Clin Invest. 1991; 87: 1681–90.
52. Wilson RF, Christensen BV, Olivari MT, Simon A, White CW, Laxson DD. Evidence for structural sympathetic reinnervation after orthotopic cardiac transplantation in humans. Circulation 1991; 83: 1210–20.
53. Buda AJ, Fowles RA, Schroeder JS et al. Coronary artery spasm in the denervated transplanted human heart. Am J Med 1981; 70: 1144–9.
54. Ducis I. The high-affinity choline uptake system. In: Whittaker VP, editor. The cholinergic synapse. New York: Springer Verlag, 1988: 409–45.
55. Zimmermann H. Cholinergic synaptic vesicles. In: Whittaker VP, editor. The cholinergic synapse. New York: Springer-Verlag, 1988: 350–82.
56. Newton MW, Jenden DJ. False transmitters as presynaptic probes for cholinergic mechanisms and function. Trends Pharmacol Sci 1986; 7: 316–20.
57. Rogers GA, Parsons SM, Anderson DC et al. Synthesis, in vitro acetylcholine-storage-blocking activities, and biological properties of derivatives and analogues of trans-2-(4--phenylpiperidino)cyclohexanol (vesamicol). J Med Chem 1989; 32: 1217–30.
58. Marshall IG, Parsons SM. The vesicular acetylcholine transport system. Trends Neurosci 1987; 10: 174–7.
59. Kaufman R, Rogers GA, Fehlmann C, Parsons SM. Fractional vesamicol receptor occupancy and acetylcholine active transport inhibition in synaptic vesicles. Mol Pharmacol 1989; 36: 452–8.
60. Brittain RT, Levy GP, Tyers MB. The neuromuscular blocking action of 2-(4--phenylpiperidino)cyclohexanol (AH 5183). Eur J Pharmacol 1969; 8: 93–9.
61. Rogers GA, Parsons SM. Persistent occultation of the vesamicol receptor. Neuroreport 1990; 1: 22–5.
62. Hicks BW, Rogers GA, Parsons SM. Purification and characterization of a nonvesicular vesamicol-binding protein from electric organ and demonstration of a related protein in mammalian brain. J Neurochem 1991; 57: 509–19.
63. Kilbourn MR, Jung YW, Haka MS, Gildersleeve DL, Kuhl DE, Wieland DM. Mouse brain distribution of a carbon-11 labeled vesamicol derivative: presynaptic marker of cholinergic neurons. Life Sci 1990; 47: 1955–63.
64. Mulholland GK, Buck F, Sherman PS et al. 4-[18F]Fluorobenzyl-ABV: a new potential marker for central cholinergic presynaptic sites [abstract]. J Nucl Med 1991; 32: 994.
65. Jung YW, Mulholland GK, Sherman PS et al. Synthesis of two chiral [C-11]Benzovesamicols for mapping heart cholinergic innervation [abstract]. J Nucl Med 1991; 32: 974.
66. Hutchins GD, Van Dort ME, Toorongian SA, Wieland DM. Evaluation of the kinetic properties of [C-11]threo-meta-hydroxyephedrine (1S,2S) in dog myocardium [abstract]. J Nucl Med 1991; 32: 928–9.
67. Gildersleeve DL, Toorongian SA, Van Dort ME et al. [C-11]Epinine: neuronal marker for heart sympathetic neurons [abstract]. J Nucl Med 1991; 32: 994.

Leukocytes, platelets, lipoproteins

32. Labeling of leukocytes, platelets, and lipoproteins: useful in clinical cardiology?

BERTHE L.F. VAN ECK-SMIT and ERNST E. VAN DER WALL

Introduction

In the detection of infectious foci, thrombo-embolic processes, and atherosclerotic plaques within the cardiovascular system, diagnostic modalities like echocardiography, computed tomography, and magnetic resonance imaging currently play a much more important role than radionuclide imaging. However, in some cases radionuclide imaging can provide important additional information or localize focal pathology at a much earlier stage than the above-mentioned modalities. In this chapter, the feasibility and limitations of radionuclide imaging with labeled leukocytes, platelets, and lipoproteins will be reviewed. Furthermore, the clinical value of these imaging procedures will be discussed. Chapters 33–35 provide detailed information of these imaging modalities.

Cardiac imaging with radiolabeled leukocytes

Mature leukocytes are very short-lived cells which disappear from the circulation as a result of pooling in spleen and destruction by the reticulo-endothelial system in about 10 hours. However, when they migrate into tissue, their survival time mounts up to about 4 days [1]. As leukocytes avidly target inflammation sites, labeled leukocytes should be the ideal modality for detection of infectious foci. Since leukocyte imaging was first described in 1977 by Thakur [2], this method has earned an important place in the detection of infectious sites. Based on a great number of clinical investigations, several

429

Ernst E. van der Wall et al. (eds), What's new in cardiac imaging?, 429–436.

authors [3, 4] have reported an overall sensitivity of about 85% and an even higher specificity for acute infections and abscesses. For several reasons, these figures are much lower in cardiovascular infection detection. Many infectious foci within the heart are too small to visualize, especially when high blood pool activity remains due to contaminating labeled red cells and platelets [3]. Additionally, cardiac infections, especially endocarditis, have the tendency to be chronic, resulting in a less avid migration of leukocytes towards the infection site [4].

Labeling procedures

Cell separation
For labeling leukocytes, cells must be isolated in vitro. In fact, there are two different cell preparation methods; (1) the simpler, mixed leukocytes which are invariably contaminated with erythrocytes and platelets, and (2) the more time-consuming pure granulocytes. The former is perfectly suitable in most clinical circumstances where patients plasma is rich in granulocytes because of neutrophilic reaction on infection. In some clinical situations, when contaminating blood components will disturb image quality, pure granulocyte suspension will be preferable.

Cell labeling
Indium-111 (In-111)-labeled compounds, when added to a cell suspension in vitro, diffuse passively through the cell membranes and transfer the radiolabel to cytoplasmatic components [5]. These lipophylic compounds show some selectivity in uptake in different cell types, resulting in a higher uptake in leukocytes and platelets compared to red cells [1].

The physical properties of In-111 (gamma-rays 171 and 245 keV, half-life 2.8 days) make this nuclide suitable for imaging with a gamma camera over a period of 3 days after injection.

For labeling leukocytes with technetium-99m (Tc-99m), this nuclide is first bound to hexamethylpropyleneamineoxime (HMPAO), a highly lipophilic compound which passes the cell membrane easily. Once intracellularly, the compound (Tc-99m HMPAO) changes in a hydrophilic state which makes radioactivity stay inside the cell [6]. Tc-99m HMPAO shows highly selective uptake in granulocytes and a more stable binding to the cell, which makes it very suitable for labeling mixed cell suspension.

Physical properties of Tc-99m (pure gamma-emitter 140 keV, half-life 6 hours) allow the administration of high amounts of radioactivity resulting in better image quality than In-111-labeled leukocytes. One disadvantage for cardiac imaging can be the more prominent uptake in bone marrow and the limited period of time for imaging, which can result in false negative findings because of high blood pool activity [6].

Clinical results

Although echocardiography has successfully visualized valve vegetations and myocardial abscesses in 80% of patients with known endocarditis [7], it has also been shown to have a low sensitivity in patients with prosthetic valves and valve calcifications. Cerqueira et al. [8, 9] and Oates et al. [10, 11] reported successful visualization and localization of infective sites by In-111-labeled leukocytes in patients with prosthetic heart valves (see Chapter 33). In all of these cases, echocardiography was nondiagnostic at the time of investigation. Marked pericardial uptake at an early stage of purulent pericarditis, even before clinical signs are present, was reported by Greenberg et al. [12] reflecting the immediate migration of leukocytes as a result of chemotactic stimuli produced by the infective organism and tissue components of the host [1, 13].

Conclusion: labeled leukocytes

Although studies are limited in number, the initial results suggest that detection of infection by labeled leukocytes is certainly not sensitive enough for screening in clinical practice, but this approach can be very useful if echocardiography is nondiagnostic.

Cardiac imaging with radiolabeled platelets

Present techniques for noninvasive diagnosis of thrombosis and atherosclerosis are based on imaging of the remaining partial or total stenosis of the impaired vessel rather than visualizing the causing thrombus or atherosclerotic plaque. Various factors control platelet-vessel wall interaction in normal hemostasis, thrombo-embolic clot formation, and genesis of atherosclerosis [14]. Thrombosis is a surface reaction and a dynamic process of embolization and fragmentation (fibrinolysis). Atherosclerosis, on the other hand, is primarily a process of the subendothelial layers of the vessel wall. The role of platelets in thrombo-embolic clot formation varies in time [14]. Since Thakur et al. [15] described the labeling of platelets with In-111-labeled compounds, several investigators [16–21] studied imaging qualities of labeled platelets both in animal models and in man.

Labeling procedures

Cell separation
Platelets, being the smallest cells in blood, can easily be separated by centrifugation. Contamination by other small cells like erythrocytes and lymphocytes is negligible [15].

Cell labeling
As previous described, lipid soluble complexes of In-111 added to a cell suspension in vitro, diffuse passively through the cell membrane and transfer the radionuclide to cytoplasmatic components. Like in leukocyte labeling, it is also possible to use Tc-99m HMPAO for labeling purposes. The avidity of this complex to enter the cell and stability of the binding in platelets is less than in leukocytes [6, 15, 16].

Clinical results
Knight et al. [17] studied in dogs the effect of aging (1–48 hours) of venous thrombi on platelet incorporation after In-111-platelet injection. A rapidly increasing thrombus/blood radioactivity ratio was found within the first 12 hours after thrombus formation. Optimal ratios were found between 12 and 15 hours, followed by a marked decrease in the activity ratio resulting in a 5:1 ratio after 48 hours post-thrombus formation. Cella et al. [18] studied the imaging possibilities of fresh pulmonary emboli induced in the canine model. Only 14 of 26 emboli (mean weight 0.65 g) could be detected by means of radiolabeled platelets. Others, like Sostman et al. [19], found imaging qualities decreasing with time after embolization rather than with age of the originating thrombus.

These studies suggest that labeled platelets can only be expected to image thrombo-embolic processes in the acute phase of embolization and thrombosis. As will be described in one of the following chapters (see Chapter 34) indeed large, hematologically active thromby located within the left ventricle can be detected some days after injection of In-111-labeled platelets. Yamada et al. [20] also diagnosed active thrombi in man. These thrombi were located in the left atrium and could only be detected after 48–96 hours due to high blood pool activity within the first days. Ezekowitz et al. [21] investigated the role of In-111 labeled platelets in a large group of patients ($n = 103$). They found that thrombi located in the deep veins of the leg could successfully be imaged in patients at risk for thrombosis and those with clinically suspected disease. However, successful imaging was not possible until blood pool activity decreased enough to visualize the process, which means 2–3 days after administration. Moreover, sensitivity dropped markedly after heparin treatment.

Conclusion: thrombo-embolic imaging

Although a great number of active thrombi can be visualized with In-111-labeled platelets, the 2-day time-lag between injection and visualization and the drop of sensitivity after heparin treatment makes this method less suitable for daily clinical practice. Moreover, echocardiography is highly sensitive in detecting thrombo-embolic processes within the heart and should be therefore the first choice in thrombo-embolic screening within the heart.

Platelet imaging in atherosclerotic plaques

As atherosclerosis is primarily a process of fibro-fatty deposition within the intima of the arterial wall, platelet activation and thrombus formation do not occur unless loss of endothelial cells and stenosis of the vessel results in local decrease of production of prostacycline substance (i.e. platelet desaggregating substance with vasodilating properties) and hemodynamic impairment [22].

Clinical results

Powers et al. [23] reported the results of In-111 platelet imaging in 100 patients with angiographically proven atherosclerotic lesions of the carotid artery. Platelet deposition was observed in only 41% of the lesions and false positive results were found in 13%. No correlation was found in platelet concentration and the severity of the atherosclerotic lesion. Lesions located within the heart will be even more difficult to visualize because of high blood pool activity and relatively small lesion size.

Cardiac imaging with radiolabeled lipoproteins

Atherosclerotic plaques may quite well develop in the vessel wall long before it results in changes of the lumen. Most noninvasive techniques deal with the space-occupying and the resulting hemodynamic impairment rather than with the primary plaque.

Atherosclerotic plaques develop as fibro-fatty deposits, mainly containing cholesterol complexed to proteins and cholesterol-esters, within the intima of the arterial wall [22]. These atheromata may be sparsely distributed at first, but as the disease advances, they can cover a great deal of the inner layer of the vessel wall. A variety of complications may occur such as calcification, internal bleedings, ulceration through the endothelial surface followed by thrombosis and embolic discharge and even rupture of the vessel. For therapeutic reasons,

identifying patients at risk for acute complications and prevention of hemodynamic disturbances can be of the utmost importance [24, 25].

As described earlier, radiolabeled platelets can, in some cases, visualize
active thrombotic plaques at the moment that complications like ulceration or
stenosis already exist. Low density lipoproteins (LDL) are abundantly present
in active atheromata. Lees et al. [24, 26] managed to isolate the substance from
plasma and they successfully labeled LDL with Tc-99m. In this way, they tried
to visualize active atherosclerotic plaques before complications may evolve.

Labeling procedures

The separation of autologous LDL from plasma is a time consuming procedure
of sequential ultracentrifugation and dialysis for almost 2 days [24, 26]. Recent
developments in preparation and modification of autologous LDL to obtain
better imaging qualities will be discussed in more detail in Chapter 35.

Clinical results

After intravenous injection, Tc-99m LDL is mainly found in the blood pool for
several hours. The half-time of clearance of LDL from plasma is approximately 30 hours. Increasing uptake is seen in organs, most prominent in liver,
adrenals, kidney, spleen, and intestine [26, 27]. Until recently, only small
groups of patients have been studied, but there is clear evidence that radiolabeled LDL is rapidly sequestrated in the abnormal arterial wall. It was also
found that the uptake of LDL is dependent on the tissue composition of the
atherosclerotic plaque. Fibrocalcificated plaques, which are regarded as non-
evolving with little risk of complications, do not take up a detectable amount of
labeled LDL in contradistinction to plaques containing macrophages, foam
cells, hematoma, and necrosis, which is regarded as evolving tissue and at risk
of complications.

The possibility to detect these plaques with a gamma camera does not only
depend on the uptake of LDL by the atheroma, but also on the radioactivity
ratio plaque/blood pool. As blood pool activity stays high for more than
several physical half-lives of the isotope, only severe atheromatous disease will
be detected [26, 27].

Conclusion: labeled lipoproteins

Because there are still many problems, like time-consuming isolation of LDL
from plasma and the long half-life of LDL in the circulation, this technique is

not yet suitable for routine patient care. Recent research results, however, appear very promising.

Clinical relevance of the use of labeled blood components in cardiology

Elaborate separation and labeling procedures, poor target to non target ratios and a time-lag of several days between the moment of injection and imaging, make these modalities less feasible for daily clinical use. Recent developments in modifying these radiopharmaceuticals to obtain better imaging properties seem, however, very promising [28]. Moreover, echocardiography, because of its continuous availability, is relatively low cost and its high sensitivity for space-occupying processes within the heart are almost ideal for screening purposes. Radionuclide imaging, however, can be very useful in the individual patient. Because of its high specificity, scintigraphy can provide important additional information in clinical practice.

References

1. Peters AM. Infection. In: Sharp PF, Gemmel HG, Smith FW, editors. Practical nuclear medicine. Oxford: IRL Press, 1989: 299–327.
2. Thakur ML. Indium-111: a new radioactive tracer for leukocytes. Exp Hematol 1977; 5 (Suppl 1): 145–50.
3. McAfee JG, Samin A. In-111 labeled leukocytes: a review of problems in image interpretation. Radiology 1985; 155: 221–9.
4. McDougall IR, Baumert JE, Lantieri RL. Evaluation of 111In leukocyte whole body scanning. AJR Am J Roentgenol 1979; 133: 849–54.
5. Johnson DG, Coleman RE. Detection of inflammatory disease using radiolabeled cells. In: Gottschalk A, Hoffer PB, Potchen EJ, editors. Diagnostic nuclear medicine. 2nd ed. Baltimore: Williams & Wilkins, 1988: 1125–36.
6. Peters AM, Danpure HJ, Osman S et al. Clinical experience with 99mTc-hexamethylpropyleneamineoxime for labelling leucocytes and imaging inflammation. Lancet 1986; 2: 946–9.
7. Melvin ET, Berger M, Lutzker LG, Goldberg E, Mildvan D. Noninvasive methods for detection of valve vegetations in infective endocarditis. Am J Cardiol l981; 47: 271–8.
8. Cerqueira MD, Jacobson AF, Matsuda M, Stratton JR. Indium-111 leukocyte scintigraphic detection of mitral valve vegetations in active bacterial endocarditis. Am J Cardiol 1989; 64: 1080–1.
9. Cerqueira MD, Jacobson AF. Indium-111 leukocyte scintigraphic detection of myocardial abscess formation in patients with endocarditis. J Nucl Med 1989; 30: 703–6.
10. Oates E, Sarno RC. Detection of a prosthetic aortic valvular abscess with indium-111 labeled leukocytes. Chest 1988; 94: 872–4.
11. Oates E, Sarno RC. Detection of bacterial endocarditis in Indium-111 labeled leukocytes. Clin Nucl Med 1988; 13: 691–3.

12. Greenberg ML, Niebulski HIJ, Uretsky BF et al. Occult purulent pericarditis detected by indium-111 leukocyte imaging. Chest 1984; 85: 701–3.
13. Riba AL, Thakur ML, Gottschalk A, Andriole VT, Zaret BL. Imaging experimental infective endocarditis with indium-111 labeled blood cellular components. Circulation 1979; 59: 336–43.
14. Dewanjee MK. Cardiac and vascular imaging with labeled platelets and leukocytes. Semin Nucl Med 1984; 14: 154–87.
15. Dewanjee MK. The chemistry of 99mTc-labeled radiopharmaceuticals. Semin Nucl Med 1990; 20: 5–27.
16. Becker W, Borner W, Borst U, Kromer EP, Gruner KR. Tc-99m-HMPAO: a new platelet labelling compound? Eur J Nucl Med 1987; 13: 267–8.
17. Knight LC, Primeau JL, Siegel BA, Welch MJ. Comparison of indium-111 labeled platelets and iodinated fibrinogen for the detection of deep vein thrombosis. J Nucl Med 1978; 19: 891–4.
18. Cella G, Tow DE, Godin P, Cunninghan T, McKracken L, Sasakara AA. Indium-111 autologous platelets in the detection of experimental pulmonary emboli [abstract]. Thromb Haemost 1981; 46: 417.
19. Sostman HD, Neumann RD, Loke J et al. Detection of pulmonary embolism in man with 111In-labeled autologous platelets. AJR Am J Roentgenol 1982; 138: 945–7.
20. Yamada M, Hoki N, Ishikawa K et al. Detection of left atrial thrombi in man using indium-111 labelled autologous platelets. Br Heart J 1984; 51: 298–305.
21. Ezekowitz MD, Pope CF, Sostman HD et al. Indium-111 platelet scintigraphy for the diagnosis of acute venous thrombosis. Circulation 1986; 73: 668–74.
22. Robbins SL. Blood vessels. In: Robbins SL, editor. Pathologic basis of disease. Philadelphia: Saunders, 1974: 581–636.
23. Powers WJ, Siegel BA. Thrombus imaging with indium-111 platelets. Semin Thromb Hemost 1983; 9: 115–31.
24. Lees AM, Lees RS, Schoen FJ et al. Imaging human atherosclerosis with 99mTc-labeled low density lipoproteins. Arteriosclerosis 1988; 8: 461–70.
25. Lees RS, Lees AM, Strauss HW. External imaging of human atherosclerosis. J Nucl Med 1983; 24: 154–6.
26. Lees RS, Garabedian HD, Lees AM et al. Technetium-99m low density lipoproteins: preparation and biodistribution. J Nucl Med 1985; 26: 1056–62.
27. Lees RS, Lees AM, Strauss HW et al. The distribution and metabolism of Tc-99m labeled low density lipoprotein in human subjects [abstract]. J Nucl Med 1985; 26: P35.
28. Schelbert HR. Current status and prospects of new radionuclides and radiopharmaceuticals for cardiovascular nuclear medicine. Semin Nucl Med 1987; 17: 145–81.

33. Indium-111 leukocyte scintigraphy for detection of valvular abscesses and vegetations

MANUEL D. CERQUEIRA

Introduction

Infective endocarditis results from colonization and invasion of the endothelial surfaces of the heart by bacterial or fungal organisms. Infection usually follows an episode of transient bacteremia from a distant source of acute infection or as a result of dental or surgical manipulation. Rheumatic heart disease, congenital cardiac abnormalities, prosthetic valves, and age-related atherosclerosis and fibrocalcification are predisposing factors. Bacterial endocarditis is classified on the basis of the infecting organism and histologic appearance into subacute and acute forms. Subacute endocarditis is histologically characterized by invasion through the endothelium and formation of vegetations consisting of a meshwork of platelets, fibrin, and bacteria, but there are usually few polymorphonuclear leukocytes. Lesions typically occur in areas of endothelial damage caused by a jet or Venturi effect that forms a sterile thrombus that becomes infected following transient bacteremia. Acute endocarditis is usually caused by highly invasive organisms that attach to endothelial surfaces and may not require a sterile platelet-fibrin thrombus for initial endothelial invasion. Histologically, there is marked destruction of the myocardium with infiltration by large numbers of polymorphonuclear leukocytes.

Given these histologic changes, it is anticipated that Indium-111 (In-111) leukocyte scintigraphy will have a useful role only in certain types of endocarditis, that is, only in the presence of increased numbers of leukocytes in association with large vegetations and extensive areas of tissue destruction will there be sufficient uptake to allow imaging. Thus, the sensitivity of this technique will be low in those cases of subacute endocarditis associated with

Ernst E. van der Wall et al. (eds), What's new in cardiac imaging?, 437–445.
© *1992 Kluwer Academic Publishers. Printed in the Netherlands.*

small surface vegetations and minimal tissue destruction. For these types of lesions, labeled platelets or fibrin specific antibodies may be useful [1]. Leuko-cyte scintigraphy will not be useful for endocarditis screening in patients with underlying cardiac abnormalities who have episodes of transient bacteremia. Such patients will have to be managed on the basis of clinical suspicion, physical examination findings, and other forms of laboratory evaluation. Gallium-67 scintigraphy has not been useful in such situations [2].

Sensitivity should be higher in patients with acute endocarditis who usually have increased numbers of leukocytes in association with extensive tissue invasion, necrosis, and abscess formation. In this situation, the question of abscess formation versus slow response to antibiotics needs to be answered in order to make a decision on surgical versus continued medical management.

Currently, In-111, radiolabeled leukocytes are used for evaluation of such patients [3, 4]. In-111 labeled nonspecific immunoglobulin imaging has been reported to accurately identify intravascular prosthetic graft material infection and this may have a role in future studies [5, 6]. Alternative methods of leukocyte labeling with Technetium-99m (Tc-99m) are available, but not frequently used [7–9]. I will review my experience using In-111 leukocyte scintigraphy in patients with endocarditis and indicate alternative methods of evaluation.

Leukocyte separation and radiolabeling

Several leukocyte separation and radiolabeling methods are available. The major factors determining which methods are used is the ease of preparation and the retained function and viability of the leukocytes following separation and radiolabeling.

Leukocyte separation

The method selected should produce the greatest number of viable, functional leukocytes with a minimal amount of red blood cell and platelet contamination. Modifications of the initial method of McAfee and Thaker using acid citrate dextrose sedimentation, hetastarch, and differential centrifugation to obtain platelet poor, leukocyte-rich plasma is most frequently used. This method is simple to perform and produces a high yield of viable leukocytes that retain chemotaxis and the ability to bind and kill bacteria. However, the ease of leukocyte separation using this method is offset by contamination with as much as $29 \pm 15\%$ of platelets and 10–20% with red blood cells. Since the In-111 radiolabeling method is very nonspecific, the final preparation consists of platelets, leukocytes, and red blood cells. We have observed contamination with approximately 18% of platelets using our method of isolation and radiolabeling [10]. Thus, in vivo uptake may be nonspecific for leukocyte accumulation and areas of thrombus formation may incorporate In-111 labeled platelets and red blood cells. In view of the histologic findings in areas of endocarditis, incorporation of In-111 platelets and red blood cells introduced as contaminants may increase the sensitivity of detection, but care must be taken to exclude hemorrhage and thrombosis occurring in the absence of infection.

Other methods of cell separation are available that produce a higher leukocyte purity, but the additional time and equipment required have limited their applicability in most clinical settings [11]. Pure populations of polymorphonuclear leukocytes can be obtained using Ficoll-Hypaque differential density centrifugation techniques, but this method requires additional preparation time. Cell sorters that separate leukocytes on the basis of size are also available.

Radiolabeling

Isolated leukocytes have been successfully labeled with Tc-99m sulfur colloid, Tc-99m hexamethylpropyleneamine (HM-PAO) and In-111 [7–9]. Despite the high energy, long halflife, and low dose of administered activity (0.5–1.0 mCi or 18.5–37 MBq), In-111 is most frequently used due to ease of labeling, high yields of viable cells, and the extensive clinical experience acquired over a 15 year period.

In-111 is attached to 8-hydroxyquinoline to form In-111 oxine, a highly lipophilic ligand that readily diffuses across cell membranes. Leukocytes are incubated with In-111 oxine which readily enters the cytoplasm and dissociates into oxine and In-111. The In-111 is retained by binding to intracellular proteins, while the oxine readily diffuses out of the cells and is removed by washing.

Following intravenous injection, the In-111 leukocytes are cleared from blood with a half life of 5–6 hours. They are normally concentrated in the spleen, liver, and bone marrow. Imaging is routinely performed at 18–24 hours and if persistent blood pool activity is observed, this may indicate contamination by large amounts of red blood cells which have a longer blood half life than leukocytes.

Clinical applications

I have found In-111 leukocyte scintigraphy to be clinically useful in 2 patient

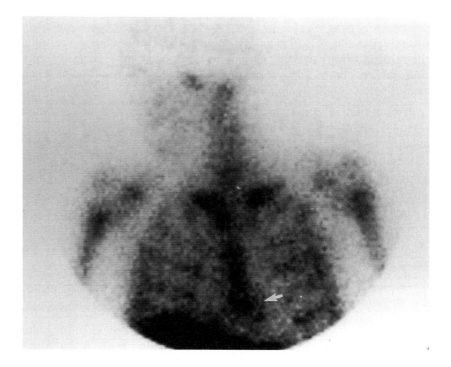

Figure 1. Anterior chest image showing a focal area of In-111 leukocyte uptake to the left of the sternum (arrow). (Cerqueira MD, Jacobson AF. Indium-111 leukocyte scintigraphic detection of myocardial abscess formation in patients with endocarditis. J Nucl Med 1989; 30: 703–6. Reprinted with permission from The Society of Nuclear Medicine.)

groups: patients with prosthetic valve endocarditis and those with heavy valvular or annular calcification where endocarditis is clinically suspected but not documented. In both these groups, transthoracic echocardiography and computerized x-ray tomography are limited in identifying abscess formation and vegetations in prosthetic or heavily calcified native valves. Frequently, the clinical decision to continue antibiotic treatment or undergo valve replacement can be aided by identification of abscess formation or the presence of large vegetations.

Prosthetic valve endocarditis

Early after starting antibiotic treatment for prosthetic valve endocarditis, persistent fevers and continued positive blood cultures may be due to treatment failure or to noncardiac sites of infection due to septic embolization. The development of congestive heart failure, usually a late finding of severe

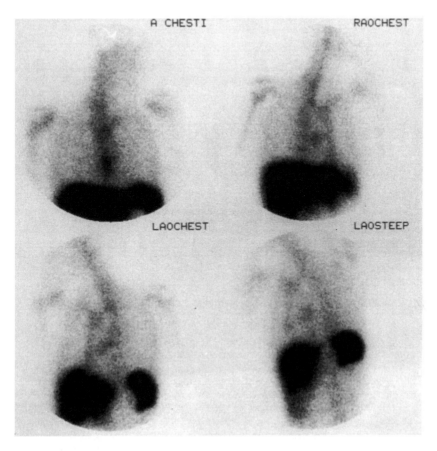

Figure 2. Four images of chest: On the anterior image, focal activity is beneath the sternum and not visualized, but oblique images separate it from overlapping sternum and allow excellent visualization. (Cerqueira MD, Jacobson AF. Indium-111 leukocyte scintigraphic detection of myocardial abscess formation in patients with endocarditis. J Nucl Med 1989; 30: 703–6. Reprinted with permission from the Society of Nuclear Medicine.)

annular destruction which makes surgery difficult, or recurrent embolization, are clear indications for surgical intervention. Thus, identification of abscess formation or large vegetations is an indication for early surgical intervention in order to prevent further deterioration and get the best operative result. Figures 1 and 2 are examples of In-111 leukocyte scans in patients with prosthetic aortic valves and *staph. aureus* bacteremia [4]. Although bone marrow in the sternum normally accumulates In-111 leukocytes, in both patients there is enhanced uptake in areas adjacent to the sternum. In Figure 2, oblique views were necessary to avoid overlap of the sternal bone marrow activity and allow visualization of a myocardial abscess. In some patients,

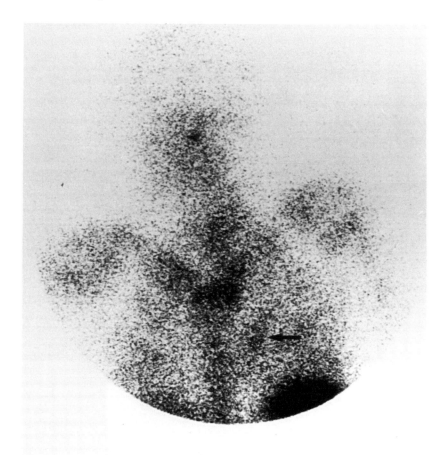

Figure 3. Anterior image of the chest showing abnormal uptake to the left of the upper portion of the sternum (arrow). (Cerqueira MD, Jacobson AF. Indium-111 leukocyte scintigraphic detection of myocardial abscess formation in patients with endocarditis. J Nucl Med 1989; 30: 703–6. Reprinted with permission from the Society of Nuclear Medicine.)

posterior views may be helpful in locating atrial or atrioventricular valve foci of infection. In theory, single photon emission computed tomography should improve sensitivity by avoiding overlap of marrow and other background activity, but the very low count rates from In-111 limit image quality and may not improve detection over planar imaging. In the patients in Figures 1 and 2, surgical exploration immediately following imaging identified sewing ring abscesses.

In-111 scintigraphy may also localize distant sites of infection caused by septic emboli that may account for continuing fevers and positive blood cultures. Some of these sites may be surgically drained by a percutaneous

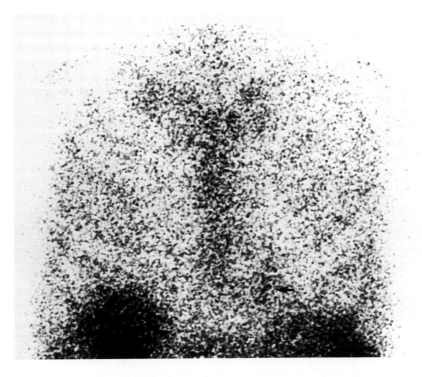

Figure 4. Anterior In-111 leukocyte scintigram showing abnormal focal accumulation in the area of the mitral valve (arrow). Normal leukocyte uptake is noted in the liver, spleen and bone marrow. (Cerqueira MD, Jacobson AF, Matsuda M, Stratton JR. Indium-111 leukocyte scintigraphic detection of mitral valve vegetations in active bacterial endocarditis. Am J Cardiol 1989; 64: 1080–1. Reprinted with permission from the American Journal of Cardiology.)

procedure to minimize possible prosthetic valve infection while antibiotic treatment is continued. In addition, In-111 leukocyte scintigraphy is extremely useful in identifying infected areas due to thrombophlebitis, intravenous catheters, or dialysis fistulas.

Native valve endocarditis

In patients with heavy calcification of valvular cusps, annulus, or leaflets, it may be difficult, if not technically impossible, to adequately visualize vegetations or abscess formation. In-111 leukocyte scintigraphy may be useful in such patients. Figures 3 and 4 are from patients with chronic renal failure and *staph. aureus* bacteremia being treated with antibiotics who continued to be febrile [3]. Echocardiography was technically difficult in both cases. Following the positive In-111 leukocyte scan in the patient shown in Figure 4, a repeat

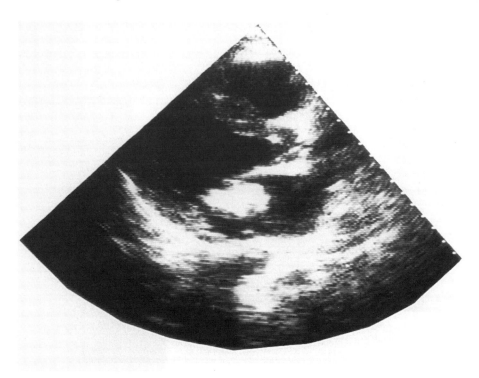

Figure 5. Parasternal long-axis two-dimensional echocardiogram, obtained immediately after the leukocyte scan, shows large vegetation attached to the posterior mitral valve leaflet that has prolapsed into the left atrium. (Cerqueira MD, Jacobson AF, Matsuda M, Stratton Jr. Indium-111 leukocyte scintigraphic detection of mitral valve vegetations in active bacterial endocarditis. Am J Cardiol 1989; 64: 1080–1. Reprinted with permission from the American Journal of Cardiology.)

echocardiogram is shown in Figure 5 [3]. It identified a large vegetation that had appeared over the 4 day interval since the initially negative echocardiogram. At autopsy, there was no evidence of abscess formation.

Other cardiac infections

In-111 leukocyte scintigraphy has been reported to be useful for the identification of purulent pericarditis, and abscess formation in areas of myocardial aneurysms of thrombi [12, 13].

In summary, In-111 leukocyte scintigraphy has an unknown, but probably low, sensitivity for detection of endocarditis. However, it is very specific and may provide diagnostic information that assists in management of prosthetic or heavily calcified native valve endocarditis where echocardiography is limited. Attention to the technical details of leukocyte separation and an aware-ness that platelet and red blood cells may be present as contaminants are necessary for optimal clinical utilization of this method.

Acknowledgement

Supported by the General Medical Research Services of the Department of Veterans Affairs, Washington, DC, USA.

References

1. Riba AL, Thakur ML, Gottschalk A, Andriole VT, Zaret BL. Imaging experimental in-fective endocarditis with Indium-111-labeled blood cellular components. Circulation 1979; 59: 336–43.
2. Wiseman J, Rouleau J, Rigo P, Strauss H, Pitt B. Gallium-67 myocardial imaging for the detection of bacterial endocarditis. Radiology 1976; 120: 135–8.
3. Cerqueira MD, Jacobson AF, Matsuda M, Stratton JR. Indium-111 leukocyte scintigraphic detection of mitral valve vegetations in active bacterial endocarditis. Am J Cardiol 1989; 64: 1080–1.
4. Cerqueira MD, Jacobson AF. Indium-111 leukocyte scintigraphic detection of myocardial abscess formation in patients with endocarditis. J Nucl Med 1989; 30: 703–6.
5. Rubin RH, Fischman AJ, Callahan RJ et al. In-111-labeled nonspecific immunoglobulin scanning in the detection of focal infection [see comments]. N Engl J Med 1989; 321: 935–40. Comment in: N Engl J Med 1989; 321: 970–2.
6. Strauss H, Fishman AJ, Khaw B et al. Detection of acute inflammation with immune imaging. In: Chatal JF, editor. Monoclonal antibodies in immunoscintigraphy. Boca Raton: CRC Press, 1989: 325–35.
7. McAfee J, Thakur M. Survey of radioactive agent for in vitro labeling of phagocytic leuko-cytes. I. Soluble agents. J Nucl Med 1976; 17: 480–7.
8. English D, Anderson BR. Labeling of phagocytes from human blood with 99mTc-sulfur colloid. J Nucl Med 1975; 16: 5–10.
9. Vorne M, Soini I, Lantto T, Paakkinen S. Technetium-99m HM-PAO-labeled leukocytes in detection of inflammatory lesions: comparison with gallium-67 citrate. J Nucl Med 1989; 30: 1332–6.
10. Gilbert BR, Cerqueira MD, Vea HW, Nelp WB. Indium-111-labeled leukocyte uptake: false-positive results in noninfected pseudoaneurysms. Radiology 1986; 158: 761–3.
11. Dewanjee M. Cardiac and vascular imaging with labeled platelets and leukocytes. Semin Nucl Med 1984; 14: 154–87.
12. Greenberg ML, Niebulski HI, Uretsky BF et al. Occult purulent pericarditis detected by Indium-111 leukocyte imaging. Chest 1984; 85: 701–3.
13. Reinke FE, Yuille DL, Jackson LJ, Zeft HJ, Mullen DC. Cardiac aneurysm complicated E. coli abscess. J Nucl Med 1983; 24: 1154–7.

34. Detection of cardiac thrombi with indium-111 platelet scintigraphy

FREEK W.A. VERHEUGT

Introduction

Thrombosis is intravascular clotting of blood due to inappropriate stimuli. In general, thrombosis can be divided in venous and arterial thrombosis. In both types of thrombosis different mechanisms initiate the clotting of the blood. In venous thrombosis, stasis of blood triggers the intrinsic pathway of the coagulation system. Arterial thrombosis is usually initiated by platelets activated by a high shear stress. Thrombin can also probably initiate thrombosis in both arteries and veins.

The left ventricle is a compartment of the cardiovascular system, in which high pressure differences are generated. Furthermore, the blood flow velocity in the left ventricle is generally high. Therefore, thrombosis in a normally functioning left ventricle is highly unlikely. However, the myocardium of the left ventricle can be damaged by ischemia, volume overload, pressure overload, or toxic agents such as viruses and chemicals (ethanol). Stroke volume will decrease and the flow patterns within the left ventricle are changed compared to the normal situation. Deterioration of left ventricular function can be divided into global or segmental dysfunction. Global dysfunction is seen in dilated cardiomyopathy and in volume overload. Segmental dysfunction is almost exclusively observed in ischemic heart disease, especially after myocardial infarction with aneurysm formation. The apex of the left ventricle is especially subject to aneurysm development. Anterior myocardial infarction due to occlusion of the left anterior descending coronary artery is the major cause of left ventricular aneurysm in the Western World. In a left ventricular aneurysm, the flow patterns can be intensively changed compared

447

Ernst E. van der Wall et al. (eds), What's new in cardiac imaging?, 447–454.
© *1992 Kluwer Academic Publishers. Printed in the Netherlands.*

to the normal situation [1] and thrombosis can easily occur. The exact mechanism of thrombus formation in a left ventricular with aneurysm is not known. Probably, two important pathways must be followed for the development of thrombosis in the dyskinetic area of the left ventricle. First, there is the necrotic endocardium, on which thrombus formation is possible due to platelet adhesion. Secondly, the severely disturbed flow pattern of the blood causes areas of stasis, by which intrinsic activation of the coagulation system occurs. After thrombus formation, the thrombus may grow during which active incorporation of fibrinogen and platelets occurs. Whether the thrombus, which can reach a size of several centimeters, stays in the aneurysm or dislodges, is unknown. When flow patterns in the aneurysm change and left ventricular function improves, which can be seen over time after infarction, the thrombus might dissolve without embolism [2].

The clinical importance of left ventricular thrombosis lies in the risk of systemic embolism. Especially, the cerebral thromboembolic stroke is a catastrophic complication of myocardial infarction in general and of left ventricular aneurysm in particular. Therefore, the diagnosis of left ventricular thrombosis is important in preventing this complication of left ventricular aneurysm. Finally, the prevention and treatment of left ventricular thrombosis is of most utmost importance, since the detection and clinical behavior of left ventricular thrombi can now be easily studied by several techniques.

The detection of left ventricular thrombosis

The considerations on the genesis of left ventricular thrombi are important in the diagnosis of left ventricular thrombus. The thrombotic process can be detected by three well defined imaging techniques in cardiovascular medicine:
(1) The detection of a filling defect within the left ventricle
(2) The detection of an echodense area by echocardiography
(3) The active incorporation of thrombus components like platelets

Left ventricular angiography and radionuclide ventriculography

A left ventricular thrombus is a space-occupying process in the left ventricle. Any imaging technique which opacifies the left ventricle is able to show a filling defect. Two techniques have been used for the detection of left ventricular thrombi, which show filling defects: left ventricular angiography and radionuclide ventriculography.

Left ventricular angiography [3] performed in the right anterior oblique projection, can indicate a filling defect in a left ventricular aneurysm. The sensitivity of this technique, when surgical verification was used, is about 50% with a specificity of about 80% [3]. Because of its high cost, routine angiography is not useful in screening patients for the detection of left ventricular thrombosis.

Radionuclide ventriculography is safer, cheaper, and more easily available. It was shown that its sensitivity is not much better than contrast ventriculography, but its specificity is nearly 100% [4]. A disadvantage of this technique is that only large thrombi can be visualized, because radionuclide ventriculography is done in the left anterior oblique position, by which the aneurysmatic apex is not very easily identified. Due to its low sensitivity, radionuclide ventriculography has not been very popular in the screening of patients at risk for left ventricular thrombosis.

Echocardiography

Echocardiography has become the standard diagnostic tool for the detection of left ventricular thrombosis [5] and it has been shown that its sensitivity is very high (90–95%), but also that its specificity was lower than that of radionuclide ventriculography. Possibly, reverberations might cause false positive echocardiograms. However, its availability, low cost, and safety has made echocardiography the almost ideal diagnostic tool for the screening and detection of left ventricular thrombosis. Furthermore, echocardiographic studies can be endlessly repeated.

Echocardiography detects thrombus mass and can also give some information about thrombus behaviour [6]. Protruding and mobile thrombi might embolize, mural and flat ones will not. These thrombus characteristics are of utmost importance in the preventive measures for embolic stroke.

Indium-111 platelet scintigraphy

The detection of incorporation of hemostatic material into the left ventricle is the most specific sign of left ventricular thrombosis. Labeling blood platelets has shown to be the most specific technique for the detection of left ventricular thrombosis [7]. However, its sensitivity is lower than that of echocardiography. Although this seems to be a shortcoming of the technique, it was clearly shown that hematologically active thrombi incorporate platelets and inactive ones do not [8, 9].

The technique is simple but laborious. Platelets are separated from platelet-rich plasma of the patient and incubated with indium-111 oxine [10]. After in vitro labeling, the platelets are washed and reinjected into the patient. Because of the long half-life of indium-111 (68 hours) the incorporation can be

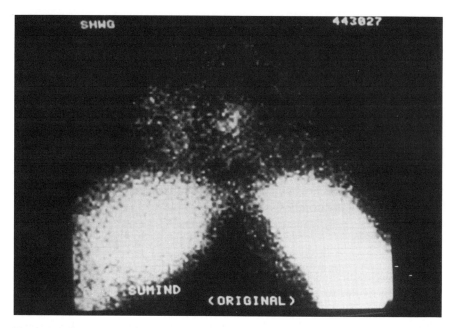

Figure 1. Indium-111 platelet scintigram of a patient with a recent anterolateral myocardial infarction 72 hours after platelet labeling. Left anterior oblique position. Note the hot spot (thrombus) in the left ventricle. At the left, the liver is seen, on the right the spleen. A faint blood pool image can be observed.

detected after a few days after injection, when the blood pool of labeled platelets has been disappeared.

Newer labeling techniques include the use of indium-111 troponolate [11] or acetylacetone [12] instead of oxine. Intriguing results have been obtained with technetium-99m platelet labeling, by which the disadvantages of indium-111 can be eliminated. For these purposes, the isotope is coupled with exametazine (technetium-99m hexamethylpropyleneamine oxime (HM-PAO), Ceretec®, Amersham, Little Chalfont, Buckinghamshire, United Kingdom) which penetrates the platelet during the in vitro labeling [13].

Platelet labeling has a potential of quantification of left ventricular platelet deposition, which makes prospective drug studies possible. It is clear, that due to its time consuming and laborious properties, indium-111 platelet scintigraphy has not become a popular tool in the diagnosis and screening of left ventricular thrombosis.

The value of indium-111 platelet scintigraphy in the prevention, diagnosis, and treatment of left ventricular thrombosis

The incidence of left ventricular thrombosis detected by indium-111 platelet scintigraphy in consecutive patients with myocardial infarction is very low [9]. It was shown, that especially anterior myocardial infarctions give rise to thrombus formation (Figure 1). By scintigraphic techniques, it became possible to quantitate platelet deposition in the left ventricle after acute myocardial infarction (Figure 2). In acute infarction, platelet deposition is higher than in remote myocardial infarction [8]. It was also shown that platelet deposition is higher in patients with transmural myocardium infarction than in those with subendocardial infarction [9]. However, for quantitative purposes indium-111 platelet scintigraphy should be combined with technetium-99m blood pool scintigraphy to subtract activity from nonthrombus bound circulating platelets. Dual isotope substraction has considerable problems, especially in the field of tissue attenuation and the places of anatomical landmarks. In rabbit carotid arteries [14] and humans [8] it was shown that quantitation of platelet deposition is possible, but in both studies anatomical validation was incomplete.

Prevention of left ventricular thrombus formation studied by indium-111 platelet scintigraphy is hardly done [15–17]. The prevention of thrombus formation can be much better studied with echocardiography. From those studies, it emanated, that high dose heparin might prevent thrombus formation in the setting of myocardial infarction [18].

Longitudinal study with indium-111 platelet scintigraphy is hardly possible because of its high radiation burden. Also in this field echocardiography has large advantages. Once a left ventricular thrombus has been detected, oral anticoagulation is advocated, although efficacy and safety in its resolution and the prevention of embolization are not fully proven [19].

Conclusion

Indium-111 platelet scintigraphy is the most specific diagnostic tool for the detection of left ventricular thrombosis. It is a laborious technique with a high radiation burden and, therefore, cannot be used as a routine test for the screening of left ventricular thrombosis. While echocardiography detects thrombus mass, platelet scintigraphy identifies its hematological activity and, therefore, its embolic potential. Dual isotope substraction using technetium-99m blood pool scintigraphy makes quantification of platelet deposition

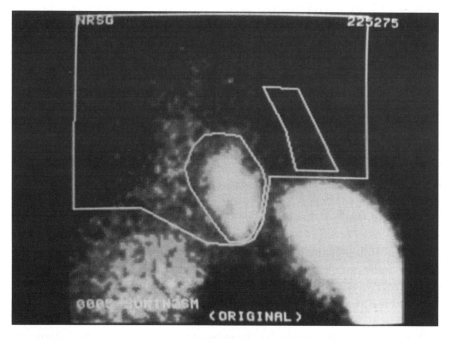

Figure 2a.

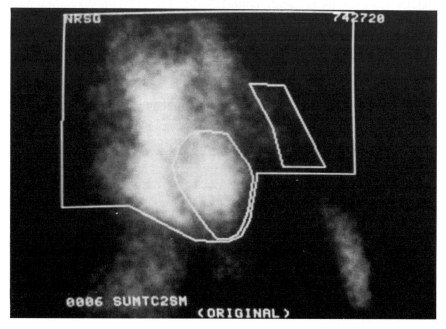

Figure 2b.

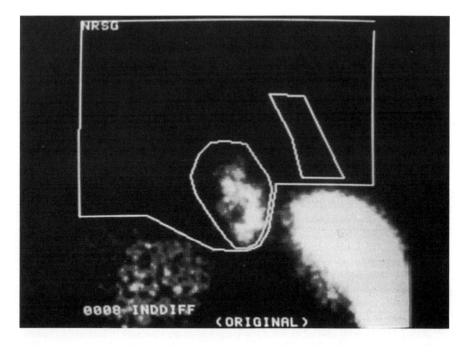

Figure 2c.

Figure 2a. Quantitation of platelet deposition in the left ventricle [8]. Indium-111 platelet scinti-gram of a patient with a recent anterior myocardial infarction 72 hours after platelet labeling. Left anterior oblique position. Note the hot spot (thrombus) in the left ventricle and a faint blood pool image. To quantify platelet deposition, areas of interest are drawn over the thorax, left ventricle (see Figure 2b) and left lung.
Figure 2b. Quantitation of platelet deposition in the left ventricle [8]. Simultaneous techne-tium-99m blood pool image of the same patient in the same position as Figure 2a.
Figure 2c. Quantitation of platelet deposition in the left ventricle [8]. Blood pool subtracted indium-111 platelet scintigram.

possible. Newer platelet imaging techniques, that are less time consuming and offer a lower radiation exposure, are eagerly awaited.

References

1. Delemarre BJ, Visser CA, Bot H, Dunning AJ. Prediction of apical thrombus formation in acute myocardial infarction based on left ventricular spatial flow pattern. J Am Coll Cardiol 1990; 15: 355–60.
2. Funke Küpper AJ, Verheugt FW, Peels CH, Galema TW, Roos JP. Left ventricular throm-bus incidence and behaviour studied by serial two-dimensional echocardiography in acute

anterior myocardial infarction: left ventricular wall motion, systemic embolism and oral anticoagulation. J Am Coll Cardiol 1989; 13: 1514–20.

3. Reeder GS, Lengyel M, Tajik AJ, Seward JB, Smith HC, Danielson GK. Mural thrombus in left ventricular aneurysm: incidence, role of angiography, and relation between anticoagulation and embolization: Mayo Clin Proc 1981; 56: 77–81.

4. Stratton JR, Ritchie JL, Hammermeister KE, Kennedy JW, Hamilton GW. Detection of left ventricular thrombi with radionuclide angiography. Am J Cardiol 1981; 48: 565–72.

5. Asinger RW, Mikell FL, Sharma B, Hodges M. Observations on detecting left ventricular thrombus with two dimensional echocardiography: emphasis on avoidance of false positive diagnosis. Am J Cardiol 1981; 47: 145–56.

6. Meltzer RS, Visser CA, Kan G, Roelandt J. Two-dimensional echocardiographic appearance of left ventricular thrombi with systemic emboli after myocardial infarction. Am J Cardiol 1984; 53: 1511–3.

7. Ezekowitz MD, Wilson DA, Smith EO et al. Comparison of indium-111 platelet scintigraphy and two-dimensional echocardiography in the diagnosis of left ventricular thrombi. N Engl J Med 1982; 306: 1509–13.

8. Verheugt FW, Lindenfeld J, Kirch DL, Steele PP. Left ventricular platelet deposition after acute myocardial infarction. An attempt at quantification using blood pool substracted indium-111 platelet scintigraphy. Br Heart J 1984; 52: 490–6.

9. Funke Küpper AJ, Verheugt FW, Jaarsma W et al. Detection of ventricular thrombosis in acute myocardial infarction: value of indium-111 platelet scintigraphy in relation to two-dimensional echocardiography and clinical course. Eur J Nucl Med 1986; 12: 337–41.

10. Scheffel U, Tsan MF, McIntyre PA. Labeling of human platelets with [111In]8-hydroxyquinoline. J Nucl Med 1979; 20: 524–31.

11. Peters AM, Saverymuttu SH, Malik F, Ind PW, Lavender JP. Intrahepatic kinetics of indium-111 labelled platelets. Thromb Haemost 1985; 54: 595–8.

12. Sinn H, Silvester DJ. Simplified cell labelling with indium-111 acetylacetone. Br J Radiol 1979; 52: 758–9.

13. Becker W, Borst U, Krahe T, Börner W. Tc-99m-HMPAO labelled human platelets: in vitro and in vivo results. Eur J Nucl Med 1989; 15: 296–301.

14. Isaka Y, Kimura K, Yoneda S et al. Platelet accumulation in carotid atherosclerotic lesions: semiquantitative analysis with indium-111 platelets and technetium-99m human serum albumin. J Nucl Med 1984; 25: 556–63.

15. Funke Kupper AJ, Verheugt FW, Den Hollander W. Failure of sulfinpyrazone to prevent left ventricular thrombosis in patients with acute myocardial infarction treated with oral anticoagulants: a randomized trial in 100 patients. In: Kessler Ch, Hardeman MR, Henningsen H, editors. Clinical application of radiolabelled platelets. Dordrecht: Kluwer, 1990: 116–27.

16. Stratton JR, Lighty GW Jr, Pearlman AS, Ritchie JL. Detection of left ventricular thrombus by two-dimensional echocardiography: sensitivity, specificity, and causes of uncertainty. Circulation 1982; 66: 156–66.

17. Ezekowitz MD, Cox AC, Smith EO, Taylor FB. Failure of aspirin to prevent incorporation of indium-111 labelled platelets into cardiac thrombi in man. Lancet 1981; 2: 440–3.

18. Turpie AG, Robinson JG, Doyle DJ et al. Comparison of high-dose with low-dose subcutaneous heparin to prevent left ventricular mural thrombosis in patients with acute transmural anterior myocardial infarction. N Engl J Med 1989; 320: 352–7.

19. Tramarin R, Pozzoli M, Febo O et al. Two-dimensional echocardiographic assessment of anticoagulant therapy in left ventricular thrombosis early after acute myocardial infarction. Eur Heart J 1986; 7: 482–92.

35. Scintigraphic detection of atherosclerosis with radiolabeled low density lipoprotein

DOUWE E. ATSMA

Summary

The noninvasive detection of early atherosclerosis can be accomplished by external scintigraphic imaging after injection of radiolabeled autologous low density lipoprotein (LDL). The radiolabeled LDL enters the forming atherosclerotic plaque, providing insight both in the localization of the lesions and the metabolic activity of the atherogenic process. Using this technique, atherosclerotic lesions have been imaged in animals and humans. This chapter discusses the present state of research with radiolabeled LDL and future developments.

Introduction

Atherosclerosis is a chronic progressive disease of the blood vessels without any clinical symptoms until late in its development. Until now, the diagnosis of asymptomatic atherosclerosis has been primarily based on the space-occupying characteristics of the well-advanced plaque, as determined by contrast angiography, ultrasound, and more recently, also by computed tomography and magnetic resonance imaging.

Since early detection of atherosclerosis is considered crucial for successful therapy [1, 2ab], the need exists for a simple noninvasive test that could be serially used to detect early atherosclerotic lesions and to monitor the effects of long-term therapy. In recent years, several researchers have been studying the possibility of scintigraphically detecting atherosclerotic plaques by demonstra-

Ernst E. van der Wall et al. (eds), What's new in cardiac imaging?, 455–464.
© *1992 Kluwer Academic Publishers. Printed in the Netherlands.*

ting the metabolic processes that take place during the formation of the plaques. Theoretically, this approach would both give information on the localization and extent of the atherosclerotic lesions, and would assess the metabolic activity of the process of atherogenesis.

Different approaches have been made, including scintigraphic imaging after intravenous administration of radiolabeled platelets [3, 4], fibrinogen [5], fibronectin [6, 7], porphyrin [8–10], monocytes [11], polyclonal antibodies [12], and LDL. Of these agents, LDL has been studied most extensively and will be discussed here.

Radiolabeled LDL as an imaging agent for atherosclerosis

It is well-known that LDL, the major cholesterol transporting lipoprotein, is involved in early atherogenesis. An increased influx of LDL into the forming plaque leads to deposition of the lipoprotein and its cholesterol either intracellularly, in macrophages and smooth muscle cells, or extracellularly, bound to proteoglycan and elastin [13–16]. Although the mechanisms involved in the LDL uptake in major arteries are not fully understood, the phenomenon is the basis for the detection of atherosclerosis by external scintigraphic imaging using radiolabeled LDL.

Since LDL is directly involved in atherogenesis, it is therefore apparently a highly suitable and specific imaging agent for atherosclerosis. However, there are also some less favorable aspects to the use of LDL in scintigraphic imaging.

First, the availability of the lipoprotein is less than optimal. The LDL must be isolated from the patient's own blood in order to prevent spread of viral infection via donor LDL. The isolation is a time-consuming process and must be repeated before each imaging session. Second, the long half-life of LDL in the circulation, especially in hypercholesterolemic patients, leads to a slow clearance of blood pool radioactivity, interfering with the identification of focal accumulation of the radiolabel in the atherosclerotic vessel wall. Third, the apoprotein B of the LDL particle, to which the radionuclide is attached, is a delicate structure easily modified by the labeling procedures. Modification of the LDL particle could lead to a different behavior of the labeled lipoprotein in circulation as compared to native LDL. Although modification of the lipoprotein is therefore undesirable in LDL metabolism studies, the consequences for imaging of atherosclerotic lesions are less clear; indeed, recent studies indicate that LDL found in the atherosclerotic plaques has experienced different forms of modification as compared to LDL in the circulation [17–20]. It is not fully understood whether the modification of the LDL particle, found in atherosclerotic lesions, has occurred after deposition in the plaque or the LDL is modified in the circulation and subsequently taken up in the plaque as a consequence of its modification. Other studies show that modified LDL is taken up faster in the atherosclerotic aorta in animal models [21, 22]. These data suggest that radiolabeled modified LDL could be a more suitable imaging agent for atherosclerosis than unmodified LDL. An additional advantage of the use of modified LDL would be an accelerated plasma clearance of circulating labeled lipoprotein as a result of increased uptake by scavenger receptors in the reticulo-endothelial system. This would lead to an improved target-to-background ratio. Some of the above-mentioned problems have already been addressed, other still need additional attention.

LDL isolation

Isolation of LDL from the patient's serum is carried out either by ultracentrifugation or by immunoaffinity chromatography. With ultracentrifugation, a serum fraction with a density of between 1.019 and 1.063 g/ml is isolated containing the LDL. With sequential ultracentrifugation, the isolation occurs in several subsequent centrifugation runs. This procedure is more elaborate and time-consuming than in gradient ultracentrifugation, whereby the isolation is achieved in just one run.

In affinity chromatography, LDL is isolated from the serum by means of polyclonal antibodies directed against apo-B, attached to a carrier material such as Sepharose. This technique provides a more rapid isolation of the lipoprotein for labeling purposes.

LDL labeling

Isotopes

Several different radionuclides have been used to label LDL in the atherosclerosis imaging studies. Although iodine-125 (I-125) labeled to LDL was successfully used in the initial report on scintigraphic imaging of atherosclerosis in humans [23], this radionuclide is not suitable for in vivo imaging because of its poor radiation characteristics. A much better radiolabel is iodine-123 (I-123) which combines high emitted energy with a short half-life of 13.2 hours, resulting in good spatial resolution and low radiation dose to the patient. The same is true for technetium-99m (Tc-99m, half-life 6 hours), while this radionuclide has advantages over I-123 in terms of availability and cost. More recently, indium-111 (In-111) has been used, which has a longer half-life of 2.83

days, allowing a longer follow-up after administration of the radiolabeled LDL. This permits imaging after substantial clearance of the blood pool radioactivity.

Labeling procedures

For labeling of the LDL particle with the different radionuclides stated above, several labeling methods have been described. Because the labeling method itself can have modifying effects on the metabolic behavior of the radiolabeled LDL, much emphasis is placed on this aspect. In our laboratory, we have recently evaluated seven different labeling techniques, using I-123 and Tc-99m, with respect to labeling yields, modification caused by the labeling techniques, and radiochemical stability of the radiolabeled LDL complex [24]. In our study it was concluded that satisfactory labeling results were achieved only when freshly isolated LDL was radiolabeled with I-123 by the iodine monochloride method, described by McFarlane [25], or with Tc-99m by the sodium dithionite method described by Lees et al. [26], or with the diamide dithiolate ligand method described by Fritzberg et al. [27], which was adapted by our group [24]. A third Tc-99m labeling technique using sodium boro-hydride and stannous chloride, recently developed in our laboratory, yields Tc-99m LDL that is stable in the circulation but is cleared much faster from circulation than native LDL [24, 28]. For In-111 labeling, the procedure described by Hnatowich et al. [29] produces stable In-111 LDL complex with a biological behavior similar to that of I-125 LDL produced by the iodine monochloride method [30, 37].

Animal studies

To validate the concept of imaging plaques using radiolabeled LDL, numerous animal studies have been carried out, most of these using a rabbit model in which the aortal endothelium was stripped by means of an embolectomy catheter [31]. Additional feeding of a cholesterol-enriched diet led to the formation of fatty streaks lesions [32]. The selective accumulation of I-125 LDL in the stripped aortas of normocholesterolemic rabbits was reported in 1983 by Roberts et al. [33], although they did not perform external imaging. Using the same radiolabel, Sinzinger and Virgolini [34] found that the uptake of radiolabel was higher at the edge of the healing aortic endothelium than in the centre of the lesions. By monitoring the kinetics of radiolabel uptake in the atherosclerotic aorta, de-endothelialized, re-endothelialized and control aorta could be distinguished. Lees et al. [26] showed the potential of Tc-99m labeled

LDL to accumulate in healing arterial wall. High-quality scintigraphic images were obtained 16 hours after administration of the Tc-99m LDL. It was found that Tc-99m LDL behaves like a trapped ligand. Following uptake by the tissue, the Tc-99m LDL remains situated at the accumulation site. This is an advantage for in vivo imaging, since it enhances development of 'hot spots' at the site of accumulation facilitating external imaging. Radioiodinated LDL is rapidly deiodinated after intracellular uptake, resulting in loss of radiolabel from the plaque, complicating scintigraphic imaging [35]. In addition, to prevent the uptake of the circulating I-123 by the thyroid gland, blocking of the gland is necessary in human studies. In our laboratory, we showed that Tc-99m LDL, labeled by a new method resulting in a shorter half-life of the radio-labeled LDL in circulation, was accumulated in the aorta of hypercholestero-lemic rabbits more than Tc-99m LDL used in previous successful imaging studies, although external imaging failed to show hot spots for both methods (Figure 1) [28].

Imaging studies after administration of LDL, labeled with the longer living In-111 in atherosclerotic rabbits, showed an increased accumulation of the In-111 LDL in the aorta, which could be externally identified by scintigraphy [36, 37].

Imaging in humans

The first to report on the scintigraphic imaging of atherosclerosis in humans were Lees et al. [23] in 1983, who used I-125 LDL in three patients with atherosclerotic lesions of the carotid arteries. Two days after reinjection of the labeled LDL, all three patients showed clear focal accumulation of the label in the neck region that corresponded well with the known localization of vessel wall lesions as found by contrast angiography. No accumulation was apparent in the carotid arteries of a control subject.

Sinzinger et al. [38] used I-123 LDL in 17 patients with clinical manifest carotid and peripheral atherosclerosis. In 10 patients accumulation of radiola-bel was observed over the carotid arteries and in six patients over the femoral artery regions, as early as 30 minutes after I-123 LDL injection. In a more recent study, 86 patients were injected with I-123 LDL [39]. Whole body scans were made up to 42 hours after injection. Some hot spots could be identified as early as 30 minutes after injection, others as late as 12 hours or more. The number and extent of the positive images correlated poorly with the clinical manifestations of atherosclerosis. Examination of surgical specimens obtained after endarteriectomy or graft implantation showed high accumulation of the label in lipid-rich lesions (almost five times more than control), while signif-

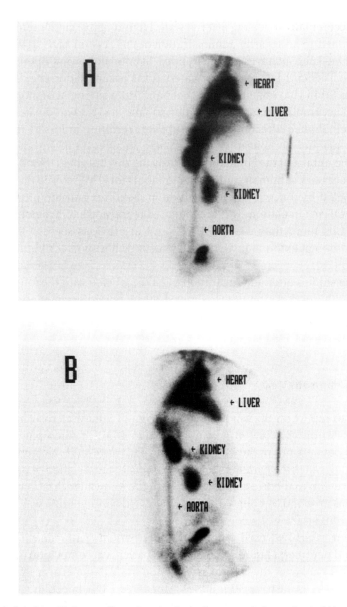

Figure 1. Scintigraphic images (lateral projection) of a normocholesterolemic (A) and a hyper-cholesterolemic (B) rabbit, 2 hours after intravenous administration of equal doses of Tc-99m LDL. Enhanced visualization of the aorta in the hypercholesterolemic rabbit as compared to the normocholesterolemic rabbit is the combined result of accumulation of the Tc-99m LDL in the vessel wall and the slower clearance from circulation of the radiolabeled lipoprotein, caused by downregulation of LDL receptors in the liver in response to the atherogenic diet.

icantly less label entered advanced lesions containing few foam cells, like fibrous plaques (only slightly more than control). Lupattelli et al. [40] studied eight patients with carotid and femoral atherosclerotic plaques, reinjecting I-123 labeled autologous LDL [40]. Immediately after reinjection of the labeled lipoprotein, accumulation over the carotid artery region was observed in six of eight patients, while in four of six patients hot spots were seen over the femoral artery region 2 to 6 hours after injection. Lees et al. [41] performed imaging of atherosclerosis in human subjects using Tc-99m LDL. Seventeen patients with documented atherosclerotic lesions were studied this way, and in four patients accumulation of radioactivity was sufficiently high to allow external imaging of the lesions 8 to 21 hours after administration of the Tc-99m LDL. Histological specimens of the atherosclerotic plaques that became available after surgery of six patients, showed that the specimens of the plaques detected by external imaging contained a large number of foam cells, whereas the undetected specimens were more mature fibrocalcific lesions.

Discussion

The concept of the noninvasive detection of atherosclerosis by means of external scintigraphy using radiolabeled LDL holds great promise for the early diagnosis of asymptomatic atherosclerosis. It is already possible to visualize experimental atherosclerosis in animals and some atherosclerotic plaques in humans. Uptake of radiolabeled LDL by the atherosclerotic plaques in humans seems to depend on the histological composition of the lesion: a much higher accumulation of the labeled LDL was observed in early atherosclerotic lesions with abundant foam cells and deposition of cholesterol, as compared to the more advanced fibrocalcified lesions. This difference in accumulation can be expected because foam cells are known to accumulate LDL in atherosclerotic plaques.

Since fatty streaks, being the most active sites in atherogenesis, are likely to respond to therapeutical intervention, such as lowering serum cholesterol levels, the serial imaging of atherosclerosis using radiolabeled LDL could be a useful tool in the monitoring of therapy. However, before imaging of atherosclerosis with radiolabeled LDL can be used on a routine basis, additional studies will be needed to further develop the procedures involved in the preparation of the most suitable imaging agent for atherosclerosis. Radiolabeled modified LDL, accumulating faster in experimental atherosclerotic lesions and clearing from circulation at an accelerated rate, might be a more suitable agent for atherosclerosis than the presently used LDL. Also, labeling of LDL with longer living radionuclides such as In-111 is likely to improve the potential to detect early atherosclerosis as a result of the higher target-to-background ratios that can be achieved.

Conclusion

Imaging of atherosclerotic lesions using radiolabeled LDL is a promising diagnostic tool, capable of providing information on the metabolic behavior of atherosclerotic plaques. Although positive imaging of atherosclerosis has been accomplished in animal and human studies, further research is needed to optimize the method for routine application in patient care.

References

1. Nikkila EA, Viikinkoski P, Valle M. Effect of lipid lowering treatment on progression of coronary atherosclerosis [abstract]. Circulation 1983; 67 (4 suppl III): III188.
2a. The lipid research clinics coronary primary prevention trial results I. Reduction in incidence of coronary heart disease. JAMA 1984; 251: 351–64.
2b. The lipid research clinics coronary primary prevention trial results II. The relationship of reduction in incidence of coronary heart disease to cholesterol lowering. JAMA 1984; 251: 365–74.
3. Isaka Y, Kimura K, Yoneda S et al. Platelet accumulation in carotid atherosclerotic lesions: semiquantitative analysis with indium-111 platelets and technetium-99m human serum albumin. J Nucl Med 1984; 25: 556–63.
4. Sinzinger H, O'Grady J, Fitscha P, Silberbauer K, Hofer R. Detection of aneurysms by gamma-camera imaging after injection of autologous labelled platelets. Lancet 1984; 2: 1365–7.
5. Mettinger KL, Larsson S, Ericson K, Casseborn S. Detection of atherosclerotic plaques in carotid arteries by the use of ^{123}I-fibrinogen. Lancet 1978; 1: 242–4.
6. Uehara A, Isaka Y, Hashikawa K et al. Iodine-131-labeled fibronectin: potential agent for imaging atherosclerotic lesion and thrombus. J Nucl Med 1988; 29: 1264–7.
7. Collins EF, Carew TE. Focal elevation of concentration of fibronectin but not of albumin in atherosclerotic lesion-susceptable sites in rabbit aorta [abstract]. Faseb J 1990; 4: A342.
8. Kessel D, Sykes E. Porphyrin accumulation by atheromatous plaques of the aorta. Photochem Photobiol 1984; 40: 59–61.
9. Palac RT, Gray LL, Turner FE, Brown PH, Malinow MR, Demots H. Detection of experimental atherosclerosis with indium-111 radiolabeled hematoporphyrin derivative. Nucl Med Comm 1989; 10: 841–50.
10. Wong DW, Hyman S, Reese I et al. Scintigraphic detection of atherosclerotic plaques in rabbits with In-111-labeled hematoporphyrin derivative. Int J Rad Appl Instrum [B] 1989; 16: 551–7.
11. Virgolini I, Fitscha P, Shiba P, Sinzinger H. Positive vessel imaging after reinjection of autologous In-111-oxine labeled monocytes to patients with atherosclerosis. In: Sinzinger H, Thakur ML, editors. Radiolabeled cellular blood elements: proceedings of the 5th In-

ternational Symposium on Radiolabeled Cellular Blood Elements, held in Vienna; September 10–14, 1989. New York: Wiley-Liss, 1990: 177–80.

12. Fischman AJ, Rubin RH, Khaw BA et al. Radionuclide imaging of experimental atherosclerosis with nonspecific polyclonal immunoglobulin G. J Nucl Med 1989; 30: 1095–100.

13. Hoff HF, Bradley WA, Heideman CL, Gaubatz JW, Karagas MD, Gotto AM Jr. Characterization of low density lipoprotein-like particles in the human aorta from grossly normal and atherosclerotic regions. Biochim Biophys Acta 1979; 573: 361–74.

14. Linden T, Bondjers G, Camejo G, Bergstrand R, Wilhelmsen L, Wicklund O. Affinity of LDL to a human proteoglycan among male survivors of myocardial infarction. Eur J Clin Invest 1989; 19: 38–44.

15. Bocan TM, Brown SA, Guyton JR. Human aortic fibrolipid lesions. Immunochemical localization of apolipoprotein B and apolipoprotein A. Arteriosclerosis 1988; 8: 499–508.

16. Smith EB, Staples HS, Dietz HS, Smith RH. Role of endothelium in sequesteration of lipoprotein and fibrinogen in aortic lesions, thrombi, and graft pseudo-intimas. Lancet 1979; 2: 812–6.

17. Steinberg D, Parthasarathy S, Carew TE, Khoo JC, Witztum JL. Beyond cholesterol. Modifications of low density lipoprotein that increase its atherogenicity. N Engl J Med 1989; 329: 915–24.

18. Shaikh M, Martini S, Quiney JR et al. Modified plasma-derived lipoproteins in human atherosclerotic plaques. Atherosclerosis 1988; 69: 165–72.

19. Ylä-Hertuala S, Palinski W, Rosenfeld ME et al. Evidence of the presence of oxidatively modified low density lipoprotein in atherosclerotic lesions of rabbit and man. J Clin Invest 1989; 84: 1086–95.

20. Boyd HC, Gown AM, Wolfbauer G, Chait A. Direct evidence for a protein recognized by a monoclonal antibody against oxidatively modified LDL in atherosclerotic lesions from a Watanabe heritable hyperlipidemic rabbit. Am J Pathol 1989; 135: 815–25.

21. Fischman AJ, Lees AM, Lees RS, Barlai-Kovach M, Strauss HW. Accumulation of native and methylated low density lipoproteins by healing rabbit arterial wall. Arteriosclerosis 1987; 7: 361–6.

22. Wiklund O, Mattson L, Camejo G, Bondjers G. Cellular uptake and degredation of LDL and modified LDL in atherosclerotic rabbit aorta. Studies in an in vitro perfusion system [abstract]. Arteriosclerosis 1989; 9: 704a.

23. Lees RS, Lees AM, Strauss HW. External imaging of human atherosclerosis. J Nucl Med 1983; 24: 154–6.

24. Atsma DE, Kempen HJ, Nieuwenhuizen W, van 't Hooft FM, Pauwels EKJ. Partial characterization of low density lipoprotein preparations isolated from fresh and frozen plasma after radiolabeling by seven different methods. J Lipid Res 1991; 32: 173–81.

25. McFarlane AS. Efficient trace-labeling of proteins with iodine. Nature 1958; 182: 53–7.

26. Lees RS, Garabedian HD, Lees AM et al. Technetium-99m low density lipoproteins: preparation and biodistribution. J Nucl Med 1985; 26: 1056–62.

27. Fritzberg AR, Abrams PG, Beaumier PL et al. Specific and stable labeling of antibodies with technetium-99m with a diamine dithiolate chelating agent. Proc Natl Acad Sci USA 1988; 85: 4025–9.

28. Atsma DE, Feitsma RI, Camps J et al. Potential of Tc-99m-low density lipoproteins labeled by two different methods for the scintigraphic detection of experimental atherosclerosis in rabbits (in press).

29. Hnatowich DJ, Childs RL, Lanteigne D, Najafi A. The preparation of DTPA-coupled antibodies radiolabeled with metallic radionuclides: an improved method. J Immunol Methods 1983; 65: 147–57.

30. Sinzinger H, Virgolini I. Nuclear medicine and atherosclerosis. Eur J Nucl Med 1990; 17: 160–78.
31. Baumgartner HR. Eine neue Methode zur Erzeugung von Thromben durch gezielte Uberdehnung der Gefasswand. Z Ges Exp Med 1963; 137: 227–47.
32. Minick CR, Stemerman MB, Isull W Jr. Effect of regenerated endothelium on lipid accumulation in the arterial wall. Proc Natl Acad Sci USA 1977; 74: 1724–8.
33. Roberts AB, Lees AM, Lees RS et al. Selective accumulation of low density lipoproteins in damaged arterial wall. J Lipid Res 1983; 24: 1160–7.
34. Sinzinger H, Angelberger P, Pesl H, Flores J, Rauscha F. Further insights into lipid lesion imaging by means of ^{123}I-labeled autologous Low Density Lipoproteins (LDL). In: Crepaldi E, Gotto AM, Manzato E, Baggio G, editors. Atherosclerosis VIII: proceedings of the 8th international symposium on atherosclerosis: Rome 9–13 October 1988. Excerpta Medica, 1989: 645–53.
35. Vallabhajosula S, Paidi M, Badimon JJ et al. Radiotracers for low density lipoprotein biodistribution studies in vivo: technetium-99m low density lipoprotein versus radioiodinated low density lipoprotein preparations. J Nucl Med 1988; 29: 1237–45.
36. Rosen JM, Butler SP, Meinken GE et al. Indium-111-labeled LDL: a potential agent for imaging atherosclerotic disease and lipoprotein distribution. J Nucl Med 1990; 31: 343–50.
37. Nicolas JM, Leclef B, Jardez H, Keyeux A, Melin JA, Trouet A. Imaging atherosclerotic lesions with In-111 labeled low density lipoproteins [abstract]. J Nucl Med 1989 (suppl); 30: 738.
38. Sinzinger H, Bergmann H, Kaliman J, Angelberger P. Imaging of human atherosclerotic lesions using ^{123}I-low density lipoprotein. Eur J Nucl Med 1986; 12: 291–2.
39. Sinzinger H, Angelberger P. Imaging and kinetics studies with radiolabeled autologous low-density lipoproteins (LDL) in human atherosclerosis. Nucl Med Comm 1988; 9: 859–66.
40. Lupattelli G, Palumbo R, Fedeli L, Deleide G, Ventura A. Radiolabeled LDL in the 'in vivo' detection of human atherosclerotic plaques. In: Crepaldi E, Gotto AM, Manzato E, Baggio G, editors. Atherosclerosis VIII: proceedings of the 8th international symposium on atherosclerosis; Rome, 9–13 October 1988. Excerpta Medica, 1989: 655–9.
41. Lees AM, Lees RS, Schoen FJ et al. Imaging human atherosclerosis with Tc-99m-labeled low density lipoproteins. Arteriosclerosis 1988; 8: 461–70.

Viability

36. Assessment of myocardial viability with scintigraphic techniques and magnetic resonance imaging: new attainments?

HUBERT W. VLIEGEN, ERNST E. VAN DER WALL,
AAF F.M. KUIJPER, PAUL R.M. VAN DIJKMAN,
ERNEST K.J. PAUWELS and ALBERT V.G. BRUSCHKE

Summary

The ability to distinguish ischemic but still viable myocardium from irreversibly damaged myocardial areas, i.e. nonviable myocardium, is of paramount importance. Myocardial ischemia may lead to contractile dysfunction in localized areas and to an increased risk of future myocardial infarction. After revascularization of ischemic areas showing contractile dysfunction, normal function can be restored. Besides, improvement of left ventricular function improves prognosis and quality of life. Both scintigraphic techniques and magnetic resonance are quite capable of characterizing myocardial tissue and to determine tissue viability. Particularly, the thallium-201 reinjection approach has given a new impetus to 'good old' thallium-201 scintigraphy.

Introduction

The ability to distinguish ischemic myocardium from areas of myocardial fibrosis in patients with coronary artery disease is extremely important. Ischemic myocardium may produce clinical symptoms such as angina and may lead to potentially life-threatening arrhythmias. Patients with myocardial ischemia are at risk for future myocardial infarction. The ischemic but viable myocardial areas are able to benefit from myocardial revascularization by coronary artery bypass surgery or by coronary angioplasty. In contrast, revascularization of fibrotic myocardium will not lead to restoration of function and improvement of prognosis.

Ernst E. van der Wall et al. (eds), What's new in cardiac imaging?, 467–478.
© *1992 Kluwer Academic Publishers. Printed in the Netherlands.*

Perfusion disturbances can lead to: (1) stunning (decreased left ventricular function as a result of acute, temporary ischemia), (2) hibernation (decreased left ventricular function resulting from chronically low oxygen supply just enough to maintain basic cell metabolism to survive but inadequate for normal function), and (3) necrosis (irreversibly damaged myocardial tissue). Rahimtoola [1] first acknowledged the existence of such a prolonged subacute or chronic stage of myocardial ischemia without pain and reduced myocardial contractility, metabolism, and ventricular function. Clinical evidence for the existence of hibernating myocardium is warranted by the improvement of contractility (e.g. increase in regional ejection fraction) of viable but dysfunctional segments after restoring adequate blood supply [2, 3]. In the clinical situation, it is important to identify severe regional myocardial asynergy as a result of hibernation, and to distinguish it from irreversible cellular injury, in order to predict which patients might benefit from revascularization. Numerous experimental and clinical studies have demonstrated that, when regional contractile dysfunction is the result of either acute or multiple intermittent episodes of ischemia, restoration of nutritive perfusion with interventions, such as thrombolytic therapy, coronary angioplasty, or coronary artery bypass grafting, will result in improvement in regional function [4, 5]. Jeopardized myocardium that manifests improved function after appropriate therapy is deemed viable in contrast to persistent dysfunctional nonviable myocardium, typically the result of completed infarction. Accordingly, definitive evidence of myocardial viability is the temporal improvement in contractile function, irrespective of the etiology of the dysfunction or the specific therapeutic interventions employed [6, 7]. To date, demonstration of temporal improvement in regional function is not practical for the prospective identification of jeopardized but viable myocardium for the purposes of guiding therapeutic interventions in individual patients; it has proven difficult to differentiate viable from nonviable myocardium.

In this chapter, an overview will be given of radionuclide assessment of viability, and assessment of viability using magnetic resonance imaging. Data from our own laboratory regarding thallium-201 reinjection imaging for detection of viability are presented. Special emphasis is given to our thallium-201 reinjection protocol, by which the relatively simple thallium imaging technique is optimized in such a way that the diagnosis viable but jeopardized can be made more accurate than it used to be. In addition, magnetic resonance imaging will be briefly discussed as this is a new noninvasive method that has been shown capable of delineating viable myocardial tissue.

Scintigraphic techniques

Radionuclide imaging allows the visualization of normal and abnormal myocardium on the basis of alteration in perfusion, metabolism or function. Medically useful radionuclides can be separated, based on their mode of decay, into two groups: single photon or positron emitters. Single photon emitters (thallium-201, technetium-99m) release gamma photons that leave the tissue in a random direction. Measurement of regional activity can be impeded by attenuation of activity from overlying tissue and the effects of scatter from photons outside the area of interest.

Positron emitting tracers (carbon-11, fluorine-18, nitrogen-13, rubidium-82) decay by the emission of a positron, a particle that has the mass of an electron but a positive rather than a negative charge. After traveling a few millimeters in tissue, the positron collides with an electron and releases two high-energy photons that go 180 degrees apart. Tracer activity can be localized and quantified using coincidence detection so that the activity is accepted only when each of the two paired detectors records the photons. The specific value of positron emission tomography (PET) in characterizing myocardial viability is discussed in Chapter 37.

Thallium-201 imaging

Thallium-201 is a diffusible cation that is taken up by myocardial tissue in proportion to flow [8]. Thallium-201 myocardial imaging has become widely used to detect coronary artery disease and to assess the significance of known coronary lesions. By comparing stress and delayed images, ischemic but viable myocardium can be differentiated from scar tissue. Ischemic regions present as reversible defects, whereas scar tissue presents as a persisting defect [9, 10]. However, conflicting reports have emerged on myocardial viability in fixed thallium-201 defects. Several studies have reported improvement of thallium-201 uptake in fixed detects after coronary artery bypass surgery [11, 12] and, in several PET studies, metabolic activity was observed in persistent thallium defects [13–15]. In patients with incomplete redistribution at 4-hour delayed thallium imaging, additional 8–24 hours delayed redistribution was frequently observed [16]. Therefore, overestimation of infarct size and underestimation of viable and potentially jeopardized myocardium may occur using the classical procedure that uses one injection and two series of images.

From animal experiments, it is known that ischemic but viable tissue can concentrate thallium-201 intracellularly as long as there is adequate residual perfusion permitting delivery of the radionuclide [17]. Myocardial thallium-201 uptake is significantly impaired when irreversible cell membrane

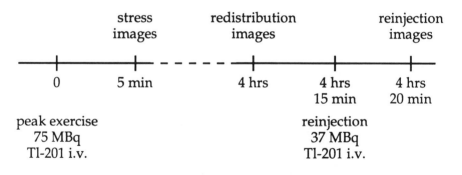

Figure 1. Thallium-201 reinjection protocol used in our laboratory.

damage is present [18]. Therefore, late thallium redistribution reflects the ability of viable myocardium to extract thallium-201 in severely hypoperfused regions with flow-limited availability of the radionuclide. Recently, Dilsizian et al. [19] underscored the value of optimizing the thallium-201 stress testing protocol by means of a second injection (reinjection) of thallium after the stress-redistribution images, followed by additional imaging. In a study, in 100 patients they found that 42 out of 85 (49%) apparently irreversible defects (after the stress-redistribution images) demonstrated improved or normal thallium uptake after the second injection of thallium. Of 15 myocardial regions with defects on redistribution studies that were identified as viable by reinjection studies before angioplasty, 13 (87%) had normal thallium uptake and improved regional wall motion after angioplasty. In contrast, all eight regions with persistent defects on reinjection imaging before angioplasty had abnormal thallium uptake and abnormal regional wall motion after angioplasty.

In our laboratory (Kuijper et al. Eur J Nucl Med, in press), we studied the impact of the thallium reinjection protocol in 203 patients with proven or suspected coronary artery disease. This technique was compared to the classic one-injection-two-imaging-series protocol. Figure 1 shows the protocol that was used. Out of 203 consecutive patients, 145 had persistent defects at the stress-redistribution images and were reinjected with 37 MBq thallium-201. In these 145 patients, the redistribution images showed a total of 386 persistent

$\longrightarrow$

Figure 2. Left anterior oblique 70° view showing thallium-201 uptake immediately post-exercise (top), after redistribution (middle) and after reinjection (bottom). Note defects in the inferior and posterior segments immediately post-exercise. After redistribution, there is partial normalization of the defect in the inferior wall without normalization of the posterior segment, and there is complete normalization of all segments after reinjection.

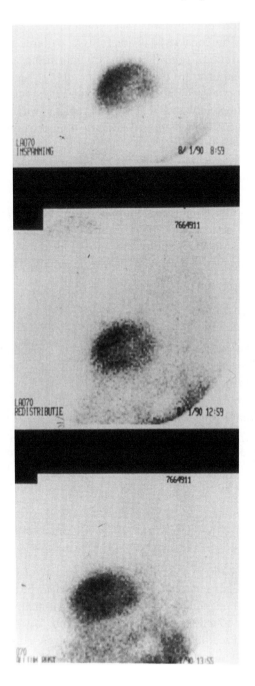

defects. From these defects, 147 (38%) filled in after reinjection, and these segments had to be considered viable. In 45 patients with only persisting defects at redistribution (and therefore thought to have only nonreversible infarct tissue), one or more defects filled in after reinjection. Therefore, in 22% (45/203) of patients submitted to thallium-201 exercise testing, reversible ischemia, indicating viable but jeopardized regions, was diagnosed only after reinjection. Figure 2 shows a typical example of improvement of thallium-201 uptake after reinjection.

Technetium-99m sestaMIBI

By using single-photon emission computed tomography (SPECT) methods, technetium-99m-labeled isonitriles (sestaMIBI) are also being used to assess myocardial perfusion and viability. Because of higher photon energies, these tracers provide images of improved diagnostic quality. The role of sestaMIBI in assessing myocardial viability is extensively addressed in Chapter 6.

Infarct avid scintigraphy

Technetium-99m pyrophosphate and indium-111 labeled antimyosin localize in regions of myocardial necrosis [20]. Unfortunately, images obtained with these tracers do not become positive until several hours after irreversible changes have occurred and the tracers require time for delivery to the damaged tissue. Dual isotope scintigraphy with thallium-201 (perfusion) and indium-111 antimyosin (necrosis) is a new approach to detect viable tissue. The antimyosin images can be superimposed on the perfusion images to distinguish between viable and necrotic tissue. In case of a mismatch, the difference is related to hypoperfused, viable myocardium. This particular issue is discussed in Chapter 22.

Positron emission tomography

Prospective delineation of viable from nonviable myocardium based on patterns of myocardial perfusion and metabolism can be obtained with PET. Myocardial ischemia induces characteristic changes in myocardial metabolism that accompany reductions in contractile function. Under physiologic conditions, myocardial metabolism is virtually exclusively aerobic [21]. The heart meets its oxygen demand largely by the oxidative metabolism of fatty acids and glucose. Even under fasting conditions, nonesterified fatty acids are the preferred energy source. With ischemia, oxidation of fatty acids is impaired and aerobic and anaerobic metabolism of glucose becomes proportionally more important. While it is felt that glucose metabolism can maintain cellular viability for a time after severe ischemia, it is unlikely that sufficient energy can be produced from anaerobic glucose metabolism to maintain viability indefinitely [22]. Nonetheless, since glucose metabolism (anaerobic and aerobic) predominates in ischemic myocardium, enhanced uptake of fluorine-18 (18F) fluorodeoxyglucose (FDG) in relation to flow has been proposed as an accurate means to identify viable myocardium [13, 23, 24].

FDG is a glucose analog that traces the initial components of the metabolic flux of glucose by the heart, including transmembranous transport and hexokinase-mediated phosphorylation. The phosphorylated FDG is trapped effectively within myocytes because the myocyte is relatively impermeable to it and because it is a poor substrate for further metabolism by either glycolytic or glycogen-synthetic pathways. Dephosphorylation of glucose-6-phosphate and presumably of FDG-6-phosphate, appears to be quite slow although not negligible [25, 26]. The regional distribution of FDG, assessed 40–60 minutes after administration of tracer (an interval sufficient for a large proportion of uptake and phosphorylation), is thought to reflect overall glycolytic flux [26]. The extent of myocardial uptake of FDG is not only dependent on the metabolic state of the tissue with respect to normoxia and ischemia, but is also sensitive to the pattern of myocardial substrate use [23, 27]. Results from several studies of patients with coronary artery disease (presenting either as unstable or stable ischemic syndromes) have suggested that PET with FDG can identify viable myocardium in zones of contractile dysfunction. In patients with stable coronary artery disease, improvement in regional function after revascularization was evident in 75–85% of dysfunctional segments that exhibited FDG accumulation. Besides, between 78 and 92% of segments with diminished flow and concomitantly reduced FDG uptake failed to exhibit functional improvement after surgery [13, 24]. In contrast, in patients studied within 72 hours of acute myocardial infarction and conservatively treated (no pharmacologic or mechanical revascularization was performed), only 50% of segments demonstrating uptake of FDG improved functionally over time [28]. These contrasting results can probably be explained by the inability of FDG to differentiate the metabolic fate of glucose in the myocardium, i.e. aerobic from anaerobic glucose metabolism or glycogen synthesis.

The temporal pattern of glucose use, which varies with time after ischemia, as well as the natural fate of jeopardized myocardium, is among other factors which are dependent on the amount of myocardium at risk, collateral flow, and loading conditions. The finding of myocardial uptake of FDG is now being suggested as the conditio sine qua non of viable myocardium. Consequently, studies designed to evaluate established as well as new diagnostic approaches for identifying viable myocardium, are incorporating PET using FDG as the gold standard for myocardial viability. This, however, is premature.

The relatively poor spatial resolution of the current generation of tomographs operated in the ungated mode, precludes delineation of transmural gradients of tracers within the myocardium. Accordingly, imaging with PET cannot distinguish FGD accumulation in metabolically active tissue within zones of infarction. These spared cells may accumulate FDG but may not be able to contribute to effective mechanical function. Further confounding factors with respect to the interpretation of enhanced uptake of FDG are data of recent experimental studies which suggest that even homogeneously infarcted myocardium can accumulate glucose [29]. Moreover, preliminary studies suggest that myocardial glucose utilization varies significantly during the time course of reperfusion [30] and that the maintenance of oxidative metabolism during ischemia, and recovery of oxidative metabolism after recanalization, may be the critical determinant of ultimate functional recovery [31, 32]. Consequently, positron emitting tracers that can measure oxidative metabolism or tissue hypoxia directly such as carbon-11 acetate or 18-fluoro-misonidazole may prove to be more useful than FDG in identifying viable myocardium. The value of the PET technique in assessing viability in patients following myocardial infarction is addressed in Chapter 37.

Gould et al. [33] described a new approach for identifying viable myocardium with PET using rubidium-82. The ability to extract and retain rubidium was used to define viability. A primary goal of cardiac PET will likely continue to focus on the metabolic abnormalities that underlie myocardial dysfunction. High costs of the equipment and radiopharmaceuticals, however, limit widespread application.

Magnetic resonance imaging

With the application of magnetic resonance imaging (MRI) techniques in clinical cardiology, an important tool has been added to the currently available diagnostic arsenal for the evaluation of patients with coronary artery disease [34]. Proton nuclear MRI is a noninvasive method which gives excellent anatomic resolution, provides contrast between tissues and flowing blood, is intrinsically three-dimensional, and can often distinguish between normal and abnormal tissue on the basis of tissue relaxation properties [35]. The identification of ischemic and infarcted tissue by MRI has been greatly improved by the use of paramagnetic contrast agents, such as gadolinium (Gd)-diethylene triaminepentaacetic acid (DTPA) [36].

Rather than aiming at competing with established imaging techniques, MRI techniques are to be used in those conditions for which they are uniquely suited, that is (1) myocardial tissue characterization, (2) assessment of regional myocardial blood-flow distribution with contrast agents, (3) noninvasive angiography, (4) flow imaging of the great vessels, and (5) in vivo myocardial biochemistry (MR spectroscopy).

The temporal resolution attained by cine MRI has extended the application of MRI to the assessment of cardiac function [37]. Cine MRI can be sequentially performed without causing harm to the patient, so that the severity of cardiac disease states can be monitored and the response to interventions determined. Since both the endocardial and epicardial borders are well defined by MRI, it is possible to assess wall thickening during the cardiac cycle and to detect regional myocardial dysfunction. The cinematic display of MR images facilitates identification of abnormal wall motion during the cardiac cycle. Regions with previous myocardial infarcts exhibit absent or severely reduced wall thickening during systole. Although there may be normal systolic inward motion, the absence of wall thickening indicates that the infarcted region is only passively pulled inward by traction of the surrounding normal myocardium [38].

The capability of MRI to provide sequential information about the state of pathologically altered myocardium in combination with assessment of diastolic wall thickness and systolic wall thickening makes it potentially suitable for identification of viability in areas previously affected by myocardial infarction. The unique features of MRI such as good anatomical and temporal resolution, three-dimensional capabilities, easy reproducibility, an unlimited field of view, and lack of radiation, render MRI an imaging modality which has the potential to assume increasing importance in the functional evaluation of myocardial viability in patients with coronary artery disease.

Conclusion

Ischemic myocardium that manifests improved function after appropriate therapy is considered viable in contrast to persistently dysfunctional, nonviable myocardium, typically the result of completed infarction. Using radionuclide techniques, an adequate distinction can be made between viable and nonviable myocardial segments, although every technique has his own drawbacks. Theoretically, the PET technique seems to be superior to the routinely applied thallium-201 imaging. Thallium-201 imaging, however, has become more reliable since the introduction of the reinjection protocol. This modification of the relatively simple thallium-201 imaging seems to be the answer to the discrepancies between thallium-201 and PET images. The relatively low cost and the large experience with thallium-201 imaging makes thallium-201 reinjection the procedure of first choice as a diagnostic test for assessing viability. MRI is a relatively new promising technique that certainly will gain a place in the analysis of viable tissue in patients with coronary disease.

References

1. Rahimtoola SH. A perspective on the three large multicenter randomized clinical trials of coronary bypass surgery for chronic stable angina. Circulation 1985; 72 (6 suppl): V123–35.
2. Bodenheimer MM, Banka VS, Hermann GA, Trout RG, Pasdar H, Helfant RH. Reversible asynergy. Histopathology and electrocardiographic correlations in patients with coronary artery disease. Circulation 1976; 53: 792–6.
3. Chatterjee K. Swann HJC, Parmley WW, Sustaita H, Marcus HS, Matloff J. Influence of direct myocardial revascularisation on left ventricular asynergy and function in patients with coronary heart disease: with and without previous myocardial infarction. Circulation 1973; 47: 276–86.
4. Serruys PW, Simoons ML, Suryapranata H et al. Preservation of global and regional left ventricular function after early thrombolysis in acute myocardial infarction. J Am Coll Cardiol 1986; 7: 729–42.
5. White HD, Norris RM, Brown MA et al. Effect of intravenous streptokinase on left ventricular function and early survival after acute myocardial infarction. N Engl J Med 1987; 317: 850–5.
6. Braunwald E, Kloner RA. The stunned myocardium: prolonged, postischemic ventricular dysfunction. Circulation 1982; 66: 1146–9.
7. Iskandrian AS, Heo J, Helfant RH, Segal BL. Chronic myocardial ischemia and left ventricular function. Ann Intern Med 1987; 107: 925–7.
8. Melin JA, Becker LC. Quantitative relationship between global left ventricular thallium uptake and blood flow: effects of propranolol, ouabain, dipyridamole, and coronary artery occlusion. J Nucl Med 1986; 27: 641–52.
9. Pohost FM, Zir LM, Moore RH, McKusick KA, Guiney TE, Beller GA. Differentiation of transiently ischemic from infarcted myocardium by serial imaging after a single dose of thallium-201. Circulation 1977; 55: 294–302.
10. Beller GA, Watson DD, Ackel P, Pohost GM. Time course of thallium-201 redistribution after transient myocardial ischemia. Circulation 1980; 61: 791–7.
11. Gibson RS, Watson DD, Taylor GJ et al. Prospective assessment of regional myocardial perfusion before and after coronary revascularisation surgery by quantitative thallium-201 scintigraphy. J Am Coll Cardiol 1983; 1: 804–15.
12. Iskandrian AS, Hakki AH, Kane SA, Goel IP, Mundth ED, Segal BL. Rest and redistribution thallium-201 myocardial scintigraphy to predict improvement in left ventricular function after coronary arterial bypass grafting. Am J Cardiol 1983; 51: 1312–6.
13. Tillisch J, Brunken R, Marshall R et al. Reversibility of cardiac wall-motion abnormalities predicted by positron tomography. N Engl J Med 1986; 314: 884–8.
14. Brunken R, Schwaiger M, Grover-McKay M, Phelps ME, Tillisch J, Schelbert HR. Positron emission tomography detects tissue metabolic activity in myocardial segments with persistent thallium perfusion defect. J Am Coll Cardiol 1987; 10: 557–67.

15. Tamaki N, Yonekura Y, Yamashita K et al. Relation of left ventricular perfusion and wall motion with metabolic activity in persistent defects on thallium-201 tomography in healed myocardial infarction. Am J Cardiol 1988; 62: 202–8.
16. Kiat H, Berman DS, Maddahi J et al. Late reversibility of tomographic myocardial thallium-201 defects: an accurate marker of myocardial viability. J Am Coll Cardiol 1988; 12: 1456–63.
17. Moore CA, Cannon J, Watson DD, Kaul S, Beller GA. Thallium-201 kinetics in stunned myocardium characterized by severe postischemic systolic dysfunction. Circulation 1990; 81: 1622–32.
18. Melin JA, Wijns W, Keyeux A et al. Assessment of thallium-201 redistribution versus glucose uptake as predictors of viability after coronary occlusion and reperfusion. Circulation 1988; 77: 927–34.
19. Dilsizian V, Rocco TP, Freedman NMT, Leon MB, Bonow RO. Enhanced detection of ischemic but viable myocardium by the reinjection of thallium after stress-redistribution imaging. N Engl J Med 1990; 323: 141–6.
20. Willerson JT, Parkey RW, Bonte FJ, Lewis SE, Corbett J, Buja LM. Pathophysiologic considerations and clinicopathological correlates of technetium-99m stannous pyrophosphate myocardial scintigraphy. Semin Nucl Med 1980; 10: 54–69.
21. Camici P, Ferrannini E, Opie LH. Myocardial metabolism in ischemic heart disease: basic principles and application to imaging by positron emission tomography. Prog Cardiovasc Dis 1989; 32: 217–38.
22. Kobayashi K, Neely JR. Control of maximum rates of glycolysis in rat cardiac muscle. Circ Res 1979; 44: 166–75.
23. Marshall RC, Tillisch JH, Phelps ME et al. Identification and differentiation of resting myocardial ischemia and infarction in man with positron emission computed tomography, 18F-labeled fluorodeoxyglucose, and N-13 ammonia. Circulation 1983; 67: 766–78.
24. Tamaki N, Yonekura Y, Yamashita K et al. Positron emission tomography using fluorine-18 deoxyglucose in evaluation of coronary artery bypass grafting. Am J Cardiol 1989; 64: 860–5.
25. Neely JR, Morgan HE. Relationship between carbohydrate and lipid metabolism and energy balance of heart muscle. Ann Rev Physiol 1974; 36: 413–59.
26. Ratib O, Phelps ME, Huang SC, Henze E, Selin CE, Schelbert HR. Positron tomography with deoxyglucose for estimating local myocardial glucose metabolism. J Nucl Med 1982; 23: 577–86.
27. Gropler RJ, Siegel BA, Lee KJ et al. Nonuniformity in myocardial accumulation of fluorine-18-fluorodeoxyglucose in normal fasted humans. J Nucl Med 1990; 31: 1749–56.
28. Schwaiger M, Brunken R, Grover-McKay M et al. Regional myocardial metabolism in patients with acute myocardial infarction assessed by positron emission tomography. J Am Coll Cardiol 1986; 8: 800–8.
29. Bianco JA, Sebree L, Subramanian R, Hegge J, Tschudy J, Pyzalski R. C-14 deoxyglucose accumulation in myocardial infarction [abstract]. J Nucl Med 1990; 31 (Suppl): 835.
30. Buxton DB, Vaghaiwalla-Mody F, Krivokapich J, Phelps ME, Schelbert HR. Quantitative measurement of sustained metabolic abnormalities in reperfused canine myocardium [abstract]. J Nucl Med 1990; 31 (Suppl): 795.
31. Brown MA, Nohara R, Vered Z, Perez JE, Bergmann SR. The dependence of recovery of stunned myocardium on restoration of oxidative metabolism [abstract]. Circulation 1988; 78(4 Suppl III): III467.
32. Gropler RJ, Siegel BA, Perez JE et al. Recovery of contractile function in viable but dysfunctional myocardium is dependent upon maintenance of oxidative metabolism [abstract]. J Am Coll Cardiol 1990; 15(2 Suppl A): 203A.

33. Gould KL, Yoshida K, Hess MJ, Haynie M, Mullani N, Smalling RW. Myocardial metabolism of fluorodeoxyglucose compared to cell membrane integrity for the potassium analogue rubidium-82 for assessing infarct size in man by PET. J Nucl Med 1991; 32: 1–9.
34. Van der Wall EE, De Roos A, editors. Magnetic resonance imaging in coronary artery disease. Dordrecht: Kluwer, 1991.
35. Herfkens RJ, Higgins CB, Hricak H et al. Nuclear magnetic resonance imaging of the cardiovascular system: normal and pathologic findings. Radiology 1983; 147: 749–59.
36. Brown JJ, Higgins CB. Myocardial paramagnetic contrast agents for MR imaging. AJR Am J Rontgenol 1988; 151: 865–71.
37. Buser PT, Auffermann W, Holt WW et al. Noninvasive evaluation of global left ventricular function with use of cine nuclear magnetic resonance. J Am Coll Cardiol 1989; 13: 1294–300.
38. Pettigrew RI. Dynamic cardiac MR imaging. Techniques and applications. Radiol Clin North Am 1989; 27: 1183–203.

37. Is it worth assessing regional myocardial viability with positron emission tomography?

CHRISTIAN DE LANDSHEERE, LUC PIÉRARD,
PIERRE MELON, DOMINIQUE COMAR,
HENRI E. KULBERTUS and PIERRE RIGO

Introduction

For many years, tracers of perfusion have been used for the diagnosis of regional myocardial ischemia. For this purpose, thallium-201 has been, by far, the most widely used tracer in single photon scintigraphy. However, thallium-201 scintigraphy – even in the tomographic mode (SPECT) – underestimates regional viability, particularly after myocardial infarction. Tamaki et al. [1, 2].

We know from the experimental work of Randle et al. [3], Neely and Morgan [4], Opie [5] and Liedtke [6] that ischemic but still viable myocardium utilizes glucose preferably to fatty acids for energy production. Glucose is first transformed in glucose-6-P under the influence of hexokinase. Later on, it is metabolized in several steps which finally leads to the production of energy, CO_2 and H_2O (aerobic conditions). In anaerobic conditions, metabolization of glucose ends up with the accumulation of lactate, with an energetic yield 19 times smaller than in the aerobic pathway. Applying these observations, Marshall et al. [7] from UCLA, initiated the concept of successively using two positron emitters: a perfusion tracer, nitrogen-13 [^{13}N]ammonia and an indicator of glucose uptake, fluorine-18 [^{18}F]deoxyglucose (analogue of glucose which is 'trapped' in the myocardial cells) for assessing regional myocardial viability. This combined study was performed in 15 patients who suffered a myocardial infarction less than 3 months before positron emission tomography (PET) observation. A pattern of 'FDG-flow mismatch' was observed in 10 cases, of whom 9 suffered from angina. Based on these results and on sub-

479

Ernst E. van der Wall et al. (eds), What's new in cardiac imaging?, 479–491.

sequent studies from other groups, the idea of utilizing PET as a clinical tool has progressively received wider acceptance.

However, several issues remain unsolved and some controversy persists. The goal of this chapter is to present the Liège experience of detecting partial regional myocardial viability in ischemic heart disease. Our results will be compared to the data published in the literature in order to better understand the significance of the various patterns of perfusion and glucose uptake regional abnormalities.

Our results have been previously reported [8–17]. They are summarized in 'Non-invasive imaging of cardiac metabolism: single photon scintigraphy, positron emission tomography and nuclear magnetic resonance', edited by E.E. van der Wall [12] and in a PhD thesis [15].

Methods

All studies were performed with a whole-body tomograph, ECAT-II (Ortec and Cy, Tennessee). This tomograph has a spatial resolution of 16 to 20 mm. It is a single-slice machine. Usually, 3 transverse planes are recorded from the base to the apex of the left ventricle.

Results are expressed in percent of perfusion (potassium-38) and in percent of [^{18}F]deoxyglucose (FDG) uptake. In addition, the ratio glucose uptake-perfusion (G/P ratio) is calculated after normalization to the reference perfusion region within the scan; the G/P ratio is an index of the extraction of glucose by myocardial cells.

Potassium-38 is injected (370 to 555 MBq) first. We wait for the physical decay of the cationic tracer (half-life? 7.7 minutes). FDG (half-life: 110 minutes) is therefore injected 30 minutes later (370 MBq, usually).

Table 1. Reference values for perfusion glucose uptake (expressed in percent) and G/P ratio ($n = 10$).

	Perfusion	Glucose uptake	G/P ratio
Segments of lateral wall	91.0 ± 4.2	99.8 ± 10.2	1.10 ± 0.11
Segments of anterior wall	80.5 ± 4.6	85.3 ± 9.9	1.06 ± 0.14
Segments of the septum	80.2 ± 9.7	77.0 ± 6.5	0.97 ± 0.10

Results

Reference values established in normal volunteers

For the determination of reference perfusion, glucose uptake and G/P ratio values, 10 normal young volunteers were studied. Results are shown in Table 1.

As a mean, perfusion is evaluated to 91% in the lateral wall. It is lower in the anterior wall and septum, due to partial volume effect. However, we did not attempt to correct for this effect which exerts the same influence on perfusion and glucose uptake: the G/P ratio is close to 1, in each region of the left ventricle.

Using these mean values and according to the method proposed by Guttman [18], reference intervals (at the level of 95%) are calculated. For example, perfusion will be considered as abnormally low if < 71.8%, in the anterior wall and mid-slice of the left ventricle. The reference interval for glucose uptake is 64.6–109.9%. The G/P ratio will be considered as abnormally high if > 1.42.

Patterns of perfusion and glucose uptake abnormalities in 'chronic' myocardial infarction and in unstable angina

(a) Group 1: chronic stage of myocardial infarction
This group is composed of 16 cases (55 ± 10 years old) all submitted to coronary angiography. In 15 cases, the left anterior descending artery (LAD)

Table 2. Perfusion, glucose uptake (expressed in %) and G/P ratio in patients who suffered a myocardial infarction and in cases with unstable angina.

	Perfusion (%)	Glucose uptake (%)	G/P ratio
Group 1: chronic infarction (anterior segments)			
– occluded artery (*n* = 7)	39 ± 12	41 ± 19	1.02 ± 0.27
– stenotic artery (*n* = 9)			
– no thrombolysis (*n* = 4)	44 ± 13	73 ± 20	1.68 ± 0.62
– thrombolysis (*n* = 5)	42 ± 19	69 ± 27	1.65 ± 0.62
	(RV: 80.5 ± 4.6)	(RV: 85.3 ± 9.9)	(RV: 1.06 ± 0.14)
Group 2: unstable angina (lateral segments)			
– stenotic artery (*n* = 7)	55 ± 11	128 ± 45	2.47 ± 1.36
	(RV: 91.0 ± 4.2)	(RV: 99.8 ± 10.2)	(RV: 1.10 ± 0.11)

RV = reference values.

is responsible for an anterior myocardial infarction (MI), whereas a severe stenosis of right coronary artery (RCA) is observed after an inferior MI.

(b) Group 2: unstable angina
Group 2 includes 7 patients. In 4 cases aged 63 ± 9 (mean $\pm$ SD) years, angor unstable is a complication of a myocardial infarction, whereas in the 3 remaining cases (58 ± 5 years old), ischemic heart disease was proved but without any history of myocardial infarction. All patients of this group present multi-vessel disease.

PET results obtained in groups 1 and 2 are shown in Table 2.

In cases belonging to group 1 with occluded artery, perfusion, and glucose uptake are similarly diminished: no residual viable myocardium seems to persist. If the artery responsible for the infarction is stenotic but not occluded – independently of the treatment applied at the acute phase of infarction – the mean result of glucose uptake is increased, compared to perfusion, suggesting that some partially viable myocardium still utilizes glucose for energy production.

In patients of group 2 (with unstable angina), there is an absolute increase of glucose uptake (more than 100%) and G/P ratio is higher than 2. These findings suggest that corresponding myocardium is ischemic and might become necrotic in the absence of any revascularization procedure (percutaneous coronary angioplasty or coronary artery bypass grafting).

Patterns of perfusion and glucose uptake abnormalities in acute myocardial infarction

Positron emission tomography was performed 12 days as a mean after the

Table 3. Characteristics of the population (patients with acute MI).

Group	n	Age (years)	Sex	Location of infarction	Coronary stenosis (expressed in %)
1. No TBL	11	56 ± 6	11M	9A; 2L	(a) 70–95%; $n = 6$ (b) 100%; $n = 5$
2. TBL	37	53 ± 11	35M; 2F	32A; 41P; 1L	(a) $< 50\%$; $n = 7$ (b) 50–85%; $n = 15$ (c) 90–99%; $n = 15$
3. TBL & PTCA	7	54 ± 10	6M; 1F	7A	$< 50\%$; $n = 7$

TBL = thrombolysis. PTCA = percutaneous coronary angioplasty. M = male. F = female. A = anterior. L = lateral. IP = infero-posterior.

admission into the coronary care unit in a group of 55 patients. Characteristics of the population are summarized in Table 3.

Patients were separated into three groups according to the treatment applied at the admission to the hospital. Patients of group 1 ($n = 11$) did not receive any thrombolytic agent. In group 2 ($n = 37$), 1.5 million units of streptokinase were administered intravenously. In group 3 ($n = 7$) PTCA was applied in addition to thrombolysis. In most of the cases, the infarction was located in the anterior wall. The residual coronary artery lesions differ in the 3 groups. In the first group, the artery responsible for the infarction was occluded in 5 cases or presented a stenosis > 70% in 6 other cases. No occlusion was observed in the second group treated by streptokinase. In this group, residual stenosis is < 50% in 7 cases, ranging from 50 to 85% in 15 patients and 90–99% in 15 other patients. As a consequence of PTCA, no significant residual stenosis was observed after the procedure in all patients of group 3.

Results obtained in these 3 groups are summarized in Table 4.

In the first group, glucose uptake is relatively increased (75%) compared to perfusion (53%) in cases with significant coronary stenosis but no occlusion. If the artery responsible for the infarction is occluded, perfusion and glucose uptake are similarly diminished, respectively to 37 and 42% (G/P = 1.13).

Table 4. Regional perfusion, glucose uptake (expressed in percent) and G/P ratio in 55 patients studied at the acute stage of a myocardial infarction.

	Perfusion (%)	Glucose uptake (%)	G/P ratio
1. No TBL			
(a) 70–95%	53 ± 14	75 ± 40	1.43 ± 60
($n = 6$)			
(b) 100%	37 ± 14	42 ± 21	1.13 ± 0.22
($n = 5$)			
2. TBL			
(a) <50%	58 ± 20	60 ± 19	1.05 ± 0.20
($n = 7$)			
(b) 50–85%	47 ± 19	67 ± 23	1.53 ± 0.65
($n = 15$)			
(c) 90–99%	38 ± 8	69 ± 28	1.83 ± 0.71
($n = 15$)			
3. TBL & PTCA			
<50%	44 ± 11	79 ± 4	1.90 ± 1.13
($n = 7$)			
	(RV: 80.5 ± 4.6)	(RV: 85.3 ± 9.9)	(RV: 1.06 ± 0.14)

TBL = thrombolysis. PTCA = percutaneous coronary angioplasty. RV = reference values.

In the second group, perfusion decreases with the severity of stenosis (from 58.2% in the subgroup without significant stenosis to 37.7% in the subgroup with severe residual stenosis). Glucose uptake is similar in subgroups (a), (b), (c). Consequently, the G/P ratio is higher in subgroup (c) in relation to a more pronounced flow deficit.

The third group (stenosis < 50%, thrombolysis and PTCA) is characterized by a diminution of perfusion which is similar to the subgroup only treated by thrombolysis, but characterized by a more severe residual stenosis (50–85%). Mean glucose uptake of the third group is 79% leading to the highest mean G/P value: 1.90.

Partial myocardial viability was demonstrated in 2 cases only out of 11 (18%), in group 1 (no thrombolysis). In group 2 (thrombolysis), viable myocardium was observed in 25 out of 37 patients i.e. 68%. Finally, myocardial viability was identified in 5 patients out of 7 who were submitted to PTCA in addition to thrombolysis (group 3).

These data suggest that the salvage of partially viable myocardium depends on the treatment applied at the admission to the hospital and on the severity of residual stenosis (which is related partly to the success of therapy) in the arterial territory responsible for the infarction. Thrombolysis seems to influence favorably the preservation of myocardial viability but it remains to be demonstrated whether this beneficial effect is persistent. We also need to know the functional status (in terms of regional contractility) of segments characterized either by a moderate perfusion and/or glucose uptake deficit or by a 'FDG-flow mismatch'. To answer these questions, we studied a group of 29 patients with anterior MI using low-dose dobutamine echocardiography in addition to positron emission tomography. Results obtained in this new group of patients are presented in the following section.

Comparative study of perfusion, glucose uptake and regional wall motion abnormalities using positron emission tomography and 2D-echocardiography at the acute stage of an anterior myocardial infarction and in a short-term follow-up observation [19]

The study group is composed of 29 patients aged 54 ± 11 (mean $\pm$ SD) years, with an anterior acute myocardial infarction. In all cases, thrombolysis was applied within 3 hours after the onset of symptoms. Streptokinase (1.5 million units) was injected intravenously in 17 patients, whereas recombinant tissue plasminogen activator (rt-PA) was the administered thrombolytic agent in the remaining 12 patients. The dose of rt-PA was 100 mg: bolus injection of 10 mg followed by 50 mg in the first hour; then, 20 mg/hr of rt-PA were infused during the subsequent 2 hours.

The initial PET study was performed within 2 weeks after the onset of infarction; the delay between coronary angiography and PET ranged 24–72 hours. In addition to these investigations, 2D-echocardiography was performed at rest, in basal conditions and during the administration of dobutamine, according to the method published by Pierard et al. [17]. Dobutamine was administered at low doses (5 μg/kg/min over 2 minutes followed by 10 μg/kg/min for 2 more minutes). After a mean delay of 9 months, all patients were submitted again to positron emission tomography and 2D-echocardiography (basal conditions).

Six comparable segments were considered for data analysis, both for PET and ECHO. A regional score of wall motion was calculated as follows: 1 for normal contractility, 2 for hypokinesia, 3 for akinesia and 4 represents dyskinesia. Normal score is therefore 6, whereas the most severe alteration of contractility would determine a score of 24.

Three groups of patients were selected according to PET classification into:
– myocardial viability characterized by the preservation of regional perfusion within normal limits, in 2 segments at least (8 patients; mean age: 49 ± 11 years);
– myocardial viability defined as an abnormally high FDG uptake relative to perfusion ('FDG-flow mismatch'), in 2 segments or more (8 patients; mean age: 59 ± 8 years);
– matched deficit of perfusion and glucose uptake in 2 segments or more (13 patients; mean age: 54 ± 11 years).

PET and ECHO results are summarized in Table 5.

Regional wall motion abnormalities decreased with dobutamine in all patients of group 1 (perfusion within normal limits) and a low score was also observed in the follow-up study.

In group 2 ('FDG-flow mismatch'), alteration of regional contractility de-

Table 5. Perfusion (P) and glucose uptake (G) expressed in %, ratio of glucose uptake to perfusion (G/P) and score of regional wall motion.

	P	G	G/P	ECHO-BC	ECHO-DB	ECHO-FU
Group 1 (n = 8)	81 ± 10	82 ± 18	1.01 ± 0.17	11 ± 2	7 ± 1	7 ± 2
Group 2 (n = 8)	38 ± 9	74 ± 26	1.95 ± 0.53	16 ± 2	12 ± 3	16 ± 2
Group 3 (n = 13)	49 ± 12	54 ± 12	1.12 ± 0.21	13 ± 3	12 ± 4	13 ± 5

BC = basal conditions. DB = dobutamine. FU = follow-up.

creased in 5 out of 8 patients under the influence of dobutamine. However, later on deterioration of regional left ventricular function was documented.

In group 3 (matched alteration of perfusion and glucose uptake), 4 cases out of 13 showed less severe abnormalities of regional wall motion during dobutamine administration. Functional recovery was observed in the follow-up observation in 3 of them.

Plate 37.1 shows an example of a study performed in a patient belonging to group 1. Mrs D, aged 65 years, suffered an anterior myocardial infarction. She was admitted to the hospital 150 minutes after the onset of symptoms. Thrombolysis (with rt-PA) was initiated rapidly after admission. She underwent coronary ventriculography on day 10. A high grade stenosis (80–90%) of the left anterior descending artery was observed after the origin of the first diagonal branch. The initial PET study was recorded on day 7 and the follow-up investigation was performed 9 months later. Perfusion (left panels) and glucose uptake (right panels) are within normal limits both in the early study and in the follow-up: no infarction is visible. Regional wall motion improves with dobutamine in the former study and is normal in the latter.

Contrasting with this illustration, Plate 37.2 presents an example of 'FDG-flow mismatch' identified in the anterior wall (one arrow) and septum (two arrows), in the early study performed on day 5, in a patient also treated by rt-PA. Echocardiography confirms the diagnosis of myocardial viability: regional contractility improves in the area of infarction, under the effect of dobutamine. Two days later, Mrs P. suffered from severe chest pain and reinfarction was documented. Coronary angiography performed on day 9 showed occlusion of the left anterior descending artery. PET was performed one month after the initial investigation. At that time, perfusion and glucose uptake are similarly decreased in the territory of infarction. Viability has turned to necrosis, in the area of infarction which is now akinetic.

Data obtained in this group of 29 patients suggest that the preservation of regional myocardial viability in the risk zone of an acute myocardial infarction is of complex nature. They also indicate the need for combined and repeated studies of perfusion, metabolism and function. The best recovery was observed in the group of patients with 'normal' perfusion, suggesting that the perfusion parameter has major importance. This conclusion has been confirmed by Grandin et al. [20].

These authors studied 14 coronary patients recovering from anterior ischemia ($n = 7$) or infarction ($n = 7$). Contrast ventriculography was performed at the time of the PET investigation and again 4 to 8 months after percutaneous coronary angioplasty. Ventriculography was used to separate patients according to end-diastolic and end-systolic volumes. In 9 patients, volumes decreased between the first and the second studies, resulting in an increase of left ventricular ejection fraction (LVEF). In the remaining 5 patients, enddiastolic and endsystolic volumes increased leading to a LVEF decrease. 'FDG flow-mismatch', defined as a ratio higher than 1.2, was observed in 8 out of the 9 cases belonging to the first group of patients. Myocardial blood flow (MBF) was 72 ± 21 ml/min/100 g. In the second group of patients, only 1 out of 5 had abnormally high FDG/MBF ratio. In this group, flow was evaluated to 49 ± 8 ml/min/100 g ($p < 0.001$). This work has been continued and presented by Melin and coworkers at the last meeting of the European Concerted Action in Cardiology, held in Brussels on 4 November 1991. The population is now composed of 21 patients: 14 with decreased volumes and 7 with increased volumes. According to a stepwise logistic regression analysis, the absolute estimation of regional myocardial blood flow in the affected segments of the left ventricle (anterior wall) is the best indicator of good functional outcome in patients with anterior wall dysfunction either related to anterior myocardial infarction or to anterior wall ischemia.

Discussion: role of PET as a clinical tool with special reference to the combined assessment of perfusion and glucose uptake

From our data presented above, we conclude that:
(1) In the *normal population*, glucose uptake is proportional to perfusion, in all studied segments;
(2) In *'chronic infarction'*, glucose uptake patterns differ in relation to coronary artery anatomy:
   • In the majority of patients who suffered a myocardial infarction, with occluded coronary artery, glucose uptake is decreased in proportion to the flow deficit: necrosis appears to be complete;
   • In some cases characterized by critical coronary artery lesions without occlusion, disproportion between glucose uptake and perfusion may be observed, even several months after the acute coronary event.
(3) In *unstable angina*, large uncoupling between glucose uptake and perfusion seems to be 'the rule'.
(4) At the *acute phase of a myocardial infarction*, the combined study of perfusion with and glucose uptake provides a means of identifying:
   – Viable myocardium characterized by a small decrease of perfusion or no perfusion abnormality. Perfusion and glucose uptake are proportional;
   – Viable myocardium characterized by 'FDG-flow mismatch', with a more profound deficit of perfusion than in the preceding pattern and a relative increase of glucose uptake;

– Necrotic myocardium with matched and severe deficits of perfusion and glucose uptake.

The two first patterns occur more frequently in patients submitted to thrombolysis than in cases who did not receive any thrombolytic agent. However, the pattern of disproportionately high FDG uptake relative to flow, observed at the acute stage of infarction, may disappear with time, together with deterioration of regional contractility. This observation indicates that utilization of glucose in the zone at risk of a myocardial infarction may correspond to transient myocardial viability. On the contrary, if perfusion has returned within normal limits, regional myocardial viability seems to persist, together with an excellent functional outcome.

Are these results supported by the literature? To answer this question, we have selected the review from Schwaiger and Hicks published in the April 1991 issue of the Journal of Nuclear Medicine entitled: 'Clinical PET: its time has come' [21] and the abstract of a communication presented by Schelbert at the third meeting of the American Institute for Clinical PET, held in Washington DC, 24–26 October 1991 [22].

Marshall et al. [7] showed that residual FDG uptake in segments with reduced flow corelated with the presence of postinfarction angina, the site of ischemic electrocardiographic changes during ischemia and the presence of severe coronary artery disease. Later on, Brunken et al. [23] studied 16 patients with Q-wave infarction. Approximately 60% of left ventricular segments with ECG or wall motion abnormality criterion of infarction had preserved FDG uptake (in our 37 cases of infarction treated by thrombolysis, 68% of the patients are characterized by PET identification of regional myocardial viability). However, they found similar regional scores of contractility in segments with and without FDG uptake, an argument in favor of the unique information provided by PET.

The predictive value of FDG uptake for tissue recovering following revascularization has been investigated by Tillisch et al. [24] and Tamaki et al. [25]. Both studies show that regional improvement in contractile function is more frequently observed in segments with FDG uptake identified before the revascularization procedure. Al-Aouar et al. [26] demonstrated in addition that the predictive value for functional recovery of areas with preserved or relatively increased FDG uptake (compared to decreased perfusion) was higher in segments with severe regional asynergy. This important observation supports the concept that PET is able to provide particularly useful information in cases with severe impairment of left ventricular function.

Brunken et al. [27, 28] and Tamaki et al. [29] have tested the additional value of PET compared to traditional techniques such as thallium-201 myocardial imaging. Their results clearly demonstrate that the standard techniques of stress-redistribution thallium-201 imaging overestimate the extent of non-viable myocardium (particularly in segments with fixed defect of thallium-201). For Tamaki et al. [29], FDG uptake is observed in 22% of the segments with persistent defects following thallium-201 reinjection, confirming the limitation of thallium-201 scintigraphy, even with a different methodology. As shown by Bonow et al. [30], the discordance between thallium-201 SPECT including reinjection and FDG results is more pronounced in segments with less than 50% reduction of regional thallium-201 activity.

In order to investigate the clinical outcome of patients submitted to PET viability studies, Eitzman et al. [31] have followed 82 out of 120 patients who underwent PET between August 1988 and March 1990, at the University of Michigan. Average time interval of follow-up was 12 months. Concordant decrease of flow and FDG was observed in 40 patients, whereas 42 patients were characterized by reduced flow but maintained metabolic activity. The incidence of cardiac events is higher in the group with PET defined ischemically compromised myocardium who did not undergo revascularization.

In the proceedings of the Third International PET Conference organized by the Institute for Clinical PET (ICP), Schelbert [22] provides the most simple definition of myocardial viability: 'reversible impairment of regional myocardial contractile function'. He also identifies cases who will benefit most from PET viability studies: 'patients in whom presence or absence of reversible dysfunction is critical for management or in whom other tests have resulted in equivocal findings' (in the presence of severe coronary artery disease).

Conclusion

Positron emission tomography allows the combined assessment of perfusion, glucose uptake and also of myocardial oxidative metabolism, with the additional possibility of expressing results in quantitative terms. Among other clinical applications of PET in cardiology, it is now well established that the 'PET viability studies' make the indications for revascularization or heart transplant more precise and more secure, in selected cases.

For the identification of regional viability after an acute myocardial infarction, two criteria can be applied. The first one is related to perfusion. It is highly predictive of functional recovery if perfusion is preserved within normal limits. However, further research is needed to establish these limits, using both assessment of perfusion in actual quantitative terms and dobutamine echocardiography.

The second criterion is metabolic: high glucose uptake relative to perfusion. From our experience, such myocardial viability may be transient; the optimal time for complementary revascularization has still to be determined in order to achieve lasting full functional recovery.

References

1. Tamaki N, Ohtani H, Yonekura Y et al. Can reinjection of thallium-201 SPECT replace FDG-PET for assessing tissue viability [abstract]? J Nucl Med 1990; 31: 742.
2. Tamaki N, Ohtani H, Yamashita K et al. Metabolic activity in the areas of new fill-in after thallium-201 reinjection: comparison with positron emission tomography using fluorine-18-deoxyglucose. J Nucl Med 1991; 32: 673–8.
3. Randle PJ, Garland PB, Hales CN, Newsholme EA. The glucose-fatty acid cycle. Lancet 1963; i: 785–9.
4. Neely JR, Morgan HE. Relationship between carbohydrate and lipid metabolism and the energy balance of the heart muscle. Annu Rev Physiol 1974; 36: 413–59.
5. Opie LH. Effect of regional ischemia on metabolism of glucose and fatty acids. Circ Res 1976; 38 Suppl I: I53–I74.
6. Liedtke AJ. Alterations of carbohydrate and lipid metabolism in the acutely ischemic heart. Progr Cardiovasc Dis 1981; 23: 321–6.
7. Marshall RC, Tillisch JH, Phelps ME et al. Identification and differentiation of resting myocardial ischemia and infarction in man with positron computed tomography, F-18 labeled fluorodeoxyglucose and N13-ammonia. Circulation 1983; 67: 766–78.
8. De Landsheere C, Raets D, Pierard L et al. Residual metabolic abnormalities and regional viability after a myocardial infarction: a study using positron tomography, F-18 deoxyglucose and flow indicators [abstract]. J Am Coll Cardiol 1985a; 5: 451.
9. De Landsheere CM, Raets D, Pierard LA et al. Fibrinolysis and viable myocardium after an acute infarction: a study of regional perfusion and glucose utilization with positron emission tomography [abstract]. Circulation 1985b; 72 (4 Suppl III): III393.
10. De Landsheere C, Raets D, Pierard L et al. Thrombolysis in anterior myocardial infarction: effect on regional viability studied with positron emission tomography [abstract]. Circulation 1987a; 76 (4 Suppl IV): IV5.
11. De Landsheere C, Raets D, Pierard L et al. Investigation of myocardial viability after an acute myocardial infarction using positron emission tomography. In Heiss WD, Pawlik G, Herholz K, Wienhard K, editors. Clinical efficacy of positron emission tomography, Dordrecht: Martinus Nijhoff, 1987b: 279–96.
12. De Landsheere C, Raets D, Pierard L et al. Viabilité myocardique après infarctus du myocarde traité par fibrinolyse: évaluation directe par tomographie à émission de positons combinant une étude régionale de la perfusion et de la captation glucidique. J Biophys Bioméc 1987c; 11 (Suppl 2): 185–7.
13. De Landsheere CM. Assessment of glucose utilization in normal and ischemic myocardium with positron emission tomography and 18F-deoxyglucose. In: Van der Wall E, editor. Noninvasive imaging of cardiac metabolism, Dordrecht: Martinus Nijhoff, 1987d: 241–63.
14. De Landsheere C, Raets D, Pierard L et al. Regional myocardial perfusion and glucose uptake: clinical experience in 92 cases studied with positron tomography [abstract]. Eur J Nucl Med 1989; 15: 446.
15. De Landsheere C. Contribution de la tomographie par émission de positons à l'étude de l'insuffisance coronarienne. Thèse d'agrégation de l'enseignement supérieur, 1990 [dissertation].

16. Rigo P, De Landsheere C, Raets D, Del Fiore G, Quaglia L, Lemaire C. Myocardial blood flow and glucose uptake after myocardial infarction. Eur J Nucl Med 1986; 12: S59–S61.

17. Pierard LA, De Landsheere C, Berthe C, Rigo P, Kulbertus HE. Identification of viable myocardium by echocardiography during dobutamine infusion in patients with myocardial infarction after thrombolytic therapy: comparison with positron emission tomography. J Am Coll Cardiol 1990; 15: 1021–31.

18. Guttman I. Statistical tolerance regions. London: Griffin, 1970.

19. De Landsheere C, Pierard L, Melon P et al. Understanding perfusion and glucose uptake patterns by the use of low-dose dobutamine in 29 patients with anterior myocardial infarction. J Am Coll Cardiol 1992 [in press].

20. Grandin C, Melin JA, Essamri B et al. Prediction of functional improvement with PET in patients recovering from acute anterior ischemia [abstract]. J Nucl Med 1991; 32: 1012.

21. Schwaiger M, Hicks R. The clinical role of metabolic imaging of the heart by positron emission tomography. J Nucl Med 1991; 32: 565–78.

22. Schelbert HR. Assessment of myocardial viability with positron emission tomography. Proceedings of the third annual international PET conference of the Institute for Clinical PET. Washington D.C. 1991: 38–41.

23. Brunken R, Tillisch J, Schwaiger M et al. Regional perfusion, glucose metabolism, and wall motion in patients with chronic electrocardiographic Q wave infarctions: evidence for persistence of viable tissue in some infarct regions by positron emission tomography. Circulation 1986; 73: 951–63.

24. Tillisch J, Brunken R, Marshall et al. Reversibility of cardiac wall-motion abnormalities predicted by positron tomography. N Engl J Med 1986; 314: 884–8.

25. Tamaki N, Yonekura Y, Yamashita K et al. Positron emission tomography using fluorine-18-deoxyglucose in evaluation of coronary artery bypass grafting. Am J Cardiol 1989; 64: 860–5.

26. Al-Aouar ZR, Eitzman D, Hepner A et al. PET assessment of myocardial tissue viability. University of Michigan experience [abstract]. J Nucl Med 1990; 31: 801.

27. Brunken R, Schwaiger M, Grover-McKay M, Phelps ME, Tillisch J, Schelbert HR. Positron emission tomography detects tissue metabolic activity in myocardial segments with persistent thallium perfusion defects. J Am Coll Cardiol 1987; 10: 557–67.

28. Brunken RC, Kottou S, Nienaber CA et al. PET detection of viable tissue in myocardial segments with persistent defects at Tl-201 SPECT. Radiology 1989; 172: 65–73.

29. Tamaki N, Yonekura Y, Yamashita K et al. Relation of left ventricular perfusion and wall motion with metabolic activity in persistent defects on thallium-201 tomography in healed myocardial infarction. Am J Cardiol 1988; 62: 202–8.

30. Bonow R, Dilsizian V, Cuocolo A, Bacharach S. Identification of viable myocardium in patients with chronic artery disease and left ventricular dysfunction: comparison of thallium scintigraphy with reinjection and PET imaging with ^{18}F-fluorodeoxyglucose. Circulation 1991; 83: 26–37.

31. Eitzman D, Al-Azouar Z, Kanter L et al. Clinical outcome in patients with advanced coronary artery disease following PET viability studies [abstract]. J Nucl Med 1991; 32: 1011–2.

38. Assessment of tissue viability after myocardial infarction with fluorine-18 deoxyglucose using planar imaging; the alternative approach

FRANS C. VISSER, JAAP J. TEULE,
JACOBUS D.M. HERSCHEID, GUIDO R. VAN LEEUWEN,
ARTHUR VAN LINGEN, HANS HUITINK and
GERRIT W. SLOOF

Introduction

Assessment of tissue viability after myocardial infarction has become an important issue in recent years because the widespread use of thrombolytic therapy in acute infarction has limited infarct size and has improved prognosis. The issue of the therapeutic management of the residual stenosis of the infarct related coronary artery is still controversial.

Multiple clinical trials have demonstrated that acute coronary angioplasty (PTCA) of the infarct-related coronary artery is obviously not the treatment of choice, as mortality and recurrent infarction was not different in PTCA patients compared to medically treated patients [1, 2]. An alternative approach may be the assessment of the presence of viable myocardial tissue in the area of infarction. If viable tissue can be demonstrated in the infarct area, then these patients might benefit from bypass surgery or PTCA while those patients with necrotic tissue might benefit from medical treatment aiming at reducing left ventricular dilation after infarction.

At this moment, tissue viability can only be reasonably assessed with fluorine-18 deoxyglucose (FDG) using positron emission tomography (PET). The increased uptake of FDG in the area of myocardial infarction suggests tissue viability. This has been demonstrated by Tillisch et al. [3] and Tamaki et al. [4], showing that patients with increased FDG uptake improve in left ventricular function after revascularization. The details of this approach are discussed in Chapter 19. The costs of the PET devices and the long acquisition period for assessing FDG uptake, however, limit the widespread use of these diagnostic tools. Recently, it has been demonstrated that FDG uptake can be visualized

Ernst E. van der Wall et al. (eds), What's new in cardiac imaging?, 493–499.
© *1992 Kluwer Academic Publishers. Printed in the Netherlands.*

with conventional gamma cameras, using a specially designed 511 keV collimator [5]. The advantage of assessing increased FDG uptake in this manner is that gamma cameras are generally available, allowing routine viability assessment after thrombolytic therapy. Moreover, the relatively long half-life of F-18 (110 minutes) allows the commercial production of FDG, transportation and off-site use of the tracer.

In this chapter, therefore, we report the initial experience of planar FDG imaging in patients after myocardial infarction. Three aspects of planar FDG imaging were studied:

(1) FDG image quality,
(2) assessment of increased FDG uptake in patients after myocardial infarction, and
(3) the influence of glucose and insulin on planar FDG uptake.

FDG imaging quality

For this purpose, 49 patients were studied after a first myocardial infarction. Patients (39 males, mean age 61 ± 12 years) were all admitted because of a recent myocardial infarction as proven by history, elevated cardiac enzymes, and development of Q waves or transient ST-T wave changes. Thirty-five patients had a transmural infarction as evidenced by pathological Q waves. All patients were studied in the afternoon after a light meal. One hour prior to FDG administration, patients were loaded with oral glucose ranging in dose from 12.5 to 50 gram glucose. After intravenous administration of 2.5–5 mCi FDG planar imaging started 45 minutes later with the patient at rest in a supine position. A specially designed 511 keV collimator was used and images were made in the three standard projections: anterior, left anterior oblique 45 and 70 degrees. A matrix of 128 × 128 pixels was chosen and the acquisition time per view was 8 minutes. An example is given in Plate 38.1. The images were projected on a monitor screen without background subtraction or threshold settings and the images were visually scored by two experienced observers as

Table 1. Target/background ratios in the anterior projection of patient images.

	Heart/lung ratios	Heart/liver ratios
Mean values	2.39	1.71
Standard deviation	0.57	0.45
Range	1.57–4.38	0.94–2.90

good, moderate, or poor. Twenty-five images of patients were classified as good, 18 as moderate and 6 as poor. Of the 43 patients with good and moderate images, 40 showed an image defect (93%).

To quantify the target to background ratios, a region of interest (ROI) was drawn in the anterior view over the myocardium with normal FDG uptake, over the lung and the liver area. From the average counts/pixel of the three ROIs the heart/lung and heart/liver ratios were calculated. Results are given in Table 1. The average heart/lung ratio was 2.4 with a range from 1.6 to 4.4. The mean heart/liver ratio was 1.7 with a range from 0.9 to 2.9. An example of a high heart/lung ratio is given in Plate 38.1, the results of a poor image with low heart/lung ratios is given in Plate 38.2. From the analysis it can be concluded that the quality of planar FDG images is such that in the majority of cases, the heart and the tracer defects can clearly be visualized. In 12% of the patients, the image quality was poor, which may possibly due to a low glucose or insulin level in these patients (see below). The favorable outcome of the results formed the basis for the subsequent studies.

Assessment of increased FDG uptake in patients after myocardial infarction

The aim of this study was to investigate whether increased FDG uptake could be demonstrated in patients after infarction. For this purpose, 41 patients (33 males, mean age 63 ± 12 years) underwent both thallium-201 (Tl-201) and FDG scintigraphy at rest. Twenty-four patients had an inferior and 17 an anterior infarction. Thirty-three were treated with thrombolytic therapy. FDG scintigraphy was performed as described above. On the same day as the FDG imaging, patients were studied with Tl-201 (2–3 mCi). The same views were used for both Tl-201 and FDG imaging. From the Tl-201 images circumferential profiles were made: after background subtraction according to Watson et al. [6], and 9 point smoothing, 60 radii were constructed and the pixel with the highest intensity per radius was plotted. The outflow tract was discarded. The countrates in the profiles were normalized to the highest pixel value (100%). The profiles were compared with a normal profile of 21 healthy volunteers and patients without coronary artery disease (mean values minus 2 standard deviations). The area in which the patient profile was lower than the profile of the normals, was assigned as the infarct defect (Figure 1). From the FDG images, circumferential profiles were made in the same manner as from the Tl-201 images. In the infarct defect, the values of the FDG were subtracted from the Tl-201 values, yielding information about the relatively increased FDG uptake in the infarct defect. The differences between normalized Tl-201 and FDG counts in the infarct defect were divided by the number of radii in the

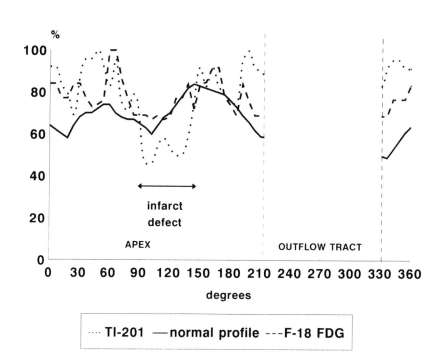

Figure 1. Analysis of the Tl-201 and FDG data. The circumferential profile of Tl-201 was compared with a normal profile. The area in which the Tl-201 counts were lower than the counts of the normal profile, was assigned as infarct defect. In this infarct defect the FDG counts were subtracted from the Tl-201 counts. In this example, a clear increased FDG uptake was seen in the infarct defect.

defect, resulting in an average increased FDG uptake in the defect. Plate 38.3 shows an example of a patient with a 'matched' defect on the Tl-201 and FDG

Table 2. Comparison between Tl-201 and FDG uptake in infarct defects.

	Tl-201	FDG
Size (radii)	56 ± 17	42 ± 12[a]
Range	1–83	0–74
% decreased uptake in defect[b]	33% ± 9%	23% ± 6%
Range	5%–49%	−3%–23%

[a] FDG uptake is only measured in Tl-201 defects.
[b] Compared to normal profiles.

image: the left image is the Tl-201 image, on the right is the FDG image. In both, a large defect is seen posteriorly. The circumferential profile of this patient is seen in Plate 38.4. Plate 38.5 shows the images of a patient with an septal infarction. A large infarct defect is seen on the Tl-201 image (left) while in the same area, FDG uptake is increased (right). The profile of this patient is given in Plate 38.6. Table 2 shows the information of the Tl-201 and FDG data. The mean size of the Tl-201 defects was 56 radii (of 180 radii analyzed) with a range between 1 and 83 radii. The average FDG uptake in the infarct defect was 10% higher than the Tl-201 uptake with a range of -3 to 23%. Six patients showed equal or higher FDG uptake compared to the normal profile of Tl-201 in the tracer defects, while the remaining patients showed lower FDG uptake compared to the normal profile. However, it is fair to state that the last-mentioned data may not be correct because normal limits of FDG uptake for planar imaging do not yet exist. Nevertheless, it can be concluded that, when comparing FDG uptake with a flow tracer such as Tl-201, relative or absolute increased FDG uptake is present in a substantial number of patients after myocardial infarction. It may indicate that tissue viability can be assessed using this approach. Although this method is, at best, a semi-quantitative approach, the diagnostic procedure can be applied in general hospitals without PET facilities and thus in a large patient population.

The influence of glucose and insulin on planar FDG uptake

Recent data [7] suggest that FDG uptake is not only dependent on glucose uptake but is also related to the circulating insulin levels. High insulin levels promote glucose uptake and therefore also FDG uptake. We therefore compared planar FDG uptake in 6 patients with both low and high insulin levels. During the low insulin protocol, insulin was infused at a rate of 20 mU/kg/hr, starting 1 hour before FDG administration. Glucose was simultaneously infused at a rate of 6 mg/kg/min and adjusted according to acutely determined glucose levels (every 5 min). In the high insulin protocol, insulin was infused at a rate of 100 mU/kg/hr and glucose also initially at a rate of 6 mg/kg/min and

Table 3. Blood level data in the low and high insulin protocol.

	Low insulin	High insulin
Glucose mmol/l	8.2 ± 1.7	7.0 ± 1.9
Insulin mU/l	31 ± 8	138 ± 9
K mmol/l	4.9 ± 0.3	5.1 ± 0.6

Table 4. Data from the heart-lung-liver ratios in six patients.

	Low insulin	High insulin
Heart/lung ratio	2.42 ± 1.03[a]	2.93 ± 0.15
Heart/liver ratios	1.99 ± 0.59[a]	2.91 ± 0.63
Defect/normal Myocardium ratio	0.88 ± 0.07	0.77 ± 0.10

[a] $p < 0.05$.

adjusted when necessary. During both protocols somatostatin was infused at a rate of $100 \, \mu g/hr$ to block endogenous insulin secretion and KCl 1 gr/hr was given intravenously to prevent hypokalemia. FDG imaging was performed as described above. From images made in the anterior projection, ROI's were drawn over myocardial area with normal uptake and over tracer defects and ROIs were drawn over the lung and liver area. From these data heart/lung, heart/liver, and tracer defect/normal myocardium ratios were calculated. The results from blood samples are given in Table 3. The high insulin protocol resulted in high insulin levels (mean 138 mU/l), while glucose levels were comparable to the low insulin protocol. An example of a patient study is given in Plate 38.7. A better FDG uptake is noted during high insulin infusion. Table 4 shows the results of the ratios. A significantly higher heart/lung and heart/liver ratio is present during high insulin infusion. Although the defect/normal myocardium ratio is lower during high insulin infusion (resulting in a better discrimination between normal myocardium and tracer defects), this difference was not significant.

Our results indicate that better target/background ratios are observed during stimulation of FDG uptake by high insulin levels. Therefore, this clamping technique should be used during FDG imaging. Somatostatin was used in our study to reach stable insulin levels, especially during the low insulin protocol, and is not necessarily needed in high insulin protocols.

Conclusion

FDG imaging is feasible using planar imaging with conventional gamma cameras. Images of the myocardium are of adequate quality, distinguishing between normal myocardium and tracer defects and resulting in favourable target to background ratios. The use of a clamping technique, which allows high insulin levels during imaging, is preferable because uptake FDG uptake in the myocardium is promoted. When combining FDG imaging with a flow tracer such as Tl-201, increased FDG uptake can be observed in the infarct defect in patients after myocardial infarction. These data therefore suggest that tissue viability can be assessed. However, further prospective studies are needed to establish the efficacy and clinical value of this diagnostic approach.

References

1. Topol EJ, Califf RM, George BS et al. A randomized trial of immediate versus delayed elective angioplasty after intravenous tissue plasminogen activator in acute myocardial infarction. N Engl J Med 1987; 317: 581–8.
2. Simoons ML, Bertrui A, Col J et al. Trombolysis with tissue plasminogen activator in acute myocardial infarction: no additional benefit from immediate percutaneous coronary angioplasty. Lancet 1988; 1: 197–202.
3. Tillisch J, Brunken R, Marshall R et al. Reversibility of cardiac wall motion abnormalities predicted by positron tomography. N Engl J Med 1986; 314: 884–8.
4. Tamaki N, Yonekura Y, Yamashita K et al. Positron emission tomography using Fluorine-18 Deoxyglucose in evaluation of coronary artery bypass grafting. Am J Cardiol 1989; 64: 860–5.
5. Hoeflin FG, Hopf M, Ledermann H, Noelpp U, Roesler H, Weinreich R. Routine detection of non-perfused but viable (hibernating or stunned) myocardium after recent infarction with 18-fluoro-deoxyglucose using a gamma camera. First results of the subsequent coronary angioplasty [abstract]. Eur J Nucl Med 1989; 15: 447.
6. Watson DD, Campbell NP, Read EK, Gibson RS, Teates CD, Beller GA. Spatial and temporal quantitation of of plane thallium myocardial images. J Nucl Med 1981; 22: 577–84.
7. Knuuti J, Nuutila P, Ruotsalainen U et al. Euglycemic hyperinsulinemic clamp and oral glucose load in stimulating myocardial glucose utilization during positron emission tomography [abstract]. J Nucl Med 1991; 32: 988.

SECTION EIGHT

Alternative stress imaging

39. New developments in pharmacological stress imaging

F. PAUL VAN RUGGE, ERNST E. VAN DER WALL
and ALBERT V.G. BRUSCHKE

Introduction

Accurate assessment of the localization, extent and severity of jeopardized myocardium is invaluable for the management of patients with coronary artery disease. Moreover, identification of viable myocardium is of major importance when angioplasty or bypass-surgery is considered. Recent development of innovative imaging strategies provided the clinical cardiologist with new diagnostic tools to determine myocardial perfusion and left ventricular function. These imaging modalities require a (sub)maximal level of stress in order to increase coronary flow and myocardial oxygen demand. Although exercise is by far the most physiological method for producing a (sub)maximal level of stress, a considerable number of patients are unable to adequately perform conventional exercise stress testing. Pharmacological stress seems to be an appropriate substitute for bicycle and treadmill exercise, and is gaining increasing popularity. In addition, pharmacologically induced stress avoids excessive chest wall motion due to high respiration frequency, thereby contributing to high quality images. Currently, several stress agents are used in conjunction with thallium-201 scintigraphy, two-dimensional echocardiography and, recently, magnetic resonance imaging (MRI). The most employed agents include vasodilators such as dipyridamole and adenosine, and catecholamines such as dobutamine.

The appearance of perfusion defects and wall motion abnormalities has been considered as both reliable and sensitive markers of myocardial ischemia, that precede the occurrence of electrocardiographic abnormalities and anginal pain during exercise. This chapter will focus on the currently available

Ernst E. van der Wall et al. (eds), What's new in cardiac imaging?, 503–537.

and applicated forms of pharmacological stress in conjunction with recently developed imaging modalities, particularly two-dimensional echocardiography and magnetic resonance imaging. The potential for qualitatively and quantitatively analyzing wall motion will be emphasized.

I. Dipyridamole

I.1. Introduction

Pharmacological stress testing has been proven to be an accepted tool in the assessment of coronary artery disease. In the past decade, myocardial perfusion scintigraphy using thallium-201 during dipyridamole stress has been extensively studied and reported for the detection of coronary artery disease [1–3], prediction of future cardiac events [4], and evaluation of perioperative cardiac risk [5, 6]. Perfusion scintigraphy during pharmacological stress is an attractive alternative for patients who are unable to perform conventional exercise. Some investigators have proposed combining the administration of dipyridamole with isometric handgrip [7] or low level treadmill exercise [8].

The basic characteristic of perfusion scintigraphy is the induction of an increase in coronary blood flow in order to demonstrate a perfusion disparity between the myocardial regions which can be detected with radioactive tracers [9]. Dipyridamole is well suited for provoking such a condition of coronary hyperemia due to its vasodilating properties. This section briefly reports the mechanism of action of dipyridamole and will focus on echocardiography and MRI during dipyridamole stress (Table 1). It will not address the value of dipyridamole in myocardial perfusion imaging.

I.2. Dipyridamole

Dipyridamole is a lipophilic pyridimine derivative and was initially introduced as a coronary vasodilator for the treatment of angina pectoris. However, when given intravenously, it provoked or aggravated anginal attacks based on the capacity to induce flow maldistribution. After investigation of this paradoxical response, dipyridamole was considered to be an adequate agent in cardiac perfusion imaging based on flow heterogeneity. Currently, it is widely prescribed as an antithrombotic drug due to its inhibiting effects on the platelet function. In the circulation, it is highly bound to plasma proteins, values ranging from 91 to 99%. Dipyridamole is metabolized in the liver and is eliminated primarily by biliary excretion as a glucuronide conjugate while it is subjected to enterohepatic recirculation. Its elimination has a tri-exponential course and its half-life is approximately 10 hours [10, 11].

1.3. Mechanism of action

Dipyridamole acts as a coronary vasodilator particularly by its effect on the level of the small resistance arterioles [12, 13]. Its dilating action has not been fully elucidated, but appears to be related to the increased plasma level of endogenous adenosine, a potent coronary arteriolar vasodilator [2, 10, 11]. Both oral and intravenous administration of dipyridamole blocks the transmembrane transport and reuptake of adenosine into myocardial, endothelial, and blood cells, thereby indirectly increasing the endogenous plasma adeno-

Table 1. Dipyridamole: dose, mechanisms of action, hemodynamic responses, side effects and antidotum.

Dose: The standard dose of dipyridamole for perfusion-scintigraphy is 0.142 mg/kg/min i.v. given for 4 minutes; two-dimensional-echo is performed using 0.84 mg/kg i.v. for 10 minutes

Coronary vasodilation accompanied with minor systemic vasodilation, mediated by the increase of adenosine at the receptor site, due to:
– inhibition of uptake of adenosine into myocardial, endothelial and blood cells
– inhibition of adenosine deaminase, the enzyme that converts adenosine into inosine
Other actions of dipyridamole include
– inhibition of phosphodiesterase activity, resulting in accumulation of cyclic adenosine 3',5'-monophosphaat (cAMP), thereby potentiating vasodilation
– stimulation of prostacyclin synthesis and release from endothelium

Hemodynamic responses:
– *regional disparity or heterogeneity of myocardial blood flow: increase of coronary blood flow up to 3–5 times baseline level in normal coronary arteries, compared with a limited increase in stenotic arteries dependent on the lumen narrowing*
– *mild reduction in systolic blood pressure*
– *slight reflex increase in heart rate*
– *insignificant alteration in myocardial oxygen demand (rate-pressure product)*

Side effects:
– angina: myocardial ischemia may occur due to an absolute decrease in endocardial blood flow (transmural or vertical steal) or when blood is shunted away through a collateral vessel (horizontal steal)
– flushing, headache, and dizziness
– nausea and epigastric pain

Antidotum: Aminophylline (60–240 mg i.v.) promptly reverses severe side effects by blocking the adenosine receptors competitively

sine level. At the receptor site, adenosine exerts a powerful vasodilating effect. In addition, dipyridamole prevents inactivation of adenosine by inhibiting the enzyme adenosine deaminase, which is responsible for its conversion. Dipyridamole also inhibits the phosphodiesterase enzyme, resulting in an accumulation of cyclic adenosine 3',5'-monophosphate (cAMP), which enhances vasodilation. Furthermore, a stimulation of the prostacyclin synthesis and release by dipyridamole has been suggested. Adenosine has several effects on the cardiovascular system, which will be discussed in the next section.

1.4. Rationale for dipyridamole in cardiac imaging

Previous reports have shown that resting coronary flow and its regional distribution are little affected by relative severe stenosis and are therefore insensitive measures for evaluating coronary disease. Gould et al. [14] demonstrated that resting coronary flow is not altered until a 85% diameter stenosis is present, whereas maximal coronary flow is affected by a 30–45% diameter stenosis. The hyperemic response was abolished when there was a ± 88 to 93% diameter narrowing. Overall, there was a marked impairment of coronary flow reserve with progressive stenosis of 65 to 95% diameter narrowing.

After administration of dipyridamole, the vasodilating effects occur predominantly in the small resistance vessels or the coronary arterioles. Consequently, the overall physiologic effect is a decrease of the vascular tone and thus a decrease of the coronary vascular resistance. As a consequence, there is a marked increase in coronary blood flow.

In patients with normal coronary arteries, the coronary blood flow during physical exercise may increase two to three times above the basal resting levels. Under normal resting conditions, coronary blood flow is adjusted by the mechanism of autoregulation to meet myocardial demand [15, 16]. The maximal amount of blood flow that can be recruited is defined as the coronary flow reserve (ratio of maximal to resting flow). The mechanism of autoregulation is abolished during vasodilation. Consequently, the coronary perfusion has become completely pressure-dependent. The relationship between coronary flow and perfusion pressure has become linear. This vasodilating reserve can be recruited with increasing myocardial oxygen demands, such as occur during exercise. Also, vasodilation can be induced pharmacologically and has been shown to exceed physiological vasodilatory reserve [16]. Infusion of dipyridamole may increase the coronary blood flow four to five times above resting levels (pharmacological vasodilator reserve) indicating a coronary flow reserve of four to five [9, 17]. In patients with significant coronary artery stenosis, the vascular bed distal to the stenosis is dilated to a certain amount such as to warrant normal resting flow. Accordingly, the coronary vasodilator reserve is limited and severe stenoses will result in an exhausted flow reserve. When dipyridamole is administered in these patients, no further significant vasodilation will occur in the distal vascular bed and subendocardial coronary flow will not rise. However, the normal coronary arteries possess the full capacity to vasodilate. Hence, a regional flow heterogeneity or perfusion maldistribution may appear. When the ratio of maximal flow in a normal to stenotic coronary artery is at least 2 : 1, the flow heterogeneity can be detected in the myocardial perfusion image of thallium-201 [9].

Thus, the basic principle of dipyridamole thallium imaging is to create a heterogeneity of coronary blood flow rather than provoking myocardial ischemia. Nevertheless, true ischemia manifested by wall-motion abnormalities, ST-T depression, or angina, may develop. There are two potential causes for ischemia after administration of dipyridamole. The first is an increase in myocardial oxygen consumption, as assessed by the rate-pressure product. However, several investigators have reported only modest increases in the double product, thereby excluding this parameter as the major cause of ischemia [18–20]. The second and most likely mechanism arises from the pressure-flow relations characterizing coronary stenoses [9, 14, 17, 21–24]. At normal resting conditions with severe stenosis, resting flow and distal perfusion pressure are reduced to stimulate compensatory subendocardial coronary vasodilation. Consequently, resting flow is maintained at the cost of vasodilatory capacity. Ultimately, with progression of the disease, the vasodilator reserve will be exhausted. Experimental studies have demonstrated that under conditions of maximal coronary vasodilation, lowered perfusion pressure is linearly related to a fall in subendocardial perfusion [25, 26]. In response to a vasodilator stimulus, such as pharmacologically induced stress by dipyridamole or physical exercise, the flow velocity through a coronary stenosis will increase. The energy or pressure loss across the stenosis due to viscous friction (f) increases in linear proportion to the flow velocity (v), whereas pressure loss due to flow separation (s: vortex shedding, turbulent eddies) increases as a function of the square of flow velocity ($\triangle P = fv + sv^2$). For a given stenosis, the pressure gradient increases in a curvilinear relation to flow velocity according to the quadratic equation [9, 14, 22, 23].

Consequently, a small increase in coronary flow through a stenotic artery after arteriolar vasodilation is associated with a large increase in pressure gradient due to the mentioned pressure losses. This increased pressure drop across the stenosis at elevated flow rates will result in a decreased distal coronary perfusion pressure, the subendocardium may become underperfused and ischemia may finally develop. Therefore, a redistribution of coronary transmural flow occurs in the presence of coronary stenosis during pharmacological vasodilation [27]. In mildly stenosed arteries, the subepicardial flow will increase proportionately more compared to the subendocardial flow, which results in an attenuated subendocardial/subepicardial flow-ratio. As a consequence, transmural blood-flow gradients may arise after vasodilation. In severely stenosed arteries, a fall in absolute subendocardial flow (in cc/min per gram endocardium) may occur after a vasodilator stimulus despite an increased subepicardial flow. In patients with severe coronary artery disease, resting flow and distal coronary perfusion pressure are reduced enough to stimulate compensatory subendocardial vasodilation and nearly exhaust maximal vasodilator reserve. Dipyridamole then induces a significantly greater vasodilation in subepicardial arterioles compared with subendocardial arterioles. As a result, subepicardial flow increases proportionately more than subendocardial flow. When absolute subendocardial coronary perfusion falls below resting levels, myocardial ischemia develops. This phenomenon is appropriately defined as 'subendocardial steal', 'endocardial-epicardial steal', 'vertical steal', or 'intracoronary steal' [17, 27–29]. Coronary 'steal' may also occur in the presence of collateral vessels. At resting conditions, collateral flow may be sufficient to warrant adequate distal coronary perfusion. During arteriolar vasodilation, the perfusion pressure at the origin of the collateral vessel may decrease, causing a fall in absolute collateral flow, despite an increase in the flow of the donor artery. This is called 'classical steal', 'horizontal steal', or 'intercoronary steal' by an adjacent perfusion bed with a proportionately greater increase in coronary flow compared with the diseased vascular bed. Although the term 'steal' remains controversial, it has been considered as an important clinical sign during cardiac imaging. It may indicate severe coronary artery disease with exhausted vasodilator reserve and ischemic but viable myocardium [27–29].

I.5. Hemodynamic effects

The vasodilation induced by dipyridamole is not restricted to the coronary vasculature. However, several investigators have shown that dipyridamole causes a more pronounced decrease in the coronary vascular resistance than in systemic resistance, indicating that dipyridamole is a rather selective coronary vasodilator [1, 2, 18–20]. The following systemic effects may occur: a mild reduction in systolic and diastolic blood pressure, a reflex increase in heart rate and a slight increase in cardiac output. Myocardial oxygen demand, as assessed by the rate-pressure product, is minimally increased.

As mentioned before, the coronary hemodynamic effects of dipyridamole are well defined by the stenosis pressure gradient and coronary flow velocity relationship: after coronary vasodilation, elevated flow through a stenotic artery is associated with an increased pressure gradient across the stenosis and a fall in distal coronary perfusion pressure. Consequently, subendocardial perfusion may be reduced despite an increased subepicardial flow and ischemia may become manifest.

I.6. Side effects

Recently, the side-effect profile of dipyridamole in a large number of patients who underwent dipyridamole-thallium imaging was reported [30]. Serious side effects were rare. In the 3911 patients who were studied by several investigators, two fatal and two nonfatal myocardial infarctions were reported. Other cardiac side effects include ST-T depression, angina, and arrhythmias. Dipyridamole-induced chest pain was a moderately specific marker and induced ST-T depression was a highly specific marker for coronary artery disease. However, both were insensitive for the assessment of significant coronary stenoses.

Noncardiac side effects occur more frequently. Headaches, flushing, dizziness, nausea, dyspepsia, and epigastric pain are not uncommon. However, most of these mild side effects do not require any treatment. Acute bronchospasm has been reported in six patients who received dipyridamole intravenously. All episodes of bronchospasm rapidly reversed after administration of intravenous aminophylline.

Intravenous aminophylline can be administered when rapid reversal of side effects is required. Aminophylline reverses serious side effects promptly by blocking the adenosine receptors [31, 32]. Therefore, aminophylline is considered as the drug of choice for treatment of severe side effects. However, a few patients have to be treated with a combination of aminophylline and nitroglycerin.

I.7. Imaging protocols

The most widely used and reported thallium protocols involve the intravenous injection of 0.142 mg/kg/min of dipyridamole for 4 minutes, as pointed out by Gould et al. [9, 17]. This optimal dose increases the coronary blood flow or velocity by three to five times above baseline value. The patient should be studied in the fasting state because nausea and emesis may occur, and to minimize splanchic blood flow which results in accumulations of thallium-201 in the liver and spleen. Furthermore, patients are instructed not to take caffeinated beverages and to discontinue xanthine- and caffeine-containing medications. Because studies have shown that the peak effect occurs 2–3 minutes after the infusion of dipyridamole, thallium in injected 7 minutes after the start of the dipyridamole infusion (or 3 minutes after the completion).

During the entire procedure, continuous electrocardiographic monitoring and blood pressure recordings are required. In order to decrease the pulmonary blood volume as well as both lung and splanchnic thallium uptake, the patient is asked to stand up and walk about before thallium injection. Subsequently, the initial (after 12–35 minutes) and delayed (after 180–240 minutes) thallium images are required and compared with each other. The presence and site of perfusion defects as well as the nature of the abnormality (transient or fixed) are determined. Reversible defects reflect ischemic viable myocardial tissue, whereas fixed defects correspond to myocardial scar.

In the beginning, *dipyridamole echocardiography* was performed using the same instructions concerning fasting, diet and medication, and dosage regimen as reported for the thallium studies. However, the initial dose of 0.56 mg/kg of dipyridamole over 4 minutes yielded a moderate sensitivity for the detection of coronary artery disease [33, 34]. Therefore, the dose of dipyridamole has been adjusted [35, 36]. The dosage regimen of the so-called 'high dose dipyridamole echocardiography test' is as follows: 0.56 mg/kg in 4 minutes followed by a 4 minutes pause in the administration of dipyridamole and then 0.28 mg/kg in 2 minutes. The cumulative dose is therefore 0.84 mg/kg in 10 minutes. Two-dimensional echocardiograms are continuously recorded during the dipyridamole infusion and up to 10 minutes after the end of the infusion. In the baseline studies, all standard echocardiographic views are obtained whenever possible. During the dipyridamole infusion, new regions of abnormal wall motion are identified on multiple views by moving the transducer in different positions. The test is considered positive when areas of transient asynergy are detected which were absent or present to a lesser degree during the baseline examinations.

I.8. Dipyridamole echocardiography

Although echocardiography during exercise has been performed succesfully [37, 38], it suffers from technical limitations due to hyperventilation and excessive chest-wall movement. Furthermore, the examinations are performed immediately after exercise. Consequently, wall-motion abnormalities may be absent at the time of delayed imaging when transient ischemia resolves rapidly.

The initial studies with dipyridamole echocardiography using a cumulative dipyridamole dose of 0.56 mg/kg over 4 minutes, reported an overall sensitivity of 56% and specificity of 100% for the presence of coronary artery disease [33]. In the same group of patients, exercise stress-testing yielded an overall sensitivity of 62% and a specificity of 80%. All the included patients were off anti-anginal therapy. In another study on 62 patients with angina at rest [39], the sensitivity was 62%. The authors suggested that dipyridamole was probably a less potent stimulus for inducing ischemia compared to conventional exercise. They also assumed that the dosage of dipyridamole was not maximal in all patients to provoke maximal vasodilation. Additionally, Margonato et al. [34] reported a 52% sensitivity in 21 patients with severe chronic stable angina pectoris with multivessel coronary artery disease. In order to solve this problem, Picano et al. [35] proposed dipyridamole echocardiography using higher doses as described in the previous section. In a study performed in 93 patients with effort angina, the overall sensitivity increased from 53 to 74%, when the higher dose of dipyridamole was given to patients with a negative low dose test. The investigators reported no loss in specificity or an increased risk. However, the sensitivity for the patients with one-vessel disease remained lower (50%) compared with exercise electrocardiography (54%); the sensitivity for two-vessel disease was 81% and for three-vessel disease 100%. In another study [40], the same authors investigated 55 patients with effort angina pectoris using echocardiography during exercise as well as during high-dose dipyridamole. For detecting angiographically assessed coronary artery disease, they reported a 72% sensitivity during dipyridamole-echocardiography and a 76% sensitivity during exercise-echocardiography. The specificity was 100 and 87%, respectively. With the high dose of 0.84 mg/kg for 10 minutes, Bolognese et al. [41] studied asymptomatic patients one week after uncomplicated acute myocardial infarction. The sensitivity of transient remote asynergy in predicting multivessel disease was 68% and specificity 100%. Pirelli et al. [42] reported a 71% sensitivity for detection of restenosis after angioplasty, which was similar to exercise electrocardiography in a population which largely consisted of patients with one-vessel disease. Masini et al. [43] performed high dose dipyridamole-echocardiography in 83 women with chest pain and found a 79% sensitivity with dipyridamole-echocardiography and a 72% sensitivity with exercise electrocardiography, whereas the dipyridamole echocardiography test had greater specificity (93% versus 52%). To evaluate the prognostic value of the dipyridamole echocardiography test, Picano et al. [44] studied 539 patients with chest discomfort or with old myocardial infarction. Prospectively, there were 118 cardiac events (cardiac death, reinfarction, revascularization procedures to treat progressive angina). Survival analysis identified a transient myocardial dyssynergy after dipyridamole infusion as the most powerful independent predictor of future cardiac events (relative risk ratio 2.7). During the 3-year follow-up, cardiac events occurred in 6% of the patients with a normal high-dose dipyridamole-echocardiography test, in 26% with a positive high-dose test and in 41% with positive low-dose dipyridamole echocardiography test. In another study, Picano et al. [45] investigated 74 patients with angina undergoing single-lesion percutaneous transluminal coronary angioplasty. Both before and after the revascularization procedure, a high dose dipyridamole echocardiography test was performed. Before angioplasty, 69 patients had a positive echocardiogram, based on abnormal regional wall motion, and five had a negative echocardiogram. There were 63 successful procedures (diameter reduction of $>20\%$ and residual stenosis $<50\%$), five unsuccessful angioplasty procedures and six major cardiac complications (death, acute infarction, emergency bypass-surgery). In the 63 patients with angiographically successful angioplasty, the dipyridamole echocardiography test was positive in 58 patients before and in only 16 after the procedure. In the five patients with an unsuccessful angioplasty, the echocardiogram was positive in all five before and in four patients after the procedure. They concluded that an excellent agreement exists between the functional improvement assessed by dipyridamole echocardiography and the anatomic results of the angioplasty.

I.9. Dipyridamole magnetic resonance imaging

Magnetic resonance imaging (MRI), as an innovative imaging modality, has the potential to provide high-quality images of the heart with excellent spatial resolution. The three-dimensional information is obtained without the need for radiation or contrast injection, the procedure is entirely noninvasive and the field of view is unlimited. Conventional spin-echo sequences provide a well-defined depiction of anatomical structures and abnormalities in a variety of cardiac disease [46]. In addition, with the development of fast imaging sequences [47], the temporal resolution improved substantially to monitor cardiac function [48, 49]. Consequently, evaluation of cardiac function has become possible using measurements of ventricular volumes [50], ejection fraction [51], qualitative wall motion dynamics [52], quantitative wall thickness and wall thickening [53–55], wall stress [56] and regurgitant volumes [57].

Dynamic exercise in a magnetic resonance scanner is precluded due to space restriction and motion artefacts. However, pharmacological stress with MRI has been reported as an adequate alternative for physical exercise. Pennell et al. [58, 59] were the first to report dipyridamole stress during magnetic resonance imaging. Magnetic resonance imaging suffers from rather long imaging times. Accordingly, the investigators modified the currently used protocols for dipyridamole echocardiography to prolong the effects of dipyridamole on wall motion: the infusion regime consisted of 0.56 mg/kg of dipyridamole over 4 minutes with a bolus of 10 mg given at 10 minutes, provided that serious side effects were absent. The study population consisted of 40 patients with chest pain and abnormal exercise test who were admitted for undergoing a coronary angiography, a dipyridamole thallium perfusion scintigraphy, and a dipyridamole magnetic resonance imaging. Thirty-nine patients had coronary artery disease, of whom 23 patients suffered a previous myocardial infarction. All 23 patients with previous myocardial infarction had fixed thallium-201 defects on the redistribution images, whereas 36 patients of the entire study group had reversible thallium perfusion defects. All 23 patients with previous infarction showed wall motion abnormalities on the magnetic resonance images. However, reversible wall-motion abnormalities were demonstrated in only 24 patients following dipyridamole infusion, which is 67% of the number of patients with reversible thallium defects.

The authors concluded that dipyridamole is not the ideal pharmacological stress agent for detecting coronary artery disease using wall-motion studies with magnetic resonance imaging.

I.10. Conclusion

Dipyridamole perfusion imaging and radionuclide angiography have become standard procedures in nuclear cardiology. New applications are the study of cardiac function during dipyridamole stress utilizing echocardiography and, recently, MRI.

Stress echocardiography has been shown to be a safe, feasible, and rather fast noninvasive method in the evaluation of patients with coronary artery disease. Advantages include its low cost, its widely availability, and the opportunity to examine critically ill patients (Coronary Care Unit) due to its portability. Furthermore, it is an imaging modality with less patient discomfort. However, two-dimensional echocardiography suffers from a number of drawbacks. The image acquisition strongly relies on adequate acoustic windows, which are not available in all patients. Also, the quality of the images is operator-dependent. Additionally, spatial resolution is limited and endocardial border definition is difficult. Obviously, important physiological parameters provided by exercise, which are known to contain prognostic information, are not available during pharmacological stress testing [60].

Although dipyridamole is well suited as a pharmacological stress agent in perfusion studies, its value for application in functional cardiac imaging using wall motion analysis is less clearly. Particularly, the reported sensitivities using dipyridamole echocardiography are not favorable, even with the high-dose infusion protocols. Dipyridamole is probably not the ideal pharmacological stressor for assessment of functional properties, due to its minimal effects on myocardial inotropy and rate-pressure product, the most important determinants of myocardial oxygen consumption. Its role in myocardial perfusion imaging, however, is invaluable.

II. Adenosine

II.1. Introduction

Adenosine has been known as a vasoactive substance with powerful vaso-dilator properties. The precise mechanism of action is still not fully elucidated, but it is suggested that adenosine exerts its vasodilating effect by acting on two different receptors: an endothelial cell receptor and a vascular smooth muscle cell receptor [61].

The mechanism of dipyridamole, as discussed in the previous section, is based on elevated interstitial adenosine concentration due to blockade of cellular reuptake of adenosine and decreased metabolism by adenosine-dea-minase. Therefore, it has been proposed to achieve the elevation of adenosine levels directly by adenosine infusion, instead of indirectly by infusion of dipyridamole [62].

Two important characteristics of adenosine for clinical and diagnostic use are its rapid onset and offset of action and its extremely short half-life. The effective half-life of 10–30 seconds of adenosine accounts for a high degree of safety, since its effects disappear rapidly after discontinuation of the in-travenous administration. Furthermore, the duration of action is very short, which allows repeated measurements during the same examination. Additionally, intravenously administered adenosine has been demonstrated to induce effectively a near-maximal coronary vasodilation, comparable to the maximal hyperemia caused by intracoronary injected papaverine. Wilson et al. [63] demonstrated a 4.4 fold increase in coronary blood flow velocity with in-travenous adenosine at a dose of $140 \mu g/kg/min$.

In the last years, there has been increasing interest in adenosine for three reasons. First, it may be a promising pharmacological stressor in performing myocardial perfusion imaging. Second, adenosine may play a key role in the generation of angina pectoris in patients with coronary artery disease as well as angina-like chest pain in normal subjects [64, 65]. Third, adenosine has been increasingly investigated for its application in the diagnosis and treatment in patients with supraventricular arrhythmias in which the atrioventricular (AV) node is part of the reentrant circuit [66, 67].

This section will focus on the applications of adenosine for myocardial perfusion imaging as an alternative for dipyridamole in provoking hetero-geneity of coronary flow.

II.2. Metabolism of adenosine

Adenosine is an endogenously produced substance that dilates the resistance vessels in all tissues, except in the kidney and in the hepatic venous system [61]. Adenosine can be formed extracellularly and intracellularly by dephosphorylation of AMP (ATP pathway) catalyzed by the enzyme 5′-nucleotidase. The ATP pathway is particularly important during myocardial ischemia, when ATP breakdown occurs and leads to the production of adenosine. Also, it can be formed intracellularly by degradation of *S*-adenosyl-homocysteine (SAH), a process belonging to the *S*-adenosylmethionine-dependent transmethylation reactions (SAM pathway) that is catalyzed by SAH-hydrolase. Consequently, AMP and SAH are considered as the precursors of adenosine. The cardiomyocytes are thought to be the major source of adenosine, whereas other sources include the cardiac vascular endothelium, blood platelets and adrenergic nerve endings [68].

After its release into the interstitial space, adenosine exerts its effects on vascular smooth muscle A_1 receptors and endothelial cell A_2 receptors, thereby inducing arteriolar vasodilation [61, 69]. Subsequently, adenosine is rapidly removed within 30 seconds by washout and by two enzymatic processes. Some of the adenosine passes through the capillary endothelial cells where a significant fraction is degraded to inosine and hypoxanthine by adenosine deaminase and nucleoside phosphorylase, respectively. Further degradation occurs in the erythrocytes by these enzymes. A large fraction of the adenosine, however, is taken up by the myocardial cells, where the nucleoside can either be phosphorylated by adenosine kinase to AMP or deaminated to inosine by adenosine deaminase in the cytosol. The rephosphorylated fraction of adenosine is then reincorporated into the myocardial adenine nucleotides (salvage pathway). Only a small fraction of the cardiac adenine nucleotides is derived by de novo synthesis.

II.3. Mechanism of vasorelaxation

The precise mechansim by which adenosine elicits relaxation of the systemic and coronary vasculature is still not completely understood, but several possibilities have been suggested. When adenosine is released from the cardiomyocytes into the interstitial space, adenosine is thought to act on two different purinoreceptors, located on the vascular smooth muscle cells and on the endothelial cells, respectively. Subsequently, adenosine probably acts directly on vascular smooth muscle receptors, and indirectly by stimulation of endothelial cell receptors. The endothelial cells then induce relaxation of the vascular smooth muscle by a still unidentified coupling mechanism [61]. The direct effects of adenosine on the vascular smooth muscle cells result from an increase in cyclic adenosine monophosphate (c-AMP), which has been reported to be associated with vascular smooth muscle relaxation [70].

Recently, it has been demonstrated that adenosine activates guanylate cyclase in membranes to increase the intracellular concentration of cyclic guanosine monophosphate (c-GMP), which ultimately leads to vasorelaxation by complex mechanisms of signal transduction [71]. Adenosine also stimulates the production of inositol phosphates, which breaks down inositol triphosphate, a second messenger mediating intracellular calcium release and smooth muscle contraction [72]. Another suggested mechanism is the influence of adenosine on cellular calcium dynamics. Adenosine may inhibit the slow inward calcium current, impair the calcium uptake, and interfere with the calcium utilization in the contractile apparatus [69, 73]. An important feature of adenosine is the attenuation of vascular tone by modulating sympathetic neurotransmission. Adenosine inhibits presynaptically the norepinephrine release from the adrenergic nerve terminals [61, 74, 75]. Finally, a physiological role for endothelium-derived relaxing-factor (EDRF) has been proposed, but could still not be established [76].

II.4. Cardiovascular effects of adenosine

Besides coronary and systemic vasodilation, adenosine exerts several cardiovascular effects [61]. These are listed in Table 2 and will be briefly discussed below. In addition, adenosine exerts many extracardiac effects, including respiratory stimulation by interaction with the carotid chemoreceptors. The well-known inhibition of platelet aggregation by dipyridamole is probably mediated by adenosine. Adenosine increases coronary blood flow, increases cerebral blood flow but causes a reduction in renal blood flow [61].

At the doses used for myocardial perfusion imaging by Verani et al. [62] and in the study for coronary blood flow velocity measurements by Wilson et al. [63], adenosine causes a reflex increase in heart rate and a decrease in systolic and diastolic blood pressure. Higher doses of adenosine have a depressant

Table 2. Cardiovascular effects of adenosine.

- coronary and systemic vasodilation
- vasoconstriction of the preglomerular arterioles in the kidney leading to a reduction in renal blood flow
- increase in cerebral blood flow
- depression of sinoatrial (SA) node activity
- impairment of atrioventricular (AV) conduction
- decrease of atrial contractility (both directly and indirectly)
- indirect decrease of ventricular contractility after catecholamine-stimulation
- modulation of vasomotor tone by presynaptic inhibition of norepinephrine release in adrenergic nerve terminals

effect on the sinoatrial SA node (negative chronotropic effect). Intravenous administration of adenosine has been shown to cause sinus bradycardia, sinoatrial exit block and sinus arrest [66, 67]. These effects are thought to be mediated at the cellular level by an increase in potassium conductance, leading to an enhanced K^+ outward current which hyperpolarizes the resting membrane potential.

Furthermore, adenosine impairs conduction of the impulses through the atrioventricular (AV) node (negative dromotropic effect), which may ultimately result in a complete AV-block [66, 67, 77]. The site of action appears to be the proximal region of the AV junction region, since adenosine increases the conduction time between the atrium and the His bundle (A–H interval), whereas it does not prolong the His bundle to ventricle (H–V) interval [61–78]. The prolongation of the A-H interval is due to a depression of the action potentials of nodal (N) cells. It has also been suggested that the impairment of the conduction through the AV node is related to an increase in potassium conductance.

In addition, adenosine decreases both atrial and ventricular contractility (negative inotropic effect). In atrial tissue, adenosine decreases the contractility directly as well as indirectly. In ventricular myocardium, however, adenosine has no direct effect and reduction of contractility occurs only by an indirect effect. This indirect negative inotropic effect can be demonstrated only when the myocardium has been previously stimulated by catecholamines, forskolin, amrinone, or histamine, e.g. agents known to increase adenylate cyclase activity and accumulation of c-AMP. Consequently, adenosine has been proposed as a negative feedback inhibitor of the stimulatory actions of catecholamines, by both presynaptic inhibition of the norepinephrine release from nerve terminals and postsynaptic attenuation of the positive inotropic action of catecholamines [61, 79–82].

Finally, adenosine has been proven to be highly efficacious in terminating supraventricular tachycardias in which the AV node is part of the reentrant circuit. However, adenosine has little effect on impulse generation and conduction in ventricular myocardium. These differing regional cardiac effects and the short half-life have resulted in the use of adenosine in the diagnosis and treatment of cardiac arrhythmias [66, 67].

II.5. Adenosine infusion protocol

Biaggioni et al. [83] reported an adenosine study using increasing infusion doses (80–180 μg/kg/min). However, infusions greater than 140 μg/kg/min in normal volunteers were characterized by a large dropout rate due to adverse effects. Consequently, in the recent reported studies, the maximal tolerated dose of adenosine was determined to be 140 μg/kg/min.

In the recently reported studies, the adenosine infusion protocol consist of intravenous adenosine administration at a rate of 140 μg/kg/min maintained for 6 minutes. In these thallium studies, thallium was injected 3 minutes after the start of the infusion. Perfusion imaging was initiated within 5 minutes of the end of the infusion and repeated 4 hours after thallium injection.

II.6. Adenosine imaging studies

Verani et al. [62] were the first to use intravenous adenosine as a pharmacological stress agent for evaluating patients with suspected coronary artery disease in conjunction with thallium-201 emission computed tomography. They studied 89 patients who were unable to perform conventional exercise and they were referred for evaluation of suspected coronary artery disease. The sensitivity assessed by quantitative tomography was 73% for patients with one-vessel disease, 90% for those with two-vessel disease, and 100% for patients with three-vessel disease. The overall sensitivity and specificity for detection of coronary artery disease was 83 and 94%, respectively. Side effects occurred in 83% of the patients, mainly consisting of chest and jaw pain. None of the patients experienced advanced AV block, hypotension, or bronchospasm.

In another study, Nguyen et al. [84] investigated 53 patients with and 7 without coronary artery disease using single photon emission computed tomography with thallium-201 during adenosine-induced coronary hyperemia. The sensitivity and specificity for detecting coronary artery disease were 92 and 100%, respectively. Twenty-five also underwent two-dimensional echocardiography. Only two of the 20 patients with coronary artery disease developed new wall motion abnormality during adenosine infusion. Side effects were reported in 88% of the patients, and were mild in nature with no occurrence of bronchospasm and second or third degree AV block. Aminophylline infusion was used in three patients for reversal of side effects.

In 100 subjects, Coyne et al. [85] compared thallium-201 scintigraphy after intravenous infusion of adenosine with conventional exercise thallium testing. Forty-seven patients with angiographically proven coronary artery disease and 53 control subjects were studied. The overall sensitivity of adenosine thallium testing for coronary artery disease was 83%, whereas it was 81% with exercise thallium testing. The specificities were 75 and 74%, respectively. Side effects were reported in 94% of the study population, but the patients never needed treatment.

Recently, Iskandrian et al. [86] reported their results of thallium imaging during adenosine infusion in 132 patients with coronary artery disease and in

16 patients with normal coronary angiograms. The sensitivity was 87% in the 54 patients with one-vessel disease, 92% in the 37 patients with two-vessel disease and 98% in the 41 patients with three-vessel disease. In the patients with normal coronary angiograms, 14 of the 16 patients showed normal thallium images (specificity 88%). Any adverse effect occurred in 91% of the patients. Transient second- or third-degree AV block developed in four patients and seven patients required aminophylline administration for reversal of the side effect.

Zoghbi [87] reported preliminary results from a study of 62 patients with suspected coronary artery disease who underwent two-dimensional echocardiography and simultaneous thallium 201 single-photon emission computed tomography (SPECT) during intravenous administration of 140 μg/kg/min of adenosine. In 49 of the 62 patients (79%), the investigator observed agreement between adenosine echocardiography and SPECT thallium imaging in discriminating normal from abnormal adenosine studies. The sensitivity for detection of coronary artery disease was 89% for adenosine echocardiography, 83% for adenosine thallium imaging, and 91% when either test was abnormal. During adenosine infusion, two patients developed second-degree atrioventricular block of the Wenckebach type, which was self-limiting. Occurrence of third-degree AV block was not observed.

II.7. Side effects

The nature of the side effects is the same as those reported after administration of dipyridamole, as can be expected. However, adverse effects occur more frequently when compared to dipyridamole. The side effects are generally mild, transient, and rarely warrant reversal with aminophylline. The most reported side effects include headache, flushing, chest pain, throat or jaw pain, dizziness, dyspnea, and abdominal discomfort [62, 84–86]. Three major side effects require further comment. First, depression of sinoatrial or atrioventricular node function can result in heart block in a dose-dependent fashion. Second, intravenous infusion of adenosine can cause a significant fall in arterial blood pressure. In patients with a reduced reflex tachycardia or with intravascular volume depletion, it may result in significant hypotension. Third, although rarely reported, administration of adenosine may elicit attacks of bronchospasm. Dyspnea during administration of adenosine may also result from stimulation of the carotid chemoreceptors leading to hyperventilation [83].

Although most of the reported severe side effects are transient and well tolerated, studies consisting of larger numbers of patients are required to fully ascertain the incidence and predisposing factors of these side effects.

II.8. Conclusion

The results of the recently reported clinical imaging studies using adenosine infusion as a pharmacological stress agent are promising regarding to the diagnostic accuracy of the test for detecting coronary artery disease. Adenosine induces a near-maximal coronary hyperemia, which is required for the assessment of coronary flow studies and myocardial perfusion imaging to identify the functional significance of coronary artery stenosis. Its extremely short half-life and rapid onset and offset of action are favorable in clinical diagnostic use. These attractive characteristics of adenosine may contribute to a high degree of safety and allow repeated measurements during examination. The relative high incidence of side effects is of concern and should be further evaluated to establish the safety and feasibility of adenosine stress imaging. Overall, the nature of the side effects of adenosine is comparable with those of dipyridamole, but they occur more frequently. Generally, after adenosine, the side effects are more short-lived, transient, well tolerated, and rarely warrant premature termination of the adenosine infusion or reversal with aminophylline.

In addition, adenosine may be of clinical value in the diagnosis and treatment of supraventricular tachycardias in which the atrioventricular junction is involved in the reentrant circuit.

The precise role of adenosine in myocardial ischemia and in the generation of angina pectoris remains to be established.

III. Dobutamine

III.1. Introduction

Catecholamines are widely used for acute inotropic support in the manage-

Table 3. Adrenergic receptor localization and effects after interaction with catecholamines.

Adrenergic receptor	Localization	Action
β_1	Myocardium	Enhance contractility
	SA node	Increase heart rate
	AV node	Increase conduction
β_2	Arterioles	Vasodilation
	Lungs	Bronchodilation
α	Arterioles	Vasoconstriction
	Myocardium	Enhance contractility

ment of severely compromised ventricular function. Substantial loss of ventricular contractility often results from myocardial injury due to atherosclerotic heart disease. Acute intravenous inotropic intervention is required to improve hemodynamics and clinical status of patients with severe heart failure.

Most catecholamines have, in common a positive inotropic effect and a positive chronotropic effect, both increasing myocardial oxygen requirements [88]. The role of dopamine and dobutamine, currently the most frequently applied parenteral catecholamines, in the treatment of severe heart failure, cardiogenic shock, and septic shock, has well been established [89–91].

At present, newly developed imaging modalities have led to an increasing search for pharmacological stress agents. Two-dimensional echocardiography and MRI are becoming extensively used and widely available. However, these techniques do not allow patient motion during image acquisition, thereby precluding dynamic exercise.

Dobutamine, as a synthetic catecholamine, seems to provide attractive opportunities to stress the cardiovascular system pharmacologically, and its main characteristics will be discussed in this section.

III.2. The catecholamines

The catecholamines are the agents most commonly used for short-term inotropic support. They consist of the natural, endogenously occurring catecholamines, (nor)epinephrine and dopamine, and the synthetic, exogenously administered catecholamines (dobutamine and isoproterenol). Depending on their structure, catecholamines may activate cardiac β_1-adrenergic receptors, β_2-adrenergic receptors and/or α-adrenergic receptors (Table 3). The predominant mechanism of action is determined by the type of adrenergic receptor that is stimulated [92] (Table 4). Stimulation of myocardial β_1-adrenergic

Table 4. Adrenergic receptor activity of catecholamines.

	α peripheral	β_1 cardiac	β_2 peripheral
Norepinephrine	+ + + +	+ + + +	0
Epinephrine	+ + + +	+ + + +	+ +
Dopamine[a]	+ + + +	+ + + +	+ +
Isoproterenol	0	+ + + +	+ + + +
Dobutamine	+	+ + + +	+ +
Methoxamine	+ + + +	0	0

[a] Also renal and mesenterial vasodilation after stimulation of dopaminergic receptors at low dose (< 5 μg/kg/min).

receptors increases the rate of discharge of the sinoatrial node resulting in an increase of the heart rate, enhances atrioventricular conduction, and augments ventricular contractility. The β_2-adrenergic receptors mediate vasodilation in the peripheral vasculature and bronchodilation in the lungs. The α-adrenergic receptors in peripheral vessels mediate arterial vasoconstriction. It has been reported, however, that some of the positive inotropic effects may also be mediated through the stimulation of myocardial α_1-adrenergic receptors [93].

Norepinephrine is the endogenous catecholamine that is synthesized and stored in the granules in adrenergic nerve endings in the myocardium. It is a powerful α_1-agonist with modest β_1-stimulating effects [94]. The administration of this drug elicits a cardiovascular vasopressor response through dose-related vasoconstriction. Although norepinephrine exerts a modest positive inotrophic effect, its strong vasoconstricting properties make it a potent vasopressor. Consequently, norepinephrine is mostly used in the clinical setting of severe hypotension and/or shock secondary to a septic or cardiogenic mechanism. Norepinephrine is started at an infusion rate of 0.01–0.02 μg/kg/min and advanced in dose every 10–15 minutes until the desired effects, i.e. a systemic pressure response, are achieved or undesirable side effects occur. The side effects are those with the other catecholamines and include tachycardia, dysrhythmias, tremor, anxiety, and headache.

Dopamine is a precursor in the synthesis route of norepinephrine and possesses combined positive inotropic and vasoconstricting properties. Dopamine powerfully stimulates α_1- and β_1-adrenergic receptors with only a mild β_2-stimulating effect. Some of the effects of dopamine are mediated through a dopamine-induced release of endogenous norepinephrine from nerve endings [92, 95]. Dopamine has some characteristics which make it a unique drug. Infusions of dopamine elicit a dose-related biphasic hemodynamic response. At lower doses (< 6 μg/kg/min), dopamine increases stroke volume and cardiac output and decreases vascular resistances with a mild increase in systemic blood pressure. At doses > 6 μg/kg/min, vasopressor effects become dominant, manifested by a substantial increase in systemic blood pressure and vascular resistance. At these dose, the overall hemodynamic effect of dopamine is almost the same as that elicited by norepinephrine, probably due to a greater recruitment of α_1-receptor stimulation and a greater release of endogenous norepinephrine. Another remarkable feature of dopamine is its capacity to stimulate the renal dopaminergic receptors [95, 96]. Dopaminergic-receptors (DA_1) activation increases renal blood flow, glomerular filtration rate, and sodium clearance. Doses > 8 μg/kg/min are often accompanied by side effects, which are the same as described for norepinephrine.

Isoproterenol, as a synthetic catecholamine, has great inotropic properties, mediated by β_1-agonism. In addition, isoproterenol exerts a strong stimulating effect on the peripheral vascular β_2 receptors, resulting in a powerful vasodilation. However, the therapeutic value of isoproterenol for the treatment of acutely depressed cardiac contractility is limited due to its chronotropic activity and considerable risk of arrhythmias [97]. Moreover, the substantial vasodilating effect of isoproterenol diverts a large portion of the cardiac output to the skeletal muscle, lowers peripheral resistance to the point of reducing diastolic arterial pressure, and may ultimately impair coronary perfusion pressure [92]. Positive inotropy is noted at a dose of $0.007–0.014\,\mu g/kg/min$ with a rather dramatic dose-related enhancement of vasodilation, chronotropy, and occurrence of dysrhythmias. Consequently, the clinical and diagnostic use of isoproterenol is limited.

Epinephrine is an endogenous catecholamine with α_1-, β_1-, and β_2-agonist properties. Unfortunately, its intravenous administration may provoke unpredictable chronotropic, vascular, and arrhythmogenic effects.

III.3. Dobutamine

Dobutamine is synthetic catecholamine developed as a relatively selective positive inotropic drug for short-term parenteral administration [98]. Dobutamine has the capacity to stimulate β_1-, β_2- and α_1-adrenoreceptors in the cardiovascular system. The heart contains predominantly β_1-adrenoreceptors that mediate positive inotropic and chronotopic effects when stimulated. However, the heart also contains a population of α_1-adrenoreceptors that, in contrast to β_1-adrenoreceptors, only mediates a positive inotropic response [93]. The peripheral vasculature contains a mixed population of postsynaptic α_1- and α_2-adrenoreceptors which both produces vasoconstriction when stimulated, and β_2-adrenoreceptors, which mediate vasodilation [98].

Dobutamine has long been considered to be a selective β_1-adrenoreceptor agonist, with relatively weak activity at the α- and β_2-adrenoreceptors. Previous studies have confirmed that the α-adrenoreceptor effects of dobutamine are confined to the α_1-adrenoreceptor subtype [99, 100]. In addition, the α_1- and β_2-adrenoreceptor effects are known to be considered more prominent than originally proposed.

The inotropic effect of dobutamine is generally attributed to stimulation of myocardial β_1-adrenoreceptors. However, several studies suggest that α_1-adrenoreceptor effects may contribute substantially to the inotopic potential of the agent [93, 99, 100]. Intravenous administration of dobutamine augments ventricular contractility with a resultant increase in stroke volume and cardiac output. In experimental animals as well as in patients with congestive heart failure, dobutamine infusion decreases central venous pressure, pulmonary artery pressure, pulmonary vessel resistance, and pulmonary capillary wedge pressure. Consequently, left-ventricular end-diastolic pressure and volume are lowered. Furthermore, the increase in stroke volume and ejection fraction results in a reduction of the left ventricular end-systolic volume. Accordingly, reduction of ventricular sizes is partly responsible for a decrease in wall stress, an important determinant of myocardial oxygen consumption [92, 101].

Considerable changes in blood pressure are relatively uncommon during dobutamine infusion. The increase in cardiac output caused by dobutamine is offset by a net reduction in total systemic vascular resistance leading to minimal changes in blood pressure. There are several factors influencing the total systemic vascular resistance [92, 93, 101]. First, a reflex withdrawal of sympathetic tone results from the increased cardiac output. Second, direct β_2-adrenoreceptor-mediated activity induces substantial vasodilation. Third, the α_1-adrenoreceptor-mediated vasopressor effect is probably offset by a postsynaptic vascular α_1-adrenoreceptor antagonism by the metabolite 3-*O*-methyldobutamine. As a consequence, the net decrease in total peripheral vascular resistance following the increase in cardiac output after dobutamine infusion, results in a relatively unaffected arterial blood pressure.

Dobutamine does not stimulate renal dopaminergic receptors [98, 102]. Therefore, the augmented renal blood flow arises secondarily from the increase in cardiac output.

Finally, administration of dobutamine is generally not accompanied by tachycardia and dysrhythmias, unless higher doses are required. However, dobutamine facilitates atrioventricular conduction [103, 104] and may, therefore, increase the ventricular rate in patients with atrial fibrillation.

III.4. Pharmacokinetics, metabolism and infusion protocol

The hemodynamic effects of dobutamine correlate linearly with plasma concentration and dose [105]. Dobutamine is administered as a continuous intravenous infusion at starting doses of 2–5 μg/kg/min with 2–5 μg/kg/min increments every 10 minutes until the desired hemodynamic and clinical status is achieved or serious side effects occur. The onset of action is within 2 minutes and the maximal effect occurs after 10–14 minutes. The mean plasma half-life in patients with low-output failure is approximately 2 minutes [106]. The short half-life is secondary to rapid redistribution and to metabolism by catechol-*O*-methyl transferase [107]. The major metabolites are 3-*O*-methyldobutamine and dobutamine glucuronide, from which the former probably is pharmacologically active. The metabolites are eliminated primarily by the kidney. Infusions lasting longer than 72 hours may be accompanied by the development of pharmacodynamic tolerance, presumably due to down-regulation of the β-adrenergic receptors [108].

III.5. Rationale for dobutamine as a pharmacological stressor

The use of catecholamines as a pharmacological alternative for physical exercise in the detection of functionally significant coronary artery stenosis is based on the concept that myocardial ischemia may result from the potent inotropic and chronotropic effects. The β-adrenergic inotropic agents are generally thought to be deleterious in the presence of myocardial ischemia because the ischemia can be intensified by oxygen-consuming effects of the agents, while oxygen supply at the same time is limited. Initially, this concept was based on the effects of isoproterenol, which has been shown to increase the extent of experimental myocardial infarction [109]. However, dopamine and dobutamine have proven to possess less pronounced chronotropic effects at intermediate dose. Moreover, Gillespie et al. [110] have shown that administration of dobutamine in doses sufficient to improve ventricular performance after myocardial infarction does not exacerbate myocardial injury or ventricular dysrhythmias. They found that dobutamine does not increase infarct size over predicted values. In a study of both anesthetized dogs with acute myocardial ischemia and conscious dogs with myocardial infarction, both groups without heart failure, Willerson et al. [111] concluded that dobutamine significantly increased regional myocardial blood flow to all areas of the heart. Vatner et al. [112] investigated the effects of dopamine, dobutamine, and isoproterenol in conscious dogs after coronary occlusion by measuring overall left ventricular function, regional myocardial wall motion, and regional myocardial blood flow. They concluded that β-adrenergic stimulation does not always exert a deleterious effect on regional function and blood flow in ischemic areas. However, when the inotropic stimulation was accompanied by tachycardia, blood flow fell and contractile function deteriorated in the ischemic myocardium during all experiments. Meyer et al. [113] examined the influence of dobutamine on hemodynamics and coronary blood flow in patients after routine cardiac catheterization. They demonstrated a great increase in coronary arterial perfusion after dobutamine in patients without coronary artery disease. However, in patients with severe three-vessel disease, dobutamine resulted in a much smaller increase in coronary perfusion, and the pattern of perfusion became heterogeneous. In a more recent study, McGillem et al. [114] studied the sensitivity of catecholamines in anesthetized dogs for the assessment of reactive hyperemia and regional myocardial function in subcritical stenoses. They demonstrated that neither dopamine nor dobutamine were capable of detecting lesions associated with $>20\%$ of control reactive hyperemia in the animal model. Also, dopamine was incapable of detecting even more severe impairments of reactive hyperemia ($<20\%$ of control). However, dobutamine was associated with depressed regional function when reactive hyperemia was impaired by more than 80% ($<20\%$ of control).

Coronary blood flow predominantly occurs during diastole and is determined primarily by the pressure gradient between the diastolic aortic pressure and the filling pressure in the left ventricle, and the time in diastole in which flow can occur [92]. In the failing heart, left ventricular filling pressure is elevated thereby reducing the gradient for diastolic coronary perfusion. Tachycardia increases myocardial oxygen demand and reduces diastolic perfusion time. Hypotension also reduces the gradient for flow [92].

Dobutamine, and the other catecholamines, increases myocardial oxygen consumption (MVO_2) by augmenting contractility [87, 92, 98, 115]. Other actions that increase MVO_2, such as increased heart rate or systolic pressure, occur to a lesser degree with dobutamine. In heart failure, dobutamine enhances contractility and reduces left-ventricular filling pressures, thereby increasing the gradient for diastolic flow. The reducing end-diastolic and end-systolic ventricular volumes and end-diastolic ventricular (filling) pressure may account for a decreasing myocardial size. As a consequence, wall stress will decrease resulting in a decreased MVO_2, since wall stress is a major determinant of MVO_2. Because dobutamine tends not to induce tachycardia at low-to-medium dose, and maintains diastolic aortic pressure while decreasing left ventricular filling pressure, it will improve coronary blood flow. The concomitant reduction in heart size compensates for the augmented myocardial oxygen consumption caused by increased contractility. However, when dobutamine is used in the presence of coronary artery disease not accompanied by heart failure, the increase in contractility that increases myocardial oxygen demand is not offset by a large reduction in filling pressure that would have reduced oxygen requirements. Since coronary artery stenosis may impede an adequate increase of coronary blood flow, ischemia may develop. In these circumstances, myocardial ischemia may become manifest when tachycardia or hypotension arise, which occurs after isoproterenol administration [92, 109, 112].

Table 5. Practical considerations of pharmacological stress using dobutamine.

– Favorable pharmacokinetic properties (short half-life)	– Operator control
– Reproducible dose-effect relation	– Detection of ischemic threshold
– High tolerance and safety	– Resemblance with physical exercise
– Mild side effects	
– Extensive clinical experience with the agent	

In summary, dobutamine appears to be a well-suited catecholamine for pharmacological stress induction, since it has shown powerful positive inotropy with relatively mild chronotropic, arrhythmogenic, and vascular effects at intermediate doses. At higher doses, the occurrence of tachycardia and the further increase in systolic blood pressure may account for the induction of myocardial ischemia. Hence, myocardial oxygen requirements may increase substantially due to augmented contractility and increase in rate-pressure product. When myocardial ischemia develops, a coronary steal effect has been proposed as a contributing factor. Additionally, the favorable pharmacokinetic properties (short half-life) and the clinical experience with the drug may contribute to its safety and feasibility (Table 5).

III.6. Dobutamine echocardiography

In one of the first echocardiography studies with dobutamine, Palac et al. [116] reported a 84% sensitivity and 86% specificity for detection of coronary artery disease. Seventeen patients (94%) with multivessel disease were identified correctly. During exercise electrocardiography, the sensitivity and specificity were 60 and 79%, respectively.

Berthe et al. [117] have shown that dobutamine stress echocardiography was superior in detecting three-vessel disease after myocardial infarction compared to pre-discharge submaximal exercise. Using dobutamine doses up to 40 μg/kg/min, the sensitivity and specificity were 85 and 88%, respectively. The overall accuracy of dobutamine stress echocardiography was 87%, which was higher than exercise electrocardiography (59%) and dobutamine stress electrocardiography (70%). No significant arrhythmias were reported.

Three weeks after myocardial infarction, Mannering et al. [118] performed dobutamine echocardiography using a maximal dose of 20 μg/kg/min. However, acceptable recordings were obtained in only 42 of the 50 patients (82%). Wall motion abnormalities were predominantly seen in the patients with three-vessel disease. Complex and frequent ventricular dysrhythmias occurred in eight patients, including one nonsustained ventricular tachycardia.

Cohen et al. [119] assessed the value of dobutamine digital echocardiography for detecting coronary artery disease in 70 patients. Dobutamine was infused up to a maximal dose of 40 μg/kg/min. Dobutamine echocardiography was positive in 44 of the 51 patients with coronary artery disease (overall sensitivity 86%). The sensitivity for identifying one-vessel disease was 69%, for two-vessel disease 89%, and for three-vessel disease and left main disease 100%. No major complications were noted during the test. Nonsustained ventricular tachycardia occurred in 5 patients. However, all were asymptomatic and hemodynamically insignificant. Additionally, the ventricular runs were transient, occurred at the higher doses of dobutamine, and never warranted reversal with a β-adrenoreceptor blocking agent.

To compare dobutamine echocardiography to dipyridamole echocardiography, Previtali et al. [120] studied 35 patients with suspected coronary artery disease. They employed the high-dose dipyridamole infusion protocol (0.84 mg/kg for 10 minutes), whereas dobutamine was infused up to 40 μg/kg per minute. The dobutamine echocardiography test was negative in all the patients with no critical coronary lesions, whereas a positive test was found in 8 of the 16 patients with one-vessel disease (50%) and in 92% with multivessel disease, resulting in an overall sensitivity of 68% and a specificity of 100%. The dipyridamole echocardiography test yielded a sensitivity of 31% in one-vessel disease and 92% in multi-vessel disease, resulting in an overall sensitivity of 57% and a specificity of 100%. Ventricular arrhythmias occurred in 11 patients during the dobutamine test and in none with the dipyridamole test. However, the arrhythmias did not require premature termination of the dobutamine infusion or any treatment with β-adrenoreceptor blocking agents. Thus, dobutamine demonstrated a slightly higher sensitivity for the detection of one-vessel disease.

Sawada et al. [121] performed two-dimensional echocardiography during dobutamine infusion to a maximum dose of 30 μg/kg per minute in 103 patients who underwent coronary arteriography. Fifty-five patients had normal wall motion at baseline. Stress-induced wall motion abnormalities developed in 31 of 35 patients (89%) who had significant coronary artery disease. The sensitivity was 81% for those with one-vessel disease and 100% for those with multi-vessel and left main disease. Forty-eight patients had abnormal wall motion at rest, including seven who had diffuse abnormalities involving all three regions of coronary perfusion. These seven patients were excluded for further analysis. Fifteen patients had coronary artery disease confined to the regions that demonstrated abnormal wall motion at rest, whereas 26 patients had one or more regions with normal rest wall motion that were supplied by significantly diseased vessels (remote disease). Twenty-one of 26 patients (81%) with remote disease developed stress-induced wall motion abnormalities in regions that correspond to the location of remotely diseased vessels. Thirteen of 15 patients (87%) without remote disease did not develop remote stress-induced wall motion abnormalities. The investigators reported arrhythmias in 15% of all patients. No patients had a ventricular tachycardia or hypotension.

III.7. Dobutamine magnetic resonance imaging

Pennell et al. [59] were the first to report MRI during dobutamine stress. They studied 22 patients with a history of angina and an abnormal exercise electrocardiogram. The imaging protocol consisted of both MRI and thallium-201 scintigraphy during dobutamine infusion to a maximal dose of 20 μg/kg/min. Of the 22 patients studied, 20 had coronary artery disease as defined by having a stenosis in a major coronary artery of at least 50% of the luminal diameter. Nineteen patients had reversible perfusion defects on the thallium scintigrams and all 19 (100%) demonstrated reversible wall motion abnormalities on the magnetic resonance images. The dobutamine tests were well tolerated. None of the patients developed ventricular tachycardia. The increase of heart rate during dobutamine is advantageous in reducing the imaging time, which is known to be rather long using MRI.

Table 6. Comparison of pharmacological stress agents.

	Dipyridamole	Adenosine	Dobutamine
mechanism/action	vasodilation	vasodilation	inotropy chronotropy
coronary/myocar dial effect	coronary flow disparity	coronary flow disparity	myocardial oxygen demand
administration	oral/i.v.	i.v.	i.v.
maximal dose	0.84 mg/kg/min (375 mg orally)	140 μg/kg/min	40 μg/kg/min
plasma half-life	$\pm$ 10 hours	< 10 seconds	$\pm$ 120 seconds
repeated measurements during one examination	no	yes	yes
preferred imaging strategy	thallium-201 scintigraphy	technetium-99m-teboroxime scintigraphy	echocardiography magnetic resonance imaging
contraindications	unstable angina, recent infarction, hypotension	2- and 3-degree AV-block, sick sinus syndrome, hypotension, bronchospastic lung disease, unstable angina, recent infarction	hypertrophic cardiomyopathy, severe hypertension
side effects	frequent, long-lasting	frequent, mild, transient	rare, mild, transient
antidotum	aminophylline	aminophylline	β-blocker
metabolism	liver	endothelium cardiomyocytes erythrocytes	liver
excretion	bile	kidney (uric acid)	kidney

III.8. Conclusion

The initial reports of pharmacological stress imaging using dobutamine are promising. The reported echocardiographic studies [116–121] demonstrate a high sensitivity and specificity for the detection of coronary artery disease. In fact, the diagnostic accuracy seems to be superior to the dipyridamole echocardiography test. Dipyridamole, as a vasodilator, primarily induces a flow maldistribution, that not necessarily results in myocardial ischemia. This creation of flow heterogeneity makes dipyridamole extremely suited for myocardial perfusion imaging [122]. Dobutamine produces a substantial increase in myocardial oxygen requirements by its positive inotropic action. At higher doses, the augmented contractility is often accompanied by tachycardia and an increase in systolic blood pressure. Consequently, a marked imbalance between myocardial oxygen demand and supply may occur, resulting in ischemia. Two-dimensional echocardiography and MRI are well suited to detect wall motion disturbances as an early manifestation of myocardial ischemia. One of the more serious side effects of dobutamine, which may limit its use is the occurrence of ventricular arrhythmias. Fortunately, ventricular tachycardia has been infrequently reported, even with doses up to 40 μg/kg. Therefore, dobutamine seems to be a potentially useful pharmacological stressor for cardiac imaging based on contractile myocardial function.

IV. Overall conclusion

The clinical usefulness of cardiac imaging modalities which rely upon the detection of perfusion defects and wall-motion disturbances requires conditions that provoke a heterogeneity of coronary flow and a myocardial oxygen imbalance, respectively. Traditionally, this has been achieved by exercise stress testing. Many patients cannot perform dynamic exercise sufficiently for various reasons. Pharmacological stress has been proven to be an attractive alternative for physical exercise. Currently, several stress agents are used in conjunction with thallium-201 scintigraphy, two-dimensional echocardiography and, recently, magnetic resonance imaging. The most employed agents include vasodilators, such as dipyridamole and adenosine, and catecholamines, such as dobutamine (Table 6).

The predominant rationale of thallium-201 perfusion scintigraphy is based on the creation of a flow maldistribution between territories supplied by normal arteries and those supplied by stenotic arteries, that does not necessarily require ischemia. Dipyridamole and adenosine, as rather selective coronary vasodilators, are well-suited to provoke such a condition and may be classified as the ideal markers of myocardial perfusion.

Two-dimensional echocardiography and magnetic resonance imaging have the potential to provide noninvasively information of cardiac dynamics and regional myocardial function. To assess the functional significance of coronary artery disease, detection of wall motion abnormalities and alterations in ejection fraction require the presence of myocardial ischemia. Dobutamine, as a widely applied inotropic agent in the management of severely depressed left ventricular contractile function, seems to be an appropriate pharmacological stressor when heart failure is absent. By increasing contractility, heart rate, and systolic arterial pressure, it is capable of inducing an imbalance between myocardial oxygen demand and supply, leading to ischemia in patients with coronary artery disease. In this manner, dobutamine can be considered as an adequate marker of cardiac function.

References

1. Albro PC, Gould KL, Ewstcott RJ, Hamilton GW, Ritchie JL, Williams DL. Noninvasive assessment of coronary stenoses by myocardial imaging during pharmacologic vasodilation. III. Clinical trial. Am J Cardiol 1978; 42: 751–60.
2. Leppo JA. Dipyridamole-thallium imaging: the lazy man's stress test. J Nucl Med 1989; 30: 281–7.
3. Gould KL, Sorenson SG, Albro PC, Caldwell JH, Chaudhuri T, Hamilton GW. Thallium-201 myocardial imaging during coronary vasodilation induced by oral dipyridamole. J Nucl Med 1986; 27: 31–6.
4. Leppo JA, O'Brien J, Rothendler JA, Getchell JD, Lee VW. Dipyridamole-thallium-201 scintigraphy in the prediction of future cardiac events after acute myocardial infarction. N Engl J Med 1984; 310: 1014–8.
5. Leppo JA, Plaja J, Gionet M, Tumolo J, Paraskos JA, Cutler BS. Noninvasive evaluation of cardiac risk before elective vascular surgery. J Am Coll Cardiol 1987; 9: 269–76.
6. Boucher CA, Brewster DC, Darling RC, Okada RD, Strauss HW, Pohost GM. Determination of cardiac risk by dipyridamole-thallium imaging before peripheral vascular surgery. N Engl J Med 1985; 312: 389–94.
7. Brown BG, Josephson MA, Petersen RB et al. Intravenous dipyridamole combined with isometric handgrip for near maximal acute increase in coronary flow in patients with coronary artery disease. Am J Cardiol 1981; 48: 1077–85.
8. Casale PN, Guiney TE, Strauss HW, Boucher CA. Simultaneous low level treadmill exercise and intravenous dipyridamole stress thallium imaging. Am J Cardiol 1988; 62: 799–802.
9. Gould KL. Noninvasive assessment of coronary stenoses by myocardial perfusion imaging during pharmacologic coronary vasodilatation. I. Physiologic basis and experimental validation. Am J Cardiol 1978; 41: 267–78.
10. FitzGerald GA. Dipyridamole. N Engl J Med 1987; 316: 1247–57.

11. Zeller FP, Blend MJ. The use of intravenous dipyridamole in thallium 201 myocardial perfusion imaging. Pharmacotherapy 1987; 7: 178–84.

12. Soloff LA, Gimenez JL, Winters WL Jr. Experimental and clinical observations on 2,6-bis(diethanolamino)-4,8-dipiperidino-pyrimido-(5,4-*d*)-pyrimidine(persantin). Am J Med Sci 1962; 243: 783–9.

13. Elliot EC. The effect of persantine on coronary flow and cardiac dynamics. Can Med Assoc J 1961; 85: 469–76.

14. Gould KL, Lipscomb K, Hamilton GW. Physiologic basis for assessing critical coronary stenosis. Am J Cardiol 1974; 33: 87–94.

15. Hoffman JI. Maximal coronary flow and the concept of coronary vascular reserve. Circulation 1984; 70: 153–64.

16. Dole WP. Autoregulation of the coronary circulation. Prog Cardiovasc Dis 1987; 29: 293–323.

17. Gould KL, Westcott RJ, Albro PC, Hamilton GW. Noninvasive assessment of coronary stenoses by myocardial imaging during pharmacologic coronary vasodilation. II. Clinical methodology and feasibility. Am J Cardiol 1978; 41: 279–87.

18. Zhu YY, Lee W, Botvinick E et al. The clinical and pathophysiologic implications of pain, ST abnormalities, and scintigraphic changes induced during dipyridamole infusion: their relationships to the peripheral hemodynamic response. Am Heart J 1988; 116: 1071–80.

19. Iskandrian AS, Heo J, Askenase A, Segal BL, Auerbach N. Dipyridamole cardiac imaging. Am Heart J 1988; 115: 432–43.

20. Beer SG, Heo J, Iskandrian AS. Dipyridamole thallium imaging. Am J Cardiol 1991; 67: 18D–26D.

21. Gould KL. Quantification of coronary artery stenosis in vivo. Circ Res 1985; 57: 341–53.

22. Gould KL, Kelley KO, Bolson EL. Experimental validation of quantitative coronary arteriography for determining pressure-flow characteristics of coronary stenosis. Circulation 1982; 66: 930–7.

23. Gould KL, Kelley KO. Physiological significance of coronary flow velocity and changing stenosis geometry during coronary vasodilation in awake dogs. Circ Res 1982; 50: 695–704.

24. Gould KL. Dynamic coronary stenosis. Am J Cardiol 1980; 45: 286–92.

25. Bache RJ, Schwartz JS. Effects of perfusion pressure distal to a coronary stenosis on transmural myocardial blood flow. Circulation 1982; 65: 928–35.

26. Hoffman JI. Determinants and prediction of transmural myocardial perfusion. Circulation 1978; 58: 381–91.

27. Meerdink DJ, Okada RD, Leppo JA. The effect of dipyridamole on transmural blood flow gradients. Chest 1989; 96: 400–5.

28. Gould KL. Assessing coronary stenosis severity – a recurrent clinical need (editorial). J Am Coll Cardiol 1986; 8: 91–4.

29. Braunwald E, Sobel BE. Coronary blood flow and myocardial ischemia. In: Braunwald E, editor. Heart disease, a textbook of cardiovascular medicine. Philadelphia: Saunders, 1984: 1235–62.

29. Gould KL. Coronary steal; Is it clinically important? (editorial). Chest 1989; 96: 227–9.

30. Ranhosky A, Kempthorne-Rawson J, and the Intravenous Dipyridamole-Thallium Imaging Study Group. The safety of intravenous dipyridamole thallium myocardial perfusion imaging. Circulation 1990; 81: 1205–9.

31. Alfonso S. Inhibition of coronary vasodilating action of dipyridamole and adenosine by aminophylline in the dog. Circ Res 1970; 26: 743–52.

32. Fredholm BB, Persson CG. Xanthine derivatives as adenosine receptor antagonists. Eur J Pharmacol 1982; 81: 673–6.

33. Picano E, Distante A, Masini M, Morales MA, Lattanzi F, L'Abbate A. Dipyridamole-echocardiography test in effort angina pectoris. Am J Cardiol 1985; 56: 452–6.
34. Margonato A, Chierchia S, Cianflone D et al. Limitations of dipyridamole-echocardiography in effort angina pectoris. Am J Cardiol 1987; 59: 225–30.
35. Picano E, Lattanzi F, Masini M, Distante A, L'Abbate A. High dose dipyridamole echocardiography test in effort angina pectoris. J Am Coll Cardiol 1986; 8: 848–54.
36. Picano E. Dipyridamole-echocardiography test: historical background and physiologic basis. Eur Heart J 1989; 10: 365–76.
37. Robertson WS, Feigenbaum H, Armstrong WF, Dillon JC, O'Donnel J, McHenry PW. Exercise echocardiography: a clinically practical addition in the evaluation of coronary artery disease. J Am Coll Cardiol 1983; 2: 1085–91.
38. Ryan T, Vasey CG, Presti CF, O'Donnel JA, Feigenbaum H, Armstrong WF. Exercise echocardiography: detection of coronary artery disease in patients with normal left ventricular wall motion at rest. J Am Coll Cardiol 1988; 11: 993–9.
39. Picano E, Morales MA, Distante A et al. Dipyridamole echocardiography test in angina at rest: noninvasive assessment of coronary stenosis underlying spasm. Am Heart J 1986; 111: 688–91.
40. Picano E, Lattanzi F, Masini M, Distante A, L'Abbate A. Comparison of the high-dose dipyridamole-echocardiography test and exercise two-dimensional echocardiography for diagnosis of coronary artery disease. Am J Cardiol 1987; 59: 539–42.
41. Bolognese L, Sarasso G, Aralda D, Bongo AS, Rossi L, Rossi P. High dose dipyridamole echocardiography early after uncomplicated acute myocardial infarction: correlation with exercise testing and coronary angiography. J Am Coll Cardiol 1989; 14: 357–63.
42. Pirelli S, Danzi GB, Alberti A et al. Comparison of usefulness of high-dose dipyridamole echocardiography and exercise electrocardiography for detection of asymptomatic restenosis after coronary angioplasty. Am J Cardiol 1991; 67: 1335–8.
43. Masini M, Picano E, Lattanzi F, Distante A, L'Abbate A. High dose dipyridamole-echocardiography test in women: correlation with exercise-electrocardiography test and coronary arteriography. J Am Coll Cardiol 1988; 12: 682–5.
44. Picano E, Severi S, Michelassi C et al. Prognostic importance of dipyridamole-echocardiography test in coronary artery disease. Circulation 1989; 80: 450–7.
45. Picano E, Pirelli S, Marzilli M et al. Usefulness of high-dose dipyridamole-echocardiography test in coronary angioplasty. Circulation 1989; 80: 807–15.
46. Higgins CB. Malcolm Hanson memorial lecture. MR of the heart: anatomy, physiology and metabolism. Am J Roentgenol 1988; 151: 239–48.
47. Haase A, Frahm J, Matthaei D, Hänicke W, Merboldt KD. FLASH imaging. Rapid NMR imaging using low flip-angle pulses. J Magn Reson 1986; 67: 258–66.
48. Higgins CB, Holt W, Pflugfelder P, Sechtem U. Functional evaluation of the heart with MRI. Magn Reson Med 1988; 6: 121–39.
49. Pettigrew R. Dynamic cardiac MR imaging. Techniques and applications. Radiol Clin North Am 1989; 27: 1183–203.
50. Sechtem U, Pflugfelder PW, Gould RG, Cassidy MM, Higgins CB. Measurement of right and left ventricular volumes in healthy individuals with cine MR imaging. Radiology 1987; 163: 697–702.
51. Utz JA, Herfkens RJ, Heinsimer JA et al. Cine MR determination of left ventricular ejection fraction. Am J Roentgenol 1987; 148: 839–43.
52. Buser PT, Aufferman W, Holt WW et al. Noninvasive evaluation of global left ventricular function with use of cine nuclear magnetic resonance. J Am Coll Cardiol 1989; 13: 1294–300.

53. Sechtem U, Sommerhoff BA, Markiewicz W, White RD, Cheitlin MD, Higgins CB. Regional left ventricular wall thickening by magnetic resonance imaging: evaluation in normal persons and patients with global and regional dysfunction. Am J Cardiol 1987; 59: 145–51.

54. Peshock RM, Rokey R, Malloy CM et al. Assessment of myocardial systolic wall thickening using nuclear magnetic resonance imaging. J Am Coll Cardiol 1989; 14: 653–9.

55. Lotan CS, Cranney GB, Bouchard A, Bittner V, Pohost GM. The value of cine nuclear magnetic resonance imaging for assessing regional ventricular function. J Am Coll Cardiol 1989; 14: 1721–9.

56. Auffermann W, Wagner S, Holt WW et al. Noninvasive determination of left ventricular output and wall stress in volume overload and in myocardial disease by cine magnetic resonance imaging. Am Heart J 1991; 121: 1750–8.

57. Sechtem U, Pflugfelder PW, Cassidy MM et al. Mitral or aortic regurgitation: quantification of regurgitant volumes in patients with cine MR imaging. Radiology 1988; 167: 425–30.

58. Pennell DJ, Underwood SR, Longmore DB. Detection of coronary artery disease using MR imaging with dipyridamole infusion. J Comput Assist Tomogr 1990; 14: 167–70.

59. Pennell DJ, Underwood SR. Stress magnetic resonance imaging in coronary artery disease. In: Van der Wall EE, De Roos A, editors. Magnetic resonance in coronary artery disease. Dordrecht: Kluwer, 1990: 217–39.

60. Wackers FJ. Pharmacologic stress with dipyridamole: how lazy can one be? [editorial]. J Nucl Med 1990; 31: 1024–7.

61. Belardinelli L, Linden J, Berne RM. The cardiac effects of adenosine. Prog Cardiovasc Dis 1989; 32: 73–97.

62. Verani MS, Mahmarian JJ, Hixson JB, Boyce TM, Staudacher RA. Diagnosis of coronary artery disease by controlled coronary vasodilation with adenosine and thallium-201 scintigraphy in patients unable to exercise. Circulation 1990; 82: 80–7.

63. Wilson RF, Wyche K, Christensen BV, Zimmer S, Laxson DD. Effects of adenosine on human coronary arterial circulation. Circulation 1990; 82: 1595–606.

64. Sylven C, Beermann B, Jonzon B, Brandt R. Angina pectoris-like pain provoked by intravenous adenosine in healthy volunteers. Br Med J 1986; 293: 227–30.

65. Crea F, Pupita G, Galassi AR et al. Role of adenosine in pathogenesis of anginal pain. Circulation 1990; 81: 164–72.

66. DiMarco JP, Sellers TD, Berne RM, West GA, Belardinelli L. Adenosine: electrophysiologic effects and therapeutic use for terminating paroxysmal supraventricular tachycardia. Circulation 1983; 68: 1254–63.

67. DiMarco JP, Sellers TD, Lerman BB, Greenberg ML, Berne RM, Belardinelli L. Diagnostic and therapeutic use of adenosine in patients with supraventricular tachyarrhythmias. J Am Coll Cardiol 1985; 6: 417–25.

68. Bardenheuer H, Whelton B, Sparks HV Jr. Adenosine release by isolated guinea pig heart in response to isoproterenol, acetylcholine and acidosis: the minimal role of vascular endothelium. Circ Res 1987; 61: 594–600.

69. Berne RM. The role of adenosine in the regulation of coronary blood flow. Circ Res 1980; 47: 807–13.

70. Triner L, Nahas GG, Vulliemoz Y et al. Cyclic AMP and smooth muscle functions. Ann N Y Acad Sci 1971; 185: 458–76.

71. Kurtz A. Adenosine stimulates guanylate cyclase activity in vascular smooth muscle cells. J Biol Chem 1987; 262: 6296–300.

72. Long CJ, Stone TW. Adenosine produces agonist-induced production of inositol phosphatase in rat aorta. J Pharm Pharmacol 1987; 39: 1010–4.

73. Fenton RA, Bruttig SP, Rubio R, Berne RM. Effect of adenosine on calcium uptake by intact and cultured vascular smooth muscle. Am J Physiol 1987; 252: H797–H804.

74. Lokhandwala MF. Inhibition of cardiac sympathetic neurotransmission by adenosine. Eur J Pharmacol 1979; 60: 353–7.

75. Wakade AR, Wakade TD. Inhibition of noradrenaline release by adenosine. J Physiol 1978; 282: 35–49.

76. Rubanyi GM, Romero JC, Vanhoutte PM. Flow-induced release of endothelium-derived relaxing factor. Am J Physiol 1986; 250: H1145–9.

77. Favale S, Di Biase M, Rizzo U, Belardinelli L, Rizzon P. Effect of adenosine and adenosine-5′-triphosphate on atrioventricular conduction in patients. J Am Coll Cardiol 1985; 5: 1212–9.

78. Clemo HF, Belardinelli L. Effect of adenosine on atrioventricular conduction. I. Site and characterization of adenosine action in the guinea pig atrioventricular node. Circ Res 1986; 59: 427–36.

79. Dobson JG Jr. Mechanism of adenosine inhibition of catecholamine-induced responses in heart. Circ Res 1983; 52: 151–60.

80. Dobson JG Jr. Adenosine reduces catecholamine contractile responses in oxygenated and hypoxic atria. Am J Physiol 1983; 245: H468–74.

81. Baumann G, Schrader J, Gerlach E. Inhibitory action of adenosine on histamine- and dopamine-stimulated cardiac contractility and adenylate cyclase in guinea pigs. Circ Res 1981; 48: 259–66.

82. West GA, Isenberg G, Belardinelli L. Antagonism of forskolin effects by adenosine in isolated hearts and ventricular myocytes. Am J Physiol 1986; 250: H769–77.

83. Biaggioni I, Olafsson B, Robertson RM, Hollister AS, Robertson D. Cardiovascular and respiratory effects of adenosine in conscious man. Evidence for chemoreceptor activation. Circ Res 1987; 61: 779–86.

84. Nguyen T, Heo J, Ogilby JD, Iskandrian AS. Single photon emission computed tomography with thallium-201 during adenosine-induced coronary hyperemia: correlation with coronary arteriography, exercise thallium imaging and two-dimensional echocardiography. J Am Coll Cardiol 1990; 16: 1375–83.

85. Coyne EP, Belvedere DA, Vande Streek PR, Weiland FL, Evans RB, Spaccavento LJ. Thallium-201 scintigraphy after intravenous infusion of adenosine compared with exercise thallium testing in the diagnosis of coronary artery disease. J Am Coll Cardiol 1991; 17: 1289–94.

86. Iskandrian AS, Heo J, Nguyen T et al. Assessment of coronary artery disease using single-photon emission computed tomography with thallium-201 during adenosine-induced coronary hyperemia. Am J Cardiol 1991; 67: 1190–4.

87. Zoghbi WA. Use of adenosine echocardiography for diagnosis of coronary artery disease. Am Heart J 1991; 122: 285–92.

88. Vasu MA, O'Keefe DD, Kapellakis GZ et al. Myocardial oxygen consumption: effects of epinephrine, isoproterenol, dopamine, norepinephrine and dobutamine. Am J Physiol 1978; 235: H237–41.

89. Leier CV, Webel J, Bush CA. The cardiovascular effects of the continuous infusion of dobutamine in patients with severe heart failure. Circulation 1977; 56: 468–72.

90. Leier CV, Heban PT, Huss P, Bush CA, Lewis RP. Comparative systemic and regional hemodynamic effects of dopamine and dobutamine in patients with cardiomyopathic heart failure. Circulation 1978; 58: 466–75.

91. Stoner JD III, Bolen JL, Harrison DC. Comparison of dobutamine and dopamine in treatment of severe heart failure. Br Heart J 1977; 39: 536–9.
92. Sonnenblick EH, Frishman WH, LeJemtel TH. Dobutamine: a new synthetic cardioactive sympathetic amine. N Engl J Med 1979; 300: 17–22.
93. Ruffolo RR Jr. The pharmacology of dobutamine. Am J Med Sci 1987; 294: 244–8.
94. Vatner SF, Higgins CB, Braunwald E. Effects of norepinephrine on coronary circulation and left ventricular dynamics in the conscious dog. Circ Res 1974; 34: 812–23.
95. Goldberg LI, Hsieh YY, Resnekov L. Newer catecholamines for treatment of heart failure and shock: an update on dopamine and a first look at dobutamine. Prog Cardiovasc Dis 1977; 19: 327–40.
96. Higgins CB, Millard RW, Braunwald E, Vatner SF. Effects and mechanisms of action of dopamine on regional hemodynamics in the conscious dog. Am J Physiol 1973; 225: 432–43.
97. Gunnar RM, Loeb HS, Pietras RJ, Tobin JR Jr. Ineffectiveness of isoproterenol in shock due to acute myocardial infarction. JAMA 1967; 202: 1124–8.
98. Tuttle RR, Mills J. Dobutamine: development of a new catecholamine to selectively increase cardiac contractility. Circ Res 1975; 36: 185–96.
99. Ruffolo RR Jr, Yaden EL. Vascular effects of the stereoisomers of dobutamine. J Pharmacol Exp Ther 1983; 224: 46–50.
100. Ruffolo RR Jr, Spradlin TA, Pollock GD, Waddell JE, Murphy PJ. α- and β-adrenergic effects of the stereoisomers of dobutamine. J Pharmacol Exp Ther 1981; 219: 447–52.
101. Leier CV, Unverferth DV. Dobutamine. Ann Intern Med 1983; 99: 490–6.
102. Robie NW, Nutter DO, Moody C, McNay JL. In vivo analysis of adrenergic receptor activity of dobutamine. Circ Res 1974; 34: 663–71.
103. Bianchi C, Diaz R, Gonzales C, Beregovich J. Effects of dobutamine on atrioventricular conduction. Am Heart J 1975; 90: 474–8.
104. Loeb HS, Sinno MZ, Saudye AL, Towne WD, Gunnar RM. Electrophysiologic properties of dobutamine. Circ Shock 1974; 1: 217–20.
105. Leier CV, Unverferth DV, Kates RE. The relationship between plasma dobutamine concentrations and cardiovascular reponses in cardiac failure. Am J Med 1979; 66: 238–42.
106. Kates RE, Leier CV. Dobutamine pharmacokinetics in severe heart failure. Clin Pharmacol Ther 1978; 24: 537–41.
107. Murphy PJ, Williams TL, Kau DL. Disposition of dobutamine in the dog. J Pharmacol Exp Ther 1976; 199: 423–31.
108. Unverferth DV, Blanford M, Kates RE, Leier CV. Tolerance to dobutamine after a 72 hour continuous infusion. Am J Med 1980; 69: 262–9.
109. Maroko PR, Kjekshus JK, Sobel BE et al. Factors influencing infarct size following experimental coronary artery occlusions. Circulation 1971; 43: 67–82.
110. Gillespie TA, Ambos HD, Sobel BE, Roberts R. Effects of dobutamine in patients with acute myocardial infarction. Am J Cardiol 1977; 39: 588–94.
111. Willerson JT, Hutton I, Watson JT, Platt MR, Templeton GH. Influence of dobutamine on regional myocardial blood flow and ventricular performance during acute and chronic myocardial ischemia in dogs. Circulation 1976; 53: 828–33.
112. Vatner SF, Baig H. Importance of heart rate in determining the effects of sympathomimetic amines on regional myocardial function and blood flow in conscious dogs with acute myocardial ischemia. Circ Res 1979; 45: 793–803.
113. Meyer SL, Curry GC, Donsky MS, Twieg DB, Parkey RW, Willerson JT. Influence of dobutamine on hemodynamics and coronary blood flow in patients with and without coronary artery disease. Am J Cardiol 1976; 38: 103–8.

114. McGillem MJ, DeBoe SF, Friedman HZ, Mancini GB. The effects of dopamine and dobutamine on regional function in the presence of rigid coronary stenoses and subcritical impairments of reactive hyperemia. Am Heart J 1988; 115: 970–7.

115. Tuttle RR, Pollack GD, Todd G, MacDonald B, Tust R, Dusenberry W. The effect of dobutamine on cardiac oxygen balance, regional blood flow, and infarction severity after coronary artery narrowing in dogs. Circ Res 1977; 41: 357–64.

116. Palac RT, Coombs BJ, Kudenchuk PJ, Crane SK, Murphy ES. Two dimensional echocardiography during dobutamine infusion: comparison with exercise testing in evaluation of coronary disease [abstract]. Circulation 1984; 70 (suppl II): II184.

117. Berthe C, Pierard LA, Hiernaux M et al. Predicting the extent and location of coronary artery disease in acute myocardial infarction by echocardiography during dobutamine infusion. Am J Cardiol 1986; 58: 1167–72.

118. Mannering D, Cripps T, Leech G et al. The dobutamine test as an alternative to exercise testing after acute myocardial infarction. Br Heart J 1988; 59: 521–6.

119. Cohen JL, Greene TO, Ottenweller J, Binenbaum SZ, Wilchfort SD, Kim CS. Dobutamine digital echocardiography for detecting coronary artery disease. Am J Cardiol 1991; 67: 1311–8.

120. Previtali M, Lanzarini L, Ferrario M, Tortorici M, Mussini A, Montemartini C. Dobutamine versus dipyridamole echocardiography in coronary artery disease. Circulation 1991; 83 (suppl III): III27–31.

121. Sawada SG, Segar DS, Ryan T et al. Echocardiographic detection of coronary artery disease during dobutamine infusion. Circulation 1991; 83: 1605–14.

122. Fung AY, Gallagher KP, Buda AJ. The physiologic basis of dobutamine as compared with dipyridamole stress interventions in the assessment of critical coronary stenosis. Circulation 1987; 76: 943–51.

Color plates

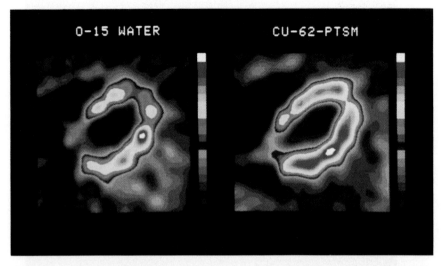

Plate 2.1. Myocardial PET image reconstructions at the mid-ventricular level obtained in a normal subject following administration of O-15 water (left panel) and Cu-62 PTSM. After correction for blood pool radioactivity, there is generally homogeneous Cu-62 PTSM activity throughout the normal left ventricular myocardium. Oxygen-15 water activity distribution is more heterogeneous in this study (see [25], reproduced with the permission of the author and publisher).

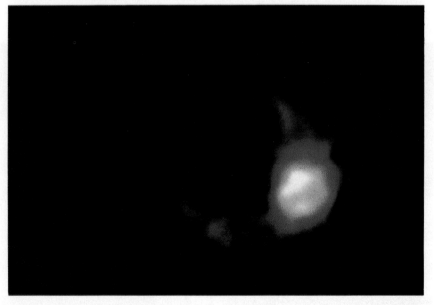

Plate 2.2. Mid chest transverse PET image of a monkey following injection of Ga-68 BAT-TECH (0.42 mCi), demonstrating excellent localization in the myocardium by 7 minutes post injection. The left ventricular cavity is appreciated, with excellent heart to background activity ratios. This unique gallium perfusion agent has a net charge of +1, and is synthesized following generation of Ga-68 from a Ge-68/Ga-68 generator (see [19], reproduced with the permission of the author and publisher).

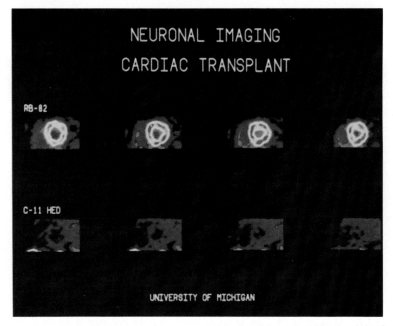

Plate 2.3. Myocardial PET images reconstructed in the short axis following injection of rubidium-82 (upper panels) and carbon-11 hydroxyephedrine (C-11 HED, lower panels). Rubidium-82 myocardial blood flow is homogeneous throughout the left ventricle in this patient with a recent cardiac transplantation. However, myocardial C-11 HED images 30 minutes following injection demonstrate markedly reduced activity in all slices as a result of cardiac denervation during transplantation. Following transplantation, an average 82% reduction in myocardial C-11 HED activity occurred at 60 minutes following injection (see [34], reproduced with the permission of the author and publisher).

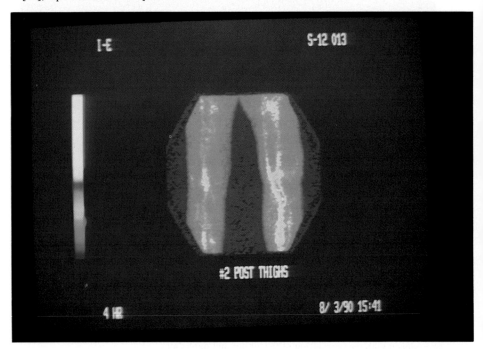

Plate 2.4. Planar posterior images of the thigh and upper calf acquired 4 hours following injection of Tc-99m S12 in a 61-year-old male immediately after right popliteal-tibial-peronial artery angioplasty. Despite the extensive area of atherosclerotic narrowing, an excellent angioplasty result occurred with a reduction of percent diameter stenosis from 90 to 10%. Corresponding Tc-99m S12 images demonstrate intense focal uptake in the right popliteal artery area with a 200% increase in local activity as compared to the contralateral unoperated artery (see [46], reproduced with the permission of the author and publisher).

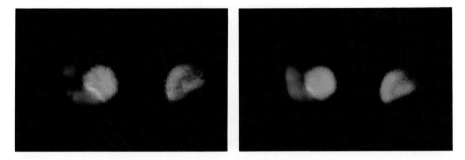

Plate 4.1. Normal (R) Dominant (L) Dominant circulations. 30° and 70° LAO projections. Right coronary artery (RCA) distribution is in red, left coronary artery (LCA) distribution in green. On the left hand side, the RCA supplies the inferior surface of the ventricle, with areas of dual supply shown in yellow. On the right hand side, the RCA supplies only the (R) ventricle and the posterior wall of the left ventricle is supplied by the circumflex coronary artery.

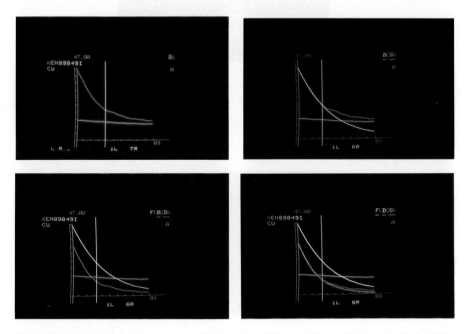

Plate 4.2. (a) Xenon washout curve (red), peak to 30 seconds (upright purple line), with background region washout curve in blue. (b) Monoexponential fit (yellow) to unsubtracted curve. (c) Background activity subtracted from xenon washout curve, with the new curve in red. (d) Monoexponential fit (purple) to background subtraced curve.

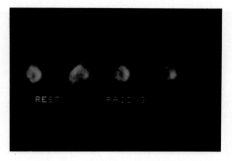

Plate 4.3. The left coronary injection in a patient with microvascular angina, at rest (left) in the 30° and 70° LAO projections, and during arterial pacing induced angina (right), demonstrating a distribution and flow defect in the lower septum.

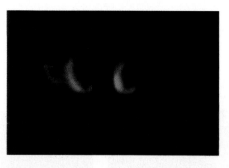

Plate 4.4. A right coronary artery injection, showing substantial collateral flow to the septum in the 30° and 70° LAO projections.

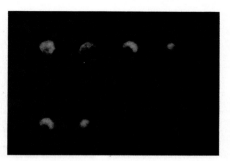

Plate 4.5. Left coronary artery injection in the 30° and 70° LAO in a patient with significant left anterior descending coronary artery disease. Top left-hand panel at rest, bottom left-hand panel, atrial pacing at 100 beats/min, top right-hand panel atrial pacing 135 beats/min, and onset of chest pain showing increasing lack of perfusion to lower septum.

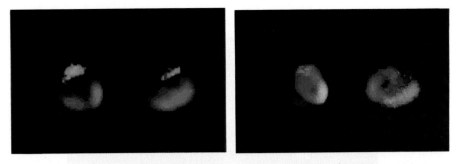

Plate 4.6. (a) Native right coronary artery in red, native left coronary artery in green. (b) Graft to the left anterior descending and obtuse marginal branch of the circumflex coronary artery in blue; total native vessel flow now in green, demonstrating perfusion to the whole left ventricle.

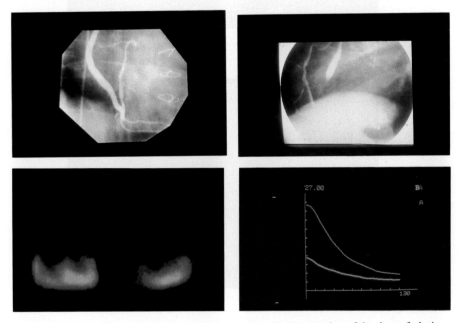

Plate 4.7. (a) Angiogram of graft to right coronary, with (b) retention of dye in graft during native right coronary artery injection. (c) Right coronary graft xenon injection, in the 30° and 70° LAO, with distribution to the inferior surface of the left ventricle. (d) Washout curves, from a normal right coronary artery in red, graft washout curve in blue, demonstrating reduced washout or flow in the left ventricular myocardium.

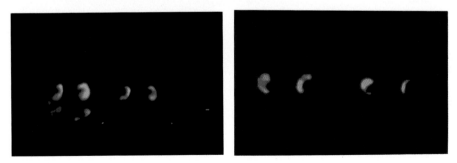

Plate 4.8. Internal mammary artery graft flow to the septum in blue, in the 30° and 70° LAO, on the left-hand side at rest and right-hand side, peak artrial pacing showing (a) flow increasing with stress, (b) decreasing with stress.

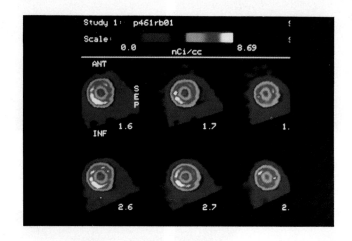

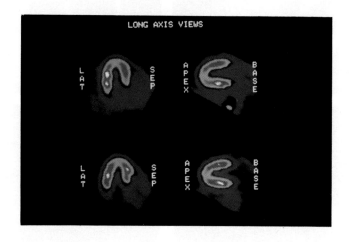

Plate 10.1. (a) Rubidium-82 PET images on a normal subject at rest (above) and with dipyridamole pharmacological stress (below) are shown in short axis, from mid-ventricle (left) to the apex (right). (b) Horizontal (left) and vertical (right) long axis images are shown. (Images courtesy of Dr Rudolph Geer, Memorial PETscan Center, Jacksonville, Florida, USA.)

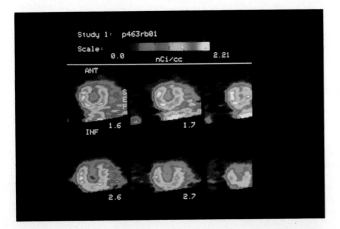

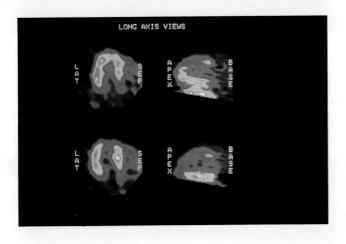

Plate 10.2. Same scheme as Plate 10.1. Images on a patient with prior myocardial infarction demonstrate anterior and apical perfusion defects at rest. These defects increase in severity and extent with dipyridamole, confirming the presence of reversible myocardial ischemia in the distribution of the left anterior descending coronary artery. (Images courtesy of Dr Rudolf Geer, Memorial PETscan Center, Jacksonville, Florida, USA.)

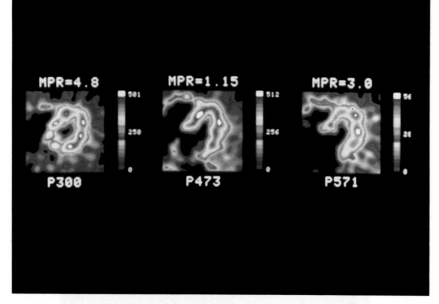

Plate 12.1.   Midventricular PET reconstruction obtained with the use of ¹⁵O-water after the injection of dipyridamole in a normal subject (left) and two patients with chest pain but angiographically normal coronary arteries. One of these patients (middle) had impaired myocardial perfusion reserve (MPR), while the other had normal perfusion reserve (right). In each patient, qualitative and quantitative assessment of myocardial perfusion indicated that perfusion was homogeneous, despite the wide differences between patients in myocardial perfusion reserve, underscoring the need for quantitative estimates in studies in which flow responses may be homogeneous. (Reproduced, with permission, from Geltman et al. [20].)

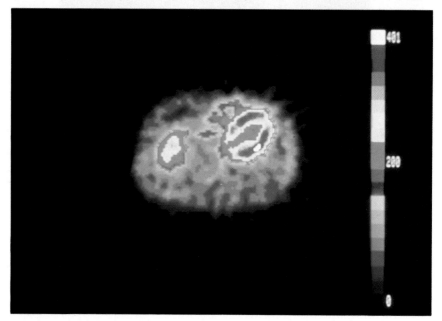

Plate 13.1.   PET image of the chest of a normal human subject reconstructed from data obtained 10–15 minutes following intravenous injection of ⁶²Cu-PTSM. (The image from 5–10 minutes post-injection is similar.) Tracer distribution in the myocardium (upper right) correlates with the distribution of myocardial perfusion seen in a ¹⁵O-water study conducted immediately prior to the ⁶²Cu-PTSM injection [5]. The top of the liver is apparent at the lower left side of the image.

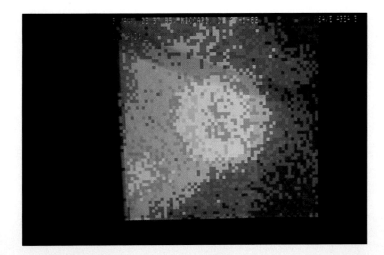

Plate 17.1. Example of an IHDA scintigram (view: LAO 45 degrees) of a patient with a posterior infarction. An area of diminished tracer uptake is seen in the posterior wall.

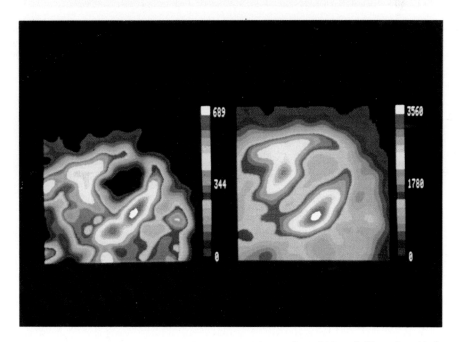

Plate 20.1. Ventricular tomographic reconstructions of perfusion (left) and oxidative metabolism (right) in a patient with acute, anterior myocardial infarction. A large anterior flow deficit is evident in the $H_2{}^{15}O$ perfusion tomogram and a concordant decrease in myocardial oxygen consumption reflected by decreased ^{11}C-acetate uptake is evident in the tomogram obtained after administration of ^{11}C-acetate. (Reproduced, with permission, from Walsh et al. [22].)

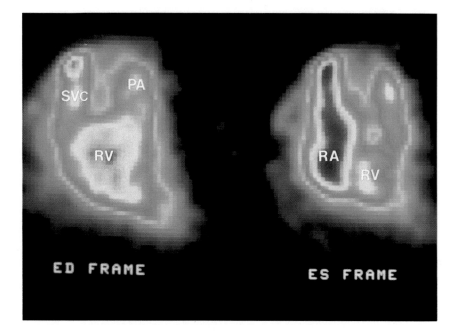

Plate 25.1. End-diastolic (ED) and end-systolic (ES) frames from a krypton-81m equilibrium ventriculographic study in the right anterior oblique projection following 'anatomical' lung subtraction (PA = pulmonary artery; RA = right atrium; RV = right ventricle; SVC = superior vena cava).

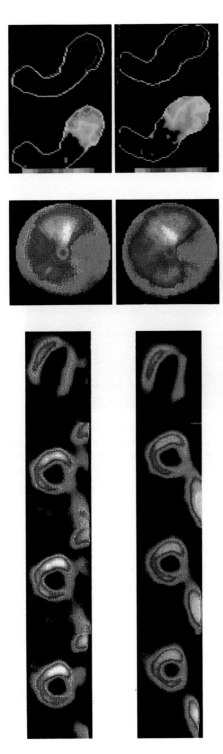

Plate 26.1. Rest (lower panel) and exercise (upper panel) sestaMIBI perfusion/function studies. The first pass studies were done with a multicrystal gamma camera during bike exercise in the upright position. The ejection fraction increased from 31% at rest to 37% during exercise. The regional ejection fraction images are also shown. The SPECT images reveal fixed defects in the anterior wall, septum, inferior wall, and apex. This is cavity dilation. The SPECT images show 3 short axis slices at apical, mid, and basal levels, and one vertical long axis slice at mid level.

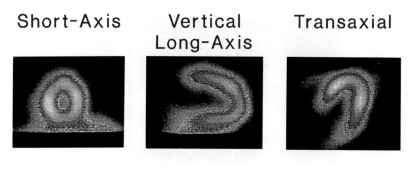

Short-Axis   Vertical
Long-Axis   Transaxial

RNA

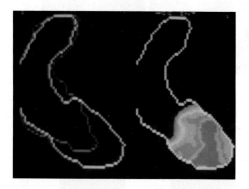

Plate 26.2. Rest sestaMIBI perfusion/function studies obtained 7 days after uncomplicated triple coronary artery bypass grafting in a 67-year-old woman with severe angina pectoris. The rest study was obtained in the supine position with a multicrystal gamma camera. The ejection fraction and wall motion are normal. The SPECT images are normal.

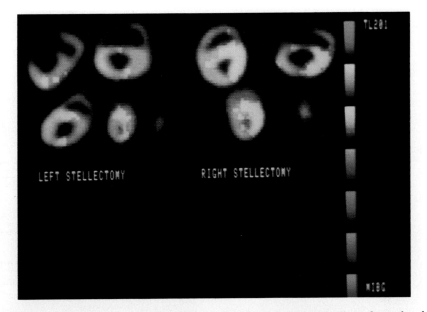

Plate 28.1. Shown are color functional maps from myocardial slices from the dog illustrated in Figure 28.1 with left stellectomy (left), and another dog with right stellectomy (right). Areas of normal innervation (balanced MIBG and thallium) are shown in red. The regions of yellow to green show decreased MIBG relative to thallium, indicating denervation. The denervated region is shown in the posterior left ventricle in left stellectomy, and the anterior left ventricle in right stellectomy. (Reproduced from *Circulation* with permission.)

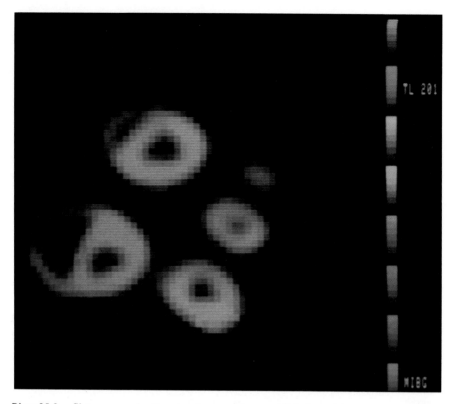

Plate 28.2. Shown are color functional maps of myocardial slices from a normal dog. The left ventricle shows a balanced distribution of MIBG and thallium. The right ventricle shows increased MIBG relative to thallium, which is occasionally seen in normal dogs. (Reproduced from *Circulation* with permission.)

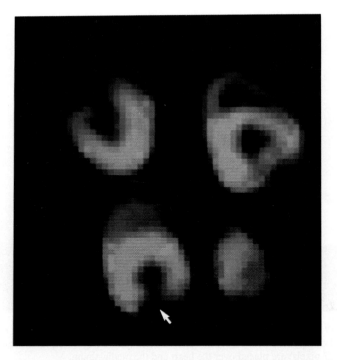

Plate 28.3. Functional maps of myocardial slices from a dog with transmural myocardial infarction. Note the area of absent activity in the slice proximal to the apex (arrow). This represents a region of transmural scar. Adjacent and distal to this region of scar is an area of denervated myocardium, represented by the yellow to green color. (Reproduced with permission from *Circulation.*)

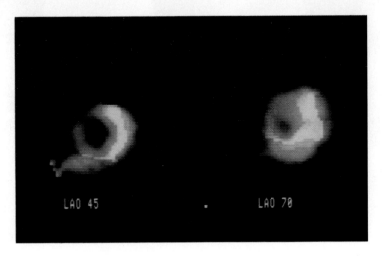

Plate 28.4. Shown are MIBG/thallium functional maps from planar images of a patient studied 2 weeks after myocardial infarction. Note the rim of denervated myocardium surrounding the region of scar.

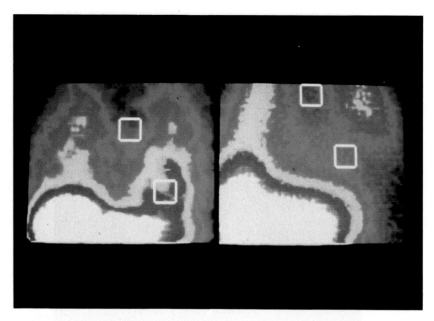

Plate 29.1. I-123 MIBG planar imaging (anterior view of the chest) of a normal subject (left) and of a patient with severe congestive heart failure (right). Squared regions of interest (7 pixels/7 pixels) are placed over the heart and the mediastinum.

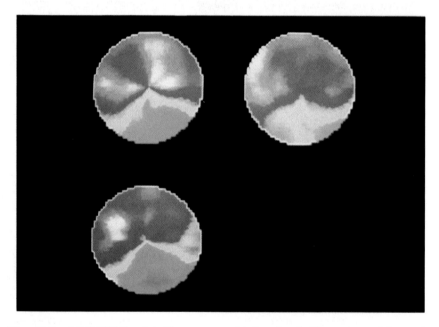

Plate 29.2. I-123 MIBG and thallium tomographic imaging (bull's eye images) in a patient with an inferior myocardial infarction. Upper row: post-dipyridamole (left) and delayed (right) thallium images. Lower row: I-123 MIBG image.

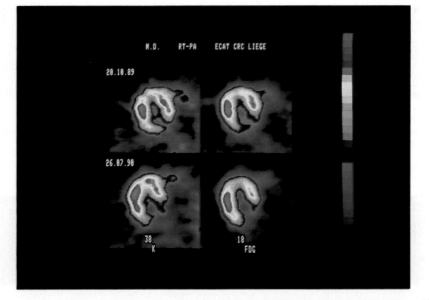

Plate 37.1. Demonstration of regional myocardial viability characterized by 'normal' perfusion and glucose uptake, in the PET studies performed 7 days after the onset of infarction and 9 months later. No infarction is visible of any of the tomograms.

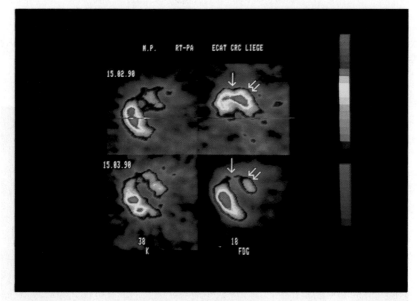

Plate 37.2. Illustration of 'FDG-flow' mismatch in a patient initially studied by PET on day 5: FDG uptake is disproportionately high compared to perfusion in the anterior wall (one arrow) and in the septum (2 arrows). A reinfarction occurs 2 days later. On day 9, coronary angiography is performed: the proximal part of the left anterior descending artery is occluded. One month later, PET shows necrosis of the anterior wall and septum: perfusion and glucose uptake are similarly depressed.

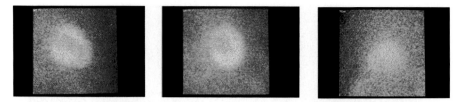

Plate 38.1. An example of the three standard views of a patient with an anterior infarction. Image quality is good and clearly an infarct defect is seen. Heart/lung and heart/liver ratios are high, being 3.4 and 2.4 respectively.

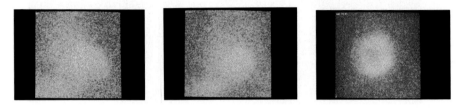

Plate 38.2. An example of a poor image with low heart/lung and heart/liver ratios. The heart region is hardly visible in the background activity. Ratios were 1.8 and 1.3 respectively.

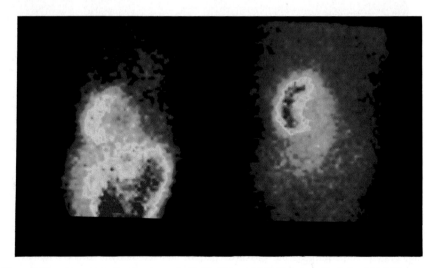

Plate 38.3. An example of a 'matched' Tl-201 and FDG defect. Left is a Tl-201 tracer defect in the posterior region. Right is the same view of FDG.

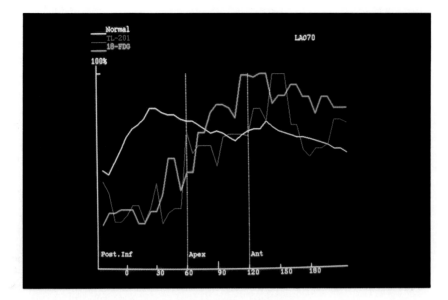

Plate 38.4.　Circumferential profile of the image in Plate 38.3.

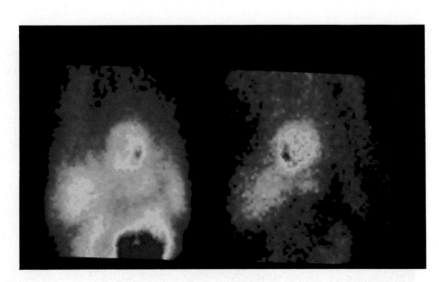

Plate 38.5.　An example of a patient with increased FDG uptake. On the left Tl-201 image a septal defect is seen. On the right FDG image the highest FDG uptake is observed in the septal region.

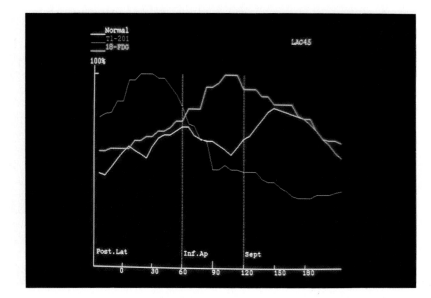

Plate 38.6. Circumferential profile of the image in Plate 38.5.

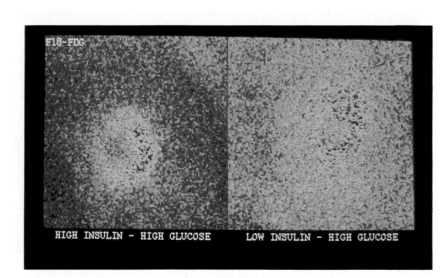

Plate 38.7. Left image shows the FDG scintigram during high insulin infusion. The right image shows the image during low insulin infusion.

Index

Developments in Cardiovascular Medicine

23. J. Roelandt (ed.): *The Practice of M-Mode and Two-dimensional Echocardiography*. 1983   ISBN 90-247-2745-6

24. J. Meyer, P. Schweizer and R. Erbel (eds.): *Advances in Noninvasive Cardiology*. Ultrasound, Computed Tomography, Radioisotopes, Digital Angiography. 1983
ISBN 0-89838-576-8

25. J. Morganroth and E.N. Moore (eds.): *Sudden Cardiac Death and Congestive Heart Failure*. Diagnosis and Treatment. Proceedings of the 3rd Symposium on New Drugs and Devices, held in Philadelphia, Pa., U.S.A. (1982). 1983   ISBN 0-89838-580-6

26. H.M. Perry Jr. (ed.): *Lifelong Management of Hypertension*. 1983
ISBN 0-89838-582-2

27. E.A. Jaffe (ed.): *Biology of Endothelial Cells*. 1984   ISBN 0-89838-587-3

28. B. Surawicz, C.P. Reddy and E.N. Prystowsky (eds.): *Tachycardias*. 1984
ISBN 0-89838-588-1

29. M.P. Spencer (ed.): *Cardiac Doppler Diagnosis*. Proceedings of a Symposium, held in Clearwater, Fla., U.S.A. (1983). 1983   ISBN 0-89838-591-1

30. H. Villarreal and M.P. Sambhi (eds.): *Topics in Pathophysiology of Hypertension*. 1984   ISBN 0-89838-595-4

31. F.H. Messerli (ed.): *Cardiovascular Disease in the Elderly*. 1984
Revised edition, 1988: see below under Volume 76

32. M.L. Simoons and J.H.C. Reiber (eds.): *Nuclear Imaging in Clinical Cardiology*. 1984   ISBN 0-89838-599-7

33. H.E.D.J. ter Keurs and J.J. Schipperheyn (eds.): *Cardiac Left Ventricular Hypertrophy*. 1983   ISBN 0-89838-612-8

34. N. Sperelakis (ed.): *Physiology and Pathology of the Heart*. 1984
Revised edition, 1988: see below under Volume 90

35. F.H. Messerli (ed.): *Kidney in Essential Hypertension*. Proceedings of a Course, held in New Orleans, La., U.S.A. (1983). 1984   ISBN 0-89838-616-0

36. M.P. Sambhi (ed.): *Fundamental Fault in Hypertension*. 1984   ISBN 0-89838-638-1

37. C. Marchesi (ed.): *Ambulatory Monitoring*. Cardiovascular System and Allied Applications. Proceedings of a Workshop, held in Pisa, Italy (1983). 1984
ISBN 0-89838-642-X

38. W. Kupper, R.N. MacAlpin and W. Bleifeld (eds.): *Coronary Tone in Ischemic Heart Disease*. 1984   ISBN 0-89838-646-2

39. N. Sperelakis and J.B. Caulfield (eds.): *Calcium Antagonists*. Mechanism of Action on Cardiac Muscle and Vascular Smooth Muscle. Proceedings of the 5th Annual Meeting of the American Section of the I.S.H.R., held in Hilton Head, S.C., U.S.A. (1983). 1984   ISBN 0-89838-655-1

40. Th. Godfraind, A.G. Herman and D. Wellens (eds.): *Calcium Entry Blockers in Cardiovascular and Cerebral Dysfunctions*. 1984   ISBN 0-89838-658-6

41. J. Morganroth and E.N. Moore (eds.): *Interventions in the Acute Phase of Myocardial Infarction*. Proceedings of the 4th Symposium on New Drugs and Devices, held in Philadelphia, Pa., U.S.A. (1983). 1984   ISBN 0-89838-659-4

42. F.L. Abel and W.H. Newman (eds.): *Functional Aspects of the Normal, Hypertrophied and Failing Heart*. Proceedings of the 5th Annual Meeting of the American Section of the I.S.H.R., held in Hilton Head, S.C., U.S.A. (1983). 1984
ISBN 0-89838-665-9

Developments in Cardiovascular Medicine

43. S. Sideman and R. Beyar (eds.): [3-D] *Simulation and Imaging of the Cardiac System.* State of the Heart. Proceedings of the International Henry Goldberg Workshop, held in Haifa, Israel (1984). 1985   ISBN 0-89838-687-X

44. E. van der Wall and K.I. Lie (eds.): *Recent Views on Hypertrophic Cardiomyopathy.* Proceedings of a Symposium, held in Groningen, The Netherlands (1984). 1985
ISBN 0-89838-694-2

45. R.E. Beamish, P.K. Singal and N.S. Dhalla (eds.), *Stress and Heart Disease.* Proceedings of a International Symposium, held in Winnipeg, Canada, 1984 (Vol. 1). 1985   ISBN 0-89838-709-4

46. R.E. Beamish, V. Panagia and N.S. Dhalla (eds.): *Pathogenesis of Stress-induced Heart Disease.* Proceedings of a International Symposium, held in Winnipeg, Canada, 1984 (Vol. 2). 1985   ISBN 0-89838-710-8

47. J. Morganroth and E.N. Moore (eds.): *Cardiac Arrhythmias.* New Therapeutic Drugs and Devices. Proceedings of the 5th Symposium on New Drugs and Devices, held in Philadelphia, Pa., U.S.A. (1984). 1985   ISBN 0-89838-716-7

48. P. Mathes (ed.): *Secondary Prevention in Coronary Artery Disease and Myocardial Infarction.* 1985   ISBN 0-89838-736-1

49. H.L. Stone and W.B. Weglicki (eds.): *Pathobiology of Cardiovascular Injury.* Proceedings of the 6th Annual Meeting of the American Section of the I.S.H.R., held in Oklahoma City, Okla., U.S.A. (1984). 1985   ISBN 0-89838-743-4

50. J. Meyer, R. Erbel and H.J. Rupprecht (eds.): *Improvement of Myocardial Perfusion.* Thrombolysis, Angioplasty, Bypass Surgery. Proceedings of a Symposium, held in Mainz, F.R.G. (1984). 1985   ISBN 0-89838-748-5

51. J.H.C. Reiber, P.W. Serruys and C.J. Slager (eds.): *Quantitative Coronary and Left Ventricular Cineangiography.* Methodology and Clinical Applications. 1986
ISBN 0-89838-760-4

52. R.H. Fagard and I.E. Bekaert (eds.): *Sports Cardiology.* Exercise in Health and Cardiovascular Disease. Proceedings from an International Conference, held in Knokke, Belgium (1985). 1986   ISBN 0-89838-782-5

53. J.H.C. Reiber and P.W. Serruys (eds.): *State of the Art in Quantitative Cornary Arteriography.* 1986   ISBN 0-89838-804-X

54. J. Roelandt (ed.): *Color Doppler Flow Imaging and Other Advances in Doppler Echocardiography.* 1986   ISBN 0-89838-806-6

55. E.E. van der Wall (ed.): *Noninvasive Imaging of Cardiac Metabolism.* Single Photon Scintigraphy, Positron Emission Tomography and Nuclear Magnetic Resonance. 1987
ISBN 0-89838-812-0

56. J. Liebman, R. Plonsey and Y. Rudy (eds.): *Pediatric and Fundamental Electrocardiography.* 1987   ISBN 0-89838-815-5

57. H.H. Hilger, V. Hombach and W.J. Rashkind (eds.), *Invasive Cardiovascular Therapy.* Proceedings of an International Symposium, held in Cologne, F.R.G. (1985). 1987   ISBN 0-89838-818-X

58. P.W. Serruys and G.T. Meester (eds.): *Coronary Angioplasty.* A Controlled Model for Ischemia. 1986   ISBN 0-89838-819-8

59. J.E. Tooke and L.H. Smaje (eds.): *Clinical Investigation of the Microcirculation.* Proceedings of an International Meeting, held in London, U.K. (1985). 1987
ISBN 0-89838-833-3

Developments in Cardiovascular Medicine

Developments in Cardiovascular Medicine

Developments in Cardiovascular Medicine

100. J. Morganroth and E.N. Moore (eds.): *Risk/Benefit Analysis for the Use and Approval of Thrombolytic, Antiarrhythmic, and Hypolipidemic Agents.* Proceedings of the 9th Annual Symposium on New Drugs and Devices (1988). 1989   ISBN 0-7923-0294-X
101. P.W. Serruys, R. Simon and K.J. Beatt (eds.): *PTCA - An Investigational Tool and a Non-operative Treatment of Acute Ischemia.* 1990   ISBN 0-7923-0346-6
102. I.S. Anand, P.I. Wahi and N.S. Dhalla (eds.): *Pathophysiology and Pharmacology of Heart Disease.* 1989   ISBN 0-7923-0367-9
103. G.S. Abela (ed.): *Lasers in Cardiovascular Medicine and Surgery.* Fundamentals and Technique. 1990   ISBN 0-7923-0440-3
104. H.M. Piper (ed.): *Pathophysiology of Severe Ischemic Myocardial Injury.* 1990
    ISBN 0-7923-0459-4
105. S.M. Teague (ed.): *Stress Doppler Echocardiography.* 1990   ISBN 0-7923-0499-3
106. P.R. Saxena, D.I. Wallis, W. Wouters and P. Bevan (eds.): *Cardiovascular Pharmacology of 5-Hydroxytryptamine.* Prospective Therapeutic Applications. 1990
    ISBN 0-7923-0502-7
107. A.P. Shepherd and P.A. Öberg (eds.): *Laser-Doppler Blood Flowmetry.* 1990
    ISBN 0-7923-0508-6
108. J. Soler-Soler, G. Permanyer-Miralda and J. Sagristà-Sauleda (eds.): *Pericardial Disease.* New Insights and Old Dilemmas. Preface by Ralph Shabetai. 1990
    ISBN 0-7923-0510-8
109. J.P.M. Hamer: *Practical Echocardiography in the Adult.* With Doppler and Color-Doppler Flow Imaging. 1990   ISBN 0-7923-0670-8
110. A. Bayés de Luna, P. Brugada, J. Cosin Aguilar and F. Navarro Lopez (eds.): *Sudden Cardiac Death.* 1991   ISBN 0-7923-0716-X
111. E. Andries and R. Stroobandt (eds.): *Hemodynamics in Daily Practice.* 1991
    ISBN 0-7923-0725-9
112. J. Morganroth and E.N. Moore (eds.): *Use and Approval of Antihypertensive Agents and Surrogate Endpoints for the Approval of Drugs affecting Antiarrhythmic Heart Failure and Hypolipidemia.* Proceedings of the 10th Annual Symposium on New Drugs and Devices (1989). 1990   ISBN 0-7923-0756-9
113. S. Iliceto, P. Rizzon and J.R.T.C. Roelandt (eds.): *Ultrasound in Coronary Artery Disease.* Present Role and Future Perspectives. 1990   ISBN 0-7923-0784-4
114. J.V. Chapman and G.R. Sutherland (eds.): *The Noninvasive Evaluation of Hemodynamics in Congenital Heart Disease.* Doppler Ultrasound Applications in the Adult and Pediatric Patient with Congenital Heart Disease. 1990
    ISBN 0-7923-0836-0
115. G.T. Meester and F. Pinciroli (eds.): *Databases for Cardiology.* 1991
    ISBN 0-7923-0886-7
116. B. Korecky and N.S. Dhalla (eds.): *Subcellular Basis of Contractile Failure.* 1990
    ISBN 0-7923-0890-5
117. J.H.C. Reiber and P.W. Serruys (eds.): *Quantitative Coronary Arteriography.* 1991
    ISBN 0-7923-0913-8
118. E. van der Wall and A. de Roos (eds.): *Magnetic Resonance Imaging in Coronary Artery Disease.* 1991   ISBN 0-7923-0940-5
119. V. Hombach, M. Kochs and A.J. Camm (eds.): *Interventional Techniques in Cardiovascular Medicine.* 1991   ISBN 0-7923-0956-1